CLINICAL
PSYCHIATRY
ESSENTIALS

CLINICAL PSYCHIATRY ESSENTIALS

Editor

Laura Weiss Roberts, MD, MA

Chairman and Charles E. Kubly Professor
Department of Psychiatry and Behavioral Medicine;
Professor
Center for the Study of Bioethics, Department of Population Health
Medical College of Wisconsin
Milwaukee, Wisconsin

Associate Editors

Jinger G. Hoop, MD, MFA

Assistant Professor
Department of Psychiatry and Behavioral Medicine
Medical College of Wisconsin
Milwaukee, Wisconsin

Thomas W. Heinrich, MD

Associate Professor
Department of Psychiatry and Behavioral Medicine
Medical College of Wisconsin;
Chief
Consultation Psychiatry Service
Froedtert Hospital
Milwaukee, Wisconsin

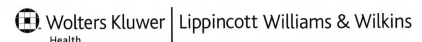

Wolters Kluwer Health | Lippincott Williams & Wilkins

Philadelphia · Baltimore · New York · London
Buenos Aires · Hong Kong · Sydney · Tokyo

Acquisitions Editor: Susan Rhyner
Managing Editor: Jessica Heise
Marketing Manager: Jennifer Kuklinski
Project Manager: Alicia Jackson
Designer: Stephen Druding
Cover Designer: Stephen Druding
Production Services: Laserwords Private Limited, Chennai, India

Library of Congress Cataloging-in-Publication Data

Clinical psychiatry essentials / editor, Laura Weiss Roberts ; associate editors, Jinger G. Hoop, Thomas W. Heinrich.
  p. ; cm.
  Includes bibliographical references and index.
  ISBN-13: 978-0-7817-7157-3 (alk. paper)
  ISBN-10: 0-7817-7157-9 (alk. paper)
  1. Psychiatry. I. Roberts, Laura Weiss, 1960– II. Hoop, Jinger G., 1958– III. Heinrich, Thomas W.
  [DNLM: 1. Mental Disorders. 2. Psychiatry. WM 140 C6408 2010]
  RC454.C5382 2010
  616.89 —dc22

                                                                    2008049174

To purchase additional copies of this book, call our customer service department at (800) 638-3030 or fax orders to (301) 223-2320. International customers should call (301) 223-2300.

Visit Lippincott Williams & Wilkins on the Internet: at LWW.com. Lippincott Williams & Wilkins customer service representatives are available from 8:30 AM to 6 PM, EST.

10 9 8 7 6 5 4 3 2 1

Together we dedicate this book to the generous and exceptional teachers of our lives. We are beholden.

For my children, Madeline, Helen, Willa, and Tom, who cause my heart to overflow with love
—Laura Weiss Roberts

For my parents and sister, who were my first teachers, and for my son, who is already my most inspiring student
—Jinger G. Hoop

To the teachers who have taught me to learn
To my family who has allowed me to learn
To the students who have motivated me to learn
To the patients who have inspired me to learn
And to the baristas who have kept me awake to learn
—Thomas W. Heinrich

CONTENTS

Danielle L. Anderson, MD
Assistant Professor
Department of Psychiatry and Behavioral
  Neuroscience
University of Chicago Pritzker School
  of Medicine
Chicago, Illinois

Jennifer A. Niskala Apps, PhD
Assistant Professor
Psychiatry and Behavioral Medicine
Medical College of Wisconsin;
Pediatric Neuropsychologist
Psychiatry and Behavioral Medicine
Children's Hospital of Wisconsin
Milwaukee, Wisconsin

Paul Ballas, DO
Fellow
Child and Adolescent Psychiatry
Thomas Jefferson University Hospital
Philadelphia, Pennsylvania

Eugene V. Beresin, MA, MD
Professor
Psychiatry
Harvard Medical School;
Director of Child and Adolescent Psychiatry
  Residency Training
Psychiatry
Massachusetts General Hospital and McLean
  Hospital
Boston, Massachusetts

Tara K. Biehl, MS
Clinical Research Manager
Psychiatry
University of New Mexico
Albuquerque, New Mexico

David Bienenfeld, MD
Professor, Director of Residency Training
Psychiatry
Wright State University
Dayton, Ohio

William V. Bobo, MD
Assistant Professor
Department of Psychiatry
Vanderbilt University School of Medicine
Nashville, Tennessee

Michael P. Bogenschutz, MD
Professor
Psychiatry
University of New Mexico School of Medicine;
Vice Chair for Addiction Psychiatry
Psychiatry
University of New Mexico Hospitals
Albuquerque, New Mexico

Robert J. Boland, MD
Associate Professor/Associate Director,
  Residency Training
Psychiatry & Human Behavior
The Warren Alpert School of Medicine
  at Brown University
Providence, Rhode Island

Juan R. Bustillo, MD
Associate Professor
Psychiatry
University of New Mexico
Albuquerque, New Mexico

Dennis S. Charney, MD
Anne and Joel Ehrenkranz Dean
Mount Sinai School of Medicine;
Executive Vice President for Academic Affairs
The Mount Sinai Medical Center;
Professor
Departments of Psychiatry, Neuroscience,
  and Pharmacology & Systems Therapeutics
Mount Sinai School of Medicine
New York, New York

Emil F. Coccaro, MD
Chair & E.C. Manning Professor
Psychiatry and Behavioral Neuroscience
University of Chicago
Chicago, Illinois

John H. Coverdale, MD, MEd, FRANZCP
Professor
Menninger Department of Psychiatry
Center for Ethics and Health Policy
Baylor College of Medicine
Houston, Texas

Deborah Anne Dellmore, MD
Director of Medical Student Education
Assistant Professor
Psychiatry
University of New Mexico
Albuquerque, New Mexico

Jennifer L. Derenne, MD
Assistant Professor
Psychiatry and Behavioral Medicine
Director of Training
Division of Child and Adolescent Psychiatry
Medical College of Wisconsin;
Child and Adolescent Psychiatrist
Children's Hospital of Wisconsin
Milwaukee, Wisconsin

Arden D. Dingle, MD
Training Director, Child and Adolescent
    Psychiatry
Psychiatry and Behavioral Science
Emory University School of Medicine
Atlanta, Georgia

Karl Doghramji, MD
Professor of Psychiatry and Human
    Behavior
Professor of Neurology
Medical Director, Jefferson Sleep Disorders
    Center
Program Director, Fellowship in Sleep Medicine
Thomas Jefferson University
Philadelphia, Pennsylvania

Hassan Fathy, MD
Psychiatry Resident
Department of Psychiatry
Faculty of Medicine
Cairo University
Cairo University Hospitals
Cairo, Egypt

Steven J. Garlow, MD, PhD
Associate Professor
Department of Psychiatry and Behavioral
    Sciences
Emory University School of Medicine;
Chief of Psychiatry
Emory University Hospital
Atlanta, Georgia

Cynthia M. A. Geppert, MD, PhD, MPH
Associate Professor
Department of Psychiatry
University of New Mexico;
Chief Consultation Psychiatry and Ethics
New Mexico Veterans Affairs Health Care
    System
Albuquerque, New Mexico

Mark J. Gorman, PhD
Instructor in Psychology
Psychiatry
Harvard Medical School;
Staff Psychologist
Psychiatry
Massachusetts General Hospital
Boston, Massachusetts

Joseph S. Goveas, MD
Assistant Professor
Psychiatry and Behavioral Medicine;
Director
Division of Geriatric Psychiatry
Medical College of Wisconsin
Milwaukee, Wisconsin

Jon E. Grant, MD
Associate Professor
Department of Psychiatry
University of Minnesota Medical School
Minneapolis, Minnesota

Patty Guedet, MD
Assistant Professor
Department of Psychiatry of Behavioral
    Medicine
Medical College of Wisconsin;
Director
Psychiatry Consultation Service
Zablocki VA Medical Center
Milwaukee, Wisconsin

Paul Haidet, MD, MPH
Associate Professor
Medicine
Houston Center for Quality of Care
    and Utilization Studies
Baylor College of Medicine;
Staff Physician
Michael E. DeBakey Veterans Affairs Medical
    Center
Houston, Texas

Pamela R. Handelsman, BA
Research Assistant
Psychiatry
Massachusetts General Hospital
Boston, Massachusetts

Thomas W. Heinrich, MD
Associate Professor
Department of Psychiatry and Behavioral
  Medicine
Medical College of Wisconsin;
Chief
Consultation Psychiatry Service
Froedtert Hospital
Milwaukee, Wisconsin

Paul E. Holtzheimer III, MD
Assistant Professor
Psychiatry and Behavioral Sciences
Emory University School of Medicine
Atlanta, Georgia

Jinger G. Hoop, MD, MFA
Assistant Professor
Department of Psychiatry and Behavioral
  Medicine
Medical College of Wisconsin
Milwaukee, Wisconsin

Waguih William IsHak, MD, FAPA
Associate Professor
Departments of Psychiatry
UCLA and USC Schools of Medicine;
Medical Director
Adult Outpatient Psychiatry
Cedars-Sinai Medical Center
Los Angeles, California

Steven M. Jenkusky, MD
Associate Professor
Psychiatry
University of New Mexico Health Sciences
  Center;
Outpatient Medical Director
University of New Mexico Psychiatric Center
Albuquerque, New Mexico

Jason E. Kanz
Clinical Neuropsychologist
Department of Neuroscience
Marshfield Clinic
Eau Claire, Wisconsin

Elizabeth Kieff, MD
Assistant Professor
Department of Psychiatry and Behavioral
  Neuroscience
University of Chicago;
Assistant Dean for Student Affairs
The Pritzker School of Medicine
Chicago, Illinois

John Lauriello, MD
Professor and Chair
Department of Psychiatry
Chancellor's Chair of Excellence in Psychiatry
University of Missouri School of Medicine
Columbia, Missouri

James L. Levenson, MD
Vice-Chair
Professor of Psychiatry, Medicine & Surgery
Department of Psychiatry
Virginia Commonwealth University
Richmond, Virginia

Richard J. Loewenstein, MD
Clinical Associate Professor
Department of Psychiatry
University of Maryland School of Medicine;
Medical Director
The Trauma Disorders Program
Sheppard Pratt Health System
Baltimore, Maryland

Michael J. Marcangelo, MD
Assistant Professor and Director of Medical
  Student Education
Department of Psychiatry and Behavioral
  Neuroscience
University of Chicago Pritzker School of
  Medicine
Chicago, Illinois

Bruce J. Masek, PhD, ABPP
Associate Professor of Psychology
Psychiatry
Harvard Medical School;
Clinical Director, Child Adolescent Psychiatry
Massachusetts General Hospital
Boston, Massachusetts

Sanjay J. Mathew, MD
Associate Professor
Psychiatry
Mount Sinai School of Medicine
New York, New York

David A. Mrazek, MD, FRC Psych
Chair
Department of Psychiatry and Psychology
Mayo Clinic;
Professor of Psychiatry and Pediatrics
Mayo Clinic College of Medicine
Rochester, Minnesota

James W. Murrough, MD
Research Fellow
Department of Psychiatry
Mount Sinai School of Medicine
New York, New York

Charles B. Nemeroff, MD, PhD
Reunette W. Harris Professor
Psychiatry and Behavioral Sciences
Emory University School of Medicine
Atlanta, Georgia

Robert F. Newby, PhD
Associate Professor of Neurology and Pediatrics
Neurology
Medical College of Wisconsin
Milwaukee, Wisconsin

Paul E. Nicholas, MD, MPH
Assistant Professor
Psychiatry and Behavioral Medicine
Medical College of Wisconsin
Milwaukee, Wisconsin

Paul Edward Quinlan, DO, MS
Associate Professor
Psychiatry
Michigan State University
East Lansing, Michigan

Madhvi Phadtare Richards, MD
Assistant Professor
Director of Child and Adolescent Psychiatry
  Residency Training
Chief of Child and Adolescent Psychiatry
  Section
Psychiatry
Michigan State University
East Lansing, Michigan

Laura Weiss Roberts, MD, MA
Chairman and Charles E. Kubly Professor
Department of Psychiatry and Behavioral
  Medicine;
Professor
Center for the Study of Bioethics
Department of Population Health
Medical College of Wisconsin
Milwaukee, Wisconsin

Steven A. Safren, PhD, ABPP
Associate Professor
Psychiatry
Harvard Medical School;
Director of Behavioral Medicine
Psychiatry
Massachusetts General Hospital
Boston, Massachusetts

Minninder J. Sandhu, MD
PGY-4 Resident Physician
Department of Psychiatry and Behavioral
  Sciences
Emory University School of Medicine;
PGY-4 Resident Physician
Department of Psychiatry and Behavioral
  Sciences
Emory University Hospital
Atlanta, Georgia

Vinay P. Saranga, MD
Psychiatry Resident
Wright State University
Dayton, Ohio

Daphne Simeon, MD
Associate Professor
Psychiatry
Mount Sinai School of Medicine
New York, New York

Brian D. Smith, MD
Assistant Professor
Psychiatry
Michigan State University
East Lansing, Michigan

Amy M. Ursano, MD
Assistant Professor
Department of Psychiatry
University of North Carolina School of
  Medicine
Chapel Hill, North Carolina

Robert J. Ursano, MD
Professor of Psychiatry and Neuroscience
Chairman, Department of Psychiatry
Uniformed Services University
Bethesda, Maryland

Nutan Atre Vaidya, MD
Professor and Chair
Psychiatry and Behavioral Sciences
Rosalind Franklin University of Medicine
  and Science
North Chicago, Illinois

Christopher H. Warner, MD
Assistant Professor
Department of Psychiatry and Behavioral
    Medicine
Medical College of Wisconsin
Milwaukee, Wisconsin;
Chief
Department of Behavioral Medicine
Winn Army Hospital
Fort Stewart, Georgia

Mark T. Wright, MD
Associate Professor
Departments of Psychiatry and Behavioral
    Medicine and Neurology
Medical College of Wisconsin
Milwaukee, Wisconsin

Joel Yager, MD
Professor
Department of Psychiatry
University of Colorado
Denver, Colorado;
Professor Emeritus
Department of Psychiatry and Biobehavioral
    Sciences
David Geffen School of Medicine
University of California at Los Angeles
Los Angeles, California;
Professor Emeritus
Department of Psychiatry
School of Medicine
University of New Mexico
Albuquerque, New Mexico

ACKNOWLEDGMENTS

Alan Stoudemire was an extraordinary psychiatrist, psychosomatic medicine physician, educator, and leader in American psychiatry who was deeply loved. He served as the original editor of Clinical Psychiatry for Medical Students, which was the starting point for this textbook project. We are grateful to follow in his footsteps, and we wish to express our appreciation to his wife, Sue, for permitting us to undertake this work.

We also wish to thank the authors whose chapters populate this text; and who generously gave their expertise and time in completing this book. Together, their chapters are a compendium of the most current knowledge in the field of psychiatry, presented in a format accessible for medical students, residents, and practicing clinicians. The chapters are arranged from specific to general-starting with a focus on understanding patients as individuals, then discussing disorders, treatments, and the care of special populations. The final chapters describe the important role of research in psychiatry and demonstrate how the practice of evidence-based medicine will enable readers to explore questions that arise in the care of patients that cannot be answered by referring to this or any textbook.

Finally, we wish to thank Lippincott Williams & Wilkins who provided helpful support and advice throughout the project, and we acknowledge sincerely the efforts of Ms. Liz Hogan Stalnaker and Ms. Jessica Heise. We thank Ms. Ann Tennier who has served as our editorial assistant. This has been a challenging and complex project and she, as always, has demonstrated competence, professionalism, and grace in every step of the way.

Understanding and Evaluating Patients with Mental Illness

CHAPTER 1

Laura Weiss Roberts

The Essential Lessons of Psychiatry

A physician's professional life, over time, becomes the accumulation of stories—stories in which the patterns and processes of illness are revealed; stories of resilience, strength, and survival; stories of near-miracles and near-misses; stories of recovery; stories of undeserved hardship and despair; stories of pain; stories of joy; stories of living, either fulfilled or not; and stories of dying, either peaceful or not. These are the stories of people, real people in whom diseases and conditions are lived experiences. These diseases and conditions have moment-to-moment importance for people, shaping their ability to love, to work, to become and do what they hoped for in their lifetimes.

In the work of psychiatry, the human stories we encounter as physicians are distinct. If you take them to heart and truly appreciate what they mean, they convey great suffering. They also can be frightening, off-putting, unsettling, intriguing, and compelling.

Consider the 47-year-old woman with terminal anorexia nervosa who weighed 47 lb at her death; or the graduate student brought to the emergency room after staying awake for 6 days, yelling and exercising nonstop, taking steroids and caffeine to enhance his body building. The 35-year-old mother of three children who acted entirely normally, volunteering at school and running errands for her ill mother, "forgetting" that her own doctor had diagnosed her with advanced malignant melanoma. The church caretaker who glued his eyelids shut, terrified that the laser beams emanating from his eyeballs would kill others. The college student secretly mutilating himself at the command of "God's voice" when he encountered certain numbers while walking along the street.

Consider the woman who owned only white shirts and navy slacks because otherwise she would take many hours to dress herself every morning, or the child who could walk into a room only after counting the objects in the room three times. The elder man who wandered and walked the streets for many hours every day, with little food and little clothing, looking for his parrot, which he believed to be poisoned, taken, or lost. The mother who placed sharpened, several-inch-long hatpins around her son's bed to protect him from menacing faces who looked at them through the windows of their home.

Consider the woman losing her marriage because of growing irritability, poor sleep and appetite, loss of daily joys, and inability to "think right." The man with extensive skin grafts, depressed and wracked with nightmares and intrusive thoughts, wanting to recover to take care of his son, the only other survivor of a family car accident in which the man was driving. The wife who, shortly after giving birth to her first child, learned that she was human immunodeficiency virus (HIV)-positive and, crying, overwhelmed in her birthing room, bound her breasts. The young man who for 6 years after "experimenting" with street drugs walked around feeling disconnected from himself, dazed, and inhuman, "like a robot," before his parents brought him for treatment.

Consider the successful businessman who, 26 hours after emergency abdominal surgery, saw flames coming out of his hospital bed. The young woman who was raped in her home and then felt "raped again" by the legal system. The young man who believed that an electronic chip had been inserted into his brain by the government when he had a computed axial tomography (CAT) scan 4 years previously. The depressed, angry girl who had sex with gang members positive for hepatitis C as an initiation rite. The middle-aged man found walking naked on the interstate who believed he was safe from harm because of the "cheetah eye" he possessed.

These are the stories of people living with mental illness or the mental health–related consequences of physical conditions and difficult life experiences. And these are just some of the stories of people I remember from my medical school and residency training.

In becoming a physician, irrespective of one's later clinical practice, there are several essential lessons to be derived from learning that occurs while "doing" psychiatry, studying the meaning of the stories told in this field. Four of the most important lessons are outlined here.

THE NATURE OF MENTAL ILLNESS

Mental illnesses are diseases or conditions that are comprised of symptoms and signs sufficiently serious, individually or together, that the affected individual is compromised in his life endeavors, including forming and sustaining good attachments to others, performing work or fulfilling a role in society, and developing strengths and capacities as a person. Mental illnesses have biological bases, underpinnings, and/or correlates, though the specific factors influencing the disease process may be unknown or uncertain. Because mental illnesses are expressed in emotions, thoughts, and behaviors and because they originate in the brain or, at the very least, affect or are directly influenced by brain processes, there is an emerging preference for the term *neuropsychiatric disease.*

Mental illnesses are not simply maladaptations or "poor coping," and they are not merely "variations" of health or simply being, let's say, an unusual style or personality. They are not natural responses to natural stresses of the everyday world. By definition, mental illnesses must substantively and adversely affect one's ways of engaging in life. Moreover, they cannot be diagnosed solely on the basis of the content of thought or observable behavior.

For example, a widower's grief may render him tearful, withdrawn, sad, and lacking energy. A soldier in an acute combat situation may be fiercely single-minded and aggressive, hyperalert and irritable, requiring little rest and sustenance, and viewing the enemy as "targets" rather than whole and complete human beings. The cancer patient who reels after a rough bout with chemotherapy may become discouraged and weepy when alone and put on a "good front" when with others. A person on a spiritual journey that fits within a particular cultural perspective may experience unusual sensory events and what may be viewed as extraordinary thoughts. Taken in context, the widower, the soldier, the cancer patient, and the spiritual person are not "ill," though the internal experience may be extremely disquieting and the observable behaviors "not normal."

On the other hand, the widower whose grief extends for years and "breaks" him from his usual life, such as quitting his job, disconnecting from his children and friends, losing interest in baseball, reading, food, and the other joys of his life in the past—this is mental illness. The soldier who returns to civilian life and for a long time is unable to focus on the broad activities of life and feel safe, have fun, sleep well, and enjoy his family, and who views all people and activities around him as "intrusions" and potential threats—this is mental illness. The cancer patient who gives up on the thus-far effective chemotherapy because she begins to see a future with no hope, finds that she cannot concentrate, and begins to think of ending her life to "preempt the cancer"—this is mental illness. The person who goes on a spiritual journey, departing from the values and experiences of his early life, and persistently has thoughts of God and the devil, leaves his usual work and relationships, and then becomes tortured about being a "bad person" who deserves punishment—this is mental illness. It is the pattern of significant compromise in a person's life that permits the diagnosis of mental illness to be given.

Interpretation of symptoms and signs in psychiatry is less straightforward than, say, the evaluation of gout or a broken bone or a "hot" appendix. The clinical data are often less clear, harder to establish, and sometimes misleading. Just as certain experiences or events can be "healthy" or appropriate in certain contexts—or pathological in other situations—clinically important data in psychiatry must be viewed in light of their potential medical and/or biological origins. The initial presentation of pancreatic cancer may be signs of depression, for instance, or for HIV-related disease, it may be neurocognitive decline and early signs of subcortical dementia. Medications for diverse conditions such as arthritis, cardiac arrhythmias, pain, asthma, and renal failure can have profound effects on the mood state and thinking of an individual with no previous psychiatric issues. Surgery, childbirth, infection, metabolic disturbances, and stroke all present primary "medical" issues, but recovery may be complicated by psychiatric considerations.

Therefore, diagnosing mental illness entails a comprehensive knowledge of the individual, his inner experience, feelings, thoughts, and views, how he behaves, the longitudinal pattern of his relationships and life, and his particular context. It also requires an understanding of biological and medical elements contributing to (causing, distorting, disguising) the clinical picture. A correct diagnosis also relies on an accurate understanding of the patient's psychological and social capacities, currently and as they have evolved over time. This can be subtle work. It involves recognition of deficits, absences, and changed "trajectories"—recognizing the importance of what is not said, the experiences and milestones that have not yet occurred, the relationships that are not enriched, the educational paths that become derailed, the potential that is not fulfilled. Many psychiatric symptoms do not arise initially in a clear and distinct manner—they declare themselves over time. In other words, diagnosing mental illness is complex and multidimensional, requiring attention to what is present and what is absent. There are very few "absolutes" or pathognomonic "signs" that in a single stroke "reveal" the existence of disease. At this point, there are no genetic "markers" of psychiatric diseases, which tend to be complex disorders resulting from the influences of many genetic and environmental factors. And, as is clear, the clinically important facts and observations may be hard to discern or interpret. For these reasons, psychiatry is a field that necessitates thoroughness, awareness of details, freedom from bias and "snap judgments," and the ability to recognize subtle patterns of things-present and things-absent.

THE SEVERITY AND PUBLIC HEALTH IMPACT OF MENTAL ILLNESS

Mental illnesses are prevalent. They are disabling and deadly. They are responsible for a large share of the disease burden throughout the world, and without significant change in clinical care systems globally, they will gain in the proportion of suffering they cause in relation to other diseases. These are strong and unfortunate statements based on strong and unfortunate evidence.

Neuropsychiatric disorders affect both genders, all ages, all cultures, and all nations through-out the world. Approximately 1% of the world's adults meet criteria for the diagnosis of schizophrenia (National Institute of Mental Health, 2008a). A recent study of data drawn from five continents indicated that lifetime prevalence for a nonpsychotic mental illness (defined as any anxiety, impulse control, mood, and substance use disorder) ranged from 1 in 8 people (Africa) to 1 in 2 people (United States) (Kessler et al., 2007). World Health Organization data suggest that neuropsychiatric diseases, including mental illnesses, substance-use disorders, and dementia, are the second leading cause of disability (behind infectious diseases, including HIV) across the world. In economically established countries, these diseases have a disproportionately higher impact because they often go untreated, or undertreated, relative to the more assertive and comprehensive treatments for less-widespread infectious diseases (Quinlan, 2009).

The vast majority of deaths worldwide are linked to medical disorders with behavioral components, including heart disease, obesity, blood-borne and sexually transmitted diseases, and primary neuropsychiatric diseases. Suicide is known as a consequence of severe, recurrent depression, but it also is strongly associated with psychosis, alcohol dependence, and anxiety disorders, among other serious illnesses. Globally, suicide alone is estimated to be the proximal cause of death for approximately 900,000 to just over 1 million people each year. Certain subpopulations and geographic regions appear to be especially vulnerable (e.g., young people in China and Europe, white elder men in US farm areas), whereas others appear less vulnerable (e.g., certain areas of Africa devastated by war and disease). Some international data almost defy belief, they are so grave—the rate of suicide among men of certain Eastern European and former Soviet countries (e.g., Lithuania, Kazakhstan, Hungary, Slovenia), for instance, was recorded as ranging from 37.9 to 70.1 per 100,000 as recently as 2004 (Caruso, 2008).

In the United States, suicide is the documented cause of death for >30,000 people each year, with a rate of 10 to 12 deaths per 100,000 across most communities. Suicide was formally listed as the 11th leading cause of death in 2004 (National Institute of Mental Health, 2008b); because it is thought to be an underestimate, the true "ranking" of suicide in comparison with other causes is unknown. Suicide attempts are far more common than is generally recognized in society, especially among young women. Completed suicides are typically preceded by prior attempts, which may be serious and cause significant illness and lasting disability (e.g., cardiotoxicity associated with tricyclic antidepressant overdoses, hepatic failure associated with acetaminophen overdoses). By way of comparison, and a surprise to many, the rate of suicide is roughly double the rate of homicide in this country. These rates of death-by-suicide are roughly comparable to the rates of death associated with chronic liver disease and cirrhosis and pancreatic cancer, better-recognized medical conditions. The suicide rate is 50 times greater than the annual death rate associated with complications of pregnancy and childbirth, and is more than twice the rate of death by acquired immune deficiency syndrome (AIDS) in the United States. Finally, the suicide death rate is half the rate of death by cerebrovascular disease, four times the rate of death associated with Alzheimer disease, and one third the rate of death associated with breast cancer (Morgan and Morgan, 2001, 2005).

While the true cost in terms of human suffering is not amenable to quantification, health economic data from a 2004 National Institutes of Health study estimated that the overall direct (e.g., cost of medications, hospitalization, disability subsidies) plus indirect (e.g., lost productivity, lost taxes) costs associated with neuropsychiatric disorders in the United States exceed $1.2 trillion annually. Analogous data for the global economic impact have not been developed at this time.

THE RELEVANCE OF MENTAL ILLNESS ACROSS CLINICAL MEDICINE

No matter what primary care field or specialty, no matter what clinical practice setting, caring for patients means caring for people with mental illness. Neuropsychiatric disease and co-occurring disorders (e.g., substance- or mental illness–related conditions) are common in clinical practice. Indeed, it is estimated that one quarter to one third of patients in ambulatory care settings have a diagnosable psychiatric disease, and nearly half of hospitalized patients on medical services have a secondary or primary psychiatric disease (Levenson, 2009).

It is especially important to recognize the interplay between certain physical and mental diseases that are at the center of current clinical practice. Two examples are cancer and cardiac disease. Several major studies over the last 12 years have shown the adverse link between depression and cancer—its incidence, its progression, and its outcome (Everson et al., 1996; Penninx et al., 1998; Watson et al., 1999; Loberiza et al., 2002; Stommel et al., 2002). Biological (i.e., medication) and psychosocial (e.g., group and individual therapy) interventions that target psychiatric symptoms have been proved to improve functional capacity, depressive symptoms, aspects contributing to a positive quality of life (e.g., coping techniques), and survival length for people living with cancer (Theobald et al., 2002; Spiegel et al., 1989; Fawzy et al., 1993). Similarly, the relationship between cardiac disease and depression has been studied. Depression occurs in 1 in 5 patients with coronary artery disease (Shapiro et al., 1996), and the presence of depression is an adverse predictive factor for measures of heart disease function and outcome (Frasure-Smith et al., 1993, 1995). Fortunately, if diagnosed and treated, depression may be treated, and improvements in morbidity and mortality have been documented with this intervention in survivors of myocardial infarctions (Glassman et al., 2002). These examples of the connections between physical health conditions and psychiatric disease suggest the exceptional importance of looking for such connections across other diseases.

People with psychiatric diseases have been identified as "high utilizers" of health care, a description that may be unfair in light of the lack of adequate access to mental health services that exists across most communities. Many neuropsychiatric diseases can be expressed in physical symptomatology, causing patients to seek physical health care. Individuals seeking medical care often may have a mental health issue that underlies the wish for treatment on that particular day. Moreover, within certain communities, the stigma of seeking mental health care directly (or even accepting and revealing that one has psychiatric symptoms) is overwhelming and shaming, driving patients into traditional medical care settings. Patients with multiple problems encompassing medical and neuropsychiatric diseases, as well as the psychosocial issues that accompany these (typically) chronic illnesses, may produce challenges in the clinical setting. These "difficult" patients may seem to seek care frequently and in a manner that causes challenges for staff and fellow patients. Recognizing the "difficulty" of patients as clinical data, usually signifying the presence of multiple diagnoses and problems that are experienced as "exponential"—not merely "additive"—is important to conscientious and compassionate care.

THE DISTINCT CLINICAL, ETHICAL, AND LEGAL SKILLS TAUGHT BY PSYCHIATRY

Psychiatry as a profession sees and honors the critical importance of the therapeutic relationship in the clinical care of *any* health issue, physical or mental in nature. The therapeutic relationship serves as the way to understanding the patient, generating an accurate diagnosis or diagnostic hypotheses, and implementing treatment. Helping a person to understand his illness, the need for certain self-care behaviors (e.g., sleep "hygiene," good nutrition), and the value of adherence to recommended therapies can all occur in the context of a positive therapeutic relationship. It is the platform for healing. Further, so many illnesses in medicine—psychiatry included—cannot yet be prevented, cured, or ameliorated fully: We as physicians and physicians-in-training can only help our patients bear their individual burdens by standing with them compassionately and with genuine knowledge of their experience. Whether our patients are newly ill or chronically so, helping them with these tasks of living with their illnesses is the core of our profession.

Psychiatry offers unique skills—clinical, ethical, and legal—in this professional endeavor and most rely on the foundation of the doctor–patient relationship. Establishing a trusting rapport—one that generates understanding, inspires confidence, demonstrates respect, and creates a safe and predictable interpersonal environment for clinical care—is perhaps the skill of utmost importance. Carefully and thoroughly exploring symptoms, signs, and experiences through the psychiatric interview is a second key skill. Related to these skills is the ability to gently work with the experience of stigma encountered by all people living with mental illness, to minimize embarrassment and provide an environment of acceptance and support. Empirical work has shown that perceptions of stigma are reduced as the biological underpinnings of disease are more fully known, so finding small ways to educate patients, families, and colleagues about neuropsychiatric disease and the connection between disorders of the brain and mental illness may be vital parts of these conversations. All subsequent clinical efforts are likely to "fail" without these safeguards in place in the therapeutic relationship.

Knowing when to look further, that is, figuring out when things are not "adding up right," is another key skill to be exercised by gathering additional data (e.g., medical chart review, from family members) and seeking laboratory testing and other clinical "collateral" information. In addition, determining barriers to optimal care in the patient's situation is important. Knowing when there are issues (e.g., in a situation involving physical risk, illicit behaviors) where consultation with another clinician or with an expert from another discipline is needed represents another key skill. Being aware of when one must alert officials, such as with threats toward specific victims or reports of sexual abuse of a child or dependent elder, is essential to appropriate clinical practice. Learning how to speak with a patient about the nature of the condition he has and its likely effects and prognosis and working together toward symptom improvement and an enhanced quality of everyday life are clinical skills that are refined over the course of time as a psychiatric practitioner.

Discerning the clinical importance of the feelings and responses elicited by the patient's behavior, good and not as good, is yet another clinical skill that "doing" psychiatry can foster. Through self-reflection and supervision, the physician learns much that can help facilitate the health and well-being of the patient. Being able to keep track of one's own biases as well as one's conflicts and impulses (e.g., to "rescue" certain patients while "rejecting" others) is critical to giving care that serves the well-being of the patient and is not driven by the clinician's own needs or desire for reward and gratification in the relationship. As with all of medicine, but especially important in psychiatry because of the rapid explosion of information in the field, a key skill is the ability to incorporate new knowledge into clinical practices to achieve higher standards of care and greater effectiveness in the treatment of people with mental illness.

Several other skills that represent a composite of clinical, ethical, and legal capacities are among those learned best in psychiatry. Examples of skills involving clinical, ethical, and legal sophistication in psychiatry are safeguarding confidentiality; obtaining informed consent or informed refusal of care; addressing situations involving physical risk (e.g., patient self-care and safety, threats of violence or harm toward others); recognizing and managing one's own responses to patients (i.e., "countertransference"); and approaching the asymmetry in power in the doctor–patient relationship.

These aspects of clinical work are more salient in the care of people with mental illness because of the stigma psychiatric disease has in most cultures, as well as the distinctly personal or intimate nature of psychiatric care. Because people living with mental illnesses sometimes are unable to care for themselves or may become a threat to others' well-being, part of the repertoire of interventions may include delimiting the freedoms and choices of the patient. Further, the relative marginalization and economic fragility of people with chronic conditions, including neuropsychiatric diseases, also contributes to the potential vulnerability of mentally ill patients in the treatment setting. Taken together, these skills enrich the abilities of practitioners from across medicine but are especially critical to the work of psychiatry.

CONCLUSION

Every medical student and early-career physician should recognize the nature of mental illness, understand its prevalence and impact throughout the world, see its relevance for clinical practice across all of medicine, and cultivate skills that address the rich clinical, ethical, and legal issues present in the lives of people with mental illness. Medical students and early-career physicians should also be attuned to the stories of their patients for whom the burden of disease is very great.

There are two final points to be made. The first is that none of us is immune to neuropsychiatric disease. We as physicians may ourselves become ill and will certainly love and work alongside people whose lives will be greatly affected by mental illness. Learning to accept this observation, with all of its implications, and making the promise to oneself to engage in active self-care and to seek or facilitate necessary care from professionals—bravely facing fears and stigma, perhaps—may help lead to a better life and better health outcome.

The second point is an invitation to understand neuropsychiatric disease and, ideally, to champion the concerns of people living with mental illness. By way of comparison, it is valuable to recall that just a few decades ago, cancer was gravely misunderstood. It was believed to be a contagious disease, a disease caused by moral infirmity, a disease that afflicted those who "deserved" it. These erroneous beliefs caused great suffering beyond the physical disability and emotional anguish of the disease processes themselves. Cancer was highly stigmatized—and yet, as scientific knowledge grew, the biases and prejudices diminished and now have nearly subsided. A similar situation to this historical example currently exists with mental illness, and particularly with certain kinds of disorders (e.g., substance-related conditions). There is hope that as psychiatric diagnoses become more clearly differentiated, their "nature" and "nurture" origins better understood, and the genetic influences upon their presentation, course, and treatment more fully determined, the burden of stigma will ease, as will the burden of suffering caused by these illnesses. It is tomorrow's physicians who will need to bring this perspective to society. Psychiatry, but more importantly, people with neuropsychiatric diseases need your understanding and your advocacy.

References

Caruso K. *International suicide statistics*. Available at suicide.org. Accessed August 11, 2008.

Everson SA, Goldberg DE, Kaplan GA, et al. Hopelessness and risk of mortality and incidence of myocardial infarction and cancer. *Psychosom Med*. 1996;58:113–121.

Fawzy FI, Fawzy NW, Hyun CS, et al. Malignant melanoma. Effects of an early structured psychiatric intervention, coping, and affective state on recurrence and survival 6 years later. *Arch Gen Psychiatry*. 1993;50:681–689.

Frasure-Smith N, Lesperance F, Talajic M. Depression following myocardial infarction. Impact on 6-month survival. *JAMA*. 1993;270:1819–1825.

Frasure-Smith N, Lesperance F, Talajic M. Depression and 18-month prognosis after myocardial infarction. *Circulation*. 1995;91:999–1005.

Glassman AH, O'Connor CM, Califf RM, et al. Sertraline Antidepressant Heart Attack Randomized Trial (SADHEART) Group. Sertraline treatment of major depression in patients with acute MI or unstable angina. *JAMA*. 2002;288:701–709.

Kessler RC, Angermeyer M, Anthony JC, et al. Lifetime prevalence and age-of-onset distributions of mental disorders in the World Health Organization's World Mental Health Survey Initiative. *World Psychiatry*. 2007;6(3):168–176.

Levenson JL. Psychiatric aspects of medical practice. In: Roberts LW, ed. *Clinical psychiatry essentials*. Baltimore: Lippincott Williams & Wilkins; 2009.

Loberiza FR Jr, Rizzo JD, Bredeson CN, et al. Association of depressive syndrome and early deaths among patients after stem-cell transplantation for malignant diseases. *J Clin Oncol*. 2002;20:2118–2126.

Morgan KO, Morgan S. *Health care state rankings 2001*. Lawrence: Morgan Kitno Press; 2001.

Morgan KO, Morgan S. *State rankings 2005*. Lawrence: Morgan Kitno Press; 2005.

National Institute of Mental Health. *The numbers count: mental disorders in America*. 2008a. Last reviewed June 26, 2008. Available at http://www.nimh.nih.gov/health/publications/suicide-in-the-us-statistics-and-prevention.shtml. Accessed August 11, 2008.

National Institute of Mental Health. *Suicide in the U.S.: Statistics and prevention*. 2008b. Last reviewed June 26, 2008. Available at http://www.nimh.nih.gov/health/publications/the-numbers-count-mental-disorders-in-america.shtml. Accessed August 11, 2008.

Penninx BW, Guralnik JM, Pahor M, et al. Chronically depressed mood and cancer risk in older persons. *J Natl Cancer Inst*. 1998;90:1888–1893.

Quinlan P. Epidemiology of mental illness. In: Roberts LW, ed. *Clinical psychiatry essentials*. Baltimore: Lippincott Williams & Wilkins; 2009.

Shapiro PA, Glassman AH, Lesperance F, et al. Treatment of major depression after acute myocardial infarction with sertraline: A preliminary study. *1996 Annual meeting new research program and abstracts*. Washington, DC: American Psychiatric Association; 1996:249–250.

Spiegel D, Bloom JR, Kraemer HC, et al. Effect of psychosocial treatment on survival of patients with metastatic breast cancer. *Lancet*. 1989;2:888–891.

Stommel M, Given BA, Given CW. Depression and functional status as predictors of death among cancer patients. *Cancer*. 2002;94:2719–2727.

Theobald DE, Kirsh KL, Holtsclaw E, et al. An open-label, crossover trial of mirtazapine (15 and 30 mg) in cancer patients with pain and other distressing symptoms. *J Pain Symptom Manage*. 2002;23:442–447.

Watson M, Haviland JS, Greer S, et al. Influence of psychological response on survival in breast cancer: A population-based cohort study. *Lancet*. 1999;354:1331–1336.

CHAPTER 2

Elizabeth Kieff and Jinger G. Hoop

The Doctor–Patient Relationship in the Context of Mental Illness

Providing excellent care to all patients, including those living with mental illness, requires thoughtful attention to the doctor–patient relationship. The ethical basis for the doctor–patient relationship is grounded in the principles of *beneficence* (to do good), *nonmaleficence* (to do no harm), *respect for autonomy* (to respect patients' ability to control their own lives and bodies), and *justice* (to treat people fairly and without prejudice) (Beauchamp and Childress, 2001; Jonsen et al., 2002). Historically, Western physicians until about the 1960s tended to act assertively and paternalistically toward those in their care, as a parent makes decisions for a child. By assuming sole responsibility for medical decision making, the paternalistic physician emphasized the ethical principles of beneficence and nonmaleficence over respect for autonomy.

Medical paternalism began to change in the United States in the 1960s and 1970s, as the civil rights movement sparked companion movements of consumer rights and patients' rights. "Patients' rights" have been described as including the right to health care and medical information, the right to accept or refuse treatment, and the right to have a voice in medical decisions. A doctor–patient relationship that is focused primarily on ensuring patients' rights upholds the principle of respect for autonomy. Without due attention to the physicians' responsibilities of beneficence and nonmaleficence, however, patients may be treated merely as consumers seeking to purchase a product or service rather than as vulnerable individuals deserving compassionate care (Dyer, 1988).

The concept of *patient-centered care* has recently gained credence as a means of fulfilling a broad scope of ethical duties within the doctor–patient relationship (see Table 2-1). The term itself originated in the 1960s to describe "how physicians should interact and communicate with patients on a more personal level" (Beach et al., 2006). In particular, "patient-centered" meant shifting the focus of care away from mere diagnosis and treatment to include views of an illness from a patient's perspective with respect to his or her preferences and needs.

In the late 1980s, the Picker Institute sought to investigate ways in which the delivery of health care could become more patient focused. The institute identified key components of patient-centered care as education and shared knowledge, involvement of family and friends, collaboration and team management, sensitivity to nonmedical and spiritual dimensions of care, respect for patient needs and preferences, and free flow and accessibility of information (The Institute for Alternative Futures on behalf of the Picker Institute, 2004). The Institute of Medicine (IOM) subsequently brought patient-centered care into the national spotlight in its 2001 report *Crossing the Quality Chasm,* which listed patient-centered care as one of the six aims of high-quality health care. The IOM defined patient-centered care as "providing care that is respectful of and responsive to individual patient preferences, needs, and values, and ensuring that patient values guide all clinical decisions" (Institute of Medicine [U.S.], Committee on Quality of Health Care in America, 2001).

The ideals of patient-centered care are particularly appropriate to the treatment of persons with mental and emotional problems. As a group, these individuals are greatly disempowered in our society and in need of comprehensive, respectful, and just health care. Furthermore, the treatment of many individuals with severe and persistent illness occurs in publically funded hospitals and outpatient centers, where physicians provide services in a context of limited time and resources. In such settings, a professional devotion to patient-centered care can provide a needed counterbalance to institutional financial pressures.

TABLE 2-1	**Three Definitions of the Patient-Centered Care**

Patient-centered care entails shifting the focus of care away from mere diagnosis and treatment to include views of an illness from a patient's perspective with respect to his or her preferences and needs (Beach et al., 2006).

Patient-centered care is respectful of and responsive to individual patient preferences, needs, and values and ensures that patient values guide all clinical decisions (Institute of Medicine [U.S.], Committee on Quality of Health Care in America, 2001).

Patient-centered care consists of six elements:
- Education and shared knowledge
- Involvement of family and friends
- Collaboration and team management
- Sensitivity to nonmedical and spiritual dimensions of care
- Respect for patient needs and preferences
- Free flow and accessibility of information

(The Institute for Alternative Futures on behalf of the Picker Institute, 2004).

Patient-centered care is also congruent with psychiatric traditions. Since the early 20th century, when psychoanalysis was a predominant mode of mental health treatment, management of the doctor–patient relationship has been considered a key aspect of psychiatric care. In traditional psychoanalysis, the psychoanalyst tends to be self-effacing in the analytic relationship, becoming something of a "blank slate" onto which the patient projects unconscious desires and conflicts. The patient's feelings about the doctor are thoroughly analyzed, and the analyst monitors his or her own reactions to the patient as a way to better understand the patient's difficulties. In this way, the analyst strives to deeply understand the patient as a unique individual and to create psychological healing through that understanding.

The aim of this chapter is to demonstrate patient-centered care as a model for the compassionate treatment of individuals with mental illness. We will present five case studies that illustrate how this approach can help physicians stay clinically and ethically grounded in the face of challenging and complex situations. Because it should be relatively easy to provide patient-centered care for patients whose values and preferences are synonymous with the physician's, we will concentrate on difficult cases, in which patients lack the capacity to make decisions for themselves, have symptoms that require involuntary treatment, or behave in ways that test the clinician's emotional resources. In some of the cases, competing ethical, legal, and cultural issues will complicate the doctor–patient relationship. Throughout the chapter, we will endeavor to show how attention to the ideals of patient-centered care can help physicians stay focused on the role as healer.

CARING FOR THE PATIENT WHO REFUSES NEEDED MEDICAL TREATMENT

> Mr. H, a 75-year-old widowed man with poorly controlled diabetes and vascular disease, presented to the emergency room with a necrotic left foot. Although delirious on presentation, Mr. H seemed to have regained his baseline mental status by day 2 of antibiotic treatment and fluid resuscitation. The consulting surgeons felt that the patient would need a below-the-knee amputation to save his life, though his death might not be imminent in the next days to weeks. In conversations with several doctors, Mr. H stated that he does not want this intervention and would like to go home to die. The patient's son disagreed and asked the doctors to let him make the decision as the patient's closest living relative. Psychiatry is consulted to determine whether the patient has the capacity to make the decision to refuse treatment.

The case of Mr. H demonstrates a common scenario in consultation-liaison psychiatry, the medical patient who refuses to consent to life-saving treatment and whose primary doctors are unsure if he is capable of making a decision with such dire consequences (Junkerman and Schiedermayer, 1998; Lo, 2005). If this were a true medical emergency, it would most likely be appropriate to proceed with surgery to preserve life because there is some doubt about the patient's ability to provide consent and insufficient time to fully evaluate it. Because it is not an emergency, the psychiatric consultants have an opportunity to meet with the patient and conduct a thorough assessment.

It is easy to see how the drama and tension inherent in such a clinical situation could cause the focus to be shifted off the patient and onto the other players. The discomfort of the medical team and the desperation of the patient's son could threaten to drown out the patient's voice. A patient-centered approach to his assessment encompasses the understanding that a decisionally capable individual has the legal and moral right to refuse medical care, even if his loved ones and the medical team feel that the decision is unwise. A patient-centered approach also suggests a compassionate stance toward the patient that will lead the consultants to probe deeply into the reasons for the treatment refusal in order to understand them and to learn whether another life-saving option might be possible (Halpern, 2001).

The process of informed consent for medical treatment can be considered to have three components: the health care providers must give information about the treatment, the patient must have decision-making capacity, and the patient must be capable of acting voluntarily and without coercion (Faden and Beauchamp, 1986). The decisional capacity of the patient has been defined as the presence of four abilities: to communicate a preference by speaking, writing, or gesturing; to comprehend information necessary to make the medical decision; to appreciate the significance of the decision in terms of the patient's own circumstances; and to use the information to reason—to weigh options and consequences to come to a considered judgment (Appelbaum and Grisso, 1995). The third feature of informed consent, voluntarism, is defined as freedom from coercion and the ability to make decisions according to one's true desires. Voluntarism is influenced by the individual's developmental stage; illness; psychology, culture, and religion; and external features such as financial pressures (Roberts, 2002).

In the course of their assessment of Mr. H, the psychiatric consultants should ask him what he understands about his condition and the proposed treatment, to learn whether sufficient information has been provided. The consultants should also talk with the patient about why he has decided to refuse treatment, to understand the decision and the reasoning behind it. During the assessment, the clinicians can rule in or out illness states that might impair an individual's ability to make decisions—such as mental retardation, dementia, delirium (which may cause waxing and waning decisional capacity), psychoses that impinge upon the patient's view of his medical condition and/or the treatment, and depression that causes irrational pessimism about the future (Leeman, 1999). Finally, factors that may impinge upon Mr. H's voluntarism should be looked for and identified if present.

During such assessments, clinicians must bear in mind that standards for informed refusal of a life-saving measure are greater than standards for consent to such a treatment. Simply put, when the risk of the patient's decision is great and the benefit is low, the patient must demonstrate a fuller and more complete understanding and appreciation of the situation. This has come to be known as the *sliding scale of informed consent* (Drane, 1984).

Once Mr. H's decisional capacity has been assessed, if he is found to be impaired, then the appropriate surrogate decision-maker should be approached. Because individuals may have the capacity to make some decisions and not others, Mr. H may have the capacity to decide who should make the medical decision for him. In other words, he may understand what it means to pick a surrogate or alternative decision-maker but not fully acknowledge how sick he is or what his treatment options are. By respecting his wishes regarding the appointment of an alternative decision-maker, his physicians demonstrate their respect for his preferences and values, even if they cannot accede to his wishes regarding the surgery. (It is worth noting that if a patient also lacks capacity to choose an alternate decision-maker, state laws typically establish who is the appropriate choice. This is usually someone within the family, a friend, or a person appointed by the state.)

If the consultants' assessment indicates that Mr. H is able to demonstrate a clear understanding of the gravity and severity of his condition and the outcome of the choice not to amputate, namely death, as well as the reasons for that choice, then his physicians must honor his choice to refuse the treatment. Rather than "writing off" the patient at this point, the physicians should try to learn what values have shaped the patient's decision and look for other options that might preserve life or reduce physical or psychological suffering while respecting those values. If religious or cultural beliefs are the basis for his refusal, for example, consultation with a chaplain or culturally knowledgeable individual might benefit the patient. If the patient wishes to die because he fears being a burden on his family, the consultants might arrange a family meeting to allow the patient to explain his concerns and the family to respond. By exploring these issues, the physicians can demonstrate true empathy for the patient rather than mere "detached concern" (Halpern, 2001).

CARING FOR THE PATIENT WHOSE CULTURAL BACKGROUND DIFFERS FROM THAT OF THE PROVIDER

> Ms. J, a 21-year-old Indian woman attending college in the United States, is hospitalized for the first time because she is hearing voices and appears delusional. Ms. J's parents immediately fly to the United States from India to be with their daughter. A careful history obtained from Ms. J, her roommate, and her parents suggests that the young woman has paranoid schizophrenia. Before the diagnosis can be shared with Ms. J, her mother pulls the treating psychiatrist aside and requests that the team not discuss the diagnosis or treatment plan with the patient. "It will devastate my daughter to be told this—please do not use the term *schizophrenia* with her. Her father and I will make all medical decisions from now on." The psychiatrist is uncomfortable with this request, as she feels it is Ms. J's right to know the details of her situation.

In multicultural societies such as the United States and Canada, it is common for cultural disparities to exist between physicians and patients. These disparities represent a gulf that must be bridged to create a therapeutic doctor–patient relationship. The notion of patient-centered care is highly appropriate to the treatment of individuals from diverse cultures because of its emphasis on understanding and respecting patients' values.

Issues of cultural competency are complex and require the treating psychiatrist to be open minded as well as humble (Department of Health and Human Services, 2000; Hoop et al., 2008). Often, a little knowledge about a particular culture can be more harmful than none at all. This is because a practitioner may base his or her sense of a patient's preferences on an incomplete or stereotyped understanding of a particular culture. It is essential that a physician who is unfamiliar with a patient's culture of origin consult with those who are more knowledgeable and talk openly about cultural issues with the patient and family.

In this case, the mother's request to make decisions for Ms. J may be based on values that the daughter also shares. A dilemma arises, however, because physicians have an ethical duty to tell the truth, and providing honest and complete information about a patient's diagnosis and treatment options is necessary to allow the patient to have an informed voice in his or her care. Most patients expect and desire their doctors to be honest with them, though some might prefer not to know all the details about poor prognoses or even rare medication side effects.

Likewise, some patients find great comfort in having a psychiatric diagnosis, while others are disturbed by being "labeled." Certainly, an individual's perception of the meaning of a diagnosis can be influenced by the larger perception of society and culture. Sharing a psychiatric diagnosis with a psychiatric patient can have important social implications. Some diagnoses carry more perceived stigma than others and may be harder to accept. There is great potential value in telling a patient about the diagnosis even when it has an associated stigma, however, as it facilitates open communication about treatment options and prognosis.

In this case, the physician must balance the duty to be truthful and the duty to honor the patient's personal preferences, which may be quite divergent from the physician's. Patients from cultures that place high value on the family as the key unit of society rather than individuals may well prefer to allow the family to make decisions about their medical care—though some patients with the same cultural background may prefer to make their own decisions.

The solution in this dilemma is for the psychiatrist to look to the patient herself for clarification: Would she prefer that the doctor speak to her parents about her diagnosis and treatment and not discuss these matters with her directly? This conversation should occur as soon as the patient is capable of participating meaningfully, but without the family being present. If the patient says she wants her parents to have control over her medical decision making, the physician should probe for the reasons for that decision, to ensure that the patient is not being coerced but is instead expressing her authentic wishes. Ultimately, the patient may express preferences that are unusual for the psychiatrist and therefore personally somewhat uncomfortable to honor. Nonetheless, it is the crux of patient-centered care for the psychiatrist to adjust personal expectations when necessary to appropriately defer to the patient's values.

CARING FOR THE PATIENT WHO POSES A DANGER TO SELF OR OTHERS

> Mr. P, an unemployed 19-year-old, is brought into a hospital emergency department by his mother, who was concerned because her son's behavior has become increasingly isolated and strange. Recently, Mr. P has begun to mutter to himself about a "plot" that he uncovered by watching television. He has accused his mother of trying to poison him and refuses to eat any food that she purchases or prepares. As a result he has lost 20 lb in the previous 4 months. The psychiatric resident interviews Mr. P privately, while his mother waits outside. Mr. P presents as a very thin, poorly groomed, and malodorous individual. He is reluctant to answer questions and refuses the resident's offer of hospitalization and pharmacologic treatment. When the resident suggests they talk with Mr. P's mother about the need for treatment, Mr. P begins to cry. He tells the resident that the woman outside is not his real mother but an imposter who looks exactly like her and is trying to kill him. He whispers that his only option is to strangle her before she succeeds.

It is a highly charged but not entirely uncommon scenario when a patient who appears severely mentally ill refuses psychiatric treatment and discloses a desire to harm a third party. Appropriately balancing the physician's responsibilities toward the patient, the threatened individual, and society may be extremely challenging. A focus on patient-centered care can provide an anchor that prevents the physician from departing too far from the primary role as healer and encourages the physician to look for ways to fulfill his or her duties toward others while treating the patient with beneficence and respect.

One important aspect of this case has to do with the confidentiality of the patient's utterance regarding the plan to kill his mother. As far back as the time of Hippocrates, the notion of privacy and confidentiality has been seen as essential to the patient–doctor relationship. Indeed, a translated excerpt of the Hippocratic oath promises, "All that may come to my knowledge in the exercise of my profession or in daily commerce with men, which ought not to be spread abroad, I will keep secret and will never reveal" (Hippocratic Writings, *The Oath*). Court rulings and regulations such as the Health Insurance Portability and Accountability Act (HIPAA) of 1996 and its interpretations by states and heath care providers are present-day reminders of the value our society places on doctor–patient confidentiality (Mosher and Swire, 2002). The social stigma that frequently accompanies mental health care adds to patients' need for confidentiality in their relationship with treatment providers.

Confidentiality is a legal privilege, however, and not an absolute right; it can be suspended in certain circumstances, such as the need to protect third parties. The landmark case *Tarasoff v Regents of the University of California, 1974 and 1976* created the legal precedent upon which most states base their expectations of a psychiatrist's "duty to warn and duty to protect" individuals who are identified as the intended victim of a patient (Anfang and Appelbaum, 1996). The duty to protect can be accomplished by warning the third party, notifying the police, or taking other steps, such as hospitalizing the patient. There is an ethical basis for the duty to warn and protect as well, in that physicians have a responsibility to act with beneficence and nonmaleficence toward individuals who are not their patients and toward society as a whole.

In the case of Mr. P, the psychiatric resident must act to protect the patient's mother from harm, which may include hospitalizing the patient against his wishes. In most states, the criteria for admitting a person against his or her wishes are high, and appropriately so. An individual must typically be deemed to be a danger to himself (either because of overt suicidal ideation or because of an inability to care for basic needs) or a danger to others. It is important for everyone involved in the process of involuntary admission to remember what is at stake. When a patient is involuntarily admitted, a health care provider is in essence overriding the individual's autonomy and depriving the individual of a basic right to liberty. This is not a procedure that should be taken lightly, although it may be required to protect a third party and the only road to initial treatment.

A patient-centered approach would cause the physician to ensure that his actions take into account Mr. P's values and preferences whenever it is possible to do so. Although he may be legally justified in suspending confidentiality and ordering an involuntary hospitalization, he is not ethically justified in excluding the patient from other aspects of medical decision making. There may be many opportunities to offer collaboration with the patient. Over time, those offers may provide a foundation for a therapeutic alliance despite the circumstances. For example, the resident may explain that he must tell Mr. P's mother about his desire to kill her and allow him to have a voice in the manner in which this information is communicated (i.e., by the resident himself or with another family member present). The confidentiality of other personal information provided by the patient should be respected if he wishes, unless it bears directly upon the threat of harm.

Once the patient is hospitalized, treatment options should be discussed with the patient as they would be for patients who are hospitalized voluntarily (Roberts and Dyer, 2004). Mr. P should be informed about psychotropic medications and anticipated side effects. The treating physician should continue to try to educate the patient about the clinical rationale for the hospitalization. If this process is conducted respectfully, some patients may choose, once they have reached a better understanding of the illness, to agree to continue the hospitalization voluntarily. Even if that does not occur, by looking for opportunities to show respect and compassion for the patient, the physician demonstrates that doctors can be trustworthy and caring. For the patient, this experience may enable him to seek and accept care in the future.

CARING FOR THE PATIENT WHO TESTS PROFESSIONAL BOUNDARIES

Mr. M, a wealthy 31-year-old businessman with bipolar disorder who is hospitalized during a manic episode, has become deeply attached to the female attending psychiatrist on the inpatient service. He frequently tells her how attractive and special she is and how grateful he is to be treated by her. On the day of his discharge, Mr. M asks to exchange home phone numbers so they can keep in touch. He suggests they meet for dinner after the physician gets off work to discuss the possibility of his making a large financial donation to further her research.

The case of Mr. M highlights the need to maintain appropriate professional boundaries in the doctor–patient relationship. Gabbard (1999) has defined therapeutic boundaries as the "edge or limit of appropriate behavior by the psychiatrist in the clinical setting." By tradition, these boundaries include limits on the appropriate time and place of doctor–patient interactions and the actions of the physician, who sets a fee for service and acts toward the patient in a manner that is exclusively devoted to providing medical care. These limits serve to protect patients, who are in a vulnerable, disempowered position relative to the provider and whose illness and dependency could otherwise be easily exploited for the physician's personal benefit.

Actions by the physician that transgress normal therapeutic boundaries and have the potential to harm the patient are considered boundary violations. Sexual activity between doctors and patients is the most well-known boundary violation. In recognition of the lasting harm that patients may suffer due to sexual exploitation, sexual contact between patients and physicians is now illegal in many states (Milne, 2002). Nonsexual boundary violations include accepting nontrivial gifts and favors from patients and participating in social and business relationships (Epstein and Simon, 1990; Gabbard, 1999).

It is helpful to think of boundaries as the "bright lines" that should not be crossed when interacting with patients. The precise location of these lines may shift slightly from specialty to specialty: in pediatrics holding a patient's hand or giving a hug is acceptable practice and, indeed, a useful intervention. In psychiatry, these same actions will frequently constitute a boundary violation. The practitioner must remember that behavior always has meaning. More importantly, the meaning a gesture has for the doctor may be imbued with something quite different by the patient. It is also worth emphasizing that some boundaries do not vary between specialties: sexual relationships with patients, accepting lavish gifts of money or goods, and behaving in a retaliatory manner toward patients are all examples of unequivocally unethical behavior.

The responsibility for maintaining therapeutic boundaries rests entirely with the clinician and not with the patient, whose illness and/or treatment may in fact encourage the development of sexual or romantic feelings toward the treatment provider. In this case, Mr. M has done nothing "wrong" or unethical by suggesting a social relationship and large financial gift, but the physician would be wrong to accept these overtures. In terms of the doctor–patient relationship, the physician's goal is to maintain appropriate professional boundaries while ensuring that the patient feels valued and respected. There is a danger that the physician's own emotional reaction to the situation (such as embarrassment or anxiety) will overwhelm her ability to focus on the patient, leading her to respond in a manner that makes the patient feel humiliated or attacked.

It would also be a serious mistake to simply take the patient's invitations at face value, without considering the many factors that may underlie his request. In this case, it may be a sign that the patient's mania is not sufficiently resolved to allow him to be discharged at this time. It might also indicate a transference reaction, in which feelings of the patient for important figures from his childhood are being enacted in the relationship with the physician. In addition, Mr. M might be anxious about his recovery and seeking continued dependency upon the physician as a way of relieving that anxiety.

Depending on the patient's capacity for this type of introspection, it may or may not be suitable for the physician to discuss these possibilities with the patient. Even if that is not possible, the physician should acknowledge the patient's wish to extend the relationship but clearly and nonjudgmentally explain that she has an ethical duty to maintain professional relationships with all her patients, and that precludes her becoming involved socially or financially with them. Conducting this conversation in a manner consistent with a patient-centered approach requires the psychiatrist to act with sensitivity, tact, and the ability to empathize with the patient's vulnerability. If the situation is well handled, the patient should leave the encounter perhaps feeling frustrated at the denial of his request but also feeling understood and respected.

CARING FOR THE "DIFFICULT" PATIENT

> A 28-year-old woman, Ms. B, is hospitalized on a medical ward for several days after attempting suicide. During her stay, she expresses strong positive and negative opinions about the medical team and staff members. She is verbally abusive to several of the nurses and technicians, whom she accuses of sloppy work or purposely trying to hurt her. She is kind and flattering to the female medical student on the team, who takes a special interest in Ms. B and spends many hours empathetically listening as the patient describes a history of childhood neglect and numerous failed relationships. The student feels they have forged a strong therapeutic alliance. But when the student returns to work after a weekend off, Ms. B calls her an "incompetent idiot" and threatens to file a malpractice lawsuit against her.

The case of Ms. B suggests the challenge of providing appropriate and compassionate care to a so-called difficult patient. Physicians may identify patients as difficult for any number of reasons that evoke a strong emotional response from the treatment provider (Groves, 1978; Robbins et al., 1988). A physician who is personally distressed by any expression of emotion may find many of his patients difficult simply because human beings tend to weep or express anger and frustration under the stress of illness. Patients may also be perceived as difficult because they have characteristics (such as wealth or fame) that evoke envy in the provider or because they are so similar to the provider in key respects that it is difficult to maintain professional objectivity. Many physicians are likely to identify patients as difficult because of personality traits that create problems in all of the patients' relationships—a propensity toward rage attacks or extreme dependency, being a "help-refusing complainer," or being seductive.

As with Ms. B, it can be especially challenging to provide patient-centered care when the patient is hostile or unpleasant, when the temptation for the physician can be to respond reflexively and nontherapeutically. Especially in these circumstances, providers can find their bearings in the ideals of patient-centered care. McCarty and Roberts (1996) have suggested a three-step process for the compassionate care of difficult patients. The first step is to identify precisely what it is about the patient that is perceived as "difficult." Then, the clinician should strive to view the troublesome behavior as a clinical sign that can provide useful clues to the patient's situation or illness. For example, Ms. B's rage may be understood as a response to the student's absence over the weekend and Ms. B's resulting feelings of abandonment. By considering this possibility, the medical student can focus on the patient's emotional state rather than being solely preoccupied by her own response to it.

The final step is to look for a way to respond therapeutically to the patient. In extreme cases, when the patient is repeatedly abusive and threatening and/or when there is no real therapeutic alliance, it may be necessary and appropriate to transfer her care to another treatment provider. This should not be done punitively, however, but out of the recognition that the patient is best served by treatment from a physician who is not frightened of or angry with the patient and whom the patient can accept. In this case involving a hospitalized patient, the entire treatment team may benefit by meeting to discuss the patient's behavior as a group and considering a range of possible responses. Without such planning, individual members of the team may become increasingly enraged at the patient and perhaps toward one another, the patient's behavior may escalate, and most importantly, the patient's care is likely to suffer.

A therapeutic response to Ms. B might include a three-pronged approach: providing her with honest but nonjudgmental feedback about the effects of her outbursts on the treatment team, encouraging her to explore possible connections between her behavior on the ward and her other relationships, and offering new strategies for coping with overwhelming feelings of rage and hurt. Lasting change for this patient is likely to require much more effort and time than is likely to occur on an acute medical ward. Nevertheless, such an approach responds to the patient in a way that not only sets limits but also demonstrates respect by viewing the behavior in terms of the patient's own life and needs.

CONCLUSION

In this chapter, we have attempted to introduce the reader to patient-centered care as a framework for the ethical and compassionate treatment of patients with mental illness. The cases presented here are examples of situations in which it may be challenging to maintain a focus on the patient's needs and preferences because of other competing demands. It would be remiss for us not to acknowledge, however, that learning about patient-centered care cannot be accomplished solely through reading about cases. Rather, we hope that this chapter will provide readers with positive examples to carry with them into future clinical encounters. It is through clinical experiences that medical professionals have the opportunity to expand their technical skills, cultural awareness, and emotional capacity for understanding others and responding compassionately. It is the teaching that is received from patients, in the context of one's own self-awareness, that helps one learn how to care for them.

Clinical Pearls

- Patient-centered care in its most basic sense means understanding and respecting a patient's values and preferences as they affect the diagnosis and treatment of illness.
- As a group, persons with mental illness tend to be socially stigmatized and marginalized. They are especially deserving of high-quality, patient-centered care.
- Ethical dilemmas in the treatment of persons with mental illness often involve a conflict between the physician's duties of beneficence and respect for autonomy.
- Decisionally capable patients can refuse treatment, even life-sustaining treatment, but the physician should work with the patient to understand the decision and look for mutually acceptable ways to prolong life or relieve suffering.
- Decision-making capacity is measured with respect to a particular decision and the patient's understanding of the risks and benefits associated with the decision.
- Therapeutic boundaries exist in every doctor–patient relationship and serve to protect patients from being exploited for the physician's personal, financial, or professional benefit.
- Becoming sexually involved with patients is never acceptable.

Self-Assessment Questions and Answers

2-1. The term *patient-centered care* means:

A. Keeping the patient at the center of every conversation
B. Focusing on what would be in the patient's best interest
C. Providing whatever care the patient requests
D. Letting the patient's needs and preferences guide clinical decisions
E. Using beneficence for the patient's good

Patient centered care has been defined as "providing care that is respectful of and responsive to individual patient preferences, needs, and values, and ensuring that patient values guide all clinical decisions" (Institute of Medicine [U.S.], Committee on Quality of Health Care in America, 2001). Choice D clearly reflects the values of patient-centered care. Certainly, keeping the patient involved in the conversation is important (choice A), but there may be times when a patient may elect not to participate in particular conversations. Choices B and C are close but too one-sided. It is the patient who decides what is in his or her best interest, and it is not the doctor's obligation to do whatever the patient asks but to consider whatever requests the patient may have. Finally, choice E is a nonsense statement; remember, beneficence means to do good. This is clearly not the correct choice.
Answer: D

2-2. The essential features of the process of informed consent are:

A. Being told about one's choices and being able to make a choice
B. Having the capacity to make a decision about medical care
C. Agreeing to do what the doctors indicate is necessary
D. The signing of a consent form by a patient
E. Information provision, decisional capacity, and voluntarism

Informed consent is not an event (the signing of a contract, for example, choice D); it is a process of exchanging information between the physician and the patient. The essential components are outlined in choice E. Choices A and B are necessary but not sufficient for informed consent to take place. Finally, choice C is certainly not correct but is included here to remind training physicians that often when patients agree with a treating physician's recommendations, practitioners become sloppy about furthering the process of informed consent.
Answer: E

2-3. Which of the following is *not* necessary for a patient to make an "informed refusal" of medical treatment?

A. The patient's decision is a good one in the opinion of the treatment team.

B. The patient has the capacity to make the medical decision.

C. The patient is free from coercion in making the decision.

D. The patient understands the risks and benefits associated with the choice.

E. The patient has the ability to communicate a choice.

All of the above except choice A are important for the refusal of care. In terms of the actual reasons, the patient's explanation may seem idiosyncratic to the physician or may not be in keeping with what seem to be generally accepted values. What is most important is that the other elements needed to refuse care are present. *Answer: A*

2-4. Physicians can suspend the privilege of patient–doctor confidentiality in which of the following circumstances? (Choose all that apply.)

A. A 20-year-old patient's mother wants to know about her son's treatment.

B. A patient has a plan to harm her husband and the means with which to do it.

C. The primary doctor of a patient with Alzheimer disorder requests the patient's psychiatric record.

D. A patient admits to feeling suicidal with plans to jump in front of a car.

E. The wife of a patient with bipolar disorder would like to discuss her husband's medications.

Circumstances in which the privilege of doctor–patient confidentiality is suspended include when patients are a danger to themselves or others (choices B and D). If a patient is a direct danger to another and the potential victim is identified, the potential victim must be directly warned about the possibility of harm. Spouses (choice E) and parents of adult children (choice A) are not allowed information regarding patients without direct consent from the patients. The rights of adolescent minors to confidentiality vary somewhat by state but often still require their consent for the disclosure of information. *Answers: B, D*

References

Anfang SA, Appelbaum PS. Twenty years after Tarasoff: Reviewing the duty to protect. *Harv Rev Psychiatry.* 1996;4:67–76.

Appelbaum PS, Grisso T. The MacArthur treatment competence study. Part I: Mental illness and competence to consent to treatment. *Law Hum Behav.* 1995;19:105–126.

Beach MC, Saha S, Cooper LA. *The role and relationship of cultural competence and patient-centeredness in health care quality.* New York: Commonwealth Fund; 2006.

Beauchamp TL, Childress JF. *Principles of biomedical ethics.* New York: Oxford University Press; 2001.

Department of Health and Human Services. *Mental health, culture, race, ethnicity supplement to mental health: A report of the surgeon general;* 2000.

Drane JF. Competency to give an informed consent: A model for making clinical assessments. *JAMA.* 1984;252:925–927.

Dyer AR. *Ethics and psychiatry toward professional definition.* Washington, DC: American Psychiatric Press; 1988.

Epstein RS, Simon RI. The exploitation index: An early warning indicator of boundary violations in psychotherapy. *Bull Menninger Clin.* 1990;54:450–465.

Faden RR, Beauchamp TL. *A history and theory of informed consent.* New York: Oxford University Press; 1986.

Gabbard GO. Boundary violations. In: Bloch S, Chodoff P, Green SA, eds. *Psychiatric ethics.* New York: Oxford University Press; 1999:141–160.

Groves JE. Taking care of the hateful patient. *N Engl J Med.* 1978;298:883–887.

Halpern J. *From detached concern to empathy: Humanizing medical practice.* Oxford: Oxford University Press; 2001.

Hoop JG, DiPasquale T, Hernandez JM, et al. Ethics and culture in mental health care. *Ethics Behav.* 2008;18:353–372.

Institute for Alternative Futures on behalf of the Picker Institute. *The doctor-patient relationship 2015: Scenarios, vision, goals and next steps;* 2004.

Institute of Medicine (U.S.), Committee on Quality of Health Care in America. *Crossing the quality chasm: A new health system for the 21st century.* Washington, DC: National Academy Press; 2001.

Jonsen AR, Siegler M, Winslade WJ. *Clinical ethics: A practical approach to ethical decisions in clinical medicine*. New York: McGraw-Hill, Appleton & Lange; 2002.

Junkerman C, Schiedermayer DL. *Practical ethics for students, interns, and residents: A short reference manual*. Frederick: University Publishing Group; 1998.

Leeman CP. Depression and the right to die. *Gen Hosp Psychiatry*. 1999;21:112–115.

Lo B. *Resolving ethical dilemmas: A guide for clinicians*. Philadelphia: Lippincott Williams & Wilkins; 2005.

McCarty T, Roberts LW. The difficult patient. In: Rubin RH, ed. *Medicine: A primary care approach*. Philadelphia: WB Saunders; 1996:395.

Milne D. Psychologists' disciplinary failure leads to new law in Ohio. *Psychiatr News*. 2002;37:18.

Mosher PW, Swire PP. The ethical and legal implications of Jaffee versus Redmond and the HIPAA medical privacy rule for psychotherapy and general psychiatry. *Psychiatr Clin North Am*. 2002;25:vi–vii, 575–584.

Robbins JM, Beck PR, Mueller DP, et al. Therapists' perceptions of difficult psychiatric patients. *J Nerv Ment Dis*. 1988;176:490–497.

Roberts LW, Dyer AR. *Concise guide to ethics in mental health care*. Washington, DC: American Psychiatric Publishing; 2004.

Roberts LW. Informed consent and the capacity for voluntarism. *Am J Psychiatry*. 2002;159:705–712.

The Psychiatric Interview

The psychiatric interview is an exceptionally important moment in the care of each patient. In this initial clinical encounter, the physician learns about the patient's life and forms an impression of the symptoms, experiences, biological influences, strengths, and relationships relevant in the presentation of the patient at that exact point in time. During the psychiatric interview, the nature of the illness, condition, or situation causing an individual to seek care is clarified. Much about the patient's future course of illness and treatment may be assessed in this early clinical interaction as well. The psychiatric interview also generates an intuitive response and "feel" in the clinician; this is crucial clinical "data" that can reveal much about the personality qualities and diagnostic considerations which may be significant in the care of the patient over time.

From the perspective of the patient, the psychiatric interview also has great importance. For a newly ill person, it may be the first time in which very difficult and very private issues are revealed to another person, the first time that an individual expresses concern that something is "wrong," and the first time that he or she is meeting a mental health provider. It may also be the first time the patient feels more fully understood and accepted with compassion and knowledge by another person, by an expert—this experience can establish rapport and trust and alleviate fears, even if it does not yield immediate answers. It is also the time when expectations for psychiatric care can be first discussed, and the clinician can address questions and worries of the patient—ranging from issues related to medication side effects to stigma and confidentiality. For individuals who are chronically ill and may have had many interactions with mental health providers, the psychiatric interview can have other importance—sorting out newly emerging symptoms or side effects, determining the need for a new treatment approach, dealing with the problems and sources of disability that can be associated with a long-standing illness, and exploring issues that relate to past experiences, positive and negative, in psychiatric treatment. Whether newly or chronically ill, however, the psychiatric interview becomes the platform for his or her future care of the patient.

For the student first learning how to perform a psychiatric interview, it will be important to keep in mind that no laboratory tests or other biological measures reliably diagnose psychiatric illnesses. The interview with the patient is therefore critical in developing diagnostic hypotheses and potential treatment approaches. Multiple sources of information aid in the evaluation of patients, including neuroimaging and laboratory testing (see Chapter 5), psychological and neuropsychological testing (see Chapter 6), medical record review, physical examination, and collateral information, but the most essential source of information, under most circumstances, remains the clinical interview. Data gathering during the psychiatric interview may be difficult because of the complexity or unusual nature of the clinical "picture" or because the patient is guarded or embarrassed or has difficulty with communication. Nevertheless, discovering information may actually be the easiest goal to attain in the interview. Building rapport, establishing expectations for care, and alleviating distress require subtle skills—active listening, tact, and interpersonal sensitivity.

Empathy is also a key factor. Imagine what it is *really* like for the patient. For instance, it is natural for people to feel discomfort and intimidation when meeting a physician, and often those feelings are magnified when meeting a psychiatrist. Owing to the stigma associated with mental illness, many people avoid psychiatric assessment. They may believe that having a psychiatric evaluation means they are "crazy" and therefore may defer evaluation despite needing help. And what if they "know" they are mentally ill, for example, because they are experiencing hallucinations or feel severely depressed and "different" from how they once were? Even after making the decision to see a psychiatrist, individuals may be reluctant to follow up as needed for treatment. This puts a large burden on the clinician to establish rapport and put the individual at ease at the very first meeting.

PUTTING THE PATIENT AT EASE

The interview may occur in a variety of settings: the emergency department, an inpatient medical ward, a psychiatric ward, an outpatient clinic, a prison, or a residential nursing or group home. The environment cannot always be manipulated in these settings, but efforts should be made to make the patient as comfortable as possible. A calm, quiet, private setting with a comfortable temperature is preferable.

Small acts of courtesy also put the patient at ease. The patient should be referred to cordially, as Ms., Mrs., or Mr. X, and interviewers should introduce themselves and explain their role in the patient's care. Patients who are not themselves medical professionals often have no conception of the differences among the terms *resident, intern, attending,* and even *medical student* (Silver-Isenstadt and Ubel, 1997), and the interviewer should make clear what his or her specific roles and responsibilities are. It is helpful to tell the patient how long the interview is expected to last and to ask if the patient needs a bathroom break or refreshment before beginning. It is very useful to have tissues available to offer patients if they begin to cry.

The patient may be accompanied by friends, family, or caregivers and should be given control over who will be present for the beginning of the interview. At some point, however, the patient should be interviewed alone to address anything that may be difficult for the patient to mention in the presence of others.

Many doctors stand while their patients sit or lie on the bed. This stance can be intimidating and may convey to patients that the clinician does not have enough time to sit down and listen to all the patient may have to say. Ideally, the interviewer should be seated at eye level with the patients, with chairs facing at an angle rather than directly opposite each other. This way, patients can look directly at the interviewer but may also comfortably avert their gaze if they prefer.

By using active listening techniques throughout the interview, the interviewer can build rapport with the patient by expressing interest and empathy both verbally and nonverbally. Active listening involves using gestures such as nodding and leaning forward, repeating the patient's own words ("So you have been feeling down ever since Ronnie died?"), and making statements that acknowledge the patient's distress ("It must be very sad to talk about your mother").

This type of listening conveys a sense that the patient is not alone in his or her experience and that the interviewer is trying to understand him or her. In many cases, these simple acts of listening and understanding are powerfully therapeutic, capable of temporarily calming anxiety and relieving despair. The phenomenon has been described in the literature on self-psychology: "Feeling understood—simple as this may sound—in reality has a profound effect on the state of the self. Feeling understood is the adult equivalent of being held" (Ornstein and Ornstein, 1996).

RECOGNIZING AND MANAGING ONE'S EMOTIONAL RESPONSES

Patients with severe psychiatric symptoms often evoke strong emotional reactions in the people who are taking care of them. Recognizing and taking stock of one's own emotional experience while seeing a patient can provide important information that will be useful in formulating a diagnosis and treatment plan.

Sometimes, the interviewer may find himself or herself experiencing the patient's emotional state. Often, simply sitting with a deeply depressed person may lead to feelings of sadness and depletion. Anxious patients may cause the interviewer to fidget along with them. While evaluating a euphorically manic patient, interviewers may find themselves smiling and feeling a little ebullient themselves. These emotional reactions to the patient are normal and can be an important aid to formulating a diagnosis.

Clinicians may also react toward patients in a manner that instructs them about the patients' interactions with others. For example, a depressed man's friends may stop calling because it takes too much effort to interact with him, and the clinician may also feel reluctant to spend time with the patient. The family of a manic woman may feel overwhelmed and annoyed with her because they feel she is self-centered and so too may the treating physician. Both the physician and the patient's family may become frustrated and confused by the poor choices and judgment of the patient with psychosis. Understanding that psychiatric illness affects patients' thinking, reasoning, and behavior allows practitioners to step away from their own emotions and view the phenomena as symptoms of the illness rather than as the patient's inherent deficits. It is always important to remember that behaviors need to be viewed as symptoms that can help the interviewer gain insight into the illness (McCarty and Roberts, 1996).

Whenever the patient elicits an emotion in the interviewer, the interviewer needs to consider why this emotion is present. Is it a normal mirroring of the patient's emotion? Is it an expected human response to the patient's behavior, which other members of the treatment team share? Or does the emotion seem to have more to do with the interviewer than the patient? In this latter case, the practitioner may be reacting to his or her own psychological issues rather than to the patient, a phenomenon called *countertransference*. For example, a medical student who grew up with an abusive, alcoholic parent may feel unwarranted irritation and anger toward patients with substance use disorders. A clinician who has suffered the suicide of a loved one may become overly anxious when evaluating a suicidal patient in the emergency department. Countertransference feelings can disrupt the therapeutic relationship, so it is essential that clinicians learn to recognize these feelings and deal with them appropriately—for example, by talking with a trusted friend, colleague, or therapist.

DATA GATHERING

A major goal of the initial psychiatric interview is to gather data that can be helpful in formulating a diagnosis and treatment plan. Adolf Meyer (Meyer and Winters, 1950) proposed that the written evaluation should reveal the patient's life story and therefore follow a more chronologic timeline: identifying information, chief complaint, family history, social history, premorbid personality, medical history, medications, past psychiatric history, history of present illness, mental status examination, and assessment and plan. As the person is understood longitudinally, the current problems become more understandable in the context of the patient's life.

Although it might be easier to organize the written documentation of the interview if the information could be gathered in the same order, this rarely occurs. Patients tend to bring up issues in an order that is logical based on their own life experiences or patterns of thought. For example, if the patient's distress is related to a medical condition, he or she may wish to begin the interview by talking about his or her medical history. An interviewer who attempts to rigidly direct the patient to answer questions that follow a preconceived format will likely appear to be a poor, uncaring listener. The task of the interviewer is to gather all the information as naturally as possible, without asking the patient to repeat himself or herself unnecessarily, and later put the data in logical order for written and oral presentations.

The process of gathering data often begins long before the interview, in the referral note from the primary care doctor or the patient's words during a phone call to make the initial appointment. Data gathering continues when the patient is first met. The manner in which the patient greets the interviewer, walks to the interviewing room, and engages in conversation offers valuable information. A brisk walk may signify energy, whereas a slow walk may be a result of pain, fatigue, or neurologic illness. If the patient comes to the interview with another person, it may indicate that the patient is too impaired to travel unaccompanied, lacks insight about the need for help, is overly dependent, and/or has strong social support.

Beginning the Interview

Most psychiatrists begin the clinical interview with an open-ended question such as, "What brought you in today?" When assessing patients as a consultant on the inpatient medical wards, it may be useful to begin the interview by asking about the patients' understanding of their medical illness and their ability to adapt to it before embarking on a psychiatric evaluation (i.e., "Why do you think your doctors wanted me to see you?"). Inquiring about this is beneficial in determining their insight into their problems or if there is some miscommunication between them and the treating team.

During the patient's response to the initial question, the clinician should listen carefully without interruption. These early moments of the interview are crucial for building rapport and relieving anxiety—by letting the patient know that he or she is in the presence of a calm, competent professional and will be heard. Furthermore, the patient's response to the first question is usually extremely informative both in content and form. The patient's verbatim answer may be quoted as the "chief complaint" for the write-up of the interview. In addition, by carefully listening to the way the patient connects one idea to another, the interviewer can detect the presence of thought disorders such as circumstantiality, tangentiality, or flight of ideas (see subsequent text). Patients who have mild thought disorders may be quite capable of coherently answering closed-ended or yes/no questions. It is only by giving them time to speak freely that the disjointed nature of their thinking becomes apparent.

Gathering the History of Present Illness and Past Psychiatric History

After several minutes of this "free speech" by the patient, the interviewer should begin to ask more specific questions to fill in details about the history of present illness. Questions regarding clarification are useful as follow-up, such as "What is it like for you to be depressed?" "In what way is your neighbor torturing you?"

The same information obtained when evaluating a physical illness is also important for evaluating a mental illness. To evaluate pain, questions about location, quality, severity, duration, precipitating causes, and alleviating factors are important. If an individual presents with depression, the interviewer will want to know the same type of information. Questions about duration of symptoms, stressors that worsen existing symptoms, and factors that have improved the patient's mood are all essential to determining the diagnosis. Does the patient's mood improve as the day progresses (diurnal mood variation)? Or when the patient is provided support by others or attends church? Does the patient feel better when taking medication? Although depression has been used here as an example, the same sort of information should be gathered for other psychiatric conditions as well. If the patient complains of poor sleep, the clinician may ask the patient to quantify how many hours he or she sleeps and whether sleep is characterized by waking up too early, nighttime awakenings, or difficulty falling asleep.

Premorbid personality should also be asked about when appropriate, although this may be best determined later, by interviewing a person who knew the patient before the illness. Many times patients who have depression will describe feeling like a different person when depressed. Determining premorbid personality gives the practitioner a perspective on the patient's baseline and possibly the goals of treatment. In other situations, knowing how the patient has deviated from baseline gives a clue as to how the illness has affected his or her behavior. This would be the case with illnesses that permanently alter personality such as traumatic brain injury, Huntington disease, and frontotemporal dementia.

After clarification is obtained, specific questions directed at assessing safety, completing the history, and determining the correct diagnosis should be asked. The past psychiatric history includes previous mental illness and any and all history of contact with psychiatry, including psychiatric hospitalizations, suicide attempts, psychotherapy, and medication. The precipitants of these past psychiatric episodes should be explored. Any psychotropic medications that have been tried should be inquired about, along with dosages and duration of treatment, the reason they were discontinued, and whether they were effective. It is not always easy to get a full history about previous medications, but knowing the maximum dosage and duration of use is helpful in determining whether a full trial of a particular medication occurred. History of electroconvulsive therapy, the number of treatments, and whether it was bilateral or unilateral should also be assessed. This information helps guide treatment.

Talking about Suicide

It is vital in any initial evaluation to inquire about suicidal ideation. Trainees often feel anxious about openly discussing this issue, fearing that they will "plant the idea in the patient's head." In fact, there is no evidence that this occurs and substantial evidence that asking about suicide can lead to appropriate clinical care and prevent premature death. A natural way of introducing this subject is to tie it to the patient's chief complaint: "Do you ever feel so sad that life does not seem worth living?" "Do the voices ever tell you to hurt yourself?" A positive answer should then be followed with questions to elicit suicidal ideation (e.g., "Have you thought about killing yourself?"), suicide plan (e.g., "How would you kill yourself?"), access or means (e.g., "Is there a gun in your home? Have you been storing pills?"), and suicide intent (e.g., "Do you intend to kill yourself?"). It is also helpful to ask about protective factors (e.g., "What has kept you going during this difficult time?").

Some patients may endorse a passive death wish by saying that they wish they would not wake up in the morning or that they were no longer alive without thinking about actively killing themselves. Previous suicide attempts are the strongest predictors of future attempts so it is important to ask about previous attempts and assess their lethality. Did the patient realize he or she would be found? Did the patient believe this attempt would result in death? Did it result in medical treatment such as intensive care unit (ICU) admission? How long did the patient think about the suicide before carrying through the attempt? Acute anxiety has also been described as a risk factor for suicide (Gonda et al., 2007). All these issues need to be explored when assessing suicide risk.

Eliciting an Accurate History of Substance Use

Because many psychiatric symptoms can be caused by intoxication or withdrawal from substances, it is crucial to gather an accurate history of patients' use of alcohol, recreational drugs, prescription drugs, herbal supplements, caffeine, and tobacco. Use of some of these substances is stigmatized or illegal in our society, so the interviewer must carefully phrase questions to exhibit a nonjudgmental and nonpunitive attitude to encourage the patient to be forthcoming. Asking the patient, "You do not use illegal drugs, do you?" clearly signals that the interviewer is not prepared to hear about drug use. Instead of referring to *illegal*, *street*, or *illicit* drugs, refer to *recreational drugs* or mention them by name. Ask about drug *use*, not *abuse*, a highly pejorative term. Useful opening questions include "What recreational drugs have you used?" or "Please tell me about your use of recreational drugs."

Other strategies for encouraging patients to accurately report drug and alcohol use include asking about how many days per week they use and then how much they drink per day. Some practitioners find that overestimating the amount of alcohol patients use normalizes heavy use and allows patients to feel more comfortable about revealing how much they are actually using. For example, the interviewer may ask, "About how much vodka do you drink per day? Three or four fifths?" The patient may respond, "Oh, no, not that much. I only have one fifth per night."

When a patient says he or she has used a substance, details about the quantity, age at first use, mode of use (e.g., intravenously, intranasal, inhaled, subcutaneously, and orally), and date and time of last use should then be elicited. Any drug treatment, involvement in treatment groups, history of withdrawal symptoms, or hospital admissions for drug intoxication or withdrawal should be noted. Common symptoms to inquire about include blackouts, seizures, and flashbacks.

If the patient reports minimal or moderate use of alcohol, a brief screen for alcoholism, the CAGE questionnaire (Ewing, 1984), can be helpful in trying to determine if the use is actually problematic (see Chapter 9). The four CAGE questions are as follows: Does the patient want to **c**ut down on drinking? Does his use **a**nnoy others? Does he feel **g**uilty about drinking? Does he use the substance early in the morning as an **e**ye opener? This set of questions has been shown to predict a diagnosis of alcohol abuse or dependence when patients answer yes to at least two of them.

Gathering Data about Medical History

Collecting the patient's medical history is relatively straightforward. All medical diagnoses of the patient should be included in the medical history, whether or not they seem related to the chief complaint or psychiatric history. Many patients are able to provide detailed medical histories after being asked a simple open-ended question about their health problems. Ask about previous diagnoses as well as current ones. Some patients do not consider themselves to have an illness after it has been adequately treated (e.g., an older female states that she used to have high blood pressure, but because on medicine she is normotensive, she believes she no longer has the diagnosis of hypertension).

Surgeries, accidents, and hospitalizations should be inquired about as well. Specific questions should be asked about history of head injury with loss of consciousness, which suggests possible brain injury. Any neurologic conditions should get close attention, such as cerebrovascular events or the type and frequency of seizures.

It is important to ask patients to list their medications with the dosages, along with any allergies. The medication list can be used as a guide to ask about any medical conditions the patient may have forgotten to mention. For example, seeing levothyroxine on the list of medications may prompt the practitioner to ask specifically about thyroid disorders.

Eliciting the Family History

Owing to the strong genetic component of psychiatric illnesses, it is important to ask about the psychiatric history of family members. Specific questions should be made about mood disorders, dementia, history of psychiatric hospitalizations, and suicides or suicide attempts. If a family member does have a psychiatric disorder, the details of the illness course and treatment are important to help guide the treatment plan for the patient. If another family member has responded to an antidepressant, it is possible that the patient may also respond to the same medication.

Gathering the Social and Developmental History

The social and developmental history details the stages of a patient's life. This portion of the history gives the clinician a picture of the patient as a human being and allows an appreciation of the patient's strengths, weaknesses, and maximum level of functioning. These data are of great importance in psychiatry, because of the field's emphasis on psychological, developmental, and social aspects of patients' lives.

Clinicians may wish to begin this part of the interview by asking patients to tell them where they were born and grew up and who was in their family. During this part of the interview, the clinician should attempt to learn whether there were any difficulties with the patient's birth, delay in milestones, or early illnesses that may give clues to developmental delay. The interviewer may also ask if the patient attended regular school or special classes. Patients should be asked about their experiences with teachers and friends, clues to social and behavioral problems. Grades in school, changes in performance, and highest grade level completed are all essential points. The reason for any stops or breaks in education should be explored. School is a stressful time for some people and may be when psychiatric problems surface.

Childhood abuse and neglect is unfortunately widespread and should be considered when interviewing any patient. Patients will often not divulge that they were abused in childhood unless the clinician asks about it directly (i.e., "Were you ever physically, emotionally, or sexually abused?"). Many patients feel ashamed and that they are to be blamed for the abuse and are reluctant to speak about it unless it is brought up in this way. If a patient is extremely distressed due to current psychiatric symptoms, it may be prudent to temporarily delay asking about abuse history to avoid worsening the distress.

If the patient says that childhood was disrupted by death, divorce, parental substance use, or abuse, the impact on the patient should be explored. Investigating adverse childhood events gives clues as to how self-reliant the patient has had to be and whether the patient was afforded adequate support growing up. This will often affect future relationships and may affect the way the patient interacts with health care providers. It is hard to accept help and support if this has not been experienced before. A person who has never had someone to depend on will believe that the practitioner will fail him or her before given a chance to fail.

The interviewer should also inquire about the patient's experiences since childhood, including military service and employment. When treating veterans, it is important to inquire about the branch, rank, years of service, discharge status, and combat exposure. Discharge status often provides clues to whether the patient developed mental illness while in the military.

The occupation history details the length and type of previous work as well as the patient's current job position. Reasons for switching jobs and any current stressors in the work environment need investigation. If the person is currently unemployed, the cause should be determined and financial means explored.

The ability to form lasting interpersonal relationships is an important issue for assessment. Those who can form relationships are likeable enough for others to tolerate being around and can tolerate other people's imperfections. To evaluate this, the interviewer should ask about past and current relationships (e.g., "Tell me about the important people in your life"). The patient should be asked about marital history, divorces, and children and grandchildren. Further questions about the quality of relationships with significant people can help clarify how the patient relates to others.

Questions about the patient's sexual history may be uncomfortable for the interviewer, but are essential to taking a complete history. Patients often expect to be asked about sexual matters during a psychiatric interview and will be prepared and perhaps eager to discuss difficulties that they have not been able to talk about with anyone else. The patient's sexual preference should be ascertained (e.g., "Do you have sex with men, women, or both?") and risky sexual practices, such as multiple partners or unprotected sex, explored. The patient will feel more comfortable responding to questions about sexual activities if the clinician is comfortable asking them.

Social, cultural, and spiritual values are also important in understanding the patient. Involvement in the community, organization membership, and extracurricular activities are extremely important to some patients, and discussion of these activities can help bolster patients' sense of themselves as worthwhile members of society. Religion is also extremely significant to many patients and should be inquired about in a nonpartisan way that encourages conversation (e.g., "Is religion or spirituality important to you? If so, please tell me about your faith.").

Finally, ask about the patient's contacts with the legal system in a nonjudgmental manner (e.g., "Have you had any legal troubles? Have you ever been arrested? Have you been involved in any lawsuits?"). These may be clues to diagnosis or current stressors. Patients who have been arrested should be asked about legal charges and whether there were convictions and jail or prison sentences. Current or past lawsuits by or against the patient should also be included. If the patient is elderly, it is important to note if there is a living will and power of attorney for health care in place.

Review of Systems

A review of systems is performed during psychiatric evaluations just as in other medical disciplines for each biologic system: head, ears, nose, throat, respiratory, gastrointestinal, cardiovascular, endocrine, neurologic, urogenital, constitutional, integumentary, and musculoskeletal. Many medical illnesses are associated with psychiatric illnesses (e.g., hypothyroid or obstructive sleep apnea with depression) or are caused by psychotropic medications (e.g., atypical antipsychotics causing metabolic syndrome). A careful review of systems can allow undetected medical conditions to be identified and treated.

Gathering Data for the Mental Status Examination

The mental status examination is the objective portion of the psychiatric interview. It provides a snapshot of the patient's current presentation and is instrumental in making a diagnosis. The mental status examination begins immediately when meeting the patient and is based primarily on the observations of the practitioner. The elements of the mental status examination are described in Chapter 6. How these elements are assessed during the interview will be the focus here.

Appearance and General Behavior

Throughout the interview, the clinician can easily take note of the patient's appearance, including body habitus, whether the patient appears his or her stated age, the level of consciousness, and any distinguishing characteristics such as tattoos or piercings. The patient's attire is notable, as is the quality of hygiene and grooming. Poor hygiene, odor, and unkempt appearance may provide insight into the patient's ability for self-care. The attitude of the patient toward the examiner should also be monitored. For example, a histrionic or manic patient may have seductive behavior, whereas a paranoid patient may be guarded and repeatedly scan the environment. The patient's eye contact should be noted as well. Normal eye contact consists of periods of meeting the other person's gaze and then looking away. People with depression, low self-esteem, schizophrenia, autism, and other conditions may make no eye contact at all. A person with paranoid psychosis may look intently into the eyes of the interviewer, described as a *paranoid stare*.

Motor Activity

Involuntary movements, such as tics, tremors, and abnormal mouth movements, should be carefully observed during the interview. Abnormal movements may be a side effect of psychotropic medications. Selective serotonin reuptake inhibitors may cause tremor or bruxism; neuroleptics can cause dystonic reactions, tardive dyskinesia, and akathisia; and lithium may cause tremor. Psychomotor agitation or retardation should also be noted. A person with psychomotor retardation tends to walk slowly and have few to no movements; this may occur with depression. Psychomotor agitation includes fidgeting and pacing.

Speech

The way patients speak provides insight into their psychopathology. A person who talks rapidly and is extremely difficult to interrupt would be said to exhibit pressured speech. A person who only speaks in response to a direct question lacks spontaneous speech. The volume of speech should be noted, particularly when the patient is loud or talks unusually softly. Fluency and articulation give insight into the presence of aphasias. The rhythm and tone of the speech should be described as well.

Mood and Affect

Mood is the patient's own subjective report of his or her current emotional state. The mood is often reported as a direct quote from the patient following a direct inquiry during the early part of the interview (i.e., "How have you been feeling lately?"). *Affect* is the clinician's objective observation of the patient's mood and is described in terms of range, congruence with mood, intensity, appropriateness, and stability. A decreased range of affect can be described as *restricted*. If a patient's affect lacks intensity, it is described as *blunted*. On the other hand, a complete lack of emotional facial expression is termed *flat*. A *labile* affect is one in which there are sudden changes in the emotions or intensity of emotion expressed by the patient. The quality of affect can be described using many terms, including *euthymic* (normal mood), *dysthymic* (visibly sad), or *euphoric* (elevated mood).

Thought Process

Thought process is a description of the patient's flow of thoughts and ideas, and it is best assessed during the early part of the interview, when the patient is encouraged to speak freely, with minimal interruptions. The authors describe thought processes below in rough sequence from normal to highly abnormal. Normal thought processes are described as *linear* and *goal directed*. People may speak in such generalities that frequent explanation is needed; this can be referred to as *vagueness*. Some patients cannot stay on the subject when speaking but gravitate further and further away from the topic in question. This type of thought process is called *tangential*. If the patient wanders away from the subject but eventually gets back to it, providing excessive details, the thought process is termed *circumstantial*.

When patients speak very briefly, using only a few words even when asked for more detail, they may be described as having *thought poverty* or *paucity of thought*. Those who speak with many words but have little content to what they say are described as having *poverty of content*. Patients who create new words to express themselves are said to use *neologisms*, words that have idiosyncratic meaning to the user but are not in standard usage. The term *flight of ideas* refers to the thoughts of a patient who quickly and repeatedly changes subjects. Repetition of thoughts, actions, or speech is described as *perseveration* and occurs in dementias, brain injury, and autistic spectrum disorders (Table 3-1). Finally, speech that appears entirely disjointed—with words having no logical relation to one another, as if tossed in the air—is described as *word salad*.

Thought Content

During the early part of the interview, when the clinician is gathering information about the patient's current symptoms and history of present illness, he or she is also collecting data regarding the content of the patient's thought. Descriptions of thought content include abnormal ideas and thoughts such as hallucinations, delusions, phobias, and obsessions. *Hallucinations* occur when there is sensory perception without the presence of stimuli and in any sensory modality (tactile, auditory, visual, gustatory, and olfactory). *Illusions* are sometimes mistaken for hallucinations but occur when the patient misinterprets stimuli that are present, such as mistaking a shadow for a person.

Hallucinations should be asked about directly (i.e., "Have you ever had the experience of seeing visions or hearing voices when no one is present?"). When asking about auditory

TABLE 3-1	Terms to Describe Thought Disorders
Circumstantial	To respond to questions in an oblique manner but eventually answer the question
Clang associations	Use of words based on their sound rather than meaning (rhyming, alliteration)
Derailment	Thoughts follow a track of thinking, then shift suddenly and follow another
Echolalia	Echoing back words that are heard
Flight of ideas	Repetitive and rapid changing of topic
Loose associations	When ideas are loosely (distantly) associated with one another
Neologism	Using words that have no meaning except to the user
Paraphasia	Substitution of the wrong word
Perseveration	Persistent repetition of words or ideas
Tangential	To respond to questions in an irrelevant or oblique manner
Thought blocking	Train of thought is interrupted abruptly without completion
Word salad	Nonsensical string of words

hallucinations, it is important to determine if the patient is hearing multiple voices, if the voices are familiar, and if the person can make out what the voices are saying. Sometimes the voices will tell the patient to do something; these are called *command hallucinations* and are important to ask about and assess. It is also crucial to learn whether the patient believes that he or she must do what the voices say, because this puts the patient at grave risk of harming self or others.

Delusions are defined as fixed false beliefs that are not supported by cultural norms. They have been put into many different descriptive categories, which are outlined in Table 3-2. Very often patients have delusional explanations as to why they experience hallucinations (e.g., that the voice being heard belongs to demons who are tormenting the patient). Hallucinations and delusions usually are mood congruent when associated with a mood disorder—that is, the emotional content of the psychotic symptom matches the mood state of the patient. For example, a depressed person may have a delusion that he or she caused the collapse of several lives through his misdeeds, whereas a manic patient may have a delusion that she possesses godlike powers.

Other psychiatric symptoms that are related to thought content include phobias and obsessions. Phobias are fears of a specific object or situation that usually lead to intense anxiety and sometimes avoidance. Obsessions are recurrent thoughts, ideas, impulses, or images that are intrusive and inappropriate and cause distress.

Insight and Judgment

In the context of a psychiatric evaluation, the assessment of *insight* is generally based on whether the patient has awareness of his or her own illness. From the beginning of the interview, the clinician is developing a sense of whether the patient has insight and, if so, how much. Patients have many different reasons to seek psychiatric care, and the way the patient comes to psychiatric attention can give clues about the degree of insight the patient has. Because of the stigma of mental illness, some patients are reluctant to accept psychiatric diagnoses and deny having a disease, signaling poor insight. Being mandated by the court system to receive treatment is also a sign that the patient lacks insight into his or her illness. Those who seek care voluntarily and are able to name their disease have better insight into their illness.

Judgment is a sophisticated concept, that can be difficult to thoroughly assess during a single interview. Some clinicians ask theoretical questions to assess judgment (e.g., "What would you do if you smelled smoke in a crowded theater?"), but many psychiatrists feel that a better assessment of judgment is based on the patient's actual recent decision making. A person in a manic state who was found walking nude in the middle of a busy street should be considered to have extremely poor judgment, no matter how he or she answers a standard question about smelling smoke

TABLE 3-2	Hallucinations and Delusions
Capgras delusion	The fixed belief that usually recognized people are not themselves, but are imposters
Cotard delusion	Belief that one is dead and does not exist
Delusion	Fixed false belief not supported by cultural norms
Delusional misidentification syndrome	The belief that the identity of a person, object, or place has been changed or altered
Delusional parasitosis	Fixed belief of infestation by parasites
Erotic delusion	The fixed belief that someone is in love with the patient
Folie a deux	A shared delusional belief between two people
Grandiose delusion	The fixed belief that one is greater than one is or has special talents that one does not
Hallucination	The experience of a sensory perception in the absence of stimuli
Hypnogogic hallucination	Hallucinations that occur as one is falling asleep
Hypnopompic hallucination	Hallucinations that occur as one is waking up
Ideas of reference	The belief that unrelated things in the world refer to or have special relevance and meaning to the patient
Passage hallucination	The feeling that someone has passed by when no one has
Presence hallucination	The feeling that someone is present when no one is
Thought broadcasting	The fixed belief that patient's thoughts are being broadcast out so that others may hear
Thought insertion	The belief that someone has inserted thoughts into one's mind
Thought withdrawal	The fixed belief that thoughts are removed from one's mind

in a theater. Similarly, a person facing adversity who has been coping by binging on alcohol demonstrates impaired judgment. A person who adheres to medication regimens, consistently attends medical appointments, and contacts supportive friends and relatives when under stress shows better judgment.

Cognition

Cognition is also assessed during the psychiatric interview to provide information on how the brain is functioning. The term *cognition* encompasses many elements of human mental processing, and there are many different ways of evaluating it (see Chapter 8). In the course of the psychiatric interview, simple tests can be administered to provide an estimate of the person's cognitive functioning and determine whether there is a clear need for additional assessments.

Patients' orientation may be evaluated by asking their full name, current location, and the date. A simple memory test can be administered by giving three to five words to remember and then asking after several minutes if the patient can recall them. Concentration and attention may be evaluated by asking the patient to spell common words backwards or say the days of the week or months of the year in reverse order. The Trails B Test (Lezak, 1995) is also a useful test of concentration. Here, the individual alternates between letters of the alphabet and numbers in increasing order (i.e., 1A, 2B, 3C, etc.). The Clock Drawing Test (Freedman, 1994) assesses patients' ability to plan, organize, and implement their visuospatial skills. Patients are asked to draw a clock with the numbers and then put in the hands to read a specific time. Folstein's Mini-Mental State Examination (Folstein et al., 1975) may also be performed. This test contains 11 questions with a maximum score of 30. It evaluates orientation, concentration, memory, agnosia, reading, writing, and visuospatial ability. Abstract thinking may be evaluated by asking the meaning of simple proverbs (e.g., "What does this saying mean: 'People who live in glass houses should not throw stones'?"). It may also be evaluated by asking patients to describe similarities between objects (e.g., eggs and seeds, apples and oranges).

CONDUCTING INTERVIEWS IN SPECIAL CLINICAL SITUATIONS

Emergency Psychiatric Evaluations

Evaluations that occur in the emergency department typically focus on determining whether the patient requires inpatient hospitalization. Evaluation for safety is crucial and includes determining whether active suicidal or homicidal ideation is present and whether patients are currently able to provide safe care for themselves. Ability to care for oneself may be influenced by severe depression, confusion, dementia, or psychosis. It is possible that patients can be too depressed to manage their diabetes appropriately, too confused to organize themselves to bathe or toilet properly, or so delusional that they believe their food is poisoned and are in danger of starvation. The psychiatrist working in an emergency department must also know what legal criteria need to be met for voluntary versus involuntary psychiatric hospitalization.

The emergency department is a setting where establishing good rapport is especially important. Patients may be brought by police or family members, particularly when they have limited insight into their condition, and may be angry and frightened to be there. The interviewer should try to gain the patient's trust by making sure he or she is comfortable and his or her dignity is respected. If criteria for involuntary admission are not met, but the physician feels that the patient is best served by hospitalization, the patient may be more likely to accept hospitalization if he or she perceives the physician as caring, sympathetic, and working in the patient's best interest (Lidz et al., 1995).

Interviewing the "Difficult" Patient

In psychiatric practice, so-called difficult patients are common and can have various presentations, including being demanding, resistant to treatment, and deceptive (Table 3-3) (see also Chapter 2). Although a great deal of energy is generally put into treating these patients, they may receive suboptimal care due to health care providers' consciously or unconsciously punishing the patient for the difficult behavior.

The psychiatric interview is the best opportunity to learn *why* the patient is behaving in a manner that may be perceived as difficult. This information can then be interpreted as a clinical sign to help the clinician refine the diagnosis and/or treatment (McCarty and Roberts, 1996). To accomplish this, clinicians must ask questions about the behavior in a nonjudgmental way (e.g., "It is often hard for patients to take their medication every day. Has it been that way for you? Why has it been so difficult?"). By asking questions in this way, one may learn that a patient was not adherent because the prescribed medication is unaffordable or because the patient is so depressed that all treatment attempts seem futile. As another example, someone who had previously been well and functioning may become intolerably anxious when in a situation in which he or she has little control. Such patients may ask what seems like too many questions of providers and second guess them as a way of reasserting control and relieving the anxiety. During the interview, the clinician may make an empathic statement that explores this possibility and brings the issue into the discussion (e.g., "For someone who has always been in charge of things, it must be really tough to be so sick").

Interviewing the Somatizing Patient

Some patients find it difficult to recognize emotional states and instead report physical symptoms. They may present to internists complaining of nausea or abdominal pain rather than anxiety. Sometimes, patients receive negative medical evaluations before referral to a mental health practitioner. When conducting the initial interview with such a patient, it is important not to dismiss patients' physical complaints and to ensure that an adequate medical workup has been done. This requires review of medical records and past evaluations and collaborative work with primary medical doctors. During the interview, a thorough psychiatric review of systems should be

TABLE 3-3	Strategies for Interviewing Patients with Specific Characteristics
Tearful	Show patience. Provide empathic comments. Offer tissues and clarify stressors
Suicidal	Assess safety, access to means, plan, and intent. Always consider hospitalization for safety
Aggressive	Use a calm, measured voice. Ask the patient to remove any weapons. Give the patient sufficient space for comfort. Terminate the interview immediately if the patient's agitation feels threatening
"Difficult"	Investigate the cause of the patient's difficult nature. Consider the patient's problematic behavior as a symptom of pathology
Psychotic	Use open-ended questions to evaluate delusions. Use direct, straightforward questions with thought disorder
Somatizing	Listen to physical complaints and provide empathy for physical pain. Ensure that a full medical workup is done. Perform a psychiatric review of systems
Elderly	Address the patient directly. Get a history from the patient and any person accompanying the patient separately. Perform a physical and neurologic examination

performed that includes symptoms of anxiety and depression. Patients may have a number of these symptoms but fail to mention them spontaneously because of their difficulty linking them to their psychological state. The interviewer should introduce the idea that stress and psychiatric illness may affect physical well-being to help them engage in treatment. Otherwise, they may be reluctant to accept treatment that fails to address what they see as the primary problem (physical impairment).

Interviewing the Tearful Patient

Every clinician, regardless of discipline, will see patients with depression. They often avert their gaze, speak softly, sit quietly, and have bouts of crying. When a patient becomes tearful during the interview, it is important for the clinician to let the patient cry. Often, the patient has been trying to hold back emotions in front of friends and family because of embarrassment at showing outward signs of weakness. Other people in the patient's life (including many doctors) may feel uncomfortable with crying and tell the patient to stop. Psychiatric interviewers must be capable of tolerating and accepting a patient's tears. They should offer tissues, remain silent for a few moments, and then inquire about what makes the patient so sad.

Interviewing the Aggressive or Hostile Patient

A patient may be aggressive or hostile for many reasons, such as a manifestation of an agitated depression, mania, paranoia, psychosis, drug intoxication, cognitive disorder, or personality disorder. Regardless of the cause, the psychiatrist must take precautions to ensure the safety of both the patient and others during the interview. The interviewer should sit (or stand if necessary) near an unobstructed, unlocked door so that a quick exit can be made. The interview room should be cleared of dangerous objects such as scissors. Offering the patient food or drink before the interview may help calm the individual. However, some patients may be so agitated that they cannot be safely interviewed without the use of physical or chemical restraints.

Throughout the interview, the clinician should remain calm and speak in an even tone. If the patient begins shouting, the clinician should inform the patient in a normal tone that he or she will have to leave if unable to control himself or herself and then should follow through if the patient remains agitated. The clinician must curb any anger he or she begins to feel toward the patient and remember that the patient is ill and anything said is not personal. Although the situation is less than ideal, the hostile patient still requires active listening and empathy while the reason for the hostility or aggression is evaluated and addressed. If the interviewer does make the mistake of responding to the patient with anger, the patient may escalate and the agitation worsen (see also Chapter 26).

Interviewing the Psychotic Patient

Psychosis can be a manifestation of many different psychiatric and medical disorders, and the clinician should always screen for it in the initial psychiatric interview. It is defined as the presence of hallucinations, delusions, disorganized speech, or grossly disorganized or catatonic behavior. The presence of psychosis does not always make the patient an unreliable historian; in fact, he or she is often able to provide a reasonable history even in the face of delusions and hallucinations. Still, a patient with psychosis by definition has difficulty in discerning reality from fantasy, and some patients may report bizarre occurrences that are obviously delusional. Patients who have thought disorders or are experiencing auditory hallucinations may be too distracted to participate fully in an interview. Short, directed questions are much easier for such patients to answer than open-ended questions.

In cases of catatonia, the patient may not be able to provide any history at all, requiring the use of collateral information. Catatonia may occur in a mood disorder, schizophrenia, or a general medical condition. Catatonic behavior is either characterized by excessive purposeless activity, *echolalia* (repeating what is said, like an echo), and *echopraxia* (imitating the observed movements of another) or by extreme negativism and posturing. Waxy flexibility, also termed *catalepsy*, may occur in catatonic individuals and is characterized by holding uncomfortable positions after the examiner has moved their limbs.

CONDUCTING THE FOLLOW-UP INTERVIEW

The follow-up psychiatric interview occurs after a diagnosis has been made and a treatment regimen has been implemented. These assessments are shorter than initial diagnostic interviews. Also, these should begin with open-ended questions about how the patient is doing overall and if any new problems have arisen. It is useful to ask about target symptoms pertinent to the patient's illness so that response to treatment may be monitored. Side effects of the medications are checked during these appointments as well. Successive visits provide more data to assist in understanding a patient's strengths and weaknesses.

CONCLUSION AND SUGGESTIONS FOR FUTURE STUDY

This chapter is but a brief introduction to the art of psychiatric interviewing. The interview is one of the most delicate and powerful procedures in all of medicine, requiring clinicians to use simultaneously their analytic skills and their ability to empathize. Becoming a good interviewer takes time, more so for some clinicians than for others, but is achievable. Numerous elegant monographs have been written about the art of psychiatric interviewing (Goodwin and Guze, 1996; MacKinnon and Michels, 1971; Morrison, 1995), and the serious student of interviewing is encouraged to read these carefully. As the authors have tried to show, careful phrasing of questions is necessary to yield answers that are a valid and reliable basis for diagnoses. Students may wish to review the validated questions in research-based diagnostic interviews such as the Structured Clinical Interview for the Diagnostic and Statistical Manual of Mental Disorders, Fourth Edition (SCID) (First, 1997) for ideas to incorporate into their clinical interviews.

Nevertheless, reading alone is likely not sufficient to learn the art of interviewing. Trainees must practice interviewing over and over again—on friends and family members before turning to patients. Ideally, many of these interviews will be observed, either live or through audio recording, by a more experienced clinician who can provide feedback. Through this process, trainees can begin to learn not just how to collect data from patients but also the subtle and profound skills of truly listening and beginning to understand.

ACKNOWLEDGMENTS

Drs. Anderson and Hoop gratefully acknowledge the intellectual contributions of their teacher, William Egan, M.D., to their understanding of the psychiatric interview.

Clinical Pearls

- If at all possible, the interviewer should be seated at eye level with the patient, not standing.
- Begin the clinical interview with an open-ended question such as, "What brought you here today?"
- Recognizing and taking stock of one's own emotional experience while seeing a patient can provide important information that will be useful in formulating a diagnosis and treatment plan.
- It is of utmost importance in any initial evaluation to inquire about suicidal ideation.
- Some patients may be so agitated or aggressive that they cannot be safely interviewed without the use of physical or chemical restraints.
- Patients may find that the experience of being listened to and understood during the interview is therapeutic.
- An ideal way to learn the art of interviewing is to conduct several interviews while being watched by an experienced clinician who can provide feedback.

Self-Assessment Questions and Answers

3-1. Which of the following is an example of an open-ended question that may be used in a psychiatric interview?

   A. Where were you born?
   B. Which medications have been prescribed for you in the past?
   C. What concerns have brought you to meet with me today?
   D. What illnesses run in your family?
   E. How old are you?

   Most psychiatrists begin the clinical interview with an open-ended question such as, "What brought you in today?" *Answer: C*

3-2. Which of the following terms or phrases refers to persistent repetition of words or ideas?

   A. Echolalia
   B. Circumstantial
   C. Loose association
   D. Perseveration
   E. Thought blocking

   Echolalia is echoing back words that are heard. Circumstantial is to respond to questions in an oblique manner but eventually answer the question. Loose association is when ideas are loosely (distantly) associated with one another. Perseveration is the persistent repetition of words or ideas. Thought blocking is when the train of thought is interrupted abruptly without completion. *Answer: D*

3-3. Which of the following interviewing techniques is recommended in establishing rapport with a paranoid patient?

   A. Directly confronting the patient on his or her paranoid thoughts
   B. Encouraging the patient in his or her paranoid thoughts

   C. Offering empathic observations and comments
   D. Discussing the paranoid beliefs and their irrationality
   E. Telling the patient that paranoia requires the administration of medication

   Empathetic comments and observations can help build rapport with any patient, and may be extremely important when talking with a person who has paranoid ideation. Directly confronting the person about his or her paranoid thoughts is likely to cause the patient to believe that the interviewer, too, cannot be trusted. At the same time, it is unwise to encourage the patient in his or her paranoia. Statements such as "It must be very hard for you to feel watched all of the time" can demonstrate empathy without colluding with the patient's paranoid ideation. *Answer: C*

3-4. Which of the following terms or phrases refers to experiencing a sensation (e.g., auditory, olfactory, tactile, visual) in the absence of an external stimulus?

   A. Delusion
   B. Hallucination
   C. Idea of reference
   D. Thought broadcasting
   E. Thought insertion

3-5. Which of the following terms or phrases refers to the belief that unrelated things in the world have special significance or relevance to the patient?

   A. Delusion
   B. Hallucination
   C. Idea of reference
   D. Thought broadcasting
   E. Thought insertion

Delusions are fixed false beliefs that are not supported by cultural norms. Hallucinations occur when there is sensory perception without the presence of stimuli and in any sensory modality. Ideas of reference are beliefs that unrelated things in the world have special significance or relevance to the patient. Thought broadcasting is the fixed belief that patient's thoughts are being broadcast out so that others may hear. Thought insertion is the belief that someone has inserted thoughts into one's mind. *Answers*: B and C

References

Ewing JA. Detecting alcoholism: The CAGE questionnaire. *JAMA*. 1984;252(14):1905–1907.

First MB. *User's guide for the structured clinical interview for DSM-IV axis I disorders SCID-I: clinician version*. Washington, DC: American Psychiatric Press; 1997.

Folstein MF, Folstein SE, McHugh PR. "Mini-mental state." A practical method for grading the cognitive state of patients for the clinician. *J Psychiatr Res*. 1975;12(3):189–198.

Freedman M. *Clock drawing: A neuropsychological analysis*. New York: Oxford University Press; 1994.

Gonda X, Fountoulakis KN, Kaprinis G, et al. Prediction and prevention of suicide in patients with unipolar depression and anxiety. *Ann Gen Hosp Psychiatry*. 2007;6:23.

Goodwin DW, Guze SB. *Psychiatric diagnosis*, 5th ed. New York: Oxford University Press; 1996.

Lezak MD. *Neuropsychological assessment*, 3rd ed. New York: Oxford University Press; 1995.

Lidz CW, Hoge SK, Gardner W, et al. Perceived coercion in mental hospital admission: Pressures and process. *Arch Gen Psychiatry*. 1995;52(12):1034–1039.

MacKinnon RA, Michels R. *The psychiatric interview in clinical practice*. Philadelphia: WB Saunders; 1971.

McCarty T, Roberts LW. The difficult patient. In: Rubin RH, ed. *Medicine: A primary care approach*. Philadelphia: WB Saunders; 1996:395.

Meyer A, Winters EE. *The collected papers of Adolf Meyer*. Baltimore: The Johns Hopkins University Press; 1950.

Morrison JR. *The first interview: Revised for DSM-IV*. New York: Guilford Press; 1995.

Ornstein PH, Ornstein A. Some general principles of psychoanalytic psychotherapy: A self-psychological perspective. In: Lifson LE, ed. *Understanding therapeutic action: Psychodynamic concepts of cure*. Hillsdale: Analytic Press; 1996:87–101.

Silver-Isenstadt A, Ubel PA. Medical student name tags: Identification or obfuscation? *J Gen Intern Med*. 1997;12(11):669–671.

Differential Diagnosis of Mental Illnesses and Case Formulation

As in all clinical medicine, the process of psychiatric diagnosis is like detective work. The clinician must gather, prioritize, analyze, and integrate the "clues," or data the clinician gathers, to solve the diagnostic puzzle. Such data include the history obtained from the patient and other corroborating sources, the mental status examination, review of medical records, and diagnostic test results such as laboratory data, imaging, and psychological testing. The relative importance, and therefore the weight, given specific clues differs from patient to patient.

Diagnostic assessment and formulation is a dynamic and continual process that begins with the first contact with a patient. As diagnostic possibilities are considered, the process of data gathering is shaped and refined. The clinician considers and reworks a series of hypotheses about the likely syndromes that could explain the patient's problems with the ultimate goal to initiate effective treatment.

This chapter presents an approach to diagnostic assessment and case formulation utilizing the biopsychosocial model. Chapters 3, 5, and 6 (covering the psychiatric interview, neuroimaging and laboratory evaluation, and psychological and neuropsychological testing, respectively) provide the foundation and framework for differential diagnosis. The diagnostic assessment and case formulation are, in essence, the funnel for the clinical data, ultimately leading to the treatment plan.

DEFINITION AND CLASSIFICATION OF PSYCHIATRIC DISORDERS

To define and classify psychiatric disorders, there must be some agreement about what constitutes a disorder. One might assume that a psychiatric disorder is any emotion, thought, or behavior that is "abnormal." However, what is considered abnormal may vary widely depending on the patient's (or clinician's) ethnic or cultural background, religious or moral values, upbringing, and age or generational cohort.

Historically in the field of medicine, *disease* has been defined a number of ways. Some disorders are defined by structural pathology (e.g., ulcerative colitis) or histopathology (e.g., adenocarcinoma); others, by pathophysiology (e.g., congestive heart failure) or etiologic agent (e.g., meningococcal meningitis). Disorders such as hypertension or hyperlipidemia are defined by deviations from physiologic norms or predefined healthy ideals.

In psychiatry, disorders are typically defined by functional impairment. The *Diagnostic and Statistical Manual of Mental Disorders*, Fourth Edition, Text Revision (DSM-IV-TR) (American Psychiatric Association, 2000), defines *disorders* as syndromes of symptoms or behaviors associated with distress or disability or with a "significantly increased risk of suffering, death, pain, disability, or an important loss of freedom."

Psychiatry, like most of clinical medicine, bases diagnostic categories on clusters of signs and symptoms that together characterize a specific syndrome. Symptoms are the patient's subjective experience and may include thoughts, feelings, behavior, and physical sensations. Signs are the clinician's objective observations of the patient. In psychiatry, virtually no behavioral symptom or mental status finding is pathognomonic for one specific diagnosis. For example, auditory hallucinations may be seen in schizophrenia, manic psychosis, psychotic depression, cocaine or stimulant intoxication, vascular dementia, or even severe borderline personality disorder. The *combination* of signs and symptoms, together with a predictable longitudinal course, prognosis, and response to treatment, best defines and classifies a psychiatric diagnosis. This approach to diagnostic classification is called *descriptive* or *empirical*, because the categories of disorders are defined by descriptive rather than etiologic factors. DSM-IV-TR uses the descriptive or criterion-based approach to diagnostic classification.

A brief history of how different theoretic orientations in psychiatry have influenced the diagnostic classification system may be helpful. Two early approaches to describing and defining abnormal behavior (psychopathology) originated in Europe in the late 1800s. One focused on the individual's inner processes, including unconscious thoughts, wishes, and mental representations. This psychological approach, widely accepted as originating with Sigmund Freud, attempts to understand, explain, and predict behavior. Since Freud's time, a myriad of psychoanalytic theories and schools of thought have been advanced. Understanding psychiatric diagnosis from the theoretic framework of psychoanalysis typically involves the intensive and detailed study of a few individuals, and the treatment focus is on change through psychotherapy.

In contrast, Emil Kraepelin, a contemporary of Freud, established a diagnostic dichotomy based on the cross-sectional appearance and longitudinal course of symptoms in large populations of the severely and chronically ill, especially patients with psychosis. Kraepelin's approach to diagnostic classification is the foundation of the empirical–descriptive approach that underlies the current DSM.

Over the last 50 years or so, theories of psychiatric assessment and their application have evolved according to widely varying, and at times contentious, perspectives. American psychiatry before the 1960s was dominated by a psychoanalytic viewpoint. Since then, many other factors, including community mental health, behaviorism, and the explosion of research and knowledge in the neurosciences, have influenced the understanding and approach to the treatment of psychiatric illness (Fink, 1988).

DSM, the so-called bible of descriptive psychiatry, was first introduced in 1952. It was the first official classification system to focus on clinical utility, rather than defining illness for statistical purposes. Subsequent revisions have been undertaken, with the most significant change occurring in 1980 with the publication of DSM-III, the first classification system to define psychiatric diagnosis using explicit criteria. DSM-III also deviated from earlier editions by maintaining an atheoretic stance and avoiding reference to etiology of psychiatric disorders. The multiaxial system of diagnosis was introduced in DSM-III, allowing other psychosocial dimensions to be recognized and documented.

This descriptive, criterion-based approach to psychiatric diagnosis was based on a growing body of research supporting the validity and reliability of disorders based on specific characteristics, including clinical description, longitudinal course (through follow-up studies), and genetic factors (through family and adoption studies) (Feighner et al., 1972; Robins and Guze, 1970; Spitzer et al., 1978). Furthermore, ensuring that a psychiatric diagnosis describes a relatively homogenous group sharing similar clinical features, longitudinal course, and family history helps clinicians more accurately predict response to treatment. Finally, DSM-III criteria allowed clinicians (even those with disparate theoretic orientations), researchers, and educators to speak the same language.

Subsequent versions, including the current DSM-IV-TR, published in 2000, have incorporated new research findings through the use of systematic literature reviews, field studies, and reanalyses of previous epidemiologic datasets. Although DSM is based on a substantial body of empirical research, it is important to remember that it is a consensus-based classification system, written by a large number of psychiatrists forming multiple work groups, each reviewing a different category of psychiatric illness. DSM is felt to reflect the best understanding and agreement about diagnosis of mental disorders at the time of publication.

DSM-IV-TR ORGANIZATION

The organization of DSM-IV-TR includes 16 sections describing major diagnostic classes and one additional section, "Other Conditions that May be a Focus of Clinical Attention." Each section includes a description of the class of disorder with a discussion of associated features; specific culture, age, and gender features; prevalence statistics; and a discussion of differential diagnosis. The specific disorders are then defined by specific inclusion and exclusion criteria. Some diagnoses, like major depressive episode, contain polythetic criteria, meaning a diagnosis is made when a patient exhibits a defined subset of possible symptoms (e.g., five of nine criteria must be met to diagnose depression). In addition, the criteria often define exclusionary criteria, such that certain diagnostic categories are mutually exclusive. For example, major depressive episode cannot be diagnosed in the presence of a general medical condition that may account for the symptoms, like hypothyroidism. Appendix A in DSM-IV-TR contains decision trees to help guide the differential diagnosis process.

The following unfolding case vignette will illustrate the process of diagnostic assessment from the perspective of a medical student evaluating a psychiatric patient. As the trainee proceeds through the evaluation, differential diagnosis, multiaxial assessment, and case formulation, each aspect of the process will be explored in more detail.

Anna is a fourth year medical student taking an elective psychiatry rotation at a large university medical school teaching hospital. The psychiatry resident has taken a call from the emergency department (ED) requesting assessment of a patient with "mental status changes." The resident asks Anna to begin the evaluation of KH, a 20-year-old college student brought to the ED by his concerned parents. Anna first reviews the ED triage nurse's note: "Parents report patient is 'not himself, acting strange' for the last 2 weeks. Patient is anxious, guarded, and minimally responsive. He denies suicidal ideation. Vital signs: blood pressure 128/84 mm Hg, heart rate 96 bpm, respirations 16. He is afebrile."

Anna begins the interview with KH, who appears unkempt, vigilant, and internally preoccupied. After some time and considerable effort and patience on Anna's part, she is able to elicit the main concern of KH. He reported that he had dropped out of school 2 weeks previously because he was convinced that the dean was planning to expel him on violation of the school's academic misconduct policy. A month previously, KH had written a paper for a literature class and incorrectly cited a reference in a footnote. The inadvertent error was pointed out by his instructor, who nonetheless gave him a passing grade. However, KH began to believe that his classmates, and eventually the entire faculty and student body, knew he had "plagiarized" his paper. He felt overwhelmed with guilt and shame. He tearfully reported to Anna that his life was over and he might as well be dead, as he would never be able to earn a degree, get a job, or support himself. He had decided to leave school after a particularly stressful night when he had heard a radio broadcast reporting the story of his plagiarized paper. In addition, he had begun to lie awake nights, overhearing students in neighboring dorm rooms whispering that he was a cheater and a fraud.

Anna completes the history of present illness and psychiatric review of systems as best she can, given the reticence and mild agitation of KH. She administers the Mini-Mental State Examination (Folstein et al., 1975). KH's responses are latent, slowed but accurate, with a total score of 30/30.

With the consent of KH, Anna next speaks with his parents, who report a change in his personality and behavior 2 months previously during the winter semester break. He had been sullen, withdrawn, and minimally communicative. His parents privately worried that he was abusing illicit drugs, although he had never been known to drink alcohol or use any drugs previously. Six weeks after returning to campus, KH called home, stating he was dropping out of school because he was the laughingstock of the campus. When his parents picked him up from his dorm, they noted he had lost weight and begun to neglect his hygiene and personal appearance.

Anna then turned her attention to obtaining a past medical and psychiatric history and social, developmental, and family history from KH's parents. KH was the full-term product of a normal pregnancy and delivery. His father is a chemical engineer, and his mother had been an elementary school teacher who quit teaching in order to raise KH and his two brothers, 3 and 6 years older. When KH was 4, his mother had a second trimester miscarriage, followed by a severe depressive episode. Although she did not require hospitalization, she was unable to function adequately, and KH's grandmother had come to live with the family and care for her grandsons while her daughter recovered.

The following year, when KH began kindergarten, his mother's depression had substantially improved, but KH developed significant separation anxiety, and his parents elected to keep him out of school until after his sixth birthday. He was described as a quiet, sensitive, and introverted child, somewhat in the shadow of his academically successful and more outgoing older brothers. KH had generally been a B average student, had a few close friends, but had never dated extensively. Despite encouragement by his parents to pursue extracurricular activities, such as the school newspaper, he resisted, stating he was not good enough. The family attended Catholic services on a regular basis when KH was young, but KH had stopped attending Mass during high school.

KH had never seen a mental health professional previously. His past medical history was notable for childhood asthma, which resolved before adolescence. He had never been hospitalized, never had surgery, was on no medications, and had no drug allergies. Anna specifically asked whether KH had a history of head injury, febrile seizures as a child, or meningitis, which his parents denied.

Anna asked about family history of psychiatric illness and substance abuse. In addition to KH's mother, who had been successfully treated for depression at age 35, KH had a maternal aunt who had been institutionalized for many years and received "shock treatments."

DIFFERENTIAL DIAGNOSIS

As the case shows, the evaluation and differential diagnosis are interconnected in a dynamic and gradually unfolding process. The first step in the differential diagnosis is identifying the principal symptoms or presenting problems, which may or may not be the patient's chief complaint. Refinements are continually made in the history-taking process to narrow down the diagnostic possibilities and establish the major diagnostic category. Once a diagnostic category is suggested (mood disorder, psychotic disorder, etc.), the clinician must begin ruling out conditions such as medical problems or substance abuse that may better account for the symptoms.

This step is extremely important because of the implications for treatment. Many medical, neurologic, and toxic conditions can mimic psychiatric illness. Missing an underlying medical illness (such as hypothyroidism in the assessment of a depressed patient) not only predicts poor response to psychiatric treatment but also can lead to significant medical complications (such as myxedema) if the underlying condition is left untreated. The relationship of medical illness to psychiatric symptoms may be causal, contributory, or coincidental. Medical history, physical examination or neurologic findings, and laboratory abnormalities all may suggest the possibility of a direct physiologic effect of a medical condition causing psychiatric symptoms. One such example of a mental disorder due to a general medical condition is psychosis arising in the course of Huntington disease.

Causal relationships are often suggested by a temporal association between the onset of psychiatric symptoms and medical illness. Sometimes, the presence of behavioral symptoms may precede the manifestations of the medical illness. For example, onset of delirium in an elderly person is commonly the first sign of a urinary tract infection.

Understanding the typical presentation of the major psychiatric disorders with respect to symptoms, longitudinal course, age and gender, and genetic influences is important in the differential diagnosis. A disorder due to a general medical condition should be considered if the psychiatric presentation is atypical, either in symptom pattern or severity, age of onset, course, or treatment response. For example, the acute onset of hallucinations in a previously highly functioning 50-year-old would not be a typical presentation for schizophrenia, and other etiologies should be investigated.

The relationship of a general medical condition to psychiatric symptoms is not necessarily causal. Psychiatric symptoms may be a reaction to the pain, disability, lifestyle changes, or psychological stress associated with a medical problem. Even when medical illness and a psychiatric disorder are etiologically unrelated, it is important to consider the impact the psychiatric disorder has on the treatment or prognosis of the medical illness. For example, the onset of depression following myocardial infarction (MI) significantly increases the 1-year mortality rate compared to nondepressed post-MI patients (Carney et al., 2003). Patients with schizophrenia who develop diabetes may have difficulty adhering to a diabetic diet, insulin regimen, or glucose monitoring due to negative symptoms.

If a medical etiology for psychiatric symptoms has been ruled out, the next consideration is a substance-induced mental disorder. History and physical examination may suggest the presence of substance abuse, intoxication, or withdrawal, but often laboratory testing, such as a urine drug assay, is necessary for confirmation. Once the presence of substance use has been established, further investigation can help determine whether the use is etiologic. Establishing a temporal association of substance use with onset and resolution of symptoms, together with knowledge of the pharmacokinetic properties of a substance, is the most reliable way to establish causality. Substance-induced mental disorders may be due to intoxication (such as amphetamine-induced psychosis), withdrawal (as in delirium tremens), or an adverse side effect of therapeutic use of a medication (as in mood disorder due to corticosteroids). It is essential to remember that alcohol and illicit drugs are not the only substances that can cause psychiatric symptoms. Prescription medications and even environmental toxins can cause mental status changes. Another diagnostic possibility when substance abuse and psychiatric illness are comorbid is that patients "self-medicate" the symptoms of their primary psychopathology, as when a patient with generalized anxiety disorder abuses alcohol or benzodiazepines.

One last consideration in the differential diagnosis is the possibility that symptoms are not genuine (First et al., 2002). Psychiatric symptoms may be the result of conscious malingering, either for an obvious external gain (e.g., to qualify for disability income) or to assume the sick role (as in factitious disorder). Unconscious assumption of symptoms, often of a neurologic nature, may enable a patient with conversion disorder to resolve an underlying conflict or stressor. Finally, psychiatric symptoms may be part of a multiorgan system somatoform disorder (see Chapter 13).

Let us now return to Anna, as she reviews the data and considers the differential diagnosis for her patient.

Having completed the psychiatric interview and mental status examination, Anna reviews her notes to present to the resident. She notes that KH's presenting complaint is a presumably delusional belief that he is being persecuted for plagiarism. She notes that KH has auditory hallucinations and delusions of reference, but no formal thought disorder. In addition, KH exhibits a number of depressive symptoms, including weight loss, sleep disturbance, diminished interest in activities and social withdrawal, impaired concentration, and feelings of guilt and worthlessness. His hallucinations and delusions are consistent with his feelings of shame and perceived punishment and therefore appear to be mood congruent. Anna notes KH's positive family history of mood disorder. KH does not have an obvious medical condition by history to explain his psychotic symptoms, but Anna has not completed a physical examination or obtained laboratory or other diagnostic testing that might reveal an unrecognized medical cause. She observes that he is taking no prescribed or over-the-counter medications and does not appear to be abusing alcohol or illicit drugs, but she makes a note to suggest a urine drug screen for illicit substances.

Figure 4-1 demonstrates how Anna might follow a decision tree to suggest a differential diagnosis, which includes the following:

- Psychotic disorder due to general medical condition
- Substance-induced psychotic disorder
- Schizoaffective disorder
- Mood disorder with psychotic features

Because KH's mood symptoms preceded the onset of psychotic symptoms, she considers the last diagnosis on her differential to be the most likely.

Anna presents the case to the resident, and they return to the ED, where the resident confirms the history and mental status findings. They ask some additional questions and conclude that KH has never had symptoms consistent with a manic episode. The resident repeats a suicide risk assessment, and KH endorses a passive death wish but again denies any suicidal intent or plans. Anna and the resident complete a general physical examination and careful neurologic examination, both of which are unremarkable.

In light of his new-onset psychosis, together with his hopelessness and death wish, they decide to admit KH to the inpatient psychiatric service. Results of admission laboratories, including complete blood count, electrolytes, and renal and liver function tests, are all normal. The urine drug screen for illicit and controlled substances is negative, and thyroid function tests, vitamin B_{12}, and serum folate levels are all normal. They order a nonemergent brain magnetic resonance imaging study to rule out a structural lesion that might account for KH's behavioral changes.

Anna notes that KH's mood symptoms preceded the onset of his psychotic symptoms and concludes that mood disorder with psychotic features should be at the top of the differential.

MULTIAXIAL ASSESSMENT

The student's methodical and sequential process of considering diagnostic possibilities and systematically revising the differential demonstrates the importance of careful and thorough data

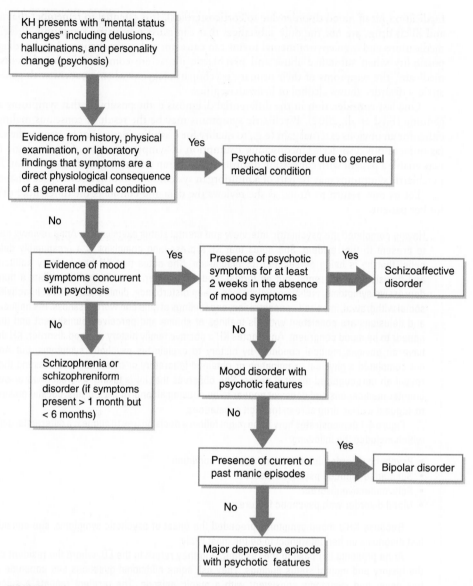

FIGURE 4-1. A decision tree to suggest a differential diagnosis

gathering. Focused diagnostic and laboratory testing with the goal of ruling out uncommon but potentially treatable medical causes is essential. Although this process may yield the most likely principal psychiatric diagnosis, the term *major depression with psychotic features* does not fully describe the depth and complexity of KH's presentation. DSM-IV-TR, like the preceding two DSM versions, uses a multiaxial system of evaluation, which allows a broader, more holistic view of an individual patient than a single diagnostic label. Recording five variables reflects a more accurate and thorough assessment of a patient, in light of the heterogeneity of patients presenting with the same diagnosis. The patient's comorbid medical illness, personality structure, environment and social support, presence of stress, and functional status all affect presentation of illness, treatment planning, and prognosis.

Table 4-1 shows Anna's DSM-IV-TR multiaxial assessment for KH. Axis I includes all the patient's major psychiatric diagnoses except for personality disorders or mental retardation and developmental disabilities, which are recorded on axis II. Axis II may also include the presence of

TABLE 4-1	**Multiaxial Assessment**

I. Major depressive episode, single, severe with mood-congruent psychotic features (296.24)
II. Rule out cluster C personality disorder (with avoidant traits)
III. History of asthma
IV. Recent departure from home to start college studies
V. GAF current 35; highest in last year 70

GAF, Global Assessment of Functioning.
(*Diagnostic and Statistical Manual of Mental Disorders*, Fourth Edition, Text Revision, American Psychiatric Association, 2000).

maladaptive personality traits not meeting the threshold for a personality disorder diagnosis. Axis III is for reporting general medical conditions that may impact a patient's presentation, treatment, or outcome. The division of the first three axes is an arbitrary and perhaps artificial distinction, and is not meant to perpetuate the false notion of "mind-body dualism." There is considerable research evidence of physiologic variables, including neurochemical, electrophysiological, and genetic factors influencing many psychiatric disorders such as schizophrenia, mood disorders, substance abuse disorders, and some anxiety disorders. Likewise, psychosocial factors clearly impact the onset, course, and response to many medical conditions.

Axis IV documents the presence and severity of psychosocial and environmental factors that may affect the diagnosis, treatment, or prognosis of axis I and II disorders. These may include factors such as the loss of a loved one or lack of social support, homelessness, educational or occupational problems, legal problems, or financial strain. Axis V is the clinician's estimate of the patient's current overall level of functioning using the Global Assessment of Functioning (GAF) scale. The GAF scale is divided into 10-point ranges of functioning, including both symptom severity and social functioning, yielding a GAF score from 0 to 100. The GAF is typically recorded on axis V for the current period, but may also be estimated over the preceding year or compared from time of admission to discharge to reflect improvement and thus justify hospitalization to third-party payors.

DIAGNOSTIC FORMULATION

The DSM multiaxial diagnosis provides a concise and objective framework for describing and classifying a patient's psychiatric diagnosis, as well as important information about pertinent medical illness, psychosocial stressors, and overall level of functioning. However, the statement that a person "meets DSM criteria" for a certain disorder does not provide adequate breadth or depth of information to fully understand a patient or develop an appropriate treatment plan. Therefore, a diagnostic formulation is ideally included as part of a psychiatric assessment. A formulation is both a process and a product. The process involves the distillation and synthesis of clinical data to plan effective treatment. The formulation has been termed the *bridge* between the diagnosis and treatment plan (Cleghorn, 1985; Jellinek and McDermott, 2004; McDougall and Reade, 1993; Mellsop and Banzato, 2006; Ross et al., 1990).

Commonly, the process of diagnostic formulation involves the application of a particular theoretic model (Sperry et al., 1992). Some of the major models of diagnostic formulation include the biomedical or disease model, the cognitive behavioral model, the psychodynamic model, and the biopsychosocial model. Depending on the presentation of the patient, one or more models may be appropriate. For example, a patient who appears to have repetitive patterns of dysfunctional interpersonal relationships, who has suffered significant developmental trauma, or who has complex family, interpersonal, or marital problems will likely require a more in-depth psychosocial assessment and the perspective of a psychodynamically oriented clinician. This typically involves examining an individual's key relationships, coping styles, strengths, and defense mechanisms (Kassaw and Gabbard, 2002; Reiser, 1988). There are different approaches to psychodynamic assessment according to theoretic orientation, including ego psychology, self psychology, and object relations (Perry et al., 1987), that are beyond the scope of this chapter.

THE BIOPSYCHOSOCIAL MODEL

The most widely known and commonly used model of diagnostic formulation is the biopsychosocial approach (Molina, 1983–1984). This paradigm was initially advocated by Engel (1977) as a new ideology for the medical profession and a shift away from the reductionist perspective of the "biomedical model." Engel was not a psychiatrist but an internist who advocated a systems approach to patient care. He noted that an individual patient is one part of an interrelated hierarchical continuum from smaller units (molecules and cells) to larger, more complex units (communities and societies). To optimally understand and treat a patient's disease, the clinician must consider the dynamic interrelationship of the different levels of the system. The biopsychosocial model requires a comprehensive and holistic perspective of a patient's condition by examining and attributing significance to each sphere of the patient's life: the biological, psychological, and sociocultural. The biopsychosocially oriented physician attempts to understand the context in which the patient experiences disease, perceives symptoms, and communicates them verbally and behaviorally. Physician attributes and values, and the physician–patient relationship itself, can influence clinical outcome (Borrell-Carrio et al., 2004). Although Engel envisioned the biopsychosocial model as the ideal for patient care across medical disciplines, it was embraced primarily by psychiatrists as a framework for diagnostic assessment and formulation. Psychiatric illness is viewed as being the multicausal result of disruption of one or more of the three systems. Illness is seen as a dynamic process, whereby alteration in one part of the system will result in disruption of another.

Biologic factors may include family (genetic) history of psychiatric illness, perinatal or childhood injuries, developmental delays, comorbid medical illness, and history of treatment response or adherence to medications. Psychological factors include the patient's personality structure, conscious and unconscious conflicts, defense mechanisms, strengths, and coping styles. Sociocultural factors include cultural and religious background, economic class, interpersonal relationships, and occupational, educational, and recreational roles.

The formulation attempts to explore, explain, and integrate factors in the biologic, psychological, and sociocultural spheres. Etiologic factors in the three spheres may be further classified into predisposing, precipitating, and perpetuating factors, the so-called three Ps of formulation (Ben-Aron and McCormick, 1980; Kline and Cameron, 1978; Sperry et al., 1992). For example, a strong family history for mood disorder is a predisposing biological factor. A precipitating factor in the psychological realm might be the acute loss of a relationship. A perpetuating social factor could be chronic unemployment and financial difficulties.

Many authors have proposed various schematic models to organize a formulation, including grids, axes, and overlapping circles typically superimposed on a chronologic time line of a patient's life (Guerrero et al., 2003; Ross, 2000; Weerasekera, 1993).

Table 4-2 is an example of how the biopsychosocial model might be applied to the diagnostic assessment and treatment plan of KH.

The ultimate goal of diagnostic formulation is to inform treatment planning, which likewise should address the biological, psychological, and social realms. The relative importance of each factor will predict the type of treatment most likely to be effective. Although a schizophrenic patient's psychotic exacerbation might be considered a direct "biologic" effect of his stopping his antipsychotic medications, effective treatment must take into consideration the patient's lack of social support, tenuous living situation, and lack of transportation to attend appointments, all of which contribute to his nonadherence.

Diagnostic assessment and formulation is one of the most complex and challenging skills, one that psychiatric residents and even experienced clinicians are continually refining and improving (McClain et al., 2004).

As shown, Anna's case formulation integrates the biological, psychological, and social factors influencing the illness, treatment, and prognosis of KH.

KH is a 20-year-old man who recently withdrew from college after developing persecutory and referential delusions that he was being harassed for plagiarizing an assigned research paper. His psychotic symptoms were accompanied by feelings of guilt and shame, as well as passive death wish. The onset of psychotic symptoms was preceded by a more subtle and gradual personality

TABLE 4-2	Applying the Biopsychosocial Model	
	Influences and Effects	**Interventions: Diagnostic and Treatment**
Bio	Family (genetic) history of mood disorders Vegetative symptoms of depression	PE and laboratory workup; neuroimaging to rule out treatable medical and neurologic etiologies Urine drug screen to assess for substance intoxication Antidepressant and antipsychotic medication Monitor longitudinally for development of bipolar cycling
Psycho	Lifelong pattern of negative self-assumptions and poor self-esteem Feelings of guilt and shame over perceived plagiarism Developmental effects of early symbolic loss of mother Childhood separation anxiety Stress of leaving home for college	Individual psychotherapy including cognitive therapy to address negative cognitions Supportive and psychoeducational therapy to educate patient about diagnosis and prognosis of depression and effects of medications Long-term insight-oriented psychotherapy
Social	Withdrawal from family and friends Chronic social inhibition and avoidance Academic struggles	Group and individual therapy to promote socialization Social skills training Referral to campus resources for academic support/tutoring

PE, preeclampsia.

change 6 to 8 weeks earlier with social withdrawal, loss of interest in appearance and usual activities, change in sleep patterns, and loss of appetite and weight.

Biological predisposing factors include genetic loading for mood disorders with a history of depression in the mother, and an unidentified chronic illness treated with electroconvulsive therapy (ECT), in a maternal great-aunt. Medical and neurologic workup for other causes of KH's symptoms (such as thyroid disease, brain tumor, cocaine or amphetamine abuse) was negative.

Although the patient attributed the onset of his symptoms to the stress and shame of being accused of plagiarism, this delusional belief appears to be an effect, and not the precipitant, of his depressive symptoms, which began approximately a month before the psychotic symptoms. However, KH tended to have chronic feelings of low self-esteem, and it is likely that he overreacted to his instructor's comment about his citation error with an exaggerated sense of failure and shame, which may have intensified his depression and provided a focus for his subsequent delusions.

Developmentally, KH had suffered the symbolic loss of his mother at age four, when his mother developed an incapacitating episode of depression following a pregnancy loss. She was unavailable to him emotionally, contributing to KH's chronic feelings of being unlovable and inadequate. He subsequently developed symptoms of separation anxiety, leading to a delay in the start of his formal education.

KH had always felt himself the subject of unfavorable comparison to his successful older brothers, and developed a pattern of negative assumptions and cognitions about his self-worth. These self-critical cognitions became more prominent in the face of the acute stress of leaving home and starting college in another town. This separation rekindled earlier fears of separating from his mother when he began kindergarten. His lifelong personality style had been one of social inhibition and avoidance of social situations. He also tended to avoid developing relationships where he might feel inadequate or be rejected.

This is the first episode of mood disorder for KH, and as such the longitudinal course of his symptoms and his functioning remains to be seen. One diagnostic possibility is that KH will develop bipolar disorder, as this diagnosis is overrepresented in patients presenting with psychotic depression (Coryell, 1996). Another diagnostic possibility is that KH will prove to have schizophrenia or schizoaffective disorder. However, his mood symptoms clearly predated the onset of psychosis, and he does not have a formal thought disorder, or first-rank symptoms such as delusions of control, thought insertion, or withdrawal. The "mood-congruent" nature of his psychotic symptoms, although not pathognomonic, is more typical of psychotic depression.

As in diagnostic assessment, treatment planning will include consideration of biological, psychological, and sociocultural factors. KH would benefit from initiation of antidepressant as well as antipsychotic medication. If KH's symptoms do not respond adequately to pharmacotherapy or he develops active suicidal ideation, ECT should be considered as a treatment option. While an inpatient, KH will be encouraged to participate in milieu therapies including group therapy, which may assist KH in improving interpersonal and social skills, as well as his coping skills. Psychoeducational and supportive therapies (individual and group) are especially important in the early phases of treatment.

Long-term treatment after hospital discharge should ideally include maintenance of pharmacotherapy and individual psychotherapy. Cognitive behavioral therapy may be useful to help KH identify and correct negative assumptions and schemata. Insight-oriented psychodynamic psychotherapy might focus on helping KH explore the developmental origins of his fear of being abandoned or rejected, as well as the recurring patterns of his avoidant behavior.

KH's response to treatment will provide further data to support or refute current diagnostic hypotheses. Fortunately, his diagnosis of major depression with psychotic features has a more favorable prognosis.

Clinical Pearls

- The approach to psychiatric assessment and differential diagnosis is the same as that for physical illness. Signs and symptoms are elicited and results of diagnostic workup are reviewed.
- It is essential to expand the clinical database by reviewing prior records and, with the patient's consent, talking to family, friends, and other health care providers.
- The process of differential diagnosis includes *ruling in* the major category of psychiatric illness and then *ruling out* other causes, such as medical illness or substance use.
- In establishing a diagnosis, the longitudinal perspective is at least as important, or more, than the cross-sectional (or snapshot) view of the patient.
- Diagnosing a DSM-IV-TR disorder requires evidence of psychiatric symptoms causing functional impairment or significant distress.
- Conditions that confer additional risk of dangerousness (such as suicidal or homicidal ideation) should not be overlooked.
- The biopsychosocial model of formulation involves examining and attributing significance to the biological, psychological, and sociocultural aspects of a patient's life and analyzing predisposing, precipitating, and perpetuating factors in each sphere.
- Even if psychosocial stressors do not directly cause psychiatric symptoms, they can affect the onset, character, and severity of symptoms or the response to treatment.

Self-Assessment Questions and Answers

4-1. A 72-year-old veteran is admitted to the inpatient psychiatric unit of the VA Medical Center with a 3-day history of confusion, visual hallucinations, and impaired sleep. Which of the following details is most important in the differential diagnosis process?

A. Educational level
B. Family history of bipolar disorder
C. History of alcohol use
D. MMSE score
E. Serum creatinine level

Although each of these factors is important in a complete diagnostic assessment and formulation, the first and most important consideration should be given to potentially treatable medical and substance-induced disorders. Because alcohol withdrawal has a high morbidity and mortality if unrecognized and untreated, evaluating the patient's history of alcohol use and risk for withdrawal is particularly urgent and salient. *Answer: C*

4-2. All of the following are reasonable steps in the initial treatment plan *except*:
A. Assessing suicide risk
B. Evaluating the patient's ability to perform activities of daily living independently
C. Obtaining corroborating history from family
D. Ordering a head CT
E. Ordering urinalysis

Again, identifying those conditions that are serious and potentially treatable is the first priority. Neuroimaging, to rule out a central nervous system hemorrhage or infarct, and urinalysis, to check for infection, are important early diagnostic interventions. Because the patient is confused, getting additional history from family, especially concerning alcohol or illicit and prescription drug use, is essential. All psychiatric patients should be assessed early on for suicidal risk. The patient's ability to perform activities of daily living (ADLs), although important information for discharge planning, is a less urgent priority at admission. *Answer: B*

4-3. The corroborating history from family, physical examination (including elevated vital signs), mental status examination, and laboratory testing all suggest that the patient is in delirium tremens. Which of the following is an accurate diagnosis as part of the patient's DSM-IV-TR multiaxial assessment?
A. Axis I: alcohol withdrawal delirium
B. Axis I: alcohol-induced dementia
C. Axis II: alcohol withdrawal delirium
D. Axis II: alcohol-induced dementia
E. Axis III: alcohol withdrawal delirium

Alcohol withdrawal delirium is the DSM-IV-TR diagnostic term for delirium tremens (DTs) and is coded on axis I, as are other cognitive disorders such as dementia and amnestic disorder. The acute onset of confusion and visual hallucinations with disturbance of sleep–wake cycle suggests delirium, as does the presence of autonomic hyperactivity (elevated vital signs). Delirium and dementia are not infrequent comorbidities, but formal assessment of the patient's baseline cognitive functioning (i.e., with neuropsychological testing) should be deferred until the patient has had adequate time and appropriate treatment to recover from acute withdrawal and other common medical complications of alcohol dependence that can impair cognition, such as dehydration and nutritional compromise. *Answer: A*

4-4. DSM-IV-TR is a diagnostic classification system that
A. Categorizes psychiatric diagnoses by etiology
B. Codes cognitive disorders such as delirium and dementia on axis II
C. Is based on empirical research and expert consensus
D. Is not utilized by psychoanalysts
E. Requires biopsychosocial formulation

DSM-IV-TR classifies diagnoses by descriptive criteria rather than etiology. It is a consensus-based classification system based on empirical research. DSM diagnoses are utilized by mental health professionals across disciplines and from different theoretic orientations, including psychoanalysts. Biopsychosocial formulation provides a more detailed and comprehensive account of a patient that is a useful complement to, but not a requirement for, the DSM multiaxial assessment. Finally, cognitive disorders, including delirium, dementia, and amnestic disorders, are coded on axis I (American Psychiatric Association, 2000). *Answer: C*

4-5. Which of the following statements about the biopsychosocial model is accurate?
A. The biopsychosocial model was designed to further refine and expand the biomedical model of illness.
B. In the biopsychosocial model all illness is viewed as the complex interaction of biological, psychological, and sociocultural factors.
C. The biopsychosocial model was studied on and applied to the chronically mentally ill.
D. All three spheres should be given equal weight in the diagnostic assessment process of the biopsychosocial model.
E. The biopsychosocial model is based on "systems theory," which was first described by George Engel.

George Engel proposed the biopsychosocial model as an alternative to the biomedical model. He based this scientific model on a systems approach, which had been described previously by biologists Von Bertalanffy and Weiss and subsequently was expanded on by numerous authors. Engel envisioned the biopsychosocial model as the ideal for all of clinical medicine, not just psychiatric populations. The biopsychosocial model challenges physicians to explore the psychosocial dimensions of illness in addition to the biological, but the emphasis and significance of the three spheres depend on the individual patient and illness (Engel, 1980). *Answer: B*

References

American Psychiatric Association. *Diagnostic and statistical manual of mental disorders*, 4th ed, text revision. Washington, DC: American Psychiatric Association; 2000.

Ben-Aron M, McCormick WO. The teaching of formulation. Facts and deficiencies. [Brief Communication]. *Can J Psychiatry*. 1980;25:163–166.

Borrell-Carrio F, Suchman AL, Epstein RM. The biopsychosocial model 25 years later: Principles, practices, and scientific inquiry. *Ann Fam Med*. 2004;2:576–582.

Carney RM, Blumenthal JA, Catellier D, et al. Depression as a risk factor for mortality after acute myocardial infarction. *Am J Cardiol*. 2003;92:1277–1281.

Cleghorn JM. Formulation: A pedagogic antidote to DSM-III. *Compr Psychiatry*. 1985;26:505–512.

Coryell W. Psychotic depression. *J Clin Psychiatry*. 1996;57(suppl 3):27–31.

Engel GL. The need for a new medical model: A challenge for biomedicine. *Science*. 1977;196:129–135.

Engel GL. The clinical application of the biopsychosocial model. *Am J Psychiatry*. 1980;137:535–544.

Feighner JP, Robins E, Guze SB, et al. Diagnostic criteria for use in psychiatric research. *Arch Gen Psychiatry*. 1972;26:57–63.

Fink PJ. Response to the presidential address: Is "biopsychosocial" the psychiatric shibboleth? *Am J Psychiatry*. 1988;145:1061–1067.

First MB, Frances A, Pincus HA. *DSM-IV-TR handbook of differential diagnosis*. Arlington: American Psychiatric Publishing; 2002.

Folstein MF, Folstein SE, McHugh PR. Mini-mental state: A practical method for grading the cognitive state of patients for the clinician. *J Psychiatr Res*. 1975;12:189–198.

Guerrero AP, Hishinuma ES, Serrano AC, et al. Use of the mechanistic case diagraming technique to teach the biopsychosocial-cultural formulation to psychiatric clerks. *Acad Psychiatry*. 2003;27:88–92.

Jellinek MS, McDermott JF. Formulation: Putting the diagnosis into a therapeutic context and treatment plan. *J Am Acad Child Adolesc Psychiatry*. 2004;43:913–916.

Kassaw K, Gabbard GO. Creating a psychodynamic formulation from a clinical evaluation. *Am J Psychiatry*. 2002;159:721–726.

Kline S, Cameron PM. I. Formulation [Clinician's view]. *Can Psychiatr Assoc J*. 1978;23:39–42.

McClain T, O'Sullivan PS, Clardy JA. Biopsychosocial formulation: Recognizing educational shortcomings. *Acad Psychiatry*. 2004;28:88–94.

McDougall GM, Reade B. Teaching biopsychosocial integration and formulation. *Can J Psychiatry*. 1993; 38:359–362.

Mellsop GW, Banzato CE. A concise conceptualization of formulation. *Acad Psychiatry*. 2006;30: 424–425.

Molina JA. Understanding the biopsychosocial model. *Int J Psychiatry Med*. 1983–1984;13:29–36.

Perry S, Cooper A, Michels R. The psychodynamic formulation: Its purpose, structure and clinical application. *Am J Psychiatry*. 1987;144:543–550.

Reiser MF. Are psychiatric educators "losing the mind"? *Am J Psychiatry*. 1988;145:148–153.

Robins E, Guze SB. Establishment of diagnostic validity in psychiatric illness: Its application to schizophrenia. *Am J Psychiatry*. 1970;126:107–111.

Ross CA, Leichner P, Matas M, et al. A method of teaching and evaluating psychiatric case formulation. *Acad Psychiatry*. 1990;14:99–105.

Ross DE. A method for developing a biopsychosocial formulation. *J Child Fam Stud*. 2000;9:1–6.

Sperry L, Gudeman JE, Blackwell B, et al. *Psychiatric case formulations*. Washington, DC: American Psychiatric Press; 1992.

Spitzer RL, Endicott J, Robins E. Research diagnostic criteria, rationale and reliability. *Arch Gen Psychiatry*. 1978;35:773–781.

Weerasekera P. Formulation: A multiperspective model. *Can J Psychiatry*. 1993;38:351–358.

Neuroimaging and Laboratory Evaluation

The clinical interview, coupled with a careful mental status examination, remains the cornerstone of a comprehensive psychiatric evaluation and treatment. This assessment also includes an in-depth review of patients' over-the-counter and prescription medications and medical and surgical histories. However, a large battery of laboratory tests and neuroimaging techniques is available to the clinician and often form an essential component in the assessment and management of psychiatric illness. These objective, biological measures are utilized for ruling out medical and neurologic illnesses that mimic psychiatric disorders; pretreatment laboratory screening; evaluating for substances of abuse; and monitoring safety and adherence for psychotropic drugs.

Despite recent advances in the innovative neuroimaging methods available for studying psychiatric disorders, their utility in routine clinical practice remains confined. The advances in biological psychiatry research have expanded the scope of laboratory testing into identifying genetic and biological markers of psychiatric disorders. However, this research does not have a major clinical application in psychiatry. Moreover, a significant amount of research is focused on defining ethical guidelines and how to interpret results from genetic testing.

This chapter will briefly discuss the commonly indicated laboratory tests, outline the historical perspective on the attempts made to correlate certain neuroendocrine measures with common psychiatric disorders, and finally describe the utility of neuroimaging techniques in psychiatry.

LABORATORY TESTS

Screening Tests

Routine Tests Indicated During the Initial Psychiatric Visit

Laboratory tests during an initial psychiatric visit are common. Some argue that the extensive battery of clinical tests provides little utility but higher health care costs when used routinely (Anfinson and Kathol, 1992). A detailed history and physical examination assists the clinician in ordering specific tests to screen for medical illnesses that may be presenting with psychiatric symptoms and signs. Table 5-1 summarizes the routinely used laboratory and imaging measures and the common medical conditions and associated psychiatric illnesses that are assessed during the initial psychiatric examination. This is not an exhaustive list; rather, it is a battery of commonly used measures in clinical psychiatric practice.

Various attempts to identify biological measures to confirm specific psychiatric disorders have lacked sensitivity and specificity. The best example is the dexamethasone suppression test (DST) that was historically used to confirm the presence of a major depressive disorder, specifically melancholic depression, and to follow a depressed patient's treatment response to medications. However, the sensitivity of DST in detecting major depressive disorder and psychotic depression was found to be only 45% and 70%, respectively. Several medical and psychiatric conditions were also noted to produce false-positive results. The specificity is 90% with controls and 77% when compared with other psychiatric diagnoses (American Psychiatric Association, 1987).

Several studies have also focused on assessment of the serotonin metabolite 5-hydroxyindoleacetic acid (5-HIAA) in major depression, impulsive aggression, and violence. Lower cerebrospinal fluid (CSF) 5-HIAA levels were observed in depressed persons who attempted suicide with higher means of lethality. Moreover, the relationship between CSF 5-HIAA and suicidal behavior was stronger in patients with melancholic depression (Roy et al., 1989; Mann and Malone, 1997). Similarly, peripheral and central serotonin measures have

TABLE 5-1   Laboratory and Neuroimaging Tests to Screen for Medical Illnesses

Laboratory Measures	Medical Conditions Screened	Associated Psychiatric Illnesses
Complete blood count with differential	Anemia, infection, leukopenia, thrombocytopenia, agranulocytosis	Depressive and psychotic disorders; psychotropic use; alcohol abuse, pre-ECT workup
Comprehensive metabolic panel		
Electrolytes	Hypernatremia/hyponatremia; hyperkalemia/hypokalemia	Pre-ECT workup, delirium workup, psychogenic polydipsia, psychotropic use, eating disorders
Glucose	Diabetes mellitus, hypoglycemia	Delirium, anxiety and panic attacks, depression, agitation
Calcium	Hyperparathyroidism/hypoparathyroidism; bone metastasis	Delirium, anxiety, depression, psychosis, eating disorders
Liver function	Hepatitis, cirrhosis, liver metastasis	Delirium, alcohol dependence, psychotropic use
Renal function	Renal disease, dehydration	Delirium, psychotropic use
Thyroid function	Hypothyroidism/hyperthyroidism	Dementia, delirium, psychosis, depression, anxiety
Urinalysis with midstream urine specimen (and urine culture if indicated)	Urinary tract infection, renal disease, urinary tract bleeding, diabetes, dehydration	Alcohol use, delirium, lithium use
Urine toxicology screen	Substance misuse	Substance use disorders, mood, anxiety, and psychotic disorders, sleep disturbance, delirium
Blood alcohol levels	Alcohol intoxication	Alcohol abuse/dependence
Serum vitamin B_{12} and folate levels	Nutritional deficiency	Dementia reversible causes workup, delirium, alcohol abuse, psychotic disorders, depression, agitation
Rapid plasma reagin (RPR)	Syphilis	Dementia reversible causes, paranoia, mood disorders
Pregnancy test	Pregnancy	Postpartum mood disorders, psychotropic use
Electrocardiogram	Cardiac conduction abnormalities	Psychotropic use, panic disorder, pre-ECT workup
Electroencephalogram (EEG)	Seizure disorder	Delirium, conversion disorder, sleep disorders
Serum medication levels (if appropriate)	Digitalis, certain antibiotics, acetaminophen, salicylate, antidepressants, lithium and anticonvulsant toxicity	Drug overdose, medication nonadherence, psychotropic drug monitoring, psychosis
Chest x-ray (for patients older than 65 yr)	Aspiration pneumonia, recurrent pneumonia, lung carcinoma, lung carcinoid tumor, and lung metastasis	Delirium, pre-ECT workup
Structural neuroimaging		
Computed tomography (CT) with or without contrast, magnetic resonance imaging (MRI) with or without contrast	History of head trauma, stroke, including brain tumors, CNS metastasis, multiple sclerosis, movement disorders and other neurologic disorders	New-onset psychosis, delirium and dementia workup, catatonia, new-onset mood and personality change, older than 50 yr, pre-ECT workup

TABLE 5-1	*Continued*	
Laboratory Measures	**Medical Conditions Screened**	**Associated Psychiatric Illnesses**
Optional tests		
Cerebrospinal fluid (CSF) analysis	CNS infection and hemorrhage, neurosyphilis	Delirium workup, dementia, depression, psychosis
Urine/serum osmolality	Hyponatremia workup, SIADH	Psychogenic polydipsia, psychotropic use
Heavy metal screen	Poisoning	Dementia, apathy, agitation, mood disturbance, psychosis
Serum amylase/lipase	Pancreatitis	Eating disorders, valproic acid therapy
Serum ammonia levels	Hepatic encephalopathy	Valproic acid therapy, alcohol dependence
Serum ceruloplasmin	Wilson disease	Psychosis, dementia
γ-Glutamyl transpeptidase	Liver dysfunction	Alcohol abuse and dependence
Polysomnography	Sleep disturbance	Sleep disorders
Serum iron, iron-binding capacity, ferritin	Iron-deficiency anemia	Depression, restless legs syndrome
Creatine phosphokinase (CPK)	Neuroleptic malignant syndrome, rhabdomyolysis	Antipsychotic use
Antinuclear antibodies (ANA)	Systemic lupus erythematosus, drug-induced lupus	Delirium, mood and psychotic disorders, dementia
Prothrombin time	Cirrhosis	Psychotropic medication use and psychotropic–warfarin drug–drug interactions
Stool phenophthalein	Laxative abuse	Delirium, eating disorders
Human immunodeficiency virus (HIV) ELISA or Western Blot[a]	HIV disease	Dementia, delirium, mood disorder, psychosis, personality changes
Hepatitis panel[a]	Hepatitis A, B, and C infection	Depression, delirium

[a]In high-risk patients.
ECT, electroconvulsive therapy; CNS, central nervous system; SIADH, secretion of inappropriate antidiuretic hormone; ELISA, enzyme-linked immunosorbent assay.

demonstrated significant correlations in individuals who exhibit impulsive aggression and violent behaviors (Lee and Coccaro, 2001). Other catecholamines and metabolites are also implicated in patients with various psychiatric disorders. However, it is imperative to understand that no specific psychiatric diagnosis can be based solely on laboratory testing.

Specific Clinical Presentation
Depression

Major depressive disorder is a common clinical condition, with a lifetime prevalence of 15% in the general population. Depressive symptoms or major depressive episodes can also be secondary to or triggered by several medications, drugs, and medical conditions, such as endocrine disorders (e.g., thyroid disease, Cushing syndrome, diabetes mellitus, parathyroid abnormalities); neurologic illnesses (e.g., cerebrovascular accident, brain tumor, epilepsy, Parkinson disease, dementia); metabolic disorders; nutritional deficiencies (e.g., vitamin B_{12}, folate, thiamine); infections (e.g., human immunodeficiency virus [HIV], neurosyphilis); autoimmune diseases (e.g., systemic lupus erythematosus); and neoplastic diseases (e.g., pancreatic cancer). During an evaluation of a depressed patient, the clinician should carefully screen for the above-mentioned disorders (Sadock and Sadock, 2003).

Anxiety

Anxiety disorders are among the most common psychiatric disorders throughout the lifespan. They can be caused by general medical conditions, including endocrine illnesses (e.g., pheochromocytoma, hyperthyroidism, hypoparathyroidism, hypoglycemia, Addison disease); electrolyte disturbances; neurologic illnesses (e.g., cerebrovascular disease, multiple sclerosis, epilepsy); cardiac and pulmonary disorders (e.g., myocardial infarction, congestive heart failure, asthma, chronic obstructive pulmonary disease, pulmonary embolism); and alcohol and illicit drug intoxication or withdrawal. Although a significant association between mitral valve prolapse and panic disorder was reported in the earlier literature, recent studies have failed to demonstrate a higher prevalence of panic disorder in patients with this form of heart valve disease when compared with patients without it.

The laboratory investigations that are commonly considered for depressive and anxiety disorders during the initial evaluation include a complete blood count (CBC), electrolytes, fasting blood glucose, liver function tests (LFTs), serum calcium levels, thyroid-stimulating hormone (TSH), urinalysis, and urine toxicology screen. If the depressed or anxious patient complains of a cardiac or respiratory symptom, has a history of coronary artery disease or cardiac arrhythmias, or raises suspicion of pulmonary embolism, a chest x-ray, cardiac enzyme panel, 12-lead electrocardiogram (ECG), and/or a computed tomography (CT) chest image may be warranted. Similarly, an electroencephalogram (EEG) or neuroimaging might be essential if a neurologic illness is suspected to be the etiology of depressive and/or anxiety symptoms. Rarely, a 24-hour screen for catecholamine or serotonin metabolites becomes essential when pheochromocytoma or carcinoid syndrome is suspected (Alpay and Park, 2004).

Psychosis

First-episode psychosis warrants a thorough diagnostic evaluation to rule out medical disorders. Psychotic symptoms might be the initial manifestation of many medical and neurologic disorders and may precede the development of other symptoms. Therefore, clinicians should evaluate for the presence of an occult medical condition especially when the patient presents with an altered mental status or an unusual (e.g., visual hallucinations) or rare (e.g., catatonia) psychiatric symptom. Differential diagnoses in a psychotic patient include neurologic disorders (e.g., complex partial seizures; trauma, tumors, or stroke affecting the frontal or temporal lobes); infections (e.g., herpes encephalitis, neurosyphilis, HIV); neurodegenerative diseases (e.g., Huntington disease); endocrine diseases (e.g., thyroid storm, myxedema madness); autoimmune diseases (e.g., systemic lupus erythematosus); and substance-induced (e.g., amphetamine, cocaine, hallucinogens, phencyclidine intoxication, alcohol hallucinosis) disorders or substance withdrawal (alcohol withdrawal delirium, barbiturate withdrawal). The initial diagnostic workup therefore should include the routine tests outlined in Table 5-1. If there is a heightened suspicion of central nervous system (CNS) pathology, lumbar puncture for CSF analysis, neuroimaging, and an EEG might be indicated (Alpay and Park, 2004; Sadock and Sadock, 2003).

Suicide attempt

More than a half-million suicide attempts occur each year, with >30,000 completed suicides annually in the United States. If a suicide attempt by drug overdose is suspected, blood levels of commonly accessible over-the-counter drugs (e.g., acetaminophen, salicylate) and serum levels (e.g., digoxin) and indirect measures of prescribed drugs (e.g., coagulation profile for suspected warfarin overdose) should be considered, along with the routinely obtained laboratory measures outlined in Table 5-1.

Substance abuse

Urine or blood drug screens are useful in detecting substance use. These screening tests are sensitive but result in false positives. Confirmatory measures are available for most drugs of abuse and may be indicated in some clinical situations. Except for alcohol and barbiturates, which are best detected in the serum, the majority of commonly abused substances are well detected in urine. Regular and excessive alcohol use can have several detrimental effects on an individual's body, which may be reflected in the commonly ordered laboratory tests. For instance, the mean corpuscular volume (MCV) is abnormally high in >50% of persons who have alcohol-related disorders and elevated *γ-glutamyl transferase* (GGT) levels are seen in >75%. Other tests to consider can include liver enzymes. Liver failure secondary to alcohol-induced cirrhosis can result in low platelet count and an abnormal coagulation profile. Furthermore, carbohydrate deficit transferrin (CDT) can be used to detect heavy alcohol consumption. Elevated levels of blood CDT suggest recent alcohol abuse. CDT is largely independent of comorbid liver disorders and therefore is considered a more efficient screening measure of alcohol abuse than the above-mentioned tests. In addition, CDT is considered superior to GGT for detecting relapse in alcoholics (Schmidt et al., 1997).

Eating disorders

Eating disorders are prevalent in up to 4% of adolescent and young adults. The CBC could show leucopenia with relative lymphocytosis. Fasting blood glucose levels are often low in the severe stages of anorexia nervosa. Mild hypothyroidism can also be present in individuals with anorexia nervosa. Purging behavior can result in hypokalemic alkalosis and elevated serum amylase levels. If laxative abuse is suspected, stool samples may be checked. Abnormal ECG findings, including ST-segment depression, prolonged QT interval, and T-wave inversion, have also been noted in these patients and are often related to electrolyte abnormalities (Halmi, 2000).

Tests for Special Populations
Children and adolescents

As in adults, clinicians need to evaluate children and adolescents for medical conditions that may mimic psychiatric illnesses before making a diagnosis of primary psychiatric disorders. Therefore, certain routine tests such as the CBC, basic metabolic panel, LFT, and TSH should be considered. In addition, total iron and total iron-binding capacity (for iron-deficiency anemia), heavy metals measurements (for exposure to toxins such as lead and mercury), CSF analysis (for CNS viral, bacterial, or fungal infections), or neuroimaging (for head injury or to rule out brain tumors) should be considered in high-risk patients. A urine drug screen should be considered for all pediatric patients who present with psychiatric symptoms, especially if they experience an acute behavioral change, psychosis, or altered mental status. In addition, high-risk adolescents (e.g., those with oppositional defiant disorder, conduct disorder), children of substance abusers, and children who have recurrent motor vehicle accidents should be screened for substance misuse. Children and adolescents who have multiple sexual partners or a history of sexual abuse should be tested for syphilis (using rapid plasma reagin [RPR]) and HIV. If the RPR is positive, the result has to be confirmed by using the fluorescent trepenomal antibody-absorption (FTA-ABS) test (Zametkin et al., 1998).

Geriatrics

In addition to environmental and physical factors, recent change in medications and various medical illnesses ranging from the benign to potentially life-threatening conditions can be associated with the onset of an anxiety and affective, cognitive, or psychotic symptomatology in the elderly. As in all clinical settings, a careful assessment should be done before ordering laboratory tests. Screening for alcohol and recreational, prescription, and over-the counter drug misuse/abuse in a geriatric patient is essential. When suspicion arises, a blood alcohol level and urine toxicology screen should be obtained. Routine measurements of CBC, comprehensive metabolic panel (CMP), and TSH are often helpful. Midstream urine for urinalysis was found to be beneficial in elderly women presenting with psychiatric symptoms. In cognitively impaired individuals, serum vitamin B_{12} and folate levels, TSH, and RPR are indicated in addition to the routine laboratory measures. Roughly 5% to 15% of patients have a reversible cause for cognitive impairment. Other tests that are not routinely indicated include chest x-ray (if pneumonia is suspected), ECG (especially before using antipsychotics), EEG (if seizures are suspected), and serum prescription drug levels (Kolman, 1984; Mookhoek and Sterrenburg van der Nieuwegiessen, 1998).

Psychotropic Medication Monitoring
Antidepressants
Tricyclic antidepressants

A baseline ECG should be obtained to monitor for conduction delays before starting tricyclic antidepressants (TCAs). Patients with cardiac conduction abnormalities are at increased risk for heart block or lethal arrhythmias, even at therapeutic TCA levels. Therefore, an annual ECG is recommended in patients who are on TCAs long term. Baseline LFT and CBC are also suggested as part of the diagnostic workup before initiating TCAs.

Blood levels are routinely monitored when using TCAs. Certain TCAs, such as nortriptyline and desipramine, have a documented therapeutic window. For instance, nortriptyline has a therapeutic window of 50 and 150 ng/mL within which the drug is most efficacious; levels above 150 ng/mL or below 50 ng/mL have demonstrated decreased effectiveness. Similarly, desipramine shows a favorable response when the blood levels are >125 ng/mL. The drugs have to be ingested at a stable dose for at least 5 days to achieve a steady state. Subsequently, the blood levels are drawn within 10 to 14 hours of the last dose. Table 5-2 summarizes the routine monitoring suggested with TCAs and antipsychotics.

Monoamine oxidase inhibitors

Serum liver enzymes have to be routinely monitored in patients on monoamine oxidase inhibitors (MAOIs) due to the potential for hepatotoxicity. Elderly individuals are more sensitive to side effects when compared with younger persons. In addition, MAOIs have been associated with lowering blood glucose concentrations and false elevations of thyroid function tests. In the elderly and medically ill patients, a baseline ECG is warranted because of the adverse cardiovascular effects of these medications.

Newer-generation antidepressants

Selective serotonin reuptake inhibitors (SSRIs) are rarely associated with hyponatremia secondary to the secretion of inappropriate antidiuretic hormone (SIADH). Serum sodium levels can fall precipitously within a few weeks of initiating SSRIs and can return to normal within days to weeks upon discontinuing the offending drug (Kirby and Ames, 2001). Hyponatremia may present a significant problem in persons who are volume depleted, elderly, or on diuretics. Therefore, serum sodium levels should be measured, especially if a patient experiences an altered mental status

TABLE 5-2   Antipsychotic and Tricyclic Antidepressants Monitoring

Laboratory Evaluation	Antipsychotics Pretreatment	12 weeks	Annually	Every 5 years	Tricyclic Antidepressants Pretreatment	Acute treatment	Annually
CBC[a]	X				X		
BMP	X						
LFT	X				X		
ECG[b]	X				X		
Pregnancy[c] test	X				X		
Fasting glucose	X	X	X				
Fasting lipid panel	X	X		X			
Blood levels (for parent drug and metabolites)						X[d]	X

[a]For clozapine, WBC should be monitored at baseline, then weekly for the first 6 months, then once every 2 weeks from 6 to 12 months, and then once every 4 weeks *ad infinitum* (if the counts are normal). If abnormal, please refer to clozapine package insert for guidelines.
[b]In high-risk patients, monitor ECG frequently and after each dose titration and steady-state levels are achieved.
[c]In women of childbearing age.
[d]Monitor frequently in patients with risk factors, medication noncompliance, poor response even after taking a therapeutic dose, and during dose titration.
CBC, complete blood count; X, routine laboratory tests recommended; BMP, basic metabolic panel; LFT, liver function test; WBC, white blood cell count; ECG, electrocardiogram.

after SSRI initiation. SSRIs can also disrupt platelet function. They reduce the platelet serotonin uptake by binding to the platelet serotonin receptors. Therefore, serotonin-mediated platelet aggregation is reduced. The net results could include patients presenting with bruising, epistaxis, prolonged bleeding time, or gastrointestinal bleeding (Serebruany, 2006). These are mostly seen as dose-related adverse effects. As a result, SSRIs may present an increased risk for inducing gastrointestinal bleeding, when used concomitantly with nonsteroidal anti-inflammatory drugs (NSAIDs), aspirin, or drugs that affect coagulation. SSRIs can also displace warfarin from the plasma protein-binding sites, thereby increasing free warfarin levels and anticoagulation effect.

Trazodone has been associated with cardiac arrhythmias, which is significant in persons with preexisting ventricular irritability and elderly patients with cardiovascular disease (James and Mendelson, 2004).

Since venlafaxine has SSRI-like properties, SIADH and associated hyponatremia may be rarely seen with its use. Mirtazapine has been linked with increased triglycerides and cholesterol in 6% and 20% or more of patients respectively, and, in rare cases, with elevation in liver enzymes. A baseline fasting lipid panel may be considered before initiating mirtazapine. Mirtazapine has also been reported to rarely cause agranulocytosis in the first 2 months of treatment, which usually resolves with the drug discontinuation. Although the rates in clinical trials are noted to be low (i.e., 1.1 per 1,000 patients), patients who develop a low white blood cell (WBC) count and fever, chills, sore throat, or other signs of infections should receive medical attention and discontinuation of mirtazapine (Montgomery, 1995).

Mood Stabilizers
Lithium

Lithium has long been shown to be effective in treating bipolar disorder and augmenting the management of depression. Lithium has a narrow therapeutic index, with therapeutic serum levels in the acute phase of treatment ranging between 0.8 and 1.2 mEq/L. Despite its benefits, lithium can cause numerous side effects. Thyroid function tests need to be monitored because diffuse, nontender goiter and hypothyroidism are associated with lithium treatment and seen more often in women than in men (Jefferson, 1990). Furthermore, lithium can cause changes on an ECG, including T-wave flattening or inversion, U waves, and first-degree atrioventricular block (Tilkian et al., 1976). Lithium is also reported to cause interstitial fibrosis, nephrogenic diabetes insipidus, nephrotic syndrome, and rarely renal failure, requiring careful monitoring of electrolytes and renal function (Raedler and Wiedemann, 2007). A CBC may reveal benign, reversible leukocytosis with lithium use. Some patients receiving lithium may exhibit elevated serum calcium secondary to increased parathyroid hormone levels. Therefore, pretreatment evaluation should include CBC, serum electrolytes, renal function tests, fasting blood glucose, TSH, and an ECG. In patients with renal disease and persistent proteinuria, a 24-hour urinary creatinine clearance might be necessary. In a healthy adult with no renal disease, steady state is achieved in 3 to 6 days on a fixed dose. Plasma levels have to be checked after an increase in daily dosage and the steady state is achieved. Blood should be drawn approximately 10 to 12 hours after the last dose of medication. During initial titration, lithium levels might need to be monitored every 3 to 4 days for earlier detection of toxic lithium levels. The maintenance level is 0.6–1.2 mEq/L, with lower levels sufficient for elderly patients and higher levels often necessary for acute mania. In women of childbearing age, a serum pregnancy test is indicated before starting lithium. During the stable maintenance phase, serum lithium levels should be monitored every 3 months, and CBC, basic metabolic panel (BMP), TSH, and ECG yearly in younger patients and once every 6 months in older adults. The cardiovascular, renal, and thyroid complications can be easily prevented if the clinician carefully follows the above-mentioned laboratory values (Jefferson and Griest, 2000; Alpay and Park, 2004) (see Table 5-3).

Carbamazepine

Carbamazepine can cause aplastic anemia, thrombocytopenia, and agranulocytosis. Carbamazepine can occasionally result in liver enzyme elevations and, very rarely, acute liver failure. As a result, a pretreatment laboratory evaluation should include CBC (including platelet count), LFTs, and a serum pregnancy test (in women of childbearing age). An ECG may be warranted in persons with cardiac disorders or those older than 40 years of age because carbamazepine

TABLE 5-3 Lithium and Anticonvulsant Drug Monitoring

Laboratory Evaluation	Lithium				Valproic Acid			Carbamazepine			
	Pretreatment	Acute treatment	Maintenance 6 months	Annually	Pretreatment	Acute treatment	Maintenance	Pretreatment	Acute treatment	Maintenance 6 mo	Annually
CBC	X			X	X	X[a]	X[b]	X	X[c]	X[b]	
BMP	X		X	X	X			X			
LFT					X	X[a]	X[b]	X	X[c]	X[b]	
Urinalysis	X				X						
TSH	X		X	X							
ECG[d]	X			X	X			X			X
Serum pregnancy test[e]	X				X			X			
Blood levels[f]	X[g]		X[b]			X[g]	X[b]		X[g]	X[b]	

[a]Monthly for 3 months, then every 3–6 months if normal; special emphasis to elderly or medically ill patients, or if delirium occurs, perform tests. If abnormal, please review guidelines.
[b]Every 3 months (for geriatric patients) to 6 months (for younger, medically healthy patients).
[c]Every 2 weeks for 2 months.
[d]At-risk patients.
[e]Women of childbearing age.
[f]Parent drug and metabolites.
[g]Obtain levels during titration, until stable dose is achieved (mostly weekly); for valproate and carbamazepine—weekly for 2 months.
CBC, complete blood count; X, routine laboratory tests recommended; BMP, basic metabolic panel; LFT, liver function test; TSH, thyroid-stimulating hormone; ECG, electrocardiogram.

may cause cardiac conduction abnormalities. Steady state is achieved after 2 to 4 days of a fixed drug dose. During the fifth day of the steady dose, serum concentrations should be determined. Frequent monitoring of carbamazepine blood levels in the first 2 months is crucial because carbamazepine can induce liver enzymes and speed up its own metabolism (autoinduction). The recommended serum level is 6 to 12 ng/mL. CBC and LFT should be repeated once every 2 weeks during the first 2 months, and once every 3 months thereafter (Zarate and Tohen, 2000).

Valproic acid

Pretreatment assessments should include CBC and hepatic function tests because valproic acid can cause thrombocytopenia, pancytopenia, and hepatic injury. The steady state of valproic acid is achieved in 2 to 4 days. Serum levels of valproic acid and divalproex sodium are therapeutic between 50 and 125 ng/mL. Serum levels of valproic acid should be done frequently until stable doses and/or adequate drug levels are achieved and then periodically during maintenance therapy. LFTs and CBC (including platelet count) should be checked every 3 to 6 months. Also, pancreatitis is rarely associated with valproic acid use, especially in the first 6 months, and serum lipase or amylase levels can be assessed to determine pancreatic function if symptoms of pancreatitis develop. Elevations of plasma ammonia levels may be seen with valproate use, and serum ammonia levels should be determined if the patient develops an altered mental status on valproic acid (Zarate and Tohen, 2000).

Other anticonvulsants

Blood dyscrasias, hyponatremia, and hepatotoxicity have been described with lamotrigine use. Baseline screening tests should include CBC and CMP, and periodic monitoring during the initial phases of the medication titration is desirable. Gabapentin is excreted through the kidneys in an unchanged state, and therefore, baseline renal function tests should be monitored. Hyponatremia is reported especially in the first 3 months of oxcarbazepine use. Gabapentin and oxcarbazepine require renal dosage adjustment in persons with renal impairment. Regardless of the anticonvulsants prescribed, pregnancy should be excluded in women of childbearing age (Wong and Lhatoo, 2000; Sommer et al., 2007).

Antipsychotics

Conventional antipsychotics especially have been associated with SIADH. Low-potency antipsychotic agents (e.g., chlorpromazine) particularly can rarely cause obstructive jaundice. Although liver problems may occur rarely with other antipsychotics, abnormal LFTs should alert the clinician to rule out a medical etiology or look for another offending drug. Agranulocytosis is also rarely caused by low-potency neuroleptics. In addition, mild elevations in serum prolactin levels are seen with conventional antipsychotics and certain atypical antipsychotics such as risperidone, clozapine, and olanzapine.

A baseline ECG should be considered in persons with known or suspected cardiac disease. Neuroleptics are associated with ECG abnormalities such as flattened, inverted, or bifid T waves and prolonged QT interval. *Torsade de pointes*, defined as polymorphous ventricular tachycardia (VT), is an uncommon variant of VT that has been reported with several conventional and novel antipsychotics. Risk factors include being a woman and/or elderly, electrolyte disturbances (e.g., hypokalemia, hypomagnesemia, and hypocalcemia), known cardiac disease, endocrine disturbances (e.g., diabetes mellitus, hypothyroidism), liver disease, prolonged QT interval, and combining antipsychotics with other medications that can prolong QT interval. Therefore, in addition to the baseline ECG, periodic ECG monitoring is also essential in high-risk patients.

Clozapine

Treatment with clozapine is associated with an increased risk of agranulocytosis (approximately 1% to 2%). Therefore, specific guidelines in monitoring the WBC and differential count exist before and after initiation of treatment with this medication. Baseline and weekly monitoring of the WBC and differential count is mandatory for the first 6 months, once every 2 weeks during 6 to 12 months of treatment, and once every 4 weeks *ad infinitum* after 1 year. Also, during discontinuation of treatment, the WBC count should be monitored weekly for at least 4 weeks. Other monitoring guidelines exist in persons with mild to severe leucopenia or granulocytopenia or if the patient develops agranulocytosis. The risk of agranulocytosis peaks in the third month of clozapine therapy, and weekly incidence rates continue to decline past 6 months. Details on the WBC and absolute neutrophil count monitoring protocol are available in the clozapine package insert.

Plasma levels of clozapine at or above 350 ng/mL may be associated with better clinical response in refractory schizophrenic patients (Kronig et al., 1995).

Antipsychotics and metabolic syndrome

Certain second-generation neuroleptics have been associated with metabolic syndrome. Clozapine and olanzapine have been linked to increased risk for diabetes mellitus and worsening of the lipid profile. In addition, clozapine and olanzapine cause significant weight gain; this side effect is also seen with risperidone and quetiapine, but at a lesser degree. Aripiprazole and ziprasidone cause minimal to no weight gain. A specific monitoring protocol is recommended with the use of antipsychotics due to the increased risk of metabolic syndrome. Weight (in respect to body mass index), waist circumference, blood pressure, fasting blood glucose, and the lipid profile should be monitored at baseline, along with family and personal history of obesity, diabetes, dyslipidemia, hypertension, or cardiovascular disease. Subsequently, weight has to be documented at 4, 8, and 12 weeks and then quarterly. The fasting plasma glucose should be repeated in 12 weeks and then annually, if normal. A fasting lipid profile should be repeated in 12 weeks and then repeated every 5 years, if within normal limits. If clinically indicated, more frequent assessments may be essential (American Diabetes Association, 2004).

Benzodiazepines

In patients with substance use disorders, urine is routinely tested for benzodiazepines. LFTs should be measured in individuals with suspected liver disease because this can assist in choosing the benzodiazepine for a particular patient. For instance, lorazepam, oxazepam, and temazepam are not dependent on the liver for their metabolism and may be better choices in patients with hepatic disease. In contrast, diazepam and chlordiazepoxide are metabolized in the liver through oxidation, and in patients with hepatic disease, their half-lives are increased, leading to toxic drug levels from drug accumulation. Before prescribing benzodiazepines, pregnancy tests should be performed in women of childbearing age.

Other Commonly Utilized Tests

Electroencephalogram

The EEG records cerebral low-voltage electrical activity detected by scalp electrodes. The EEG is performed with the person motionless to avoid muscle artifact, and the activity immediately below the scalp contributes most to the recording. Four bands of frequency measured in hertz (Hz) are produced. They are named with Greek letters: alpha (8 to 13 Hz), beta (>13 Hz), theta (4 to 7 Hz), and delta (1 to 3 Hz) waves.

Normal

Alpha rhythm dominates posteriorly and is detectable over the occipital lobe. Beta activity overlies the frontal lobe, and theta waves predominate the frontotemporal region. Alpha waves form the dominant EEG activity in a normal condition when the person is relaxed with eyes closed. The alpha rhythm disappears when the individual opens his or her eyes, becomes anxious, falls asleep, or takes medications that affect mental function.

Epilepsy

During seizure activity, the EEG consists of bursts of spikes, slow waves, or spike-and-slow-wave complexes, which may be organized in a rhythmic pattern. If this abnormal pattern is localized to one region of the brain, that area is considered a potentially epileptogenic focus. If a focal seizure spreads to the neighboring brain regions or throughout the cerebral cortex, it is said to be a generalized seizure.

Generalized seizures consist of bilateral, symmetric, synchronous paroxysmal spike-and-slow-wave discharges. Absence seizures, commonly seen in children, may occur several times daily and consist of generalized 3-Hz spike-and-slow-wave complexes. Partial complex seizures, the most common type, appear as unilateral or bilateral paroxysms of spikes, polyspikes, or slow-wave abnormalities over the temporal or frontotemporal regions.

Conversion disorder with seizures or convulsions (better known as *nonepileptic seizures* or *pseudoseizures*) will show a normal EEG pattern.

Dementia and delirium

In Alzheimer disease, alpha activity slows down from 10–13 Hz to 8 Hz. The background EEG slows down further and finally becomes disorganized in the severe stage of the illness. In vascular dementia, an EEG shows abnormalities with asymmetric discharges seen over brain areas with infarctions. Despite these EEG changes, using this tool clinically is limited in differentiating these two types of dementias. In patients with subacute sclerosing panencephalitis and Creutzfeldt-Jakob disease, the EEG shows periodic complexes (burst-suppression).

In delirium, alpha activity disappears, and the patient develops diffuse theta and delta activity, suggesting generalized slowing. In hepatic or uremic encephalopathy, the EEG may display triphasic waves.

Medications

Benzodiazepines and barbiturates produce beta activity on an EEG. Conventional antipsychotics may produce sharp waves. Antidepressants result in nonspecific abnormalities, and lithium toxicity causes spikes and sharp waves in EEGs.

Utility in clinical psychiatry

An EEG is not routinely recommended in clinical psychiatric practice. Studies have shown low clinical yield when psychiatric services have referred patients for EEG, except when the patient is on clozapine, has a known history of epilepsy, or a convulsive seizure is suspected (O'Sullivan et al., 2006). In most clinical situations, the EEG is normal or shows subtle, nonspecific abnormalities. EEG is used to differentiate between nonepileptic and "true" seizure disorders. EEG may differentiate dementia from pseudodementia (cognitive deficits secondary to depression). In most patients, depression results in normal EEG activity, whereas dementia reveals slow-wave patterns.

EEG monitoring is used during electroconvulsive therapy (ECT). ECT induces EEG changes and resembles generalized tonic-clonic seizures. Post-ECT, slow waves predominate the EEG patterns. EEG slowing is associated with memory impairment and is less pronounced with unilateral ECT treatment (Isenberg and Zorumski, 2000; UK ECT Review Group, 2003).

Polysomnography

A polysomnogram (PSG) is used to monitor the various stages of sleep. PSG simultaneously records cerebral activity (EEG), ocular movement (electrooculogram), muscle movement and tone (electromyogram), and oxygen saturation (pulse oxymetry). PSG distinguishes two phases of sleep: rapid eye movement (REM) and nonrapid eye movement (NREM) sleep. During REM sleep, EEG detects low-voltage, fast-wave patterns with ocular movement artifacts. During NREM sleep stage 1, disappearance of alpha activity during drowsiness and onset of beta activity over frontal and temporal regions are noted. During sleep stage 2, sleep spindles and K complexes are present, and during sleep stages 3 and 4 (or slow-wave), delta activity predominates (Kaufman, 2006). PSG may assist in diagnosing the various types of sleep disorders (Moore et al., 2000; Smallwood and Stern, 2004). The various changes seen on PSG in patients with psychiatric and alcohol-related disorders are explained in Chapter 17.

NEUROIMAGING IN PSYCHIATRY

The field of neuroimaging in psychiatric disorders continues to evolve and has made tremendous advances. Until recently, brain imaging in psychiatry was limited to structural imaging techniques: CT and magnetic resonance imaging (MRI). These techniques continue to assist in the differential diagnoses of neuropsychiatric disorders. They are noninvasive tools that provide images of neuroanatomical structures with excellent spatial and contrast resolution. In addition to the structural neuroimaging methods, functional neuroimaging techniques that include positron emission tomography (PET) and single photon emission computed tomography (SPECT) have been available. Although primarily research tools, innovative functional neuroimaging techniques including functional magnetic resonance imaging (fMRI) and magnetic resonance (MR) spectroscopy have received increased attention in psychiatric disorders.

Structural Neuroimaging Techniques

Computed Tomography

To generate an image using CT, an x-ray beam passes through the patient's head and is recorded by the CT detectors. The image produced depends on the degree of x-ray attenuation achieved (e.g., dense structures such as bone and acute blood lead to higher attenuation, compared with less dense material such as CSF or air resulting in lower attenuation). Higher attenuation appears brighter/whiter, whereas lower attenuation appears darker/blacker. In CT with contrast, iodine-based contrast material is introduced and increases the attenuation of blood vessels and abnormal vasculatures (e.g., arteriovenous malformations) and structures that lack an intact blood–brain barrier (BBB), and they appear white. For example, iodinated contrast assists in better visualization of brain lesions such as a tumor, abscess, bleed, or stroke that can compromise the integrity of the BBB (see Figs. 5-1 and 5-2).

Magnetic Resonance Imaging

With or without contrast, MRI produces superior images when compared with CT. MRI uses no ionizing radiation but, rather, involves a complex interaction between external magnetic fields and tissues within the patient. In other words, MRI involves the energy exchange between an external magnetic field and certain atomic nuclei. Nuclei give off energy and are used to construct the anatomic images. The appearance of images depends on specific imaging properties and is chosen per the specific clinical situation: T1-weighted images help in optimal visualization of normal anatomic structures; T2-weighted images are used to detect areas of brain pathology.

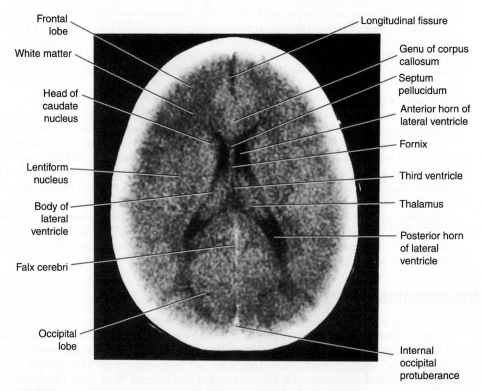

FIGURE 5-1. Horizontal (axial) computed tomographic (CT) scan of the brain.

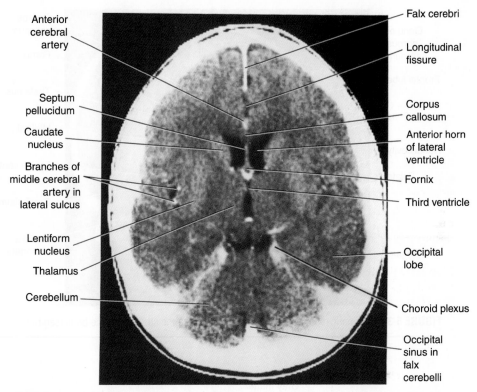

FIGURE 5-2. Horizontal (axial) computed tomographic (CT) scan of the brain (contrast-enhanced).

Contrast material (gadolinium is commonly used) results in increased T1 signal intensity of venous structures and those with a compromised BBB (see Figs. 5-3 and 5-4).

The advantages and limitations of CT and MRI are outlined in Table 5-4.

Indications for Structural Neuroimaging in Psychiatry

Structural neuroimaging techniques should be considered as part of the diagnostic workup for patients with new-onset psychosis, dementia, delirium, catatonia, anorexia nervosa, new-onset personality or mood symptoms after 50 years of age, head trauma, abnormal neurologic examination, and when a neurologic disorder is suspected (Weinberger, 1984).

As part of the pre-ECT evaluation, neuroimaging may be indicated to identify organic brain lesions such as tumors, aneurysms, arteriovenous malformations, hydrocephalus, or cerebrovascular accident.

Functional Neuroimaging

Positron Emission Tomography

PET is based on positron-emitting, biologically active radioisotopes that have to be prepared by onsite cyclotron. When inhaled or injected intravenously, radioisotopes or radioligands are metabolized in the brain and release positrons. The collision of positrons and electrons produces photons that are detected and transformed into images. The most commonly used radioligand is fluorine-18, labeled fluorodeoxyglucose (FDG), and measures glucose metabolism. FDG-PET is beneficial in studying brain function because increased glucose metabolism is seen in areas of brain activity. PET uses other radioligands that also allow noninvasive study of cerebral blood flow, oxygen metabolism, and psychotropic medication concentrations in specific brain regions (e.g., assessment of receptors for specific neurotransmitters). For instance, regional cerebral metabolism has been studied in various neurodegenerative disorders, including Alzheimer disease

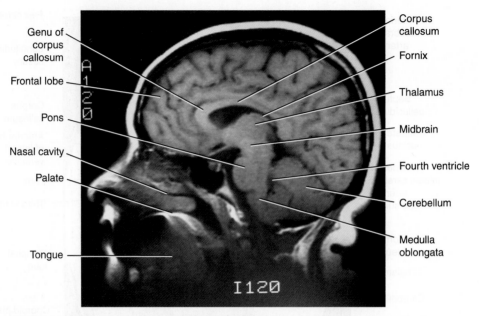

FIGURE 5-3. Magnetic resonance imaging (MRI) showing the structure of the brain (sagittal).

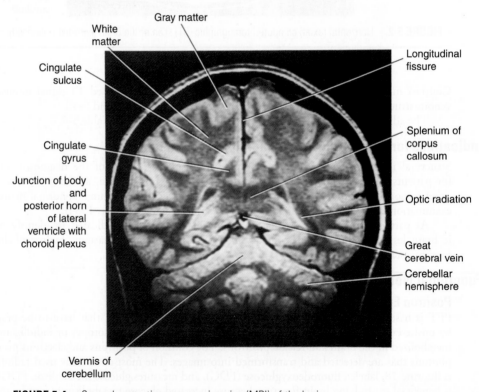

FIGURE 5-4. Coronal magnetic resonance imaging (MRI) of the brain.

TABLE 5-4	Structural Neuroimaging Differences	
Neuroimaging Type	**Advantages**	**Disadvantages**
Computed tomography (CT)	Less expensive than MRI Easily accessible Less likely to trigger anxiety than MRI; better tolerated by claustrophobic patients Detect gross pathology in a rapid and efficient manner Superior in detecting acute hemorrhage and bony or calcified lesions or skull fractures First choice in an acute trauma or uncooperative patient Recommended if MRI is contraindicated	Contraindicated in pregnancy Iodinated contrast allergic reaction may occur Less efficient in detecting posterior fossa and brainstem lesions Less helpful in assessing white matter lesions
Magnetic resonance imaging (MRI)	More sensitive than CT in detecting white matter lesions (e.g., from multiple sclerosis) Superior to screen for intracranial metastasis Superior in separating gray and white matter in both cortical and subcortical regions Does not use ionizing radiation; safer in pregnant women or young children Superior to detect posterior fossa and brainstem lesions Superior in subacute or chronic bleed	More expensive than CT Takes longer time to perform Contraindicated in patients with cardiac pacemakers, non–MRI-compatible aneurysm clips, brain stimulators, cochlear implants, and other metallic or electronic devices within the body Less well tolerated by patients with claustrophobia or anxiety disorders

(Dubois et al., 2007). PET imaging techniques have also advanced the study of the central serotonin system in mood disorders.

Medicare has approved the use of a PET scan to differentiate Alzheimer disease and frontotemporal dementia. A PET study can demonstrate changes in the brain areas vulnerable to Alzheimer disease neuropathology. This could possibly lead to detection of Alzheimer disease several years before onset of symptoms.

Single Photon Emission Computed Tomography
SPECT uses manufactured radioactive single photon–emitting isotopes to measure changes in the cerebral blood flow and, like PET, specific radioligands to assess receptor activity. When compared with PET, SPECT is less expensive, but the resolution worsens as the attempt is made to visualize deeper brain structures.

Functional Magnetic Resonance Imaging and Magnetic Resonance Spectroscopy
fMRI and MR spectroscopy are innovative imaging techniques currently used extensively in psychiatric research (Honey et al., 2002; Pearlson and Calhoun, 2007; Mitterschiffthaler et al., 2006; Smith et al., 2007). These neuroimaging tools may end up being available clinically in the future.

Clinical indications for functional neuroimaging are limited to the use of PET in Alzheimer disease. The functional imaging research findings in various psychiatric disorders are beyond the scope of this chapter.

CONCLUSION
Laboratory evaluation of patients presenting with psychiatric symptoms is an essential component for the successful diagnosis and treatment of neuropsychiatric illness.

> **Clinical Pearls**
>
> - The clinical interview remains the cornerstone of a comprehensive psychiatric assessment; laboratory measures are considered routinely to screen for medical illnesses that can mimic psychiatric disorders.
> - Currently, there are no biological measures available to confirm a specific psychiatric disorder.
> - Commonly obtained laboratory tests during the initial psychiatric visit include complete blood count, serum electrolytes, liver function tests, blood urea nitrogen and creatinine levels, TSH, urine toxicology screen, RPR, serum pregnancy (in women of childbearing age), and urinalysis. Several other measures should be considered depending on the respective patient's presentation.
> - A thorough medical and neurologic evaluation is warranted in a patient with an atypical presentation of an anxiety or mood disorder, and in persons with first-episode psychosis.
> - Psychotropic medication monitoring guidelines should be adhered to, in order to minimize the potential for adverse events.
> - Electroencephalography is not routinely recommended in clinical psychiatric practice.
> - Structural neuroimaging (i.e., CT head or MRI brain) is indicated during the workup for new-onset psychosis, dementia, delirium, catatonia, new-onset personality or mood symptoms after age 50 years, head trauma, and during clinical suspicion of a neurologic disorder.

Self-Assessment Questions and Answers

5-1. Prolonged PR, QRS, or QT intervals on electrocardiography are most commonly associated with:

A. Anxiolytics
B. Lithium
C. Sedatives
D. Tricyclic antidepressants
E. Anticonvulsants

Prolonged PR, QRS, or QT interval on ECG is commonly associated with tricyclic antidepressants. Lithium may cause T-wave flattening or inversion, U waves, and first-degree atrioventricular block. Certain antipsychotics can also prolong QT interval. *Answer: D*

5-2. A patient presents to the emergency department after having had a sudden onset of headache and syncope. The patient is noted to have altered mental status upon presentation. Physical examination shows that the neck is rigid, but otherwise there is no papilledema, and there are no focal neurologic signs. The initial investigative procedure for this presentation should be:

A. Carotid ultrasound
B. Magnetic resonance imaging (MRI) of the brain
C. Lumbar puncture
D. Electroencephalography
E. Computed tomographic (CT) scan of the head

CT, in comparison to MRI, is less expensive, quicker, more available, and more sensitive in detecting acute hemorrhage and brain calcification. CT is the study of choice in an acute trauma patient, an uncooperative patient, a suspected intracranial hemorrhage, and an acute neurologic emergency. *Answer: E*

5-3. Which of the following laboratory test results is consistent with a history of alcohol abuse?

A. Increased magnesium
B. Increased mean corpuscular volume
C. Increased ESR
D. Decreased glutamyl transaminase
E. Decreased calcium

Mean corpuscular volume is abnormally high in >50% and elevated γ-glutamyl transferase (GGT) levels are seen in >75% persons with alcohol-related disorders. *Answer: B*

5-4. A 65-year-old patient with bipolar disorder who is stable on lithium presents to the psychiatrist with mild confusion, tremors, and ataxia. The patient reports recently having a "stomach flu." The most useful laboratory test in this situation is a:

A. Liver function test
B. Thyroid-stimulating hormone (TSH) level
C. Lithium level
D. Complete blood count
E. Creatinine level

The above-mentioned symptoms in this patient are most likely secondary to lithium toxicity. *Answer: C*

References

Alpay M, Park L. Laboratory tests and diagnostic procedures. In: Stern TA, Herman JB, eds. *Massachusetts general hospital psychiatry update and board preparation*, 2nd ed. New York: McGraw-Hill; 2004:249–262.

American Diabetes Association. Consensus development conference on antipsychotic drugs and obesity and diabetes (Consensus Statement). *Diabetes Care*. 2004;27:596–601.

American Psychiatric Association. The dexamethasone suppression test: An overview of its current status in psychiatry. The APA task force on laboratory tests in psychiatry. *Am J Psychiatry*. 1987;144:1253–1262.

Anfinson TJ, Kathol RG. Screening laboratory evaluation in psychiatric patients: A review. *Gen Hosp Psychiatry*. 1992;14(4):248–257.

Dubois B, Feldman HH, Jacova C, et al. Research criteria for the diagnosis of Alzheimer's disease. Revising the NINCDS-ADRDA criteria. *Lancet Neurol*. 2007;6:734–746.

Halmi KA. Eating disorders. In: Sadock BJ, Sadock VA, eds. *Kaplan and Sadock's comprehensive textbook of psychiatry*, 7th ed., Vol. 2. Baltimore: Lippincott Williams & Wilkins; 2000:1663–1676.

Honey GD, Fletcher PC, Bullmore ET. Functional brain mapping of psychopathology. *J Neurol Neurosurg Psychiatry*. 2002;72:432–439.

Isenberg KE, Zorumski CF. Electroconvulsive therapy. In: Sadock BJ, Sadock VA, eds. *Kaplan and Sadock's comprehensive textbook of psychiatry*, 7th ed., Vol. 2. Baltimore: Lippincott Williams & Wilkins; 2000:2503–2515.

James SP, Mendelson WB. The use of trazodone as a hypnotic: A critical review. *J Clin Psychiatry*. 2004;65:752–755.

Jefferson JW. Lithium: The present and the future. *J Clin Psychiatry*. 1990;51(Suppl 8):4–19.

Jefferson JW, Griest JH. Lithium. In: Sadock BJ, Sadock VA, eds. *Kaplan and Sadock's comprehensive textbook of psychiatry*, 7th ed., Vol. 2. Baltimore: Lippincott Williams & Wilkins; 2000:2377–2390.

Kaufman DM. *Clinical neurology for psychiatrists*, 6th ed. Philadelphia: WB Saunders; 2006.

Kirby D, Ames D. Hyponatremia and selective serotonin reuptake inhibitors in elderly patients. *Int J Geriatr Psychiatry*. 2001;16:484–493.

Kolman PB. The value of laboratory investigations of elderly psychiatric patients. *J Clin Psychiatry*. 1984;45:112–116.

Kronig MH, Munne RA, Szymanski S, et al. Plasma clozapine levels and clinical response for treatment-refractory schizophrenic patients. *Am J Psychiatry*. 1995;152:179–182.

Lee R, Coccaro E. The neuropsychopharmacology of criminality and aggression. *Can J Psychiatry*. 2001;46:35–44.

Mann JJ, Malone KM. Cerebrospinal fluid amines and higher-lethality suicide attempts in depressed inpatients. *Biol Psychiatry*. 1997;41:162–171.

Mitterschiffthaler MT, Ettinger U, Mehta MA, et al. Applications of functional magnetic resonance imaging in psychiatry. *J Magn Reson Imaging*. 2006;23:851–861.

Montgomery S. Safety of mirtazapine: A review. *Int Clin Psychopharmacol*. 1995;10(Suppl 4):37–45.

Mookhoek EJ, Sterrenburg van der Nieuwegiessen IM. Screening for somatic disease in elderly psychiatric patients. *Gen Hosp Psychiatry*. 1998;20:102–107.

Moore CA, Williams RL, Hirshkowitz M. In: Sadock BJ, Sadock VA, eds. *Kaplan and Sadock's comprehensive textbook of psychiatry*, 7th ed., Vol. 2. Baltimore: Lippincott Williams & Wilkins; 2000:1677–1700.

O'Sullivan SS, Mullins GM, Cassidy EM, et al. The role of the standard EEG in clinical psychiatry. *Hum Psychopharmacol*. 2006;21:265–271.

Pearlson GD, Calhoun V. Structural and functional magnetic resonance imaging in psychiatric disorders. *Can J Psychiatry*. 2007;52:158–166.

Raedler TJ, Wiedemann K. Lithium-induced nephropathies. *Psychopharmacol Bull*. 2007;40:134–149.

Roy A, De Jong J, Linnoila M, et al. Cerebrospinal fluid monoamine metabolites and suicidal behavior in depressed patients. A 5-year follow-up study. *Arch Gen Psychiatry*. 1989;46:609–612.

Sadock BJ, Sadock VA. *Kaplan & Sadock's synopsis of psychiatry: Behavioral sciences, clinical psychiatry*, 9th ed. Philadelphia: Lippincott Williams & Wilkins; 2003.

Schmidt LG, Schmidt K, Dufeu P, et al. Superiority of carbohydrate deficit transferrin to gamma glutamyltransferase in detecting relapse in alcoholism. *Am J Psychiatry*. 1997;154:75–80.

Serebruany VL. Selective serotonin reuptake inhibitors and increased bleeding risk: Are we missing something? *Am J Med*. 2006;119:113–116.

Smallwood P, Stern TA. Sleep disorders. In: Stern TA, Herman JB, eds. *Massachusetts general hospital psychiatry update and board preparation*, 2nd ed. New York: McGraw-Hill; 2004:173–178.

Smith GS, Gunning-Dixon FM, Lotrich FE, et al. Translational research in late-life mood disorders. Implications for future intervention and prevention research. *Neuropsychopharmacology*. 2007;32:1857–1875.

Sommer BR, Fenn HH, Ketter TA. Safety and efficacy of anticonvulsants in elderly patients with psychiatric disorders: Oxcarbazepine, topiramate and gabapentin. *Expert Opin Drug Saf*. 2007;6:133–145.

Tilkian AG, Schroder JS, Kao J, et al. Effect of lithium on cardiovascular performance: Report on extended ambulatory monitoring and exercise testing before and during lithium therapy. *Am J Cardiol*. 1976;38:701–708.

The UK ECT Review Group. Efficacy and safety of electroconvulsive therapy in depressive disorders: A systematic review and meta-analysis. *Lancet*. 2003;361:799–808.

Weinberger DR. Brain disease and psychiatric illness: When should a psychiatrist order a CAT scan? *Am J Psychiatry*. 1984;141:1521–1527.

Wong IC, Lhatoo SD. Adverse reactions to new anticonvulsant drugs. *Drug Saf*. 2000;23:35–56.

Zametkin AJ, Ernst M, Silver R. Laboratory and diagnostic testing in child and adolescent psychiatry: A review of the past 10 years. *J Am Acad Child Adolesc Psychiatry*. 1998;37:464–472.

Zarate CA, Tohen M. Anticonvulsants. In: Sadock BJ, Sadock VA, eds. *Kaplan and Sadock's comprehensive textbook of psychiatry*, 7th ed., Vol. 2. Baltimore: Lippincott Williams & Wilkins; 2000:2282–2299.

CHAPTER 6

Jennifer A. Niskala Apps, Jason E. Kanz, and Robert F. Newby

Psychological and Neuropsychological Testing

Over the last several decades, medical technologies have marched forward at a rapid pace, providing physicians with many additional tools to evaluate and treat their patients. During the same period, face-to-face contact with patients has decreased, necessitating the rapid application of these technologies in assisting accurate differential diagnosis. During medical school and residency, trainees are exposed to these technologies and encouraged to utilize them in clinical practice. However, when it comes to human behavior, mental abilities, or emotions, many physicians may feel unclear about what options for psychological assessment are available.

In this chapter, the focus will be on psychological assessment (the informed evaluation of human behavior) and testing (measuring behavior as a component of psychological assessment). Arthur Benton, a prominent figure in the genesis of neuropsychology, described neuropsychological assessment as "a *refinement* and *extension* of clinical observation—a refinement in that it describes a patient's performances more precisely and reliably, and an extension in that, through instrumentation and special test procedures, it elicits types of performance that are not accessible to the clinical observer" (1991, p. 507). The same may be said in general for psychological assessment or evaluation. This chapter will provide an overview of statistical basics and other considerations to help physicians conceptualize referral questions and understand, use, and interpret the domains of assessment generally encompassed by both psychological and neuropsychological testing.

STATISTICS AND TESTING BASICS

A psychological test is an instrument that provides a measure of human behavior and mental capacities. However, how is the accuracy of a measurement determined? Several statistical issues need to be considered, including standardization and score reporting, reliability, validity, sensitivity and specificity, and positive and negative predictive value.

Test scores may be reported in a number of ways. A simple raw score may be presented; however, it is rarely meaningful unless the test enjoys widespread familiarity. For example, most psychiatrists understand that a score of 29 out of 30 on the Mini Mental Status Examination (MMSE) is normal, whereas a score of 5 out of 30 likely represents severe impairment (Folstein et al., 1975).

Psychologists are likely to present test scores using one or more common metrics. Several methods of reporting assume that test scores are normally distributed (i.e., bell shaped) in the general population. Showing where a score is relative to a normal distribution can demonstrate how far that score is above or below normal. Common scores based on a normal distribution include z-scores (mean = 0, standard deviation = 1), T-scores (mean = 50, standard deviation = 10), and standard scores (mean = 100, standard deviation = 15).

Tests are not always normally distributed, however; sometimes they are *skewed*. On some tests most people are expected to perform near perfect levels, and when they do not, it suggests impairment. For example, on certain language comprehension tests, everyone is expected to perform flawlessly, so missing even a few items may indicate a significant deficit. It will not be obvious from how the test scores are reported whether tests are skewed, so other reporting methods may be implemented. In particular, the psychologist will often utilize descriptive terms, such as *mildly impaired*, in the written report of findings to interpret results.

Test score reporters may also utilize percentile ranks, which tell how many people would be expected to perform below that score in the general population. If a person is at the 63rd percentile on a test, 63 out of 100 individuals from the normative sample would have performed below that score.

Perhaps of greatest use to most clinicians are the interpretive labels that are also given. In addition to numeric scores, psychologists commonly provide a descriptive interpretation. For example, a psychologist may report that a child's verbal intelligence quotient (IQ) is 75 (fifth percentile). Those numbers provide some useful information, but the label "borderline impaired" provides another level of interpretation. In summarizing how test results may be reported, it is essential to remember that different numbers may be shown with various meanings, distributions, and so forth. Learning to understand the interpretive statements will be essential as well.

Standardization

Standardization refers to the development of a psychological test or the rules by which test administration is governed. Ideally, when test developers design a new test, they will administer the test to a large number of individuals from a variety of backgrounds, so that the test can be generalized when applied to various clinical populations. Often, standardization samples are chosen based on census data in the country where normative data are collected. It is important for the administering clinician to know how a test was developed in order to ensure it is appropriate for use with his or her patient population. It is also important that during the development of a new instrument, the test is administered in precisely the same way each time to ensure consistency to the greatest degree possible. Once a test is marketed for general use, it should be administered in the same, or standardized, way each time.

Reliability

Reliability essentially refers to the consistency of a test. Test authors work to establish a test that produces the same results over repeated administrations. If someone stepped on a bathroom scale at home three times and it read 122, 296, and 10 on each try, that scale would be considered unreliable. Similarly, test developers want to ensure that they are getting comparable results between testing administrations (test-retest reliability), between raters or test administrators (inter-rater reliability), between forms (alternate forms reliability), or even within the same test (internal consistency reliability).

Validity

Clinicians want to know how well the test measures what it is supposed to measure, or its validity. To go back to the previous example, a bathroom scale that provides the same weight each time can be assumed to be reliable, but it would not be a valid measure of hair color, though one would hope that it is a valid measure of weight. A valid psychological test measures what it is supposed to measure. Therefore, the clinician wants a measure of depression to measure depression, a measure of IQ to measure intellect, and so forth.

Subsumed under validity are whether a test adequately samples the domain being assessed (content validity); whether it is thought to measure a theoretic construct or trait, such as psychopathology as opposed to other traits (construct validity); and whether it is related to current or future behavior (concurrent and predictive validity, respectively).

Sensitivity and Specificity

Sensitivity and specificity are often overlooked but equally important to the above statistical concepts. Sensitivity refers to the proportion of people with a condition who have a positive test result. Conversely, specificity refers to the proportion of people without disease who have a negative result. Therefore, a test with high sensitivity may be useful for ruling out a condition, but only if the test is negative. A test with high specificity may be useful for ruling in a condition, but only if the test is positive.

Alone, sensitivity and specificity are quite useless because they do not account for prevalence rates of an illness. Even with reasonable sensitivity and specificity, a low base rate illness will lead to an overabundance of false-positive findings, such that many normal individuals would be identified as having a disease when in fact no disease was present. Knowing the prevalence rates for a given illness is important. For example, assume a test has 90% sensitivity and 90% specificity for attention-deficit/hyperactivity disorder (ADHD) in children, but that the *Diagnostic and*

Statistical Manual of Mental Disorders, Fourth Edition, Text Revision (DSM-IV-TR; American Psychiatric Association, 2000) identifies the maximum prevalence rate in the general population as 5%. If this test is administered to 1,000 random children, 45 out of the 50 who actually have ADHD would have a positive test result, but 95 out of the 950 who do not have the diagnosis would also have a positive test result. In other words, more than twice as many children as actually had ADHD would be incorrectly diagnosed. This illustrates that even when measures appear to have good sensitivity and specificity, the information they provide can still have serious limitations when the disease has a low base rate.

Positive and Negative Predictive Values

Positive predictive values (PPVs) and negative predictive values (NPVs) provide a different method for understanding sensitivity and specificity. PPV refers to the proportion of people with a positive test result who have the disease. NPV refers to the proportion of people with a negative test result who do not have the disease. Using the above-mentioned ADHD example, PPV would be approximately equal to 32% and NPV would be >99%. Unlike sensitivity and specificity, predictive values depend on prevalence rates for an illness. As prevalence rates increase, PPV goes up and NPV goes down. (Note that if a practitioner has knowledge of prevalence rates for a particular illness, that information can be combined with these values to calculate a likelihood ratio, which is the post-test probability of having, or not having, a disease, but that is beyond the scope of this chapter.)

Although this is just a statistics primer as applied to psychological testing, several key points are evident. First, a test needs to be consistent (reliable). Second, tests must measure what they claim to measure (valid). Third, reported numbers may be misleading. Sensitivity, specificity, PPV, and NPV mean little without knowledge of illness prevalence, which may vary from setting to setting. Finally, performance on a test, or series of tests, is just one bit of information that is limited if not considered in the context of a detailed clinical history. Psychologists are experts at integrating all these aspects of the information, which is why they provide physicians with *assessments* rather than just test scores.

A final word of caution regarding statistical concepts: researchers and those with a proprietary investment in the development of psychological tests can make their data look much better than they actually are. For example, the original studies on the MMSE by Folstein et al. (1975) demonstrated 100% sensitivity and 100% specificity to dementia; however, the study compared severely demented individuals with normal controls, rather than mildly impaired individuals and normal controls. Although this information does not imply that Folstein was attempting to make his test look better than it actually was, this study makes the point that knowing just how a test was developed is important. During the last several years, proprietary testing companies have been marketing cognitive tests (typically computer based) directly to physicians. However, the studies on these direct-to-market instruments have not met the academic rigor of some of the more established tests and batteries. More importantly, some of these tests do not consider clinical contexts that may influence the outcome of testing. Informed clinical judgment must be combined with test results in a comprehensive evaluation.

DEMOGRAPHICS

Demographic characteristics must also be considered during both test selection and interpretation.

Age

Types of assessment instruments across domains often vary based on age. Developmental assessment tools designed to measure motor skills and early cognitive development are obviously not appropriate for fully grown individuals, nor would they be useful for assessing dementia in the elderly. Even measures within the same domain will vary by age, such as intellectual tests for which questions and stimuli vary across three primary, slightly overlapping age bands: infant and preschool (1 to 6), childhood (6 to 17), and adult (older than 16 years). Each of those measures then also utilizes both age-appropriate item selection and age-based normative values for scoring. In other words, within a child-aged intellectual measure, different items would be administered to a 6-year-old child than to a 16-year-old. Similarly, different beginning points are used on adult intellectual measures for teen, young, mid, and oldest of adults. Scoring also will be based on a specific cohort of normative values based on the person's age, sometimes to the month. Even before testing, age may also play a role in the referral question. Again, certain forms of cognitive or emotional disability would be more likely to occur in older populations, making similar questions inappropriate for children. With the breadth of tools available currently, similar domains of both psychological and neuropsychological functioning can be assessed in almost any age.

Level of Education

Level of education should always be considered when interpreting assessment results. Of the many psychosocial factors that affect development, education is relatively formal and well defined. As was mentioned during the discussion of standardization, each assessment tool created should articulate the characteristics of its normative sample. Would it be fair to administer a test originally designed and standardized on a sample of people with college educations to an adult who finished only sixth grade? Different assessment measures require varying levels of education in order for the participant to understand the instructions and complete the test appropriately.

Level of education also plays a role when scoring various instruments. In many cases, particularly any measure of academic achievement, grade-related normative data are available. Although this can be difficult to interpret, it allows the psychologist to choose whether comparing a patient to same-aged or same-educated peers is more appropriate. Further, many of these measures, even if scored using age-related norms, also provide grade-equivalents. Such scores can provide an estimation of a patient's current level of academic skills acquisition (or educational equivalent).

Region

The region of the country in which a person lives can also be an important demographic variable affecting performance. Regional dialects can influence a person's word choice, articulation, and even awareness of certain formal English terms. Not only should the patient's current geographic region be considered, but a thorough history can reveal other significant parts of a patient's life spent in different geographic regions that could impact development. Although language development is generally considered most heavily impacted by the area where an individual has lived, geographic locale can also impact other psychosocial opportunities. Individuals spending critical periods of development in remote, rural, or economically disadvantaged areas may not have the same educational opportunities as others. Formal education may not be provided in the same manner or may not be valued culturally. For example, individuals living in agricultural communities may have an extensive repertoire of farming skills but limited exposure to the types of questions often found in formal intellectual testing. Further, with increases in immigration and international adoption, it is important to consider a person's country of origin when interpreting responses to standardized testing in the United States.

Gender

An individual's gender can also impact testing performance. In fact, significant differences are found so often in standardized performances that this factor is almost always analyzed when performing normative studies. If significant sex differences are found at that time, then different normative tables for males and females will be provided for scoring interpretation. Sex differences in performance on test measures occur due to complex interactions between neurologic and psychosocial factors. Additionally, the content of a test itself may be interpreted differently by men and women intentionally. For example, on the Minnesota Multiphasic Personality Inventory (MMPI), the "Masculinity-Femininity" scale is utilized to indicate how strongly an individual identifies with same- or opposite-sex interests. The same questions are administered to every user; therefore, quite obviously different scoring criteria must be used for men and women in order to reach appropriate interpretations.

DOMAINS OF ASSESSMENT

Each area for which psychological tests have been constructed can be broken down into sub-areas and sub-sub-areas, depending on what is being assessed. For instance, most personality inventories

TABLE 6-1	Examples of Psychological Tests for Various Functions

Intelligence
Wechsler Intelligence Scales (preschool, child, adult, abbreviated)
Kaufman Brief Intelligence Test – Second Edition
Leiter International Performance Scales – Revised

Personality
Minnesota Multiphasic Personality Inventory – Second Edition Restructured Form
Beck Depression Inventory – Second Edition
Rorschach Inkblot Test
Thematic Apperception Test
Sentence Completion Survey

Academic Achievement
Woodcock-Johnson Tests of Achievement – Third Edition
Wechsler Individual Tests of Achievement – Second Edition
Wide Range Achievement Test – Fourth Edition

Memory
Wechsler Memory Scale – Third Edition
Wide Range Assessment of Memory and Learning – Second Edition

Language
Clinical Evaluation of Language Fundamentals – Fourth Edition
Peabody Picture Vocabulary Test – Third Edition
Boston Naming Test

Visual and Motor
Beery Buktenika Test of Visual-Motor Integration – Fifth Edition
Grooved Pegboard Test

Attention and Executive Functions
Conners' Continuous Performance Test – Second Edition
Gordon Diagnostic System
Delis Kaplan Executive Function Scale
Tower of London
Wisconsin Card Sorting Test

contain scales measuring depression, and then there are specific questionnaires designed just for depression by itself, many of which in turn include scales for different aspects of depression, such as dysphoric mood and self-critical thinking. Similarly, there are hundreds of commonly used published tests, some names of which are provided as a few common examples (see Table 6-1). This section provides a broad overview with some examples of specific tests, rather than presuming to condense the field into a cookbook list.

Screening

Many tests are considered screening instruments, which, by their nature, have reasonably good sensitivity but limited specificity. Perhaps the best example in psychiatry is the MMSE, a brief, 30-item instrument often used to assess cognitive ability. Most physicians are familiar with this instrument, and, in fact, many have it memorized for administration at the bedside. Screening instruments play an important role in psychiatry because they quickly provide information about cognitive or emotional functioning and help guide diagnosis and treatment. Unfortunately, some practitioners equate normal screening test scores with normal cognitive functioning. Demographic variables, lesion location, and many other variables may affect the scores. Although these instruments provide useful clinical tools, most were not designed to accurately capture the nuances or range of human behavior that a comprehensive examination might uncover.

Therefore, caution and clinical judgment must come into play when considering what to do with screening results.

Neuropsychology

Neuropsychology represents a unique branch of psychology. Neuropsychologists combine their knowledge of neuroscience and psychology, utilize a variety of psychological instruments when conducting evaluations, and combine test results with clinical information to make informed statements regarding brain–behavior relationships. Despite common thinking, there is no such thing as a neuropsychological test. Rather, it is the interpretation of test results, taking brain–behavior relationships into context, which makes an evaluation neuropsychological. Because of this distinction, it is important to clarify that all neuropsychologists are trained as psychologists, but the inverse is not true. Not all psychologists can perform neuropsychological evaluations; specialized training, typically involving a postdoctoral fellowship, is essential.

Historically, tests used by neuropsychologists included those sensitive to brain dysfunction, or organicity. Perhaps the best example is the Bender Visual-Motor Gestalt Test, which involved a series of drawings sensitive to brain damage. This test is less commonly used now.

A typical neuropsychological assessment may include tests of attention and concentration, processing speed, memory, language production and comprehension, visual-spatial perception and construction, problem solving, abstract reasoning, motor functioning, multimodal sensory perceptual functioning, and emotion designed to adequately sample the patient's functioning so that statements may be made regarding the patient's current strengths and weaknesses from a neurobehavioral perspective.

The most common approach is for the neuropsychologist to choose tests based on the referral question, data obtained during the interview, and other contextual factors, commonly referred to as a *flexible approach* (e.g., Iowa-Benton approach; Boston process approach). Some neuropsychologists still practice a fixed battery approach (e.g., Halstead Reitan Neuropsychological Battery; Luria Nebraska Neuropsychological Battery), whereby all patients receive the same set of tests irrespective of the clinical question. Whatever method of testing is chosen, the results obtained often allow the neuropsychologist to make statements regarding lesion localization, differential diagnosis, or patient strengths and weaknesses. The information is often extended to help referring doctors and patients make decisions regarding vocation, academic functioning, driving, or independent living.

Personality

Personality assessment is a careful method of analyzing a person's emotional state and manner of interacting with the world. The methods a clinician utilizes to evaluate a patient's personality will vary based on the clinician's theoretic approach and training. Generally, an assessment of personality will lead to a formulation of a person's emotional state and coping mechanisms, as well as an interpretation of self-image and of others and reality testing. Often the terms *emotional* or *psychological* testing are used interchangeably with personality assessment among medical professionals. However, psychologists will make distinctions among these terms based on their theoretic orientation.

Objective personality measures include those that have been standardized. In other words, these measures have been designed to be administered the same way every time, and normative data have been collected on a population sample. Such measures are generally formatted as questionnaires that either the clinician administers or the patient completes independently. Results are obtained by scoring the way in which the patient responded to the questions, often using computerized software. Objective measures of personality often focus on identified symptoms of emotional disorders, following the guidelines set by the DSM-IV-TR.

One example of a widely used objective personality measure would be the MMPI, which has been revised several times and currently has an adolescent version (MMPI-A) and a recently updated adult version referred to as the *Second Edition, restructured form* (MMPI-2 RF). The MMPI-2 RF is a self-administered questionnaire in which patients answer 338 true or false statements about themselves. Scoring provides 50 scales of emotional functioning and behavioral tendencies, which the clinician can utilize in the overall interpretation of the patient's personality.

A CASE OF DEPRESSION AND SUBSTANCE ABUSE

A supervisor threatened to terminate a 44-year-old woman for performance issues if she did not get some help. A psychiatrist performed a comprehensive evaluation and tentatively diagnosed major depressive disorder and alcohol abuse. To obtain additional information regarding the woman's psychological and emotional functioning, the psychiatrist requested personality testing.

The woman completed the MMPI-2, the Beck Depression Inventory, Second Edition (BDI-II), and the Beck Anxiety Inventory (BAI) and answered all the questions in a reasonable amount of time. Her F-scale (infrequency) was mildly elevated, suggesting that she might be exaggerating her symptoms, perhaps as a cry for help. On the primary clinical scales, she had significant elevations on the 2 scale (depression) and 4 scale (psychopathic deviate), a constellation of scores common in individuals with significant frustration, anger, and hostility who are prone to significant substance abuse, job loss, and family discord. Supplementary scale analysis revealed elevations on the MacAndrew Alcoholism Scale, Revised, and the Addiction Potential Scale, further raising concern regarding substance abuse. Although her BAI scores were not elevated, scores on her BDI-II revealed moderate depression.

The referring psychiatrist incorporated the information from the psychologist in supporting initial impressions regarding depression and substance abuse. After further examination, the patient began psychiatric care and entered a 2-week alcohol rehabilitation program, with ongoing psychotherapeutic support following discharge.

Projective personality assessment measures are generally associated with more psychodynamic approaches to testing. Projective measures are ambiguous stimuli administered to individuals with the assumption that they will "project" their personality into their responses. Each person must use his or her own coping skills to manage the stress induced by the presentation of an indefinite stimuli, generally in the form of a picture or inkblot. As a result, an appropriately trained clinician can learn how to interpret these responses to decode a person's emotional state.

Though there are many projective measures of varying levels of formality, the measure most often referenced, likely due to its extensive attempts at standardization, is the Rorschach Inkblot Test. Many years ago, John Exner developed a method for scoring and interpreting a person's responses to indistinct inkblots. The method of using inkblots was first published in the book *Psychodiagnostik* in 1921 by Hermann Rorschach, a Zurich psychiatrist who developed the technique while working in Switzerland, where he met Hans Huber, who designed the inkblots still used currently. Exner's scoring system, which is currently in its Fifth Edition, is extremely complex, often taking years to learn and perfect, but has a significant amount of research to support its use.

Semistructured interviews or rating scales can also be used to assess emotional states. Often these are not scored against normative data in the same manner as other measures. Rather, scales such as the Schedule for Affective Disorders and Schizophrenia (SADS), or Kiddie-SADS for children and adolescents, are designed to be administered through interview with the patient and/or family or caregivers. Scoring involves endorsing items based on DSM-IV-TR criteria at thresholds to determine current and past pathology.

Intelligence

Intelligence has been defined in many ways since serious attempts to measure it using psychometric methods were started about a century ago. A recent conceptualization by the noted cognitive psychologist Sternberg and his colleagues (1998) is particularly apt. It describes intelligent behavior as a balance among analytic, creative, and practical abilities. These various abilities work in synchrony to allow a person to perform or behave in a successful manner within his or her culture.

Tests of intelligence in clinical usage yield summary scores called *intelligence quotients* (*IQs*). IQ scores are computed in reference to the general population at a given age, not to some standard or ideal. Half of people have average IQ, one quarter above average, and one quarter below average. The latter range of scores is of most importance clinically, and the easiest way to understand below average IQ is to break it into three parts.

IQ <70 represents the lowest 2% of the population in intelligence. This range is traditionally referred to as *mental deficiency* or *mental retardation*, although newer synonymous terms with less pejorative connotations are emerging, including intellectual disability or cognitive disability. There are various levels of severity within this range, usually referred to as *mild, moderate, severe*, and *profound*. Not everyone with an IQ below 70 carries an actual diagnosis of mental retardation, because there are important additional criteria for this diagnosis, most notably significantly impaired adaptive skills, such as daily living skills. Note that the lowest 2% of the population is a lot of people, 1 out of 50.

IQ from 70 to 80 is referred to as *borderline*, and represents the 2nd to 10th percentile of the population. The mythic movie figure Forrest Gump was portrayed in this range.

IQ from 80 to 90 is called *low average*. This range is particularly relevant clinically in certain contexts, such as evaluation for the emergence of dementia in a person with previously above average functioning or in challenging school settings.

IQ represents one of the strongest correlates or predictors of school achievement and serves as an important psychometric marker in evaluation for dementia, but there are important caveats to these usages.

First, an individual's IQ is generally stable if measured reliably and validly after preschool years, but there are well-known, relatively common conditions in which IQ often gradually declines in the absence of acquired neurologic insult or disease, including some learning disabilities and mental illnesses such as schizophrenia. Conversely, enriched educational experiences, as well as quality and quantity of exposure to reading or other activities that enhance vocabulary knowledge, can yield modest increases in scores on IQ-type tests.

Second, different IQ tests in the mainstream of psychometric usage do not have identical theoretic bases or content; therefore, scores from these different tests do not always correspond exactly. Also, an individual's performance on a more recent edition of the same test generally produces scores a few IQ points lower than the previous edition, because every few years renorming by test publishers from population changes reflects the gradual gain in mental skills in the general population from decade to decade in recent history—a happy fact, but one necessitating careful updates in test norms. Comparing the score from one IQ test to a different or earlier test requires careful recalibration, consideration of "apples and oranges," and/or a margin of error beyond the usual margin of change in scores expected on psychological tests given to an individual at different times.

Third, if there is a substantial difference between the intellectual subskills within a person's IQ profile, the interpretation of the summary or full scale IQ score is often an artificial averaging of different abilities and can be overshadowed by the pattern of strengths and weaknesses. For instance, a difference of 20 points or more between the verbal and perceptual (sometimes referred to as *visual-spatial*) portions of an IQ test only occurs in small percentages of the general population, varying slightly based on age, and the difference may mean more than the summary (or full scale) score for clinical interpretation. In addition, it usually is considered invalid to interpret at face value the summary or full scale scores from traditional IQ tests (e.g., the various Wechsler scales) given to people who are not native English speakers or who have certain kinds of impairments, notably hearing or receptive/expressive language. Alternative formats for testing reasoning skills that do not involve understanding or producing speech have been developed for these situations (e.g., the Leiter International Performance Scales).

Finally, the subtle to not-so-subtle fundamental differences between definitions of intelligence end up being reflected in scores. Should IQ be measured in a way that best predicts a person's achievement in school, accomplishments in occupations, or social success? In recent decades, for instance, Sternberg has fleshed out the definition of intelligence cited in the first paragraph of this section by developing and validating tests that divide intelligence into areas called *analytic intelligence* (which is most of what traditional IQ tests measure), *practical intelligence*, and *creative intelligence*, which represent a significantly broader array of cognitive and adaptive abilities than the predominance of verbal and performance IQ (perceptual/nonverbal/spatial) in the Wechsler scales of intelligence most commonly used by clinical psychologists (Sternberg et al., 1998).

None of these caveats represents a fatal or prohibitive critique of IQ scores, which are among the most well-researched, reliable, and valid of psychological test instruments. The caveats merely guard against an overly simplistic interpretation of intelligence test results and remind physicians that this type of testing should routinely be administered and interpreted by licensed psychologists.

Rather than methodically list names and descriptions of the different sections or subtests from an example of a mainstream IQ test in clinical use, we suggest that the best learning experience can be finding an opportunity to observe a psychologist actually giving an intelligence test to a patient. The types of tasks typically incorporated into intelligence tests, such as defining increasingly difficult vocabulary words or assembling block patterns to mimic a diagram in a booklet, cannot be described in words with the same salience as actually watching the test administration. It can be beneficial to get a "bird's eye view" of other important aspects of psychometric testing, such as the psychologist's technique for not giving away whether the patient has responded correctly or incorrectly to a given item, the carefully chosen role of time limits in some but definitely not all subtests, and the common approach in individually administered tests (as opposed to most of the tests taken in group or classroom formats) of gradually increasing the difficulty of items across a subtest and then stopping when a carefully defined *ceiling* of a specified number of items failed is reached, to avoid undue time or frustration for the subject.

Achievement

Achievement generally refers to acquired skills taught in school. The most notable and commonly measured areas of achievement at elementary school age are various aspects of reading, math, and written language, although the federal definition of learning disabilities also includes aspects of oral language as areas of achievement; the eight areas are oral expression, listening comprehension, written expression, basic reading skill, reading fluency skill, reading comprehension, mathematics calculation, and mathematics problem-solving.

In secondary and postsecondary school, additional academic areas such as social studies, science, and critical thinking rise in importance within the broad definition of achievement. Some overlap exists between what is measured by intelligence and achievement tests, particularly general verbal skills such as vocabulary. The idea that intelligence, as measured by IQ tests, essentially determines or constrains achievement is a myth, even though the two are highly correlated. A significant minority of the general population develops either stronger or weaker academic skills than their intelligence would predict, traditionally referred to as *overachievement* and *learning disabilities*, respectively. It is also well established that some academic skills are more closely determined by other modules of cognitive functioning, most importantly reading by phonologic processing skills.

Most achievement test publishers present several types of scores, which can be confusing if the type of score referenced is unknown. Standard scores are the IQ-type scales explained in the previous section. Also commonly used are percentiles, stanines, and benchmarks set by organizations such as state public school departments. Grade- or age-equivalent scores from achievement tests, although intuitively appealing because they lend the impression of measuring how many years ahead or behind a person is, are notoriously unstable psychometrically and should generally be avoided in interpreting achievement tests.

As an aside, various college entrance exams have been designed to reflect more or less a balance of intelligence versus achievement, but all of them can be fairly characterized as a mixture of both. The numeric scores on such tests, of course, differ from the scales used in the clinical testing outlined above. These types of issues lead to the same advice to physicians mentioned earlier in the intelligence section, which is to seek the interpretation of a psychologist in understanding achievement scores.

Effort or Malingering

Psychologists are increasingly called upon to assist in determining symptom exaggeration. Gone are the days when it was assumed that all patients put forth consistently strong effort. Patients have many reasons to exaggerate their symptoms. In many cases, it may simply be a cry for help. Some may exaggerate their symptoms to be certain that their treating providers are aware of the degree of their distress. Sometimes secondary gain may be at stake. Personality inventories such as the MMPI-2 RF and the Personality Assessment Inventory (PAI) include multiple scales to determine whether a person is exaggerating. They also include scales examining whether a person is minimizing symptoms. Psychologists may use performance on these validity scales,

A CASE OF AMNESTIC MILD COGNITIVE IMPAIRMENT

A 77-year-old woman complained to her doctor about getting more forgetful over the last 2 years. Her doctor suggested that her memory concerns were due to anxiety, in part because her MMSE was 27/30. At her family's insistence, however, she was referred for a neuropsychological evaluation.

She presented as a pleasant woman who claimed forgetfulness and repetitiveness, which was supported by her daughter who accompanied her to the appointment. She denied feeling anxious or depressed. She completed cognitive and emotional tests, and the results were interpreted in the context of her age and education.

Although she demonstrated average or better speech production and language comprehension, spatial perception and construction, problem solving, processing speed and basic attention, performance on multiple memory measures suggested a profound memory deficit. For example, on the California Verbal Learning Test, Second Edition, a test of her ability to learn and retain a list of 16 words, she showed no evidence of learning, despite good attention to the list. After a brief distraction, she was unable to recall or recognize any of the words she had been asked just moments earlier. Similar patterns of impairment were observed on other memory tests. Emotional testing was not at all consistent with generalized or situational anxiety.

The presumptive diagnosis was amnestic mild cognitive impairment, and she was started on a cognitive enhancing medication.

in combination with relevant clinical information and history, to inform the interpretation of clinical scales regarding malingering or symptom exaggeration.

Along the same lines, the literature examining cognitive symptom exaggeration is expanding rapidly. Particularly in medicolegal settings, psychologists are asked to perform evaluations to document the presence and degree of cognitive impairment resulting from acquired injuries. Unfortunately, the individuals being seen for these evaluations have significant motivation for looking impaired and may, intentionally or not, perform suboptimally on cognitive tests. Although malingering of cognitive symptoms in a medicolegal context seems to be the setting where effort is most often at issue, there may be many other reasons for poor effort on cognitive tests, including emotional factors and fatigue. Because of the frequency of suboptimal effort, psychologists have developed cognitive tests that are sensitive to whether patients are trying their best.

When cognitive or emotional symptom exaggeration is evident, interpreting the results is quite difficult for the psychologist because it is nearly impossible to determine what represents true impairment and poor effort. The clinician must rely on clinical judgment and context in addition to test scores.

Competency

Questions of competency often come to the attention of psychologists and will briefly be considered here. For example, psychologists are asked to provide their opinions regarding a person's ability to manage finances, make medical decisions, stand trial, or parent adequately. The answers to these difficult questions must take into consideration not only an intimate knowledge of human behavior and how it affects these competencies but also a working knowledge of the law behind these issues. Although many instruments have been developed to help practitioners, it is important to note that how one scores on a test or series of tests does not render one competent or incompetent for a particular matter. The clinician must incorporate the information gathered from any tests with information from the interview and other background material in making recommendations to the court, which is ultimately responsible for deeming someone competent or incompetent.

HOW TO FORMULATE A REFERRAL OR ORDER A TESTING CONSULT

Referrals for psychological and neuropsychological evaluation occur in all settings and with all types of patients, but learning when and how to ask for such a referral can be challenging.

Unlike some medical procedures, which are circumscribed and completed the same way every time regardless of the referral source or identified patient, psychological and neuropsychological evaluations vary from patient to patient and question to question. Therefore, conscientious articulation of the referral question is vital.

Here are some examples of well-formed referral questions for psychological evaluation:

- Is Carrie showing sufficient delay in any important developmental areas to recommend treatment at this time? What kind of treatment?
- Please conduct a comprehensive baseline (i.e., repeatable battery that can help monitor change over time) neuropsychological evaluation in reference to Charley's seizure disorder. Are there any cognitive, behavioral, or emotional problems at present for which treatment would be advised, and what kind of treatment?
- Is Sally showing any cognitive or behavioral difficulties associated with her traumatic brain injury? If so, what interventions would be recommended at or outside of school?
- Does George have a learning disability that needs to be taken into account in treating his school avoidance?

When requesting an emotional or cognitive evaluation, it is important to articulate the referral question clearly, providing enough background for the testing clinician to understand what he or she is to uncover. Indicating a few key points on the referral can help the psychologist understand how to be most helpful to the referring clinician and the patient. When formulating the referral, it is often helpful to remember how the test results are intended to inform the treatment plan for the patient. Most referrals will include the following:

- The patient's chief complaint, in the patient's terms as well as the clinician's
- The frequency and severity of the problem
- Any pertinent past psychiatric or medical history (such as if the patient has received any prior or particularly recent cognitive evaluations, indicators of premorbid functioning, or background on medical issues that may be related to cognitive changes)
- The key question the clinician would like addressed

Asking a referral question can be like playing darts. If a broad target is provided by too vague a referral question, the dart may end up landing far from the spot anticipated to be the bull's eye. However, if only the bull's eye is provided, without any accompanying board around it, the dart may end up hitting something else. If there is uncertainty how to provide the information needed for a referral question, contact the psychologist directly to discuss the case. The psychologist will know what questions to ask to find out what the clinician wants to know. At times, a brief consultation with the referring clinician and/or the family may be all that the psychologist requires, possibly to understand test results provided from another source or to determine if additional testing will add to the formulation and treatment plan.

TESTING ENVIRONMENTS

Psychological testing may be performed either with inpatients or outpatients. Outpatient assessment generally affords the luxury of a quieter environment and patients who are not as sick, though it is sometimes necessary to evaluate patients when they are hospitalized. For example, when questions about imminent medical decision-making ability arise, psychologists may be asked to see someone emergently. Psychologists may also be asked to evaluate cognitive status or emotional functioning so that appropriate treatments may be enacted.

The challenges of testing inpatients are many, however. Patients often feel uncomfortable or may be in pain. They may have spent the better part of the day being poked, prodded, and examined by clinicians of every known subspecialty. They may not be sleeping because nurses wake them up every 3 hours to draw blood. They may feel self-conscious about their lack of dress and have tubes coming in and out of them. Further, there may be a loud roommate and aides or staff interrupting the examination. Attempting to retain a long series of digits is difficult enough in a quiet environment but even more challenging with all of these potential distracters. When possible, outpatient evaluation is preferred, but when inpatient testing is required (even administering the MMSE), it is important to think about the degree to which these factors may interfere.

A CASE OF TRAUMATIC BRAIN INJURY

Sally, a 5-year-old girl, was in a car crash 6 months ago and spent a week in a coma. Although she made a remarkable recovery from her injury and was discharged from rehabilitation therapies 2 months later, her kindergarten teacher now raises several concerns: Sally was previously reported to be energetic but well behaved; now she occasionally gets into conflicts with peers, at times impulsively hitting and then feeling anxiously remorseful. She knew her alphabet during preschool but now inconsistently reads letters. Her attention wanders during story time and longer academic work sessions.

Her pediatrician requested neuropsychological evaluation, which showed a contrast between average verbal reasoning skills and low average perceptual reasoning on the Wechsler Preschool and Primary Intelligence Scale, Third Edition, as well as slow mental processing speed and unexpectedly high errors on several tests sensitive to attention, including the Gordon Diagnostic System.

The neuropsychologist suggested that Sally was still recovering from her injury and recommended updated assessment by speech/language, occupational, and physical therapists at school. An Individualized Education Program for students with traumatic brain injury was started, including spending only mornings at school (to be reevaluated every 2 months, with the plan of expanding again to the whole school day), classroom placement to optimize attention, careful behavioral programming to reinforce impulse control and organization, and daily occupational therapy to strengthen visual-spatial skills.

FEEDBACK

Once the testing has been completed and interpreted, it is essential that the information gleaned from the testing be provided to the relevant parties. Providing feedback is an interactive process in which all concerned parties discuss the findings, their meanings, and the limitations of the results (Pope, 1992). The format and content of the communication of test findings vary, depending on the referral source, the questions being addressed, and the person(s) to whom the results are being presented. In addition to verbal feedback for the patient and/or family, psychologists typically communicate test results to the physician through a testing report. The testing report involves analysis, synthesis, and integration of the material gathered during the testing (Tallent, 1993) and typically includes identifying information, reason for referral, pertinent background information, behavioral observations, test findings, summary, and recommendations.

Clinical Pearls

- Screening results (e.g., MMSE) are not equivalent to comprehensive psychological evaluation and should be considered with caution and clinical judgment.
- Context is important; consider the variables relevant to the psychological assessment, including patient demographics, testing variables, and the type of testing employed.
- To have specific questions answered, ask specific questions.
- Establish trusting relationships with testing psychologists to be confident in their evaluations.
- If something about the evaluation is unclear or if it did not completely answer the questions, ask the psychologist for clarification.
- All neuropsychologists are trained psychologists; however, not all psychologists are trained to administer and interpret assessment measures as neuropsychologists.
- The terms *emotional* and *psychological* are often used interchangeably when requesting personality assessment, which can lead to confusion. Make the referral question specific.
- If a testing professional reports that a patient is below average, double check if this simply means the patient's score is below the mean. For each person on the upper half of the normal curve, there is one on the bottom half.

Self-Assessment Questions and Answers

6-1. A 12-year-old girl presents with various physical complaints for which she has been requesting to stay home from school. Following an appropriate medical evaluation, the girl appears to be medically healthy, and the physician suspects emotional issues may be playing a role in the child's behaviors. Her parents have recently separated, and there is significant stress within the household. The physician decides to refer the girl for a psychological evaluation. When writing out the referral questions, the physician indicates a desire to better understand the girl's emotional functioning and requests what form of assessment?

A. Structured personality measures and objective emotional measures

B. Structured personality measures and projective emotional measures

C. Objective and projective emotional measures

D. Structured personality measures and objective and projective emotional measures

Children can exhibit both internalizing and externalizing symptoms during emotional difficulties. Internalizing symptoms are best revealed by the child using either objective or projective measures, and externalizing symptoms by parents or teachers using structured rating scales. Therefore, it is important to request a broad assessment approach (Sattler, 2002). *Answer: D*

6-2. A 63-year-old attorney who has seen the same physician for many years recently started making uncharacteristic errors in her work, and her husband reports that her previously meticulous painting when redecorating rooms in their house has become slightly sloppy. Neither the physician nor people in her daily life detect any change in her warm, jovial personality, and she brushes off the concerns as evidence of aging. The physician requests intellectual and memory testing, which comes back normal. Which is the best next step?

A. Consider dementia or mild cognitive impairment, double-checking DSM-IV-TR clinical criteria.

B. Diagnose dementia because premorbid functioning would presumably have been above average.

C. Reassure her husband to stop worrying.

D. Refer her for further testing to rule out depression.

When psychological test results do not fit a straightforward clinical profile or contain contradictions, neither jump to a conclusion nor assume more testing is needed. All psychological assessment has meaning only within thorough clinical evaluation. *Answer: A*

6-3. A 9-year-old boy is starting to show frustration and wandering attention during reading and writing activities at school, in contrast with his conscientious approach during other subjects and earlier grades. Everyone is surprised when he obtains a score in the deficient range on the standardized reading test given to all third graders by the state department of education. His parents are dismayed that school staff are recommending an evaluation for possible special education services, because they feel he is very smart. What do you advise?

A. Complete the evaluation; they do not have to agree to special education and an independent psychologist could conduct a further review if needed.

B. Enroll him at a different school with a better reading instruction program.

C. Try stimulant medication to improve his attention.

D. Watch his progress over the next couple of years, because the group-administered test at school may not have been accurate due to his inattention.

Federal and state laws require that public school districts provide comprehensive evaluations for students with suspected learning disabilities (whether the student attends the public school or not), using methods that will provide a thorough picture (including sound testing). The timing and settings of the attention problems in this case make a diagnosis of attention-deficit/hyperactivity disorder (ADHD) less likely than a learning disability, for which testing of academic skills and other mental processing skills is relevant (Newby, 2006). *Answer: A*

6-4. When requesting emotional or personality assessment, which of the choices given provides objective measures of a wide variety of emotional states?

A. Beck Depression Inventory—Second Edition

B. Children's Depression Inventory

C. Minnesota Multiphasic Personality Inventory—Second Edition, Restructured Form

D. Rorschach Inkblot Test

Objective measures of personality focus on identified symptoms of emotional disorders, following DSM-IV-TR guidelines. The Minnesota Multiphasic Personality Inventory, Second Edition, Restructured Form, is a self-administered questionnaire on which patients endorse 338 true or false statements about themselves. Scoring provides 50 scales of emotional and behavioral tendencies, which the clinician can utilize in the overall interpretation of the patient's personality. *Answer: C*

6-5. True or False: A patient has passed the Mini Mental Status Examination (MMSE) without difficulty; therefore, a more formal assessment of memory is not required.

A. True

B. False

Patients with significant deficits in the memory systems can still appear functionally "normal" on simple screening measures. *Answer: B*

References

American Psychiatric Association. *Diagnostic and statistical manual*, 4th ed., *text revision*. Washington, DC: American Psychiatric Association; 2000.

Benton, AL. Basic approaches to neuropsychological assessment. In: Steinhauer SR, Gruzelier JH, Zubin J, eds. *Handbook of schizophrenia*, Vol. 5. Amsterdam: Elsevier Science; 1991:505–523.

Folstein MF, Folstein SE, McHugh PR. Mini-mental state. A practical method for grading the cognitive state of patients for the clinician. *J Psychiatr Res*. 1975;12(3):189–198.

Newby RF. *Your struggling child: A guide to diagnosing, understanding, and advocating for your child with learning, behavior, or emotional problems*. HarperCollins Publishers; 2006.

Pope KS. *Responsibilities in providing psychological test feedback to clients. Psychol Assess*. 1992;4: 268–271.

Sattler JM. *Assessment of children: Behavioral and clinical applications*, 4th ed. San Diego, CA: Jerome M. Sattler, 2002.

Sternberg RJ, Kaufman JC. Human abilities. *Annu Rev Psychol*. 1998;49:479–502.

Tallent N. *Psychological report writing*, 4th ed. Englewood Cliffs: Prentice Hall; 1993.

Mental Disorders

SECTION

II

Mental Disorders

CHAPTER 7

Arden D. Dingle

Disorders Usually First Diagnosed in Infancy, Childhood, or Adolescence

Many children and adolescents have diagnosable psychiatric disorders, with even more having symptoms but not meeting the criteria threshold for a disorder. There is increasing recognition of these disorders, their associated morbidity and mortality, the need for intervention, and the benefits of treatments. Psychosocial and environmental interventions continue to be primary therapies, but as the biological foundations of psychiatric disorders become clearer, other treatments, such as psychopharmacology, are becoming essential aspects of care. This chapter addresses the identification, evaluation, and treatment of psychiatric disorders as they occur in youth and common problems or situations that affect children and adolescents.

GENERAL CLINICAL ISSUES

Development

Development describes the emergence and procession of an individual's physical and mental abilities that result from interactions between the individual's intrinsic capabilities and the environment. Culture, socioeconomic factors, or other environmental issues may influence the manifestations of developmental stages/tasks. Many theories and descriptions of development are based on observations and research on individuals or groups in the westernized world, often middle class, and tend to assume the highest level of achievement. However, they still can provide useful guidelines when evaluating children and adolescents. Youth may progress differently developmentally, but the expected norms for activities and behavior for a given age can indicate whether a specific child or adolescent is within the range of what is considered typical.

The symptoms of many psychiatric disorders in youth are characteristic of normal children at earlier developmental stages or appear occasionally in many normal children. Aspects of development may be off track in psychiatrically or medically ill children and adolescents either due to the disorder or its influence. Understanding typical development is essential for the assessment and treatment of psychiatric disorders in children and adolescents (see Tables 7-1 and 7-2) (Gemelli, 1996; Davies, 2004).

Risk/Resilience

Many children and adolescents are at increased risk to develop psychiatric disorders from biological causes with significant or permanent effects such as genetic or chromosomal abnormalities or diseases, insults, or substances affecting the central nervous system (CNS). There is growing evidence that early attachment between infants and caretakers has significant implications for later development and behavior, both normal and problematic. Additional risk factors for psychopathology include trauma, stress, and unsupportive or aversive environments.

Resilience is a dynamic process in which an individual is able to adapt in the context of significant adversity. Certain youth clearly have characteristics or strengths that make it less likely for them to develop psychiatric disorders, even when dealing with extremely problematic events or circumstances. It has been proposed that resilient children and adolescents are characterized by biological and psychological flexibility. Protective factors include easygoing temperament, secure attachment with a caretaker, good parenting, higher intelligence, and supportive relationships.

TABLE 7-1	Developmental Tasks	
Age	**Overall Tasks**	**Functions of Environment**
0–12 mo	Develop and maintain attachments Gradually gain control over motor skills Develop an ability to regulate arousal and affect	Provide information about infant's body and surrounding world Provide stimulus modulation and protection Provide encouragement, support, and admiration
1–3 yr	Balance attachment, exploration, and autonomy Internalize parental values and standards Develop ability to symbolize mentally	Protect child so that the child is not too distressed from stimulation Teach child to gratify innate needs while following limits and rules Support autonomy while teaching that there are limits
3–6 yr	Develop play as vehicle for exploring reality Transition from egocentric/magical thinking to more logical and reality-based view	Provide greater access to world with adequate structure/supervision Model/support skills promoting self-regulation and self-sufficiency Reinforce logic, reality-based thinking, language, play acquisition
6–12 yr	Develop/utilize a calm, stable capability to learn Develop self-control, real-world skills, competence Establish self in world of peers	Provide secure base for more time/involvement in outside world Model and reinforce learning self-control/skills Support mastery of various academic, social, and emotional skills
13–19 yr	Establish and consolidate identity Transition to adulthood Establish realistic goals and prepare for future Establish strong peer relationships Explore intimate and romantic relationships	Provide secure base for exploration of self and role in world Model/reinforce skills of independence and self-sufficiency Support involvement with peer group, transition to adulthood Provide consistent limits and standards Accept/respect differences; tolerate youth's devaluing/criticizing

Recent research has found that certain gene constellations may confer resiliency (Kim-Cohen, 2007).

Continuity between Childhood and Adulthood Psychiatric Disorders

Children and adolescents with significant psychiatric illness are at increased risk for psychopathology as adults. However, it has been difficult to show the connection between disorders in childhood and those in adulthood because of limited information demonstrating any continuity. Both data from and analysis of recent longitudinal studies have provided increased evidence of the connections and different ideas about how to consider these issues. One approach is to examine homotypic continuities: disorders occurring in children and adults in whom the core abnormalities are similar but the presentations may vary developmentally (e.g., phobias, reading disorders, mental retardation [MR], severe autism spectrum disorders, and adolescent-onset depression). Another perspective is to examine heterotypic continuity: individuals who are impaired both as children and adults but have different problems. Individuals who develop schizophreniform disorders as adults demonstrate consistent and persistent abnormalities in childhood, such as impaired attention, early motor development delays, receptive language problems, and cognitive

TABLE 7-2 Characteristics of Developmental Periods

Age	Motor/Physical	Social	Communication	Emotional	Cognitive
0–1 yr Infancy	Rapid growth More self-initiated movements	Orientation to people Relationships with caretakers	Different sounds/cries Convey states of being Can respond to sounds	Initial self-regulation Connect to caretakers	Learning difference between new and familiar stimuli
1–3 yr Toddler	Slower growth More self-initiation Better control	Preferred relationships Reciprocal behaviors	Reciprocal Greater variety of sounds	Better self-regulation Reciprocal caretaker interactions	Exploration Observe and imitate Make goals and plans
3–6 yr Preschool	More skeletal growth Independent, controlled behaviors Better coordination and strength More adept	Develop social skills More peer interactions Verbal approaches to social interactions More adult modeling Interest in rules	Larger, increasing vocabulary Speech clear and understandable Uses language to direct behavior	Voice out needs better Separations easier Attach to noncaretakers Initial self-esteem/identity	Distinguish reality Better memory Interest in causality Classify Egocentric, magical thinking
7–12 yr School age	Consolidation and mastery of skills Improved coordination Slowest period of skeletal growth CNS maturation	More social awareness Group, peer interest Competition Realize adult fallibility Recognition of privacy Collecting/categorizing	Increasing language skills and ability to communicate verbally	Uses autonomous coping skills Attachment rituals persist Attachment to peers	Thinking more systematically, logically, realistically Greater intellectual capacity
13–19 yr Adolescence	Rapid, significant biological changes More physical activity Decreased metabolic rate (boys < girls) More physical strength (boys > girls) CNS synaptic pruning	Shift in role status More autonomy Authority conflicts Alliance shift to peers More consolidated sexual orientation Explore romantic/sexual relationships Most share parental values	Increasing use of language to interact with others, deal with emotions, stress More complicated use of language, more articulate More able to discuss abstract topics	Exploration/consolidation of personal and group identity	Increasing capability for abstract thought

CNS, central nervous system.

difficulties. Childhood anxiety disorders appear to be a significant risk factor for adult depression. Questions still to be resolved include describing the underlying mechanisms, understanding the effect of environmental or other factors, and explaining why only some individuals who have problems in childhood are affected as adults and why children with similar problems have various adult outcomes (Rutter et al., 2006).

PSYCHIATRIC EVALUATION

Diagnosis

Most child and adolescent psychiatric researchers and practitioners utilize the *Diagnostic and Statistical Manual of Mental Disorders*, Fourth Edition, Text Revision (DSM-IV-TR) (American Psychiatric Association, 2000), diagnostic criteria despite concerns that the criteria for most of the disorders are not developmentally sensitive. Other diagnostic classifications exist for specific populations or disorders but are not used systematically. DSM-IV-TR details the disorders that most commonly present in childhood and adolescence, though children and adolescents may also be diagnosed with disorders in other categories. Developmental characteristics may influence symptom presentations at various ages; children and adolescents may be diagnosed with any psychiatric disorder for which they meet criteria. They may also have significant symptoms but not meet criteria for any specific disorder. Chapter 27 details the special considerations during the assessment process for children and adolescents.

TREATMENT

Treatment Planning

Treatment should be based on a comprehensive understanding of the child, family, and environment so that a multidimensional plan can be developed. Besides focusing on the significant problems and issues, treatment planning should include personal and environmental strengths, protective factors, and any other characteristics that would promote resilience. General and specific goals should be chosen with realistic and attainable outcomes and range from relief of suffering to acquisition of "normality" to restoration of or increased functioning. Chapter 27 offers further information specific to children and adolescents during treatment planning.

Children and adolescents are usually best served by a combination of treatment modalities. An essential aspect is obtaining parental understanding and consent, as well as patient understanding and assent. It is important to provide information about the probable course of the disorder if untreated and to describe available treatments with estimates of the potential benefits and risks. The child or adolescent patient should be included in this discussion, as appropriate. With a few exceptions, all the treatments used for adults may be used for children and adolescents, with modifications for the patient's developmental status. In most cases, coordination with the parents, school, pediatrician, child welfare agency, courts, and/or recreation leader will be part of the treatment plan. It is vital to periodically discuss progress or its lack, possible alternatives, and pros and cons of various options. Good treatment plans have flexibility so that changes in functioning or environment can be incorporated and interventions modified if no longer necessary or not adequate (Dingle and Lee, 2005).

Psychiatric Interventions

Psychotherapies

Most psychiatrically ill children requiring treatment can benefit from psychotherapy. A number of psychotherapies are utilized with children, adolescents, and families; many have been developed from adult models (see Chapters 21 and 23). They vary in their theoretical approach with some differences in the identified patient and format. However, all are based on the premise that relationships between patients and therapists can provide the support and context for changes in behaviors, attitudes, and beliefs. The focus is on some aspect of how patients feel, think, or act. These factors are evaluated and addressed in the context of the youth's developmental level and environment. Psychodynamic, supportive, and cognitive therapies are most commonly utilized in individual treatment where most of the intervention is with the child or adolescent, though the caretaker has some consistent involvement. However, all of these theoretical orientations can be utilized in group and family therapies or parent training. Most behavior management is directed toward the caretakers and other involved adults (parent training), though the child participates more with increasing age. Regardless of the therapeutic approach, behavioral interventions are incorporated into most treatments. Play is often a component of therapy, either as a strategy to help the child talk or as a nonverbal expression of internal issues. Several psychotherapies have been modified to be brief interventions with evidence of effectiveness. Meta-analysis of studies (a range of therapies, problems, populations) has demonstrated that psychotherapy is helpful.

Multimodal Interventions

Multiple intervention strategies, which utilize aggressive case management, comprehensive psychiatric services, and targeted family interventions, have been demonstrated to have positive outcomes with youths who have conduct or substance use disorders or are in psychiatric crisis. Multisystemic therapy (MST) focuses on the systems that influence adolescents and their families and attempts to alter these systems in concrete ways that improve current behavior and risk factors. Combined medication and intensive psychosocial behavioral interventions have demonstrated benefits for attention-deficit/hyperactivity disorder (ADHD), particularly for associated problems with mood, anxiety, behavior, social skills, and academic performance. School-based programs with interventions designed for children, teachers, and parents have been shown to be helpful. Additional interventions can include identifying problems such as parental psychiatric illness or substance abuse, lack of basic resources such as housing, or need for additional services at school and utilizing appropriate resources for these issues.

Psychopharmacotherapy

Psychopharmacotherapy is effective in the treatment of children and adolescents especially when used as part of a planned, organized, multimodal treatment approach. When using psychopharmacological agents with children and adolescents, important general principles include minimizing the use of multiple medications and rarely using medication as the only form of treatment. Medications target specific symptoms and seldom eradicate problematic feelings, thoughts, and actions. Children, adolescents, and their families usually require additional interventions to help alleviate and prevent persistent symptoms and associated difficulties. Studies have demonstrated that integrated therapies are effective for youth with various problems.

It is important to educate the family regarding the medication and to actively evaluate the benefits, risks, limitations, and side effects. There is a need to balance the potential risks of the medication with the prognosis of the untreated disorder and what is known about the relative efficacy of medication. Most psychopharmacological agents and indications lack pediatric labeling and are unapproved ("off label") for children as a consequence of the paucity of adequate research in child and adolescent psychopharmacology. Lack of approval for an age-group or a disorder does not imply improper or illegal use, but clinicians should inform families of this fact and discuss the relevant research and clinical data. Additionally, it is important to remember that although medications tend to be associated with certain disorders, it is most effective to choose medications based on specific, targeted symptoms. Understanding target symptoms in the context of a diagnosis is important because individual target symptoms (e.g., hyperactivity) can represent multiple conditions, such as ADHD, bipolar disorder, or psychosis, for which medication approaches differ significantly. Clearly defined target symptoms help parents focus on pertinent behaviors that will be important for assessing medication effectiveness and help the clinician track and document changes during treatment. Familiarity with the pharmacokinetic and pharmacodynamic properties of various medications is helpful. Knowledge of side effect profiles is essential to maximize safety, minimize nonadherence, assess clinical response, and determine titration strategies (Dulcan, 2007). See Chapter 22 for more information.

Before initiating pharmacotherapy, the physician should perform a baseline assessment so that there can be subsequent comparison. Target symptoms can be characterized by repertoire, intensity, frequency, duration, and associated factors. If appropriate, laboratory tests should be obtained both to identify contraindications for medication and to establish baseline values of parameters that may be affected by medication. Titration, monitoring, and medication maintenance are also important. Starting with a low initial medication dose can be advantageous to minimize side effects and potentially maximize adherence. Children and adolescents may be more sensitive to the adverse effects of medication. It is important to appreciate that effective doses are very individualized. Just as psychiatric assessment should be continued during maintenance treatment, so should appropriate laboratory testing. When more than one condition or spectrum of symptoms exists, multiple medications may be required. It is important to have clearly defined target symptoms and goals and to prioritize which condition needs to be stabilized first. When multiple medications are prescribed, adjustment of one medication at a time can minimize confusion should an adverse reaction arise. The clinician also needs to know potential medication–medication interactions. Medications with equivocal or no responses should be discontinued (Lee and Cummins, 2005).

Other Therapies

Other interventions have been tried for mentally ill youth (Chapter 24). Alternative and complementary medicine (e.g., herbs, vitamins, massage, acupuncture, aromatherapy, and homeopathy) increasingly have become options sought by patients and their families for medical and psychiatric disorders, despite limited information on their use and effectiveness in children and adolescents. Dietary strategies (primarily exclusion of particular foods and substances) have been promoted as effective interventions for psychiatric disorders without significant empirical support. The diets are difficult to maintain and resisted by children and adolescents.

Electroconvulsive therapy (ECT) can be a treatment modality for some adolescents who generally have to meet the same criteria as adults. There is insufficient information and clinical experience on the use of ECT in school-aged or younger children; the data on adolescents indicate that ECT can be an effective, well-tolerated treatment intervention, though use in adolescents is uncommon because ECT tends to be a treatment of last resort. There are a few studies but no controlled ones. Some countries and states have various laws limiting the use of ECT in children and adolescents or requirements for independent second opinions.

Milieu Treatments

Children and adolescents can benefit from treatment interventions such as inpatient, partial hospitalization, day treatment, and intensive care programs. These generally are utilized when children and adolescents would benefit from more intensive care, usually on an acute basis. For those requiring more intensive care chronically, a variety of programs with a range of services provide care that either maintain youth at home with families or place them in out-of-home residential facilities.

Community Services

Comprehensive treatment plans should include maximum use of existing community resources as appropriate. For many children and adolescents, providing structured and supervised activities during non–school time can be very beneficial. After-school and weekend programs can include tutoring, general activities, or sports offered by schools, churches, and community agencies. Group or individual mentoring and activity programs can be valuable. Summer camp, school, or work programs can provide similar benefits. In many areas, similar programs are designed with therapeutic components for children and adolescents who cannot manage in regular programs.

DISORDERS USUALLY FIRST DIAGNOSED IN INFANCY, CHILDHOOD, OR ADOLESCENCE

Developmental Disorders

Developmental disorders are a heterogeneous group of conditions with physical, cognitive, psychological, sensory, or speech impairments that range in severity. These disorders may be global, affecting multiple domains of function, or specific, with only one or two areas affected. They are associated with social, educational, cognitive, and psychiatric difficulties. The prevalence ranges from approximately 1.5% for severe developmental disorders to approximately 17% for the entire spectrum of developmental delay seen in childhood. Physicians commonly see patients with MR and pervasive developmental disorders (PDDs), which affect individuals' global functioning, and specific developmental disorders such as learning disabilities in which the deficits are selective.

Although MR and PDD are distinct disorders, they share common characteristics in diagnostic criteria, assessment, and treatment.

Epidemiology

MR is one of the most common developmental disorders, with an estimated prevalence of 2.5% in school-aged children, with more males than females. Incidence of MR related to biologic causes is equal across socioeconomic groups; the milder forms of nonbiological MR occur more often in lower socioeconomic classes. Severe forms tend to be diagnosed earlier, with the milder types often identified once children start school (King et al., 1997; State et al., 1997).

Recently, the prevalence of autism and other PDDs has increased significantly. Studies have reported that from 1 to almost 7 children per 1,000 are autistic. The reasons for this increase are not clear; the best explanation appears to be changes in methodical factors: broadening the diagnosis, improved screening/diagnosis, and identification at earlier ages. Some believe that toxin exposure is responsible, but no toxins have been identified. Rett syndrome occurs in 1 of 10,000 to 15,000 female births and childhood disintegrative disorder in approximately 1.7 in 100,000 births (Wazana et al., 2007).

Etiology

The extent of the influence of genetics versus environment in causing MR, particularly for the less severe forms, is still debated. There is agreement that intelligence level is highly heritable, though environmental factors appear to be significant. Inadequate environmental stimulation during early childhood appears to be an issue for some individuals with mild MR. More severe MR is more likely to be biologically caused. The etiology is unclear in approximately 30% to 40% of cases. Some syndromes (e.g., Down, fragile X, fetal alcohol) account for about 30% of cases. Causes of MR include genetic or chromosomal abnormalities, infections, abnormal brain architecture, inborn errors of metabolism, toxins, delivery complications, physiological problems (e.g., maternal-fetal blood group incompatibilities), trauma, endocrine abnormalities, and psychosocial factors (e.g. malnutrition, deprivation). These factors can also be classified depending on whether they occur prenatally, perinatally, or postnatally.

PDDs share some common characteristics, though they probably have a number of different etiologies. PDD can be associated with various medical conditions, including tuberous sclerosis, fragile X syndrome, Down syndrome, cerebral palsy, untreated phenylketonuria, and Williams syndrome. Although the exact etiology is not clear, there appears to be a significant genetic risk with increased rates in families with autism and a high concordance rate between monozygotic twins. A multigene diathesis appears most likely. An abnormal gene has been identified in individuals with Rett syndrome. Neuroimaging and postmortem studies have demonstrated structural abnormalities in autistic individuals, and functional neuroimaging indicates that these individuals process information differently (Tanguay, 2000).

Phenomenology

MR describes a set of conditions in which an individual has global deficiencies in intellectual and adaptive functioning with an onset before age 18 (see Table 7-3). This disorder is coded on axis II of the DSM. There are various forms of MR, which are classifications of severity based on the level of cognitive and adaptive functioning. The level of severity is generally predictive of ultimate functioning, though individual, family, and community strengths and characteristics have considerable influence. Some mildly retarded individuals will no longer meet the criteria for the disorder as adults because their adaptive skills have improved and they are in environments with expectations that match their abilities (AACAP, 1999).

PDDs are a set of disorders that now are often called the *autism spectrum disorders*. The core symptoms are abnormality or delay in the ability to appropriately socially interact with others, inflexible language or behavior, and repetitive sensory and motor behaviors. Characteristic signs and symptoms include communication delay or abnormality, problems in social interactions, and stereotypic, rigid behaviors. These disorders are coded on axis I. The level of functioning of individuals with these disorders varies considerably; many who are severely affected also have MR. Autism generally is considered the most severe, with children and adolescents having problems with communication, social interactions, and aberrant behavior, though symptom severity varies widely. Asperger disorder is characterized not only by problems in these areas

TABLE 7-3	Mental Retardation: Categorization and Ultimate Functioning			
	Mild	**Moderate**	**Severe**	**Profound**
IQ	50–69	35–49	20–34	<20
Incidence	85%	10%	4%	1%
Socioeconomic class	Low	Low	No difference	No difference
Developmental year	7–11	3–7	1–3	<3
Academic level	6th Grade	2nd Grade	1st Grade or below	Preschool
Learning	Educable	Trainable	Basic skills	Nontrainable
Living as adult	Community	Sheltered	Supervision	Supervision

IQ, intelligence quotient.
(Lee and Gopalakrishnan, 2005).

but also by normal language development and average or above-average intelligence quotient (IQ) scores. PDD not-otherwise-specified (NOS) is used in cases where individuals have some of these difficulties but do not meet full criteria. A number of individuals with these disorders improve with interventions (particularly early in development) and age. Usually, the bizarre behaviors improve while the social impairment persists. Rett syndrome and childhood disintegrative disorder are rare, and Rett syndrome is the only PDD that occurs primarily in females.

Both MR and PDD often are comorbid with other psychiatric conditions or symptoms. Many individuals with autism also have MR. Common psychiatric symptoms in children and adolescents with PDD or MR include problems with attention, activity, oppositional behavior, aggression (toward self and others), mood, anxiety, feeding, and psychosis. The evaluation for these disorders should be multidimensional, with an emphasis on identifying both biological and psychosocial factors and determining the developmental status or issues. Several interview and screening instruments exist to aid in the recognition and assessment of the autism spectrum disorders. Vision and hearing screening always should be done. Psychological testing is necessary to diagnose MR and usually is indicated for PDD. Children and adolescents with visual or sensory impairments sometimes can appear to be cognitively or socially impaired, but appropriate

Clinical Characteristics of Mental Retardation

- Significantly below average intellectual functioning (IQ <70)
- Onset before age 18
- Concurrent deficits or impairment in present adaptive functioning in at least two areas:
  - Communication
  - Self-care
  - Home living
  - Social/interpersonal skills
  - Use of community resources
  - Self-direction
  - Functional academic skills
  - Work
  - Leisure
  - Health
  - Safety

Clinical Characteristics of Autistic Disorder

- Six or more symptoms:
  - Qualitative impairment in social interaction (at least two symptoms)
  - Qualitative impairment in communication (at least one symptom)
  - Restricted, repetitive, and stereotyped patterns of behavior, interests, and activities (at least one symptom)
- Delays or abnormal functioning in one or more areas with onset before age 3: social interaction, language as used in social communication, symbolic or imaginative play
- Not Rett syndrome or childhood disintegrative disorder

Clinical Characteristics of Asperger Disorder

- Qualitative impairment in social interaction (at least two symptoms)
- Restricted, repetitive, and stereotyped patterns of behavior, interests, and activities (at least one symptom)
- Impairment
- No clinically significant general delay in language
- No clinically significant delays in cognitive development, age-appropriate self-help skills, adaptive behavior (except social interaction), curiosity about environment
- Not another PDD or schizophrenia

Clinical Characteristics of Rett Syndrome

- Apparently normal prenatal and perinatal development
- Apparently normal psychomotor development from birth through first 5 months
- Normal head circumference at birth
- After period of normal development, onset of the following:
  - Head growth deceleration between ages 5 and 48 months
  - Loss of previously acquired purposeful hand movements between ages 5 and 30 months, with subsequent development of stereotyped hand movements
  - Early loss of social engagement (may develop later)
  - Poorly coordinated gait or trunk movements
- Severely impaired expressive and receptive language development with severe psychomotor retardation

screening should identify them. Individuals with learning or communication disorders can appear mentally retarded or socially impaired but are not globally affected. Youth with PDD can have symptoms that resemble psychosis or anxiety, but individuals with these other disorders do not have the ongoing, intrinsic social abnormalities of PDD. It can be difficult to decide whether children and adolescents with MR also have PDD, especially if the MR is severe. However, individuals with MR interact socially at a level that is consistent with their development and cognition.

Clinical Characteristics of Childhood Disintegrative Disorder

- Apparently normal development from birth for at least 2 years
- Age-appropriate verbal and nonverbal communication, social relationships, play, adaptive behavior
- Clinically significant loss of previously acquired skills in at least two areas before age 10:
  - Expressive or receptive language
  - Social skills or adaptive behavior
  - Bowel or bladder control
  - Play motor skills
- Abnormalities in at least two areas:
  - Qualitative impairment in social interaction
  - Qualitative impairment in communication
  - Restricted, repetitive, and stereotyped patterns of behavior, interests, and activities, including motor stereotypies and mannerisms
- Not another PDD or schizophrenia

Treatment

Psychotherapies and other somatic therapies

Behavioral, educational, psychological, and pharmacological interventions help children and adolescents and their families with the problems associated with MR and PDD. There is no cure for the core abnormalities. Treatment aims to minimize distress and maximize the child's functioning; for individuals with PDD, improving social skills is emphasized in addition to general functioning. Integrating and coordinating treatment between providers and other systems (e.g., schools) is essential. Education about the characteristics of these disorders and potential difficulties can help families plan and be proactive. Obtaining detailed information about problematic behaviors and symptoms is essential so that effective behavioral and environmental interventions can be designed and implemented. Psychological interventions to teach social skills, provide support to the family, and help higher functioning individuals cope with their distress have been found to be helpful. These children and adolescents should have educational plans and interventions to address their specific needs. Nontraditional therapies have not been found to be effective (AACAP, 1999).

Pharmacotherapy

Psychopharmacology can be useful in improving specific targeted symptoms; no medications act on the core deficits. Medications are used for the same indications as in non–developmentally delayed individuals. Often these youth respond to lower doses than typical individuals and may have more problems with side effects. Stimulants are generally used for attentional and activity difficulties, with some studies demonstrating efficacy. Different selective serotonin reuptake inhibitors (SSRIs) have been used to treat anxiety and mood symptoms, aggression, and repetitive thoughts and behaviors in these children and adolescents, with reports of success. Mood stabilizers such as sodium valproate, lithium, and carbamazepine have been employed to treat mood lability, but most of the controlled studies of these medications have focused on managing aggression. Typical and atypical neuroleptics also have been used to manage aggression and overactivity, with some controlled studies demonstrating improvement (Handen and Gilchrist, 2006; King and Bostic, 2007).

Prognostic Factors

Individuals with less severe forms of MR and PDD achieve higher levels of functioning, though environmental support is a crucial factor. Moderately impaired individuals can work and live somewhat independently with some support. Intelligence (IQ) predicts the functioning

A CASE OF PERVASIVE DEVELOPMENTAL DISORDER NOS

A 9-year-old boy is brought for an evaluation by his parents due to concern about his school performance. He is getting poor grades on group projects with teacher comments that he does not listen, dominates the group discussion, and only works on what interests him. Further questioning reveals that he has one friend with whom he spends time; their main activity together is researching dinosaurs. He has not been interested in sports or other extracurricular activities. In the interview, he describes in great detail recent discoveries about dinosaur fossils, returns to the subject even after the topic has been changed, and looks confused when asked what he talks about when others are not interested in dinosaurs. He is unable to explain what is happening in school other than "group projects are stupid" because his classmates do not have good ideas; he reports that his behavior is fine because he is the one who has the right answer. He is unable to think of any reasons for doing group activities or why the teacher is giving him poor grades. His solution is for the teacher to let him work on his own.

of lower-functioning autistic individuals. Verbal and cognitive abilities are the most accurate indicators of those with higher-functioning autism.

Specific Developmental Disorders (Learning Disorders)

Epidemiology

Learning disorders (LD) appear to have 2% to 10% prevalence in the population. More than 10% of school-aged children have significant academic difficulties, although many do not meet the criteria for LD. More males than females have been identified with these disorders in clinic and school settings, though these samples are probably not representative, because studies indicate equal prevalence in males and females. Approximately 80% to 90% of children identified with learning disabilities have reading disorders. Frequently, children have more than one learning disability (Abramowitz, 2005).

Etiology

The etiology of LD has not been determined, but there appears to be a significant genetic component, particularly for reading problems. These disorders appear to be the result of atypical brain maturation and function that may be exacerbated by adverse environmental factors. Preliminary neuroimaging of children with reading disorders indicates that the functional brain connections account for the differences in brain activation, rather than there being specific areas of the brain responsible for reading.

Phenomenology

LDs are a heterogeneous group manifested by difficulties in communication, motor skills, reading, writing, or mathematics. Youth are diagnosed with LD when they have specific deficits in their achievement in one or more areas below what would be expected on the basis of their intellectual abilities, age, and education. There also must be problems with academic performance or daily living skills. These disorders are coded on axis I. Comorbidity with LDs is common, with

Clinical Characteristics of Specific Developmental Disorders

- Academic achievement below expectation for age, schooling, intellect; impairment
- Communication and motor skills disorders require that certain other disorders not be present (e.g., PDD) or symptoms be in excess of usual presentation (e.g., MR)

several children having more than one learning disorder. Many have ADHD. Other issues can include adjustment, mood, anxiety, and demoralization problems due to academic failure. To be diagnosed, youth must have psychological testing that includes IQ and achievement assessments. Other tests may determine specific deficits in academic skills, language, speech, or motor abilities. Patients should have their vision and hearing evaluated (AACAP, 1998).

Treatment

The main focus of treatment is obtaining appropriate educational placement and services. Physicians often can be very influential advocates for these youth. It is important to educate the parents, affected children, and other involved adults. Comorbid medical, psychiatric, and psychological symptoms should be addressed with appropriate treatments. Depending on the learning disorder, physical, occupational, and speech therapy may be helpful. These children and adolescents should be reassessed on a regular basis to ensure that their education services remain appropriate.

Prognostic Factors

Children and adolescents with LD can do well if they are identified in a timely manner and receive appropriate services. Functioning and outcome improve upon treating comorbid conditions. Although LD do not resolve, affected youth can learn successfully by developing strategies to utilize and exploit their strengths.

Disruptive Disorders

Disruptive disorders are characterized by externalizing behaviors coded on axis I, including ADHD, oppositional defiant disorder (ODD), and conduct disorder (CD), each of which will be described in the following text.

Attention-Deficit/Hyperactivity Disorder
Epidemiology

Estimates of the prevalence of ADHD vary; recent data indicate a rate of about 8%. Boys outnumber girls, and girls are more likely to have the inattentive subtype. ADHD has been identified in various industrialized countries across the world. The higher rates in the United States compared with other countries is thought to be due to differences in diagnostic practices, cultural views, and study methodology (AACAP, 2007).

Etiology

ADHD is a heterogeneous syndrome with various etiological factors. Individuals with ADHD appear to have executive functioning deficits as evidenced by problems with response inhibition, vigilance, working memory, and some aspects of planning. Structural studies have revealed involvement of frontal lobes, basal ganglia, corpus callosum, and cerebellum. Dynamic imaging studies have found circuit dysfunction between the prefrontal cortex, striatum, and cerebellum. ADHD appears to have a significant genetic aspect; affected youth have more biologic relatives with the disorder. Several possible chromosomes and genes have been identified. Biological and environmental substances, such as excessive lead exposure, abnormal zinc levels, allergies, and food intolerance, also have been linked to ADHD symptoms, with lead having the strongest evidence. Prenatal nicotine exposure has been implicated, as has low birth weight, traumatic brain injury, and severe early deprivation.

Phenomenology

Individuals with ADHD have core deficits in attention, level of activity, or impulsivity. They may have abnormalities in all or some of these areas of functioning. Their behavior may vary in different environments, depending on familiarity, expectations, structure, and supervision. Often children and adolescents can have more symptoms in situations characterized by high expectations for sustained attention, prolonged physical inactivity, poor structure, inadequate supervision, or uninteresting activities. These children and adolescents can appear unimpaired when engaged in activities that are novel, engrossing, or involve individual interactions with an attentive adult. Associated problems include difficulty learning and following rules, distractibility, poor motivation, disorganization, inadequate task completion, low frustration tolerance, tendency to

Clinical Characteristics of Attention-Deficit/Hyperactivity Disorder

- Six or more symptoms from lists of inattentive, hyperactive, or impulsive symptoms:
  - Inattention
    - Fails to attend to details, makes careless mistakes
    - Difficulty sustaining attention in tasks or play activities
    - Does not seem to listen when spoken to directly
    - Does not follow through with instructions or finish tasks (not oppositional/defiant)
    - Difficulty organizing tasks and activities
    - Avoids/dislikes/hard to engage in tasks requiring sustained mental effort
    - Loses things necessary for tasks or activities
    - Easily distracted by extraneous stimuli
    - Forgetful in daily activities
  - Hyperactivity
    - Fidgets or squirms
    - Often leaves seat in situation where sitting is expected
    - Runs about or climbs excessively when inappropriate
    - Difficulty playing or engaging in leisure activities quietly
    - Often "on the go" or acts like "driven by a motor"
    - Talks excessively
  - Impulsivity
    - Blurts out answers before questions have been completed
    - Difficulty awaiting turn
    - Interrupts or intrudes on others
- Clinically significant impairment in social, academic, or occupational functioning
- Duration of at least 6 months
- Symptoms maladaptive and inconsistent with developmental level
- Some symptoms before age 7
- Impairment from symptoms in two or more settings

seek immediate gratification, and oppositional behavior. Poor peer relationships frequently occur because children and adolescents with ADHD are perceived as immature, irritating, intrusive, bossy, and socially inept.

DSM-IV-TR identifies three subtypes of ADHD: combined, predominantly inattentive, and primarily hyperactive-impulsive. Children and adolescents with the combined type tend to present most often for clinical care. Those with the primarily inattentive type have fewer behavioral problems. The primary hyperactive-impulsive subtype has been mostly used for young children in whom it is difficult to accurately assess their attention.

The presentation of ADHD varies with age. Preschool children tend to be impulsive, overactive, and aggressive. School-age children have inattention and hyperactivity. Impulsivity and hyperactivity usually improve after puberty. Problems with attention and organization continue to be significant and impairing in adolescence and adulthood for many individuals.

Children and adolescents with ADHD often have comorbid psychiatric disorders, such as LD, ODD, CD, anxiety disorders, and mood disorders. Many children who have Tourette syndrome (TS) also have ADHD. Children with neurological or other chronic medical conditions can have problems with attention and activity regulation. ADHD is diagnosed clinically by interviewing the child or adolescent and caretakers and obtaining information from other involved adults (e.g., teachers). A variety of standardized behavioral rating scales have been used to diagnose ADHD, supplementing the clinical interview and assessment. Psychological testing is beneficial to identify LD or deficits in academic achievement.

Inattention, overactivity, and impulsivity can be symptoms of other psychiatric disorders; however, the youth also have the core symptoms of the other disorder. Children and adolescents from chaotic homes or who have suffered neglect or abuse may have difficulty with goal-directed behavior, demonstrate increased activity, or exhibit attentional dysfunction. Medical conditions and drugs can also produce inattention and hyperactivity.

Treatment

Youth with uncomplicated ADHD may just need medication treatment with stimulants. For many patients, optimal treatment involves several interventions such as psychosocial treatments, medication, and environmental adjustments. It is essential to evaluate the patient's functioning across many domains and then determine the most appropriate interventions. Frequently, initial treatment focuses on deciding if medication would be beneficial, starting medication, and implementing some basic behavioral management strategies so that the child or adolescent can be more successful at home and school. After stabilization and the patient and family are more functional, other forms of psychotherapy may be helpful, depending on the issues.

Psychotherapies and other somatic therapies

Parent training can help modify and improve the patient's behavior at home and school. Behavioral techniques improve academic performance more than medication does and can decrease the dose of medication necessary for school. They can also help increase motivation to complete tasks but are less likely to improve attentional capacity. Cognitive behavioral therapies (CBTs) can be helpful in addressing problems associated with ADHD, such as poor social skills, problematic peer relationships, inadequate self-regulation, aggression, and low self-esteem. Children and adolescents with ADHD may qualify for special educational services.

Pharmacotherapy

Stimulants are the most frequently prescribed medicines for ADHD and the most effective. They are class II drugs. The stimulants have slightly different mechanisms of action but do not appear to differ significantly in efficacy. Common forms include methylphenidate (MPH), dextroamphetamine (DEX), and mixed amphetamine salts (MAS). All of these medications come in various formulations (e.g., short, intermediate, and long acting) with different time spans of efficacy. They last between 4 and 10 hours and take approximately 20 to 30 minutes to work. There is substantial evidence that stimulants significantly improve attention, motor overactivity, impulse control, and aggression; these effects lead to more organized behavior, greater task completion, and increased self-regulation. Social skills and academic productivity also can improve. Although most of the studies have been done with school-aged children, there is evidence that stimulants can be helpful across the life span. If an individual does not respond to one stimulant, another one should be tried. Children and adolescents can go off medication on nonschool days, though many are more successful with peers and extracurricular activities on medication. Most children and adolescents tolerate these medications well. Common side effects include headache, abdominal pain, decreased appetite, weight loss, and initial insomnia. These effects tend to improve with continued use of the medication. There can be slight increases in blood pressure and pulse, which may be significant for some individuals. There has been concern about the cardiovascular effects of these drugs; currently, they are not recommended for youth with cardiac problems. Irritability, affective blunting, and mood lability can occur at peak levels or as the medication is wearing off. The longer-acting preparations tend to have fewer such effects. Tics can develop or be exacerbated, though many youth with tics do well on stimulants. Psychotic symptoms can occur; they are rare and appear to be related to excessive doses or the presence of other psychiatric disorders. Weight, height, pulse, and blood pressure should be monitored regularly because long-term stimulant treatment may negatively affect ultimate height (AACAP, 2002).

Other medications used to treat ADHD include atomoxine, tricyclic antidepressants (TCAs), bupropion, venlafaxine, and α_2 agonists (e.g., clonidine). All must be taken daily. The U.S. Food and Drug Administration (FDA) has approved only atomoxine for ADHD and use in adults; it has been shown to improve attention and hyperactivity, though clinically it appears to improve activity more than attention. The other nonstimulants for ADHD are off label and generally

A CASE OF ATTENTION-DEFICIT/HYPERACTIVITY DISORDER

An 8-year-old boy's school has asked his parents to bring him for evaluation due to his ongoing problems with listening to the teachers, not completing schoolwork, and disrupting the classroom. The teacher's report describes him as engaging but irresponsible and difficult to manage because he is constantly trying to be the class clown. His parents admit that previous teachers had complained about similar behavior but this year seems worse. He has always been energetic and very active ever since he could walk. At home they have had problems with him forgetting things, losing his belongings, and not doing household chores without multiple reminders. There have been no other problems, and the family denies any significant stresses. During the interview, the boy admits that he has trouble sitting in his seat at school and that he tries to listen but that he ends up talking to his friend or playing with something in his desk.

not as effective as stimulants. They should be considered for cases in which the FDA-approved medications have failed or cannot be tolerated (Prince, 2007).

Prognostic factors

Most children with ADHD also have the disorder as adolescents. Data indicate that many will still be symptomatic as adults, although there are diagnostic issues related to the DSM criteria not being developmentally appropriate for adults and less use of other informants for adults. Adults with childhood ADHD tend to have more problematic lives than their peers. Data indicate that children with ADHD tend to do worse than their unaffected siblings or peers, even with long-term treatment, though treatment does seem to have a positive effect. Having comorbid CD predicts a worse outcome, with an increased rate of antisocial behavior and substance abuse. Youth with comorbid internalizing disorders also seem to be at higher risk for substance abuse.

Oppositional Defiant Disorder

ODD has a reported prevalence from 1% to 6% in community samples, with higher rates in boys, prepubertal children, and lower socioeconomic groups. There is considerable debate about the diagnostic construct of and criteria for ODD. The etiology is not known, but ODD appears to be best explained by the interaction of multiple individual and environmental factors. It is characterized by excessive arguing, misbehavior toward adults, poor temper control, irritability, anger, and excessive defiance of authority. The usual onset is ages 6 to 10 years; it rarely occurs before age 3 or after adolescence. The child mostly challenges parents and other involved adults and is not particularly aggressive. Parents of affected children usually model similar behavior, provide inconsistent discipline, inadequate structure or supervision, or lack the time and energy to parent appropriately. Children with ODD tend to have other psychiatric disorders such as ADHD or affective disorders. Given the significant comorbidity, it is important to diagnose and assertively treat any other psychiatric disorder. Data suggest that ODD is best treated with individual and family therapy, which emphasizes educating parents and other involved adults on good behavioral management techniques and parenting approaches. Consistent structure, expectations, and consequences in all environments are essential. Individual psychotherapy such as CBT can help children understand their behaviors and reactions to stimuli and the reactions of others to their actions. It is also helpful to involve the child in structured, prosocial activities after school and on weekends. Efforts to prevent ODD have included early childhood and other school-based programs and parent training. Some children with ODD will subsequently develop CD (approximately 30%), especially those with an earlier onset (AACAP, 2007).

Conduct Disorder
Epidemiology

Prevalence estimates of CD in the United States range from 1% to 10%, with more boys than girls, though the prevalence in girls is increasing. Cultural attitudes about race, gender, and class may influence whether a child is labeled with CD. Boys usually present at earlier ages than girls and may have more violent or aggressive traits. CD tends to occur over time, with increasing symptoms and severity.

Etiology

A cumulative risk model of risk factors appears to be the best explanation of the behaviors described by CD: the greater the number of risk factors and the earlier they appear, the higher the chance that the individual will be aggressive and have serious psychopathology. The biological vulnerabilities for aggressive behavior appear to include genetic factors, CNS insults, nervous system underarousal, neurotransmitter aberrations, and difficult temperament. Neuroimaging has demonstrated frontal and prefrontal dysfunction. Psychological factors include learning problems, language deficits, and personality traits. Important social factors appear to include family, peers, and the environment. Neglect, abuse, poor communication, and members with criminal histories often characterize the families. Parenting tends to be typified by parental conflict, absence, inadequate supervision, and ineffectiveness. In adolescence, personal characteristics such as restraint, psychological distress, and peer relationships become more important. Environmental issues include high unemployment, crime, community violence, low socioeconomic class, and poor schools (Loeber et al., 2000; Burke et al., 2002).

Phenomenology

CD is diagnosed if the child or adolescent exhibits a certain number of antisocial behaviors within a specific time frame. The context or potential etiology of the behaviors is not considered. Children and adolescents with CD tend to come from chaotic, nonfunctional families. Interactions between the family environment and the child's characteristics reinforce aggression, impulsiveness, and disregard for the rights of others. The child's behavior tends to evoke rejection by others, thereby maintaining a negative cycle of interactions. Complaints about defiance and aggression in childhood and adolescence are very common. An essential aspect of the evaluation is differentiating normal from pathological disruptive behavior and deciding whether the symptoms are related to another psychiatric disorder. Medical disorders (e.g., CNS injuries or lesions) should be ruled out. Obtaining information on the patterns, percipients, and degrees of disruptive behavior is helpful. It is also useful to ask about the extent of the problems that the disruptive behavior causes and the typical response of the adults involved. CD tends to be comorbid with a number of other psychiatric disorders such as ADHD, affective disorders, LD, and substance abuse (AACAP, 1997a).

Treatment

It is important to diagnose and assertively treat any other psychiatric disorders. The approaches used for ODD, parent training, and pronged approaches that target the individual as well as all relevant dimensions and environments are the most successful. Programs such as MST that work with the individual, family, school, and any other relevant adults or agencies have demonstrated results. Educational interventions are usually necessary. Medication may be helpful, though it is important to remember that no class of medication has demonstrated consistent efficacy against

---

Clinical Characteristics of Oppositional Defiant Disorder

- Pattern of negative, hostile, and defiant behavior
- Duration of at least 6 months
- Four or more symptoms (losing temper, arguing with adults, defying adults, deliberately annoying others, touchy, angry/resentful, spiteful/vindictive)
- Excessive for age/developmental level
- Impairment
- Not psychotic, mood disorder, or CD

Clinical Characteristics of Conduct Disorder

- Repetitive and persistent behavior pattern that violates the basic rights of others or major age-appropriate societal norms/rules
- Three or more symptoms in the last 12 months (aggression to people and animals, destruction of property, deceitfulness or theft, serious violations of rules)
- Impairment
- Childhood, adolescent, or unspecified onset
- Mild, moderate, or severe

---

aggression. Medication is more likely to be effective if the aggressive behavior is impulsive and environmentally reactive. Mood stabilizers or anticonvulsants have been used successfully, with valproic acid and lithium the best studied. Antipsychotics are also reported to be effective. Issues of nonadherence need to be addressed proactively and throughout treatment (Jensen et al., 2007).

Prognostic factors

Many individuals with CD do not develop into antisocial adults. Risk factors for the persistence of CD and progression to antisocial personality disorder include a low IQ score, parental antisocial personality disorder, early onset CD, comorbid ADHD, and more severe, frequent, and varied symptoms. Those with higher verbal IQ scores, less severe CD, fewer symptoms of ADHD, better socioeconomic status, and non–antisocial biological parents have better outcomes. More adaptive social skills, more positive peer experiences, and adolescent onset also predict a better outcome.

Feeding and Eating Disorders of Infancy and Early Childhood

Eating issues in infants and toddlers are problematic for multiple reasons in addition to the obvious ones of growth and nutrition. Feeding promotes social development, interactions, and motor development. Learning to eat requires a reciprocal interaction between the child and caretaker, and disruptions can put an infant at risk for multiple difficulties. Types of problems include mismatch between the feeding styles of the child and caretaker, caretaker difficulty adjusting to the child's increased independence and assertions of preferences, and changes in the child's normal growth rate with age and development.

Research on feeding disorders has been limited by a lack of a consensus about diagnostic criteria and classification systems. Practitioners use several systems with different organizational

---

A CASE OF CONDUCT DISORDER

A 15-year-old boy has been referred for psychiatric evaluation by the juvenile court after release from the juvenile detention center. He was arrested when police found him in a stolen car. He states that he was with a friend and did not know the car was stolen. Previous involvement with juvenile court includes charges of assault after a fight with a peer at school and truancy after he missed most of school last year. He explains that the boy at school disrespected him, which precipitated the fight. He is not sure why he stopped going to school; he was in the 7th grade after failing several grades, and he thought he was too old to be there. He lives with his grandmother, who has raised him since he was 4 after several foster care placements. Child protective services became involved after he went to preschool with multiple bruises. His grandmother describes him as being difficult and angry since early childhood. She has multiple medical problems and has been on disability for several years. His father lives with them sometimes but also stays with a girlfriend. He is unemployed with a history of drug use and prison. The boy is not sure where his mother lives but thinks she is in another state.

schemes and labels, making comparisons difficult. None adequately describe all of the possible disorders. Various approaches have used etiologies, descriptions of the feeding problems, or a combination. DSM-IV-TR uses a descriptive approach and includes three eating disorders of early childhood: pica, feeding disorder of infancy or early childhood, and rumination disorder. The most common term used medically is *failure to thrive* (FTT), a disorder with poor weight gain accompanied by problems with social and emotional development in the first 3 years of life. It is associated with increased risk for chronic deficits in growth, cognition, and socioeconomic functioning. Its etiology is multifactorial, with both organic and psychosocial components. It is also descriptive and often does not adequately capture all of the pathways to growth failure. Both feeding disorder of infancy or early childhood and rumination disorder can be associated with FTT (Chatoor, 2002).

The evaluation of a feeding disorder requires a multidisciplinary approach. Assessment of the child's motor abilities is essential because chewing and swallowing are complex coordination tasks that may be impaired. The infant and caretaker's social and feeding interactions also should be evaluated. Most of the feeding disorders involve an impaired relationship between the child and the caretaker. Caretakers with inadequate parenting knowledge or skills, significant psychopathology, major stresses, or poor environmental support can have difficulty managing the care of and relating to their infants. A psychosocial and psychiatric evaluation of the caretaker should be included in the assessment. Observing feeding interactions and other interactions between the child and caretaker provides essential information on the relationship and issues. Children with various medical conditions may have feeding problems due to excessive calorie needs, physical or mechanical difficulty with eating, or inadequate absorption of nutrients.

Treatment requires a comprehensive approach that addresses the needs and issues of the child, the caretaker, and their relationship. Any medical or psychiatric disorders should be treated appropriately. Children may require extra nutrition to catch up or specific interventions to help with feeding and eating (e.g., swallowing training). Children with developmental delays may require occupational, physical, or speech therapy. Providing education on appropriate parenting is helpful, with demonstration and reinforcement of various techniques. Helping the caregiver and child develop an adequately supportive, nurturing relationship is vital. Caretakers may need their own psychiatric treatment.

Pica

There is limited information on pica, which is defined as craving and/or eating non-nutritive substances. It can occur in young children, individuals with MR, people who are chronically anxious, and women who are pregnant. In certain cultures, it is considered normal. Often, children with pica seek treatment for other behavior and medical problems. Up to one third of children may exhibit pica at some point, and it can be normal in children younger than 3 years. Associated factors include low socioeconomic status, environmental deprivation, and parental psychopathology. Possible etiologies include nutritional deficiencies, insufficient stimulation, caretaker–child relationship difficulties, or cultural practices. Pica generally begins at ages 12 to 24 months and resolves by school age. In people with MR, it may persist into adulthood. Common substances include ice, paint, clay, or soil. Possible medical complications include heavy metal poisoning, parasitic infections, or intestinal obstruction. Education on appropriate diets combined with behavior management to reinforce appropriate eating and discourage eating non-nutritive items can be effective. Providing adequate supervision and environmental stimulation is also beneficial.

Feeding Disorder of Infancy

Feeding disorder of infancy was first described in DSM-IV (1994) and is used to diagnose infants who consistently do not eat and either fail to gain weight or lose weight. These infants have access to enough food and do not have another explanatory psychiatric or medical condition. Although this classification has been useful in providing a standard definition, there have been difficulties because it is too broad and does not account for the range of feeding problems that may have this symptom constellation. These diagnostic criteria do not include feeding disorders characterized by specific nutritional deficiencies rather than general growth failure. As a result, many infants with significant feeding problems do not meet diagnostic criteria, and it has been difficult to study this disorder systematically.

Rumination Disorder

Rumination disorder is a rare, potentially fatal problem characterized by repeated voluntary regurgitation and rechewing of food, without apparent nausea or associated gastrointestinal illness, accompanied by weight loss or failure to make expected weight gain. Often, there are associated self-stimulatory behaviors such as sucking on a thumb or cloth, head banging, and body rocking. The etiology is unknown, though most theories consider adverse psychosocial factors important, with the infant using rumination for self-stimulation or social reinforcement. However, some infants appear to be happy and have supportive and interactive parents. Genetic factors have not been established. Research has indicated a relationship between maternal eating disorders and childhood feeding problems, though it is unclear whether this association is environmental or genetic. Rumination is strongly associated with gastroesophageal reflux. It tends to occur in the first year of life and usually resolves by the second year. Spontaneous remission is common. Indigestion, halitosis, tooth decay, FTT, dehydration, electrolyte disturbances, and malnutrition can occur. Reassurance, support, and parental education are helpful. Behavioral techniques can help the parents positively interact with the child and not reinforce ruminating behavior.

Tic Disorders

Epidemiology

Tic disorders frequently occur in childhood. Transient tic disorder is the most common, with approximately 5% of children having transient and simple tics. The prevalence of chronic tic disorder in schoolchildren is estimated to be between 2% and 6% and that of TS is 4 to 6 per 1,000 in certain populations (Swain et al., 2007).

Etiology

The variable expression of tic disorders appears to be best explained by an interaction of genetic and environmental factors with increased symptoms related to stress. Research indicates that patients with TS may have increased reactivity of the hypothalamic-pituitary-adrenal and noradrenergic systems. Family studies support the genetic transmission of TS and the theory that some variants of obsessive-compulsive disorder (OCD) and ADHD are etiologically related to TS. Several chromosomal regions and cytogenic abnormalities have been implicated. Multiple genes appear to produce vulnerability to TS and related disorders. Other possible factors include gestational or perinatal insults, androgen exposure, heat, fatigue, psychosocial stresses, and postinfectious autoimmune mechanisms. Other data indicate abnormalities in the γ-aminobutyric acid (GABA) systems and neurons.

Phenomenology

Tics are sudden, repetitive, discrete, nonrhythmic, stereotypic movements or vocalizations, which can be motor or vocal, simple or complex. Typically, tics are episodic and fluctuate over time in number, severity, and location. They wax and wane and tend to worsen during transitional periods with stress, fatigue, and relaxation. They decrease during distraction or concentration. Tics diminish during sleep but may not disappear completely. It is common for tics to be preceded by uncomfortable sensations or urges. Resisting tics aggravates these sensations, and performing a tic transiently reduces this sense of internal pressure (Gaytan et al., 2005).

The same DSM criteria are used for children, adolescents, and adults. DSM-IV-TR has several tic disorders, which are classified on the basis of symptom duration and tic type. Transient tic disorder can be motor, vocal, or both. For chronic tic disorder, tics must be present at least 1 year; they can be either vocal or motor but not both. If both chronic vocal and motor tics are present (not necessarily at the same time), TS is diagnosed. Motor tics tend to appear from ages 3 to 8 and vocal tics several years later. Functional impairment is not required. Other conditions with tic-like symptoms may result from infections, toxins, medications, drugs, developmental disorders, chromosomal or genetic abnormalities, neurodegenerative disorders, neurocutaneous disorders, head trauma, and cardiovascular accidents.

Comorbid conditions are common and often more impairing than the tics. ADHD symptoms often appear before the tic disorder. Most children seen clinically for TS have ADHD, and a significant number have OCD. Behavioral problems tend to occur in patients with comorbid

---

Clinical Characteristics of Transient Tic Disorder

- Single or multiple motor or vocal tics, not both
- Tics occur many times during the day, almost every day
- Duration of at least 4 weeks; no longer than 12 consecutive months; onset before age 18
- Not due to a medical condition or substances
- Never had Tourette syndrome or chronic motor or vocal tic disorder
- Single episode or recurrent

Clinical Characteristics of Chronic Motor or Vocal Tic Disorder

- Single or multiple motor or vocal tics, not both
- Tics occur many times during the day, almost every day
- Duration of longer than a year; tic-free periods less than 3 months; onset before age 18
- Not due to a medical condition or substances; never had Tourette syndrome

---

Clinical Characteristics of Tourette syndrome

- Multiple motor tics; one or more vocal tics; tics do not have to be concurrent
- Tics occur many times during the day, almost every day
- Duration of longer than a year; tic-free periods less than 3 months; onset before age 18
- Not due to a medical condition or substances

ADHD. OCD is associated with more severe TS. Anxiety disorders and LD are also common. Social impairment, low self-esteem, and peer teasing may complicate the clinical picture. Diagnosis of tic disorder is based on history and observation. It may be helpful to ask parents to video record the child having tics because children may suppress the movements in the office. Specific tic rating scales can be used to document and monitor tic severity. No specific laboratory tests or imaging studies are indicated, unless needed to rule out other comorbid conditions.

Tics need to be differentiated from other abnormal movements. The presence of premonitory urges, the involuntary nature, and the ability to transiently suppress tics are distinguishing features. Compulsions tend to have a more elaborate cognitive component and prominent anxiety symptoms. Other abnormal movements may look like tics superficially but may be distinguished on closer examination. Chorea is composed of dance-like, chaotic movements. It is less suppressible, not stereotyped, and lacks a premonitory urge. Myoclonus is a brief, shock-like movement that is not suppressible, may result in loss of control, and may increase with activity. Stereotypies are rhythmic movements performed in a patterned way and usually seen in children and adolescents with PDD or MR. They are not distressing; children are frequently unaware of performing them and cease doing them once distracted.

Treatment

Reassurance and education can be enough to manage transient tic disorder. Chronic tics and TS may require treatment. Observation is necessary to establish the severity of tics. Treatment is warranted when tics interfere with peer relations, social interactions, academic performance, or activities of daily living and may also be indicated for significant patient distress. Often, the major source of impairment is due to comorbid conditions that should be treated first. After these conditions are under control, the tics should be reassessed to determine the need for specific treatment directed at them. It is important to remember that tics wax and wane.

Psychotherapies and other somatic therapies

Habit-reversal therapy is a form of behavioral treatment for tics. The focus is on the use of a competing muscle contraction or behavioral response opposing the tic movement along with self-monitoring and awareness training. Individual therapy may help a child cope with the stigma of illness, improve self-esteem and relationships, and reduce anxiety. Behavior modification is recommended for behavioral problems associated with ADHD and ODD. CBT may be helpful for those children and adolescents with OCD.

Pharmacotherapy

Often, the goal of medication treatment is not tic elimination but reduction to a level that does not interfere with the child's development and functioning. The first-line agents for tics are α-adrenergic agonists (e.g., clonidine and guanfacine). These agents may not be more effective than antipsychotics but have a better side effect profile and tolerability. Compared to clonidine, guanfacine causes less sedation and hypotension and can be taken less frequently. Antipsychotics have a well-documented efficacy in tics. Both typical and atypical antipsychotics have been used with positive results; generally, atypicals are preferred due to their side effect profile. In general, antipsychotics should be reserved for severe and treatment refractory tics causing significant functional impairment that fail to respond adequately to the α-adrenergic agents. Many youth do not like taking antipsychotics due to cognitive effects.

Prognostic Factors

Tics usually appear in the first decade of life. In TS, tic severity generally peaks in early adolescence, with many having decreased severity by adulthood. Approximately 20% still have moderate impairment by age 20. The severity of tic disorders reaches its peak around ages 10 to 12, and by age 18, 50% of those with chronic tics are tic free.

Elimination Disorders

Elimination disorders are diagnosed when children and adolescents have urination and defecation patterns (timing and location) that are abnormal based on their developmental stage. These disorders are coded on axis I. More boys than girls are diagnosed with these disorders. Generally, children by the developmental age of 5 years should be continent. Most children accomplish toilet training (defecation first) between ages 2½ and 4 years, though nighttime bed wetting is common until age 5. Obtaining detailed information on the process of toilet training, the onset and course of the enuresis or encopresis, and the current toileting practices and hygiene, behavior, and consequences after episodes is essential. Potential medical causes should be ruled out and any comorbid psychiatric disorders identified. Additionally, clinicians should screen for sources of stress or trauma because many children may respond to stress with regressive behavior, losing acquired developmental milestones temporarily (Mikkelsen, 2001).

Enuresis

Enuresis is very common in pediatric age-groups and has a significant spontaneous remission rate with each year of age; only a small percentage still have nocturnal enuresis by age 18. Enuresis runs in families; most affected children have first-degree relatives who were also enuretic. Enuresis can be involuntary or intentional. It can be diurnal, nocturnal, or both and primary (voluntary bladder control never attained) or secondary (voluntary bladder control attained but then lost). Most children and adolescents with enuresis do not have associated psychopathology, though they can develop self-esteem and shame issues if they are stigmatized and humiliated about wetting the bed. There appears to be an increased rate of enuresis in children with ADHD and some medical problems. Occasionally, children will be seen for enuresis related to failure to pay attention to physiological signals (e.g., too busy playing to take a bathroom break) or psychological issues (e.g., too afraid to get up at night to use the bathroom). Diurnal enuresis tends to have a higher association with other psychiatric disorders.

Generally, a mixture of education, psychological support, and behavioral intervention is the most effective intervention. Explanations and reassurance that enuresis is a common problem which resolves spontaneously for most youth can be helpful. It is essential that the parents and others do not blame or stigmatize the child. Strategies may help such as restricting caffeine, limiting fluid intake later in the day, scheduling toilet use during the night, using plastic materials to protect the bed, having a routine to deal with wet bedding and pajamas, and taking a bath in the morning. Arousal systems (i.e., urine or bladder alarm systems) are the most effective nonmedical interventions, with reported success rates of 40% to 75% after 12 months. They require very motivated children and families. Voiding completes a circuit that sets off an alarm, waking the child, who then completes voiding in the toilet. A conditioned response eventually occurs so that the physiological stimuli preceding urination become the inhibitors of voiding. Psychotherapy is not effective for enuresis but may be beneficial for any relevant stress, associated psychological difficulties, or comorbid psychiatric disorders. Medications include imipramine (25–50 mg at night) and desmopressin acetate (DDAVP; 10 μg per spray, two sprays per nostril at night). Both medicines tend to be tolerated well and are fairly effective in reducing the number of wet nights, though rarely eliminate them. Most children and adolescents with nocturnal enuresis do well (AACAP, 2004).

Encopresis

Encopresis has been found in up to 3% of a general pediatric population and 25% of pediatric gastroenterology referrals. There is a high rate of spontaneous remission with age and it is rare after age 16. Most of affected youth have had a period of continence (at least a year) before the soiling began. Poor toilet training or constipation is thought to cause encopresis. It is often associated with other psychiatric disorders, particularly ODD and CD, as well as significant social problems. Encopresis can be involuntary or intentional and is subtyped based on whether there is associated constipation and overflow incontinence. Encopresis with constipation and overflow incontinence involves stool seepage around a rectal fecal mass caused by constipation. Stool leakage stops after the constipation has been treated. In encopresis not involving constipation, the fecal material is typical in content and consistency for the individual and soiling occurs irregularly. This type is more common in children and adolescents with disruptive disorders. Delayed bowel training and inappropriate bathroom habits can occur in children with MR, children who are developmentally delayed, and those with psychosis. Anxious children may resist using public restrooms, and impulsive, inattentive children may not anticipate their need for toileting or may ignore physiological cues. Also, they may not sit on the toilet long enough to complete defecation and may have incomplete postdefecation hygiene, with smearing in their underwear.

Providing education about the pathophysiology and self-perpetuating nature of encopresis is essential. Helping the adults not blame and criticize the child is important. Treatment programs generally include treating any constipation or fecal masses if present and then teaching and implementing a regular toileting practice or protocol that becomes part of the child's daily routine so that healthy and regular bowel and bladder habits are learned and encouraged. Often the parents and other involved adults benefit from parent training or behavioral management. Children should be involved in any required cleanup of continued episodes. Diets emphasizing adequate amounts of fiber and water are promoted. Stool softeners, laxatives, and bulking agents may be necessary for maintenance therapy. Day care and schools should participate in the treatment plan for consistency. Psychotherapy may be beneficial for any comorbid psychiatric disorders or trauma and any psychological issues associated with the encopresis, such as poor self-esteem, peer difficulties, family conflict, and communication problems. Behavioral management may be helpful in promoting consistency and appropriate consequences. Biofeedback has demonstrated some treatment success with this disorder. No medication has been identified to treat encopresis.

OTHER DISORDERS OF INFANCY, CHILDHOOD, OR ADOLESCENCE
Reactive Attachment Disorder of Infancy or Early Childhood

Considerable literature based on various theoretical perspectives and observations of parent–infant bonding exists on the development and types of attachment in infants. Attachment is considered a fundamental aspect of development; ideally, infants become securely attached, viewing themselves as safe in the world and their caretakers as reliable. Secure attachment provides infants with the foundation to grow and develop successfully. Children with nonsecure attachments are at risk for psychopathology. There is considerable interest in understanding how the process of attachment works after infancy and how to intervene later in life when the initial attachment did not go well and the youth continues to have poor attachments. There is one attachment disorder listed in the DSM, reactive attachment disorder (RAD). This diagnosis requires the child to have severely disturbed social relatedness before age 5 and very pathogenic care (i.e., abuse or neglect). Children with RAD have been described as having significant behavioral and emotional problems. The data on treatment approaches are limited; the best studied are models focused on the parent–child relationship (AACAP, 2005).

Stereotypic Movement Disorder

Stereotypies are repetitive, nonfunctional movements such as hand waving, head banging, body rocking, or hitting oneself, which can be simple or complex. DSM-IV-TR criteria require that these behaviors interfere with normal activities, result in self-injury, have a certain level of severity, are not due to other psychiatric disorders or medical issues, and have a certain duration. There is a subtype for self-injurious behavior. Rhythmic stereotypies occur in normal infants during the first year of life, after which they decline. Community and clinical surveys have found that normal adults demonstrate a number and range of stereotypies, though these behaviors are usually not impairing. These behaviors are very common in children with MR, PDD, and various medical or genetic syndromes. Behavioral management is the primary intervention. Various medications, mostly antipsychotics and SSRIs, have also been employed with variable results (Stein et al., 1998; Stein and Simeon, 1998).

OTHER DISORDERS SEEN IN CHILDREN AND ADOLESCENTS

Substance Use Disorders

Annual surveys of teenagers reveal ongoing experimentation and regular use of multiple drugs, with most using alcohol and drugs occasionally and without negative consequences (AACAP, 1997b). Risk factors for adolescent substance abuse include genetic, constitutional, psychological, and sociocultural (family, peer, school, and community) factors. There are some data that youth start with tobacco, alcohol, and marijuana and then progress to other substances. Other risk factors include externalizing disorders, early substance use, and certain types of family and peer behaviors. These disorders are primarily seen in adolescents and have been associated with multiple problems including delinquency, aggression, early sexual activity, truancy, and school failure. Most have other comorbid psychiatric disorders. Substance use should be routinely addressed with all adolescents. Substance abuse or dependence in adolescents is diagnosed using the same DSM criteria as for adults (Chapter 9). All adolescents with substance problems should be evaluated psychiatrically. Interventions vary, depending on the scope and severity of the drug problems, presence of other psychiatric disorders, and family functioning (Hopper and Riggs, 2007). Substance use disorders tend to be chronic and relapsing. Youth do worse when there is early onset, more severe use, and comorbid conditions.

Psychotic Disorders

Psychotic disorders are rare in children and adolescents. They are extremely rare in those younger than 10 years and more common with increasing age, particularly for males. Schizophrenia has been the most studied and appears to have a strong genetic component. Psychotic symptoms occur more commonly as manifestations of other disorders such as depression and anxiety (Volkmar, 1996). Psychotic symptoms can be difficult to identify accurately in children due to their developmental stage and abilities. Children and adolescents who are chronically psychotic tend to be significantly thought disordered. Those with schizophrenia tend to be predominately male, and the disorder has an insidious onset, with severe negative symptoms and greater cognitive impairments. Youth who have a psychotic disorder commonly have comorbid disorders such as substance abuse, ADHD, ODD, depression, and anxiety (AACAP, 2001; Masi et al., 2006). Some longitudinal studies indicate that youth with childhood-onset schizophrenia remain impaired in adolescence but are no longer psychotic. Treatment should be multidimensional and target all areas of the child's life. Interventions generally include pharmacotherapy, psychoeducation, psychotherapy, educational modifications, and rehabilitation. Atypical antipsychotics are the first choice for medications, with some controlled studies demonstrating efficiency. Youth appear to be more treatment refractory than adults. Schizophrenia is a chronic disorder that tends to be more severe and treatment resistant the earlier in life it occurs. Although the data are limited, children and adolescents who develop schizophrenia tend to become impaired adults.

Mood Disorders

Children and adolescents are diagnosed with mood disorders using the same criteria as for adults (Chapter 11), though there are some minor developmental modifications. Most investigators believe that multiple interactive factors lead to depressive disorders such as genetic predisposition, environmental stressors, and biologic concomitants. Children and adolescents with major depressive disorder appear to have specific biologic and anatomical abnormalities, many of which are similar to those found in adults with major depressive disorder (AACAP, 1998; Zalsman et al., 2006). Research suggests that there may be significant differences between those who are depressed before puberty and those who become ill as adolescents. Environmental factors appear to be a primary influence in prepubertal depression whereas genetic issues appear to be more significant in adolescents. Common comorbid disorders include disruptive behavior disorders, ADHD, and anxiety disorders. Many have multiple comorbid diagnoses. Suicidal ideation and behavior are frequently the issues.

Bipolar disorders appear to have a genetic etiology, and studies have found more psychopathology in families of affected youth, with younger affected children being more likely to have bipolar relatives. Neuroimaging studies of bipolar youth have revealed various structural and physiologic abnormalities (Pavuluri et al., 2005). There is considerable debate about what bipolar disorder looks like in prepubertal children. The DSM-IV criteria for mania were developed from adult data and do not consider developmental differences. Bipolar youth often present with mixed symptoms characterized by frequent short periods of intense mood lability and irritability rather than classic euphoric mania. Most bipolar children and adolescents have another psychiatric disorder, most often ADHD, anxiety disorders, ODD, and CD (AACAP, 2007).

The psychosocial management of children and adolescents with mood disorders, both depressive and bipolar, should be multifocal. Possible psychotherapeutic interventions include behavioral, familial, psychotherapeutic, environmental, and pharmaceutical strategies. Family, cognitive behavioral, interpersonal, and dialectical behavior therapies have been studied and found effective. Medication is generally not adequate as the sole intervention. SSRIs are considered the first line of treatment for depression; several controlled trials have shown them to be effective in children and adolescents (Moreno et al., 2006). Open-label studies, case reports, and a few controlled studies of mood stabilizers and antipsychotics have suggested that these medications are effective in treating children and adolescents with bipolar disorders (Kowatch et al., 2005). The limited data about the outcome of children and adolescents with mood disorders indicate that a high number of them continue to have symptomatic periods with a high rate of relapse after recovery. A significant number, particularly those with adolescent onset of these disorders, will remain symptomatic in adulthood.

Anxiety Disorders

Anxiety disorders are common in children and adolescents who are diagnosed using the same criteria as for adults (Chapter 12) with some minor modifications for some of the disorders. Children and adolescents with one anxiety disorder often have another one, as well as problems with mood, learning, and attention (AACAP, 2007). Genetic factors appear to be influential; youth with anxiety have significantly more anxious relatives. For generalized anxiety disorder (GAD), children and adolescents only have to have one somatic symptom during anxiety episodes instead of the three required for adults. The diagnosis of panic disorder can be difficult to make due to normal developmental fear responses to novel situations and the occurrence of panic attacks in other anxiety disorders. The same diagnostic criteria for phobias are used for children, adolescents, and adults, with some minor modifications. The criterion of recognizing the fear as

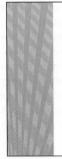

Clinical Characteristics of Separation Anxiety Disorder

- Anxiety concerning separation from home or major attachment figures
- Three or more symptoms related to excessive distress or worry associated with separation from, anticipated separation from, or harm to major attachment figures
- Duration of at least 4 weeks; onset before age 18
- Excessive and developmentally inappropriate; impairment
- Not another psychiatric disorder

unreasonable is dropped for young children, and the duration of these symptoms only needs to be 6 months for children.

Separation anxiety disorder and selective mutism are mostly diagnosed in children and adolescents. Separation anxiety disorder is characterized by developmentally inappropriate anxiety and excessive fear during real or anticipated separations from the home environment or primary attachment figures. Some separation anxiety is a normal response in children. However, children with normal levels of anxiety will tend to accommodate to novel situations after a variable amount of time. Children with separation anxiety disorder will instead experience persistent and excessive anxiety over the separation, which generally leads to consistent functional impairment. Although the remission rate is high, the course of this disorder tends to wax and wane, with symptoms recurring after stressful life events and times of transition. Selective mutism is diagnosed when a child fails to speak in specific social situations where speech is expected. Children with this diagnosis are reported to speak freely at home, may speak less to family and friends socially, and are often mute when speaking situation with adults at school and with strangers in public. The onset of the illness is often in the preschool years but may not be a problem until a child begins kindergarten.

The level of functional impairment or distress dictates the interventions for anxiety disorders. Minor, transient symptoms may not require any treatment and warrant only education and observation. Mild to moderate symptoms should first be treated with psychotherapeutic and environmental interventions. Methods with the greatest empirical support are educational, behavioral, and cognitive behavioral interventions. Medication for these disorders should be an adjunct to psychotherapeutic interventions. SSRIs are the first-line agents for all anxiety disorders. Various agents have been found to be helpful in clinical trials involving children and adolescents with various anxiety disorders. Having a childhood anxiety disorder increases the risk of having an anxiety disorder or other psychiatric disorders in adulthood.

Obsessive-Compulsive Disorder

Most individuals with OCD have the onset of their symptoms before age 18 (AACAP, 1997c; Geller, 2006). Twin and family studies indicate a strong genetic component. Increasing evidence indicates that OCD and TS may share a common genetic etiology. Pediatric autoimmune neuropsychiatric disorder associated with streptococcal infections (PANDAS) is a syndrome in which OCD and tics develop in association with a streptococcal infection. There is some debate about whether this disorder is valid. Children and adolescents are diagnosed with OCD using the same DSM-IV-TR criteria as for adults (Chapter 12), with some minor modifications. Insight into the excessiveness and unrealistic nature of obsessions and compulsions is not a requirement to make the diagnosis in children. The most commonly observed comorbid conditions include tic and anxiety disorders and depression. Other comorbid conditions are LD, language disorders, ADHD, ODD, eating disorders, and trichotillomania. The recommended treatment is CBT alone or in combination with an SSRI. Comorbid psychiatric disorders also should be treated. It appears that a number of children with OCD do not continue to have the full disorder into adolescence or adulthood.

Posttraumatic Stress Disorder

Youth primarily experience interpersonal types of trauma and most commonly are exposed to war, child maltreatment, domestic abuse, and community violence. The rates of posttraumatic stress disorder (PTSD) in children and adolescents are thought to be similar to or higher than in adults, given that youth appear more vulnerable to PTSD. Youth are diagnosed with these disorders using the same criteria as for adults, with some minor modifications (Chapter 12). These children and adolescents have high rates of mood, anxiety, and disruptive disorders, with adolescents also having substance use disorders. Traumatized youth require multidimensional treatment that targets the issues and symptoms related to the trauma and that intervenes with any comorbid medical or psychiatric disorders, psychosocial issues, and environmental situations. Psychological debriefing, CBT, and therapies utilizing the relationship between the child and caretakers have been adapted to treat youth with PTSD. SSRIs are the most commonly used medications and appear to be effective (AACAP, 1998).

Disorders with Physical Symptoms

Unexplainable physical symptoms are common in children and adolescents; they tend to be identified in medical settings after receiving a workup that demonstrates no obvious organic disease. In this category are somatoform disorders, psychological factors affecting a medical condition, factitious disorders, and malingering. Children and adolescents are diagnosed using the adult DSM criteria (Chapter 13). Data suggest that unexplained childhood physical symptoms predict emotional disorders in adults. Most studies have examined the presence or absence of a physical symptom rather than functional or psychiatric status. Conversion disorder has been studied the most in children and adolescents. It most commonly presents in school-age patients. The course is thought to be brief, and most resolve. Children and adolescents often do not have the symptom duration or variability to meet the criteria for somatization disorder, though they may meet the criteria for undifferentiated somatoform disorder. Hypochondriasis and pain disorder have not been well studied in children and adolescents. There has been no systemic study of body dysmorphic disorder in children and adolescents, though some data indicate that the onset for many individuals occurs in adolescence. Symptoms in youth appear to be similar to those in adults. Factitious disorder, also termed *Munchausen syndrome*, has been described in the pediatric literature, though more attention has been devoted to the proxy form. There is little information on factitious disorders in youth. In the proxy form, a caretaker of an individual is producing or falsely reporting symptoms in that individual. It is considered a medically focused type of child abuse. Older children and adolescents may collude actively with their caretakers. Morbidity and mortality can occur as a result of the caretaker's actions or the physicians' interventions. The outcome of factitious disorder by proxy has been described as variable, depending on severity of the symptoms and the treatment provided. There is little literature or data on malingering in youth in medical situations. The child or adolescent must be deliberately lying about or producing the symptoms with the knowledge that he or she is not ill and the objective of obtaining some benefit or avoiding some aversive situation. The inducement is not related to the perceived benefits of being sick. Generally, malingerers tend to feign symptoms rather than produce disease or injury. There are case reports in the literature involving parents instructing their children to malinger (malingering by proxy) for financial and other reasons.

It is essential to design a treatment plan that includes coordination and collaboration among medical providers, the family, the patient, and other involved organizations. Often other agencies need to be involved such as schools, child protective services, the juvenile justice system, and other community institutions. Various forms of psychotherapies, psychosocial interventions, and supportive medical care (e.g., physical therapy) can be helpful. Medication may be appropriate for specific psychiatric symptoms and body dysmorphic disorder (Dingle, 2005).

Dissociative Disorders

Considerable controversy exists about whether children and adolescents can have dissociative disorders. There is consensus that significant dissociative symptoms can occur in children and adolescents, usually as a response to trauma. Many deem it more appropriate to consider dissociation as a symptom of other disorders rather than a separate disorder. The same criteria used to diagnose adults with these disorders are used for children and adolescents (Chapter 14). Most of the literature has been on dissociative identity disorder; there have been case reports on depersonalization disorder, dissociative amnesia, and dissociative fugue. All of the children and adolescents had histories of trauma. Some investigators argue that the DSM criteria are not applicable and have developed more developmentally sensitive diagnostic standards. Treatment emphasizes establishing a safe environment, replacing dissociation with other strategies to manage stress, and educating and supporting the caretakers (Silberg, 2000).

Sexual and Gender Identity Disorders

The same criteria used to diagnose adults with sexual and gender identity disorders are used for children and adolescents (Chapter 15). Most research and clinical practice have involved patients who have gender identity issues or disorders. Boys are referred for treatment more than girls. Various etiologic factors have been explored, both psychological and biological. Treatment recommendations emphasize helping the child cope with associated problems, educating and supporting the parents, and treating any other psychiatric disorders. Currently, there is controversy about whether gender identity disorder is an actual diagnosis. Some advocate for its removal from DSM-V and argue that only a small number of children with gender identity disorder persist in the desire to be the opposite sex as they become older. Most of them resolve their gender identity issues and have a homosexual or bisexual orientation in adolescence and adulthood (Zucker, 2004).

Eating Disorders

Adult concerns about the eating habits of children and adolescents are common. In early childhood, this concern focuses on the toddler's habit of periodically eating only select foods, changing preferences frequently, and eating different amounts daily. In later childhood and adolescence, the concern relates to the amount of "junk" food eaten and preferences to eat only certain meals or at nonmeal times. Eating disorders are relatively uncommon, but problematic eating behaviors are not. Many youth voice concern about their weight and engage in various behaviors in an attempt to be thin. In addition to adolescent females, increasing numbers of males and school-aged children are affected. A number of children and adolescents have subclinical syndromes and other types of eating problems such as food avoidance emotional disorder, selective eating, and phobias related to eating. In the United States, many children and adolescents have eating habits that lead them to be significantly overweight. Problematic family patterns and relationships are often found in these conditions (Waller, 2005). Eating disorders and obesity in children and adolescents are diagnosed using the same criteria as those used with adults (Chapter 16). Youth with these disorders demonstrate similar behaviors, attitudes, and problems as adults. For many affected children and adolescents, treatment has been more successful with family involvement (Zametkin et al., 2004).

Sleep Disorders

Concerns and complaints about the quality and quantity of sleep in youth are quite common. Sleep abnormalities can be indicative of a primary sleep disorder or associated with psychiatric or medical disorders; however, they often are the result of developmental or lifestyle issues. Most childhood sleep problems are age specific and time limited. Multiple factors such as temperament, nutrition, physical discomfort, allergies, marital conflict, and parental psychopathology have been implicated. Family and cultural values and behaviors significantly determine and influence sleep habits.

DSM-IV-TR describes several sleep disorders with criteria applicable to children, adolescents, and adults (Chapter 17). The diagnostic criteria for some of these disorders do not fit children and adolescents well because they were developed on the basis of adult data. Also, some of the most common sleep problems of children and adolescents are not described in the DSM classification. One of the most commonly reported sleep disturbances is when infants, toddlers, or preschoolers have difficulty going to sleep and staying asleep unless parents are present. The child associates parental contact and interaction with sleeping and has not developed adequate skills to go to sleep on his or her own or is not using them. Another frequent sleep difficulty is due to inadequate limit setting and parental structure around helping children and adolescents go to bed (Meltzer and Mindell, 2006).

Dyssomnias

Insomnia is a common complaint and usually is secondary to another psychiatric disorder, a medical condition, a medication, stress, environmental issues, or changes in routines. Hypersomnia, excessive sleeping, can occur in children and adolescents, usually in association with depression.

Interventions should be targeted toward the underlying problems. Narcolepsy often begins in late adolescence and may be underdiagnosed in childhood. Stimulants and modafinil are used to manage the sleepiness. Cataplexy is treated with clomipramine and monoamine oxidase inhibitors (MAOIs). The most common cause of breathing-related sleep disorder (obstructive sleep apnea) in children and adolescents is hypertrophy of the tonsils and adenoids. Depending on the etiology, recommendations include surgery and weight loss. Some children may require supplemental oxygen and noninvasive ventilatory support. Protriptyline has benefited adults, but there are no data on its use in children. Circadian rhythm sleep disorder commonly occurs in adolescents who preferentially stay up late, do not get enough sleep during the week, and then sleep late on the weekends. The adolescent then is unable to fall asleep at the assigned bedtime during the week or get up at the expected time in the morning. The adolescent is tired during the day and often takes an afternoon nap. This condition can last for years; medications tend to be ineffective. Treatment consists of developing a consistent and appropriate routine and schedule. If behavioral strategies are ineffective, chronotherapy can be done.

Parasomnias

Nightmares occur in approximately 50% of children between ages 3 and 6 and are part of normal development. Nightmare disorder is diagnosed when nightmares occur frequently enough to affect functioning, primarily through sleep deprivation and anxiety. Limiting certain types of media can be helpful in addition to implementing reassuring routines that target the child's concerns. Discussing nightmares during the daylight can be useful. A significant number of all children have at least one night terror, with a smaller number having two to three per week. This phenomenon is more common in boys. Up to 75% of affected children have first-degree relatives with night terrors or sleepwalking. Children with night terrors should just be observed and monitored for safety. There is no evidence that sleep terrors are associated with psychopathology, and they usually resolve by adolescence. All children are likely to have at least one episode of sleepwalking, and some have more frequent episodes. There appears to be a genetic contribution. Onset usually is between ages 6 and 8, with a peak at approximately 12 years of age and then resolution in adolescence. Sleep terrors and sleepwalking may be comorbid; they are thought to share common genetic and neurophysiological characteristics.

For most sleep disorders, behavioral management and environmental manipulation are essential aspects of treatment. Having consistent evening schedules and routines are key to developing appropriate sleep hygiene. There are no good data on medication, especially for long-term use. Medications that have been used include antihistamines, benzodiazepines, chloral hydrate, clonidine, and melatonin. Medications developed to treat adult sleep problems have been given to youth, but no studies have been done on their use.

Impulse-Control Disorders Not Elsewhere Classified

Intermittent Explosive Disorder

DSM-IV-TR criteria for intermittent explosive disorder (IED) are the same for children, adolescents, and adults (Chapter 18). There is limited information on this disorder in children and adolescents; a preliminary study indicates that they have a high rate of mood and other symptoms. Adult data indicate that many patients report the onset of IED in childhood or adolescence (Olvera et al., 2001).

Trichotillomania

Individuals with trichotillomania exhibit recurrent hair pulling from their bodies that causes noticeable hair loss. Most of the literature on affected children and adolescents consists of case reports. The incidence appears to be higher in children (reported to be 1%) than adolescents and adults. Possible medical etiologies should be ruled out, and comorbid psychiatric conditions are common. The literature suggests that behavioral management is the most successful intervention, with some positive reports from SSRI use (Bruce et al., 2005).

Personality Disorders

Personality disorder diagnoses (Chapter 20) are used sparingly for patients younger than 18 years because personality development is not considered to be complete. Much debate exists about

---

Clinical Characteristics of Trichotillomania

- Recurrently pulling out hair with noticeable hair loss
- Increasing sense of tension before pulling or when attempting to resist
- Pleasure, gratification, or relief when pulling
- Not due to another psychiatric disorder or medical condition
- Causes significant distress or impairment

---

the diagnosis of these disorders in youth due to the developmental insensitivity of DSM criteria, ongoing developmental changes during childhood, the lack of empirical data supporting the validity and reliability of these diagnoses, and the associated stigma. Some practitioners think that youth can be appropriately diagnosed with these disorders when they demonstrate inflexible, maladaptive, and chronic patterns of coping and interacting. Children and adolescents can be diagnosed with any of the personality disorders except antisocial personality disorder, which specifically requires the patient to be an adult. Borderline personality disorder has been the most studied; these patients demonstrate problems in multiple arenas (Sharp and Bleiberg, 2007).

OTHER CLINICAL CONDITIONS OR SITUATIONS

Early Childhood

Examining and understanding infant mental health to promote healthy development is an area of intense research and clinical interest. Although DSM-IV-TR criteria for psychiatric disorders can be used to diagnose disorders in this age-group, the criteria are often difficult to apply. Other classification models have been developed that emphasize infant–caregiver relationships, infant self-regulatory characteristics, and environmental variables. Prematurity, infant or caretaker illness, poor match between infant and caretaker, neglectful or abusive parenting behavior, lack of resources, unsupportive environments, and extreme deprivation increase the likelihood that infants will have difficulty. Prenatal exposure to drugs of abuse, alcohol, tobacco, and prescribed medications may be a significant risk factor for later physical, cognitive, or behavioral abnormalities. It is also essential to consider the effect of the environment upon the infant's postnatal development, given the very problematic caretaking that tends to be associated with drug use (Talmi and Harmon, 2005).

Family Constellations

A significant number of children and adolescents grow up in families that are not the traditional model of biological parents. Many youth are raised by single parents, extended family members, adopted parents, homosexual parents, or parents of a different race. Children and adolescents who originally were in traditional households can experience other family constellations due to parental death, divorce, dating, and remarriage. Regardless of the family organization, children and adolescents generally do well if the environment is stable and nurturing. Divorce is best conceived as a process with changes and stages that can occur over many years. The best predictor of how children will do after divorce is the level of conflict in the parental relationship. Adjustment is dependent upon several variables, though having reliable parents or adult mentors appears to be important. The vast majority of adopted children thrive, though they appear to have a higher risk for psychopathology depending on their genetic background, prenatal and early childhood medical care, early life experience, and temperament match with their adoptive parents. In general, children adopted at a later age tend to have more problems. Children adopted by single parents, homosexual couples, or individuals of a different race do not appear to have any more problems than others if the parents are good caregivers and there is attention and support around potential issues. Youth in single-parent households have a higher risk for a range of difficulties; in general, single-parent families tend to be poorer and have limited social support (Schor, 2003; Kelly, 2003; Nickman et al., 2005).

Bereavement

Most children and adolescents will experience the death of someone important to them during childhood. Many symptoms of grief and bereavement overlap with those of depression. Children vary in their understanding of death, depending upon their prior personal experience and cognitive levels. However, even very young children recognize when close caretakers are missing or distressed. How children and adolescents cope with the death of someone close depends on how well they were prepared, the ability of their caretakers to be supportive and cope, the opportunities for open, healthy grieving, and the stability of their environment. Children and adolescents should be told about the death and what will happen to the body in a developmentally appropriate manner that is consistent with the family's religious and cultural beliefs. Most youth benefit from participating in the funeral or remembrance ceremony as long as there has been adequate preparation and a supportive adult is also in attendance. Children and adolescents generally do not need psychiatric treatment for simple bereavement. Significant losses may exacerbate existing psychological or psychiatric problems or precipitate the onset of such problems. Children and adolescents may need help adjusting to the death and accompanying changes in their lives (Swick and Rauch, 2006).

Homosexuality

Most gay and lesbian individuals are aware of their sexual orientation in adolescence. They may experience considerable distress and problems related to the stigma associated with being homosexual. Studies have found that homosexual youth have problems with physical and mental health, sexual risk-taking, running away, truancy, and drug use. Psychiatric assessment and therapy are focused on helping adolescents work through any issues related to their sexual orientation and treating any psychiatric disorders (Carter and Herbert, 2005).

Violence

Many children and adolescents have exhibited violent behavior by age 17, and homicide remains a major cause of death for adolescents and young adults, particularly minority males. Children and adolescents exhibit a range of aggressive behaviors from bullying to murder. Youth generally become violent in adolescence; those who start in childhood tend to be more severe. Both types appear to start with less severe crimes and progress to more severe, violent crimes. Most of these youth do not continue to be violent in adulthood. Relevant influences include poor parenting, substance abuse, and peer relationships. There is increasing evidence that genetic factors are important, though the risk appears to result from the interaction of a genetic vulnerability with adverse environmental influences. Some clinicians and researchers consider it most useful to classify aggressive behavior along the characteristics of impulsive/reactive and predatory/proactive. In addition to CD, many of these children and adolescents have other psychiatric disorders. Psychiatric symptoms that often are associated with aggression include impairments in impulse control, affective reactivity, and management of anxiety. Psychiatric care emphasizes identification and treatment of any identifiable psychiatric disorders. Successful psychosocial interventions have focused on family and parent training and increasing environmental support and structure. Many psychotropic medications have been used to manage aggression with variable results (Snyder and Sickmund, 2006; Jensen et al., 2007).

Studies of adult sex offenders indicate that a significant number of them started offending before age 18. Adolescent sex offenders and violent, nonsexual adolescent offenders appear to share the same characteristics of poor social skills, previous delinquent behavior, psychopathology, low academic performance, and poor impulse control. Many, but not all, have histories of being sexually or physically abused. They tend to come from families with significant problems including domestic violence and instability. Interventions include identifying and treating any psychiatric disorders, working to improve self-control and empathy, developing socially appropriate behaviors and coping strategies, and reinforcing appropriate sexual behavior (AACAP, 1999).

Problematic Parenting

Families with child or parental psychopathology tend to have parenting problems. There is consensus that the relationship between parents and children is a reciprocal one, with children's difficulties influencing parental behavior and vice versa. Parenting attitudes and approaches have multiple determinants, both genetic and environmental. Two global domains of parenting have been evaluated: parental warmth and parental control. Warmth refers to the ability of the parent to be nurturing, supportive, emotionally sensitive, and available. Control is defined as the ability of the parent to provide appropriate discipline: teaching children to follow the rules, setting consistent and appropriate limits, having age-appropriate expectations, and monitoring activities and location. Adolescents with parents who are adequate in both areas were better adjusted than those with parents who had problems in either or both areas. Research on the parenting practices of psychiatrically ill parents has found that they tend to be less skilled, sensitive, and child focused. The child's functioning appeared to be more related to the parenting skills than the severity of the parent's illness. Families with a psychiatrically ill parent or child tend to have dysfunctional parenting exemplified by negativity and ineffective discipline. Interventions have emphasized identifying and treating the psychopathology and parenting education (Berg-Nielson et al., 2002).

Suicide

Suicide is the third leading cause of death for youth in the ages 10 to 19, with most of them being male and with Native Americans having the highest rate. Children and adolescents exhibit suicidal behavior along a continuum of ideation, attempts, and suicide. Clinically, it is generally best to consider self-injurious ideas or behaviors as potentially suicidal and intervene to ensure safety. Approximately 90% of children and adolescents who have committed suicide had a psychiatric disorder, with most having mood disorders, many having substance abuse, and a significant number having both. The major risk factor for suicide for adolescent males is a prior attempt; for females it is a current diagnosis of major depressive disorder. In addition to identifying any psychiatric disorders and determining relevant risk and protective factors, assessment focuses on current and past suicidal behavior, plans, access to methods, alternative coping strategies, and family response and capabilities. Treatment emphasizes safety, repeated reassessment, psychiatric treatment, and therapy that includes exploring and dealing with the suicidal behavior (AACAP, 2001).

High-Risk Behavior

Engaging in high-risk behaviors is frequent in adolescence, and psychiatrically ill youth have higher rates than typical teens. Some degree of risk taking appears to be part of normal development, but a number of youth are excessively involved in such behaviors with significant degrees of morbidity and mortality. Possible problematic activities include drug use beyond experimentation, repeated unprotected sex, reckless driving, and stunts or extreme physical activities. Participation in one type appears to increase the likelihood of participating in others. Most of these youth are not aiming to hurt themselves or others. Associated psychiatric symptoms include impulsivity, affective instability, mania, depression, irritability, anxious hyperarousal, and cognitive disorganization. Assessment of these behaviors should include suicide intent, substance use, and psychiatric symptoms (Mullen and Hendren, 2005).

Abuse and Neglect

Child maltreatment remains a major public health problem in the United States. In 2005, an estimated 899,000 children and adolescents were victims of abuse or neglect (substantiated by child protective services), and 3.6 million children and adolescents were investigated by child protective services. Most (more than 60%) were neglected. Approximately 17% were physically abused, and approximately 9% were sexually abused. Definitions of neglect and abuse vary among states, though generally neglect is when caretakers fail to adequately provide for and protect children, physical abuse involves the intentional injury of a child by a caretaker, and sexual abuse refers to sexual behavior between a child and an adult. Children and adolescents often experience more than one form of maltreatment. Abuse and neglect often occur in situations where domestic violence and parental substance abuse are occurring. These children and adolescents are at high risk for multiple forms of psychopathology and poor functioning. Interventions have focused on treatment for individual children and adolescents as well as efforts targeted at prevention, prosecution of perpetrators, improving the family's functioning, and improving the foster care system to promote stable, single placements (AACAP, 2007).

CONCLUSION AND FUTURE DIRECTIONS

Working with children and adolescents who experience adversity or have psychiatric conditions is challenging but rewarding. Expanding knowledge and information on the characteristics of child and adolescent psychiatric disorders and possible treatments are providing increased options for successful identification and interventions with these children, adolescents, and families. This increased body of knowledge is also enhancing the understanding of psychopathology and therapy in adults.

Clinical Pearls

- Diagnosing and treating psychiatric disorders in children and adolescents require a thorough and comprehensive understanding of normal development.
- Assessment and treatment of children and adolescents require information from and the involvement of their caretakers and other significant adults/systems.
- Inattention, abnormal activity levels, distractibility, oppositional behavior, and developmentally inappropriate behavior occur in many psychiatric disorders in children and adolescents.
- The psychiatric treatment of children and adolescents should include psychotherapeutic and environmental interventions and may include medication.
- Treatment should target all domains of functioning.
- The use of medication should be carefully considered, with significant attention paid to the benefit/risk ratio.
- Many children and adolescents with psychiatric disorders will continue to have disorders in adulthood.

Self-Assessment Questions and Answers

7-1. The parents of a 9-year-old boy bring him for a psychiatric evaluation with concerns that he is excessively active, rarely listens to his teachers, does not complete his schoolwork, and is very distractible and impulsive. He has behaved this way at home and school since age 4. The psychiatrist does not find any comorbid conditions during the evaluation. Which of the following is essential to make this child's diagnosis?

A. Classroom observation of the child
B. Clinical interview of parents and child
C. Computer-based test of impulse control
D. Psychological testing of the child
E. Self-report measures completed by the child

Obtaining information from a variety of sources and informants is important, and testing, observation, and self-reports can be helpful, but attention-deficit/hyperactivity disorder is a diagnosis made clinically. *Answer: B*

7-2. For several months, an 8-year-old girl has been having episodes of prolonged crying and sobbing when reprimanded for misbehavior. Additionally, she has been refusing to go to bed at night, insisting that she is not tired and that the light stay on. Her parents are mystified because she is generally a well-behaved child whose infractions are minor. She is doing well academically and socially. During the psychiatric interview, the child admits that she sees something in her bedroom closet. She perceives the figure as threatening and is convinced that it wants to take her away because she is a bad person. Her thought processes are linear, organized, and coherent. The girl is *most* likely to be

A. Anxious
B. Defiant
C. Inattentive
D. Oppositional
E. Psychotic

Isolated psychotic symptoms such as hallucinations are common in children with anxiety disorders. It is unlikely that she is psychotic because she is doing well academically and socially and is not thought disordered. There is no information indicating that she is argumentative, defiant, or inattentive. *Answer: A*

7-3. During a psychiatric assessment of an 8-year-old boy for behavior problems, he reveals that he has witnessed his stepfather hit his mother. Of the following, which must be explored before ending the evaluation session?

A. Association of his behavior to this trauma
B. Extent of his mother's injury and suffering
C. His mother's reaction to being physically abused
D. Possibility of child abuse and neglect
E. Symptoms of posttraumatic stress disorder

Domestic violence is a significant risk factor for child maltreatment. Although the other options are important and should be assessed, child maltreatment should be evaluated immediately because it is a safety issue. *Answer: D*

7-4. The parents of a 10-year-old boy bring him for treatment of chronic tics because they believe that his peers will start rejecting him soon because of his twitches and abnormal behavior. During the assessment, it becomes clear that the boy is very inattentive, overactive, and distractible. Additional history reveals that his teachers have been complaining about similar behavior since he started school and that he is frequently in trouble for not completing his work, listening to the teacher, or taking turns and interrupting others and cutting in line. His teachers have repeatedly told his parents that his grades would be better if his behavior were not so disruptive. Of the following, which is the best treatment recommendation?

A. Explain that tics improve in adolescence for many individuals so the best strategy is observation and monitoring.
B. Review medication options and start clonidine, given the cognitive effects of atypical antipsychotics.
C. Explain that no medications induce remission so it would be better to try habit-reversal training.
D. Explain that attentional issues are more problematic and that a stimulant should be started first.

E. Review his adjustment and social issues and the family's distress and suggest family therapy.

Often, the comorbid conditions associated with Tourette syndrome (TS) are more impairing than the tics and should be treated first. This child appears to have TS and attention-deficit/hyperactivity disorder (ADHD); the ADHD appears to be significantly impairing his functioning. His academic and social difficulties are probably mostly related to his ADHD. Individuals with tic disorders can be treated with stimulants effectively, with variable effects on the tics. Once the ADHD is under control, the effect of the tics could be assessed and treated, if necessary. *Answer: D*

7-5. A 16-year-old girl is diagnosed with moderate major depressive disorder. Her family and friends are supportive. She is cooperative and agrees that she needs treatment, though she is pessimistic, because she believes that depression is punishment for not being a good person. Given the severity of the depression, it is decided to start her on fluoxetine and therapy. Of the following, which is the most appropriate psychotherapeutic intervention?

A. Behavioral management
B. Cognitive behavioral therapy
C. Dialectical behavior therapy
D. Family therapy
E. Interpersonal therapy

For depressed adolescents, both interpersonal therapy (IPT) and cognitive behavioral therapy (CBT) have demonstrated effectiveness. In this scenario the girl seems to have significant cognitive distortions about her illness, making CBT the best choice. IPT would be more appropriate if the depression is related to interpersonal issues. Family therapy and behavioral interventions do not seem to be indicated at this point because the family is supportive and the girl is cooperative. The girl is not described as having the behaviors for which dialectical behavior therapy is generally used. Currently, research indicates that SSRIs are the first choice for pharmacological treatment of adolescent depression, and fluoxetine has FDA approval for the treatment of depression in adolescents. *Answer: B*

References

AACAP. AACAP practice parameters for the assessment and treatment of children and adolescents with conduct disorder. *J Am Acad Child Adolesc Psychiatry*. 1997a;36:4S–25S.

AACAP. AACAP practice parameters for the assessment and treatment of children and adolescents with substance use disorders. *J Am Acad Child Adolesc Psychiatry*. 1997b;36(Suppl):140S–156S.

AACAP. AACAP practice parameters for the assessment and treatment of children and adolescents with obsessive-compulsive disorder. *J Am Acad Child Adolesc Psychiatry*. 1997c;37:27S–45S.

AACAP. AACAP practice parameters for the assessment and treatment of children and adolescents with depressive disorders. *J Am Acad Child Adolesc Psychiatry*. 1998;37(Suppl 10):63S–83S.

AACAP. AACAP practice parameters for the assessment and treatment of children and adolescents with language and learning disorders. *J Am Acad Child Adolesc Psychiatry*. 1998;37(Suppl 10):46S–62S.

AACAP. AACAP practice parameters for the assessment and treatment of children, adolescents, and adults with mental retardation and comorbid mental disorders. *J Am Acad Child Adolesc Psychiatry*. 1999;38:1606–1610.

AACAP. AACAP practice parameters for the assessment and treatment of children, adolescents, and adults with autism and other pervasive developmental disorders. *J Am Acad Child Adolesc Psychiatry*. 1999;38(Suppl):32S–54S.

AACAP. AACAP practice parameters for the assessment and treatment of children and adolescents who are sexually abusive of others. *J Am Acad Child Adolesc Psychiatry*. 1999;38(12):55S–76S.

AACAP. AACAP practice parameters for assessment and treatment of children and adolescents with schizophrenia. *J Am Acad Child Adolesc Psychiatry*. 2001;40(Suppl 7):4S–23S.

AACAP. AACAP practice parameters for the assessment and treatment of children and adolescents with suicidal behavior. *J Am Acad Child Adolesc Psychiatry*. 2001;40(Suppl 7):24S–51S.

AACAP. AACAP practice parameters for the use of stimulant medications in the treatment of children, adolescents, and adults. *J Am Acad Child Adolesc Psychiatry*. 2002;41(Suppl 2):26S–49S.

AACAP. AACAP practice parameter for the assessment and treatment of children and adolescents with enuresis. *J Am Acad Child Adolesc Psychiatry*. 2004;43(12):1540–1550.

AACAP. AACAP practice parameters for the assessment and treatment of children and adolescents with reactive attachment disorder. *J Am Acad Child Adolesc Psychiatry*. 2005;44(11):1206–1219.

AACAP. AACAP practice parameters for the assessment and treatment of children and adolescents with bipolar disorder. *J Am Acad Child Adolesc Psychiatry*. 2007;46(1):107–125.

AACAP. AACAP practice parameters for the assessment and treatment of children and adolescents with oppositional defiant disorder. *J Am Acad Child Adolesc Psychiatry*. 2007;46(1):126–141.

AACAP. AACAP practice parameters for the assessment and treatment of children and adolescents with anxiety disorders. *J Am Acad Child Adolesc Psychiatry*. 2007;46(2):267–283.

AACAP. AACAP practice parameter for the assessment and treatment of children and adolescents with attention-deficit/hyperactivity disorder. *J Am Acad Child Adolesc Psychiatry*. 2007;46(7):894–921.

Abramowitz A. Developmental disabilities: Learning disorders. In: Sexson SB, ed. *Child and adolescent psychiatry*. Malden: Blackwell Science; 2005:79–90.

American Psychiatric Association. *Diagnostic and statistical manual of mental disorders, DSM-IV TR*, Text Revision. Washington, DC: American Psychiatric Association; 2000.

Berg-Nielson TS, Vikan A, Dhal A. Parenting related to child and parental psychopathology: A descriptive review of the literature. *Clin Child Psychol Psychiatry*. 2002;7(4):529–552.

Bruce TO, Barwick LW, Wright HH. Diagnosis and management of trichotillomania in children and adolescents. *Pediatr Drugs*. 2005;7(6):365–376.

Burke JD, Loeber R, Birmaher B. Oppositional defiant disorder and conduct disorder: A review of the past 10 years, part II. *J Am Acad Child Adolesc Psychiatry*. 2002;41:1275–1293.

Carter DR, Herbert S. Child and adolescent sexuality. In: Sexson SB, ed. *Child and adolescent psychiatry*. Malden: Blackwell Science; 2005:287–302.

Chatoor I. Feeding disorders in infants and toddlers: Diagnosis and treatment. *Child Adolesc Psychiatr Clin N Am*. 2002;11(2):163–183.

Davies D. *Child development: A practitioner's guide*. New York: The Guildford Press; 2004.

Dingle AD. Disorders with physical symptoms. In: Sexson SB, ed. *Child and adolescent psychiatry*. London: Blackwell Science; 2005.

Dingle AD, Lee DO. Strategic treatment planning and therapeutic interventions. In: Sexson SB, ed. *Child and adolescent psychiatry*. Malden: Blackwell Science; 2005:37–59.

Dulcan MK, ed. *Helping parents, youth, and teachers understand medications for behavioral and emotional problems*. Arlington: American Psychiatric Publishing; 2007.

Gaytan O, Giorgadze A, Croft S. Anxiety disorders. In: Sexson SB, ed. *Child and adolescent psychiatry*. London: Blackwell Publishing Ltd; 2005:113–131.

Geller D. Obsessive-compulsive and spectrum disorders in children and adolescents. *Psychiatr Clin North Am*. 2006;29(2):353–370.

Gemelli R. *Normal child and adolescent development*. Washington, DC: American Psychiatric Press; 1996.

Handen B, Gilchrist R. Practitioner review: Psychopharmacology in children and adolescents with mental retardation. *J Child Psychol Psychiatry*. 2006;47(9):871–882.

Hopper C, Riggs P. Substance use disorders. In: Martin A, Volkmar FR, eds. *Lewis's child and adolescent psychiatry: A comprehensive textbook*. Philadelphia: Lippincott Williams & Wilkins; 2007:615–624.

Jensen PS, Buitelaar J, Pandina GJ, et al. Management of psychiatric disorders in children and adolescents with atypical antipsychotics. *Eur Child Adolesc Psychiatry*. 2007;16:104–120.

Jensen P, Youngstrom E, Steiner H, et al. Consensus report on impulsive aggression as a symptom across diagnostic categories in child psychiatry: Implications for medication studies. *J Am Acad Child Adolesc Psychiatry*. 2007;46(3):309–322.

Kelly JB. Changing perspectives on children's adjustment following divorce: A view from the United States. *Childhood*. 2003;10(2):237–254.

Kim-Cohen J. Resilience and developmental psychopathology. *Child Adolesc Psychiatr Clin N Am*. 2007; 16(2):271–283.

King BH, Bostic JQ. An update on pharmacologic treatments for autism spectrum disorders. *Child Adolesc Psychiatr Clin N Am*. 2007;15(1):161–175.

King B, State M, Shah B, et al. Mental retardation: A review of the past 10 years. Part I. *J Am Acad Child Adolesc Psychiatry*. 1997;36:1656–1663.

Kowatch R, Fristad M, Birmaher B, et al. Treatment guidelines for children and adolescents with bipolar disorder. *J Am Acad Child Adolesc Psychiatry*. 2005;44:213–235.

Lee DO, Cummins TK. Psychiatric evaluation: Biomedical assessment. In: Sexson SB, ed. *Child and adolescent psychiatry*. Malden: Blackwell Science; 2005:31–36.

Lee DO, Gopalakrishnan D. Developmental disabilities: Mental retardation and pervasive developmental disorders. In: Sexson SB, ed. *Child and adolescent psychiatry*, 2nd ed. London: Blackwell Publishing Ltd; 2005:63–78.

Loeber R, Burke JD, Lahey BB, et al. Oppositional defiant disorder and conduct disorder: A review of the past 10 years, part I. *J Am Acad Child Adolesc Psychiatry*. 2000;39:1468–1484.

Masi G, Mucci M, Pari C. Children with schizophrenia: Clinical picture and pharmacological treatment. *CNS Drugs*. 2006;20(10):841–866.

Meltzer LJ, Mindell JA. Sleep and sleep disorders in children and adolescents. *Psychiatr Clin North Am*. 2006;29:1059–1076.

Mikkelsen EJ. Enuresis and encopresis: Ten years of progress. *J Am Acad Child Adolesc Psychiatry*. 2001; 40(10):1146–1158.

Moreno C, Roche AM, Greenhill LL. Pharmacotherapy of child and adolescent depression. *Child Adolesc Psychiatr Clin N Am*. 2006;15(4):977–998.

Mullen DJ, Hendren RL. Risk-taking and dangerous behavior in children and adolescents. In: Sexson SB, ed. *Child and adolescent psychiatry*. Malden: Blackwell Science; 2005:303–310.

Nickman SL, Rosenfeld AA, Fine P, et al. Children in adoptive families: Overview and update. *J Am Acad Child Adolesc Psychiatry*. 2005;44(10):987–995.

Olvera RL, Pliszka SR, Konyecsni WM, et al. Validation of the interview module for intermittent explosive disorder (M-IED) in children and adolescents: A pilot study. *Psychiatry Res*. 2001;101:259–267.

Pavuluri M, Birmaher B, Naylor M. Pediatric bipolar disorder: A review of the past 10 years. *J Am Acad Child Adolesc Psychiatry*. 2005;44:846–871.

Prince JB. Pharmacology of attention-deficit hyperactivity disorder in children and adolescents: Update on new stimulant preparations, atomoxetine, and novel treatments. *Child Adolesc Psychiatr Clin N Am*. 2007;15(1):13–50.

Rutter M, Kim-Cohen J, Maughan B. Continuities and discontinuities in psychopathology between childhood and adult life. *J Child Psychol Psychiatry*. 2006;47(3/4):276–295.

Schor EL. American Academy of Pediatrics Task Force on the Family. Family pediatrics: Report of the task force on the family. *Pediatrics*. 2003;111:1541–1571.

Sharp C, Bleiberg E. Personality disorders in children and adolescents. In: Martin A, Volkmar FR, eds. *Lewis's child and adolescent psychiatry: A comprehensive textbook*. Philadelphia: Lippincott Williams & Wilkins; 2007:680–691.

Silberg JL. Fifteen years of dissociation in maltreated children: Where do we go from here? *Child Maltreat*. 2000;5(2):119–136.

Snyder H, Sickmund M. *Juvenile offenders and victims: 2006 national report*. Washington, DC: Office of Juvenile Justice and Delinquency Prevention; 2006.

State M, King B, Dykens E. Mental retardation: A review of the past 10 years. Part II. *J Am Acad Child Adolesc Psychiatry*. 1997;36:1664–1671.

Stein DJ, Niehaus DJ, Seedat S, et al. Phenomenology of stereotypic movement disorder. *Psychiatr Ann*. 1998;28(6):307–312.

Stein DJ, Simeon D. Pharmacotherapy of stereotypic movement disorder. *Psychiatr Ann*. 1998;28(6):327–331.

Swain JE, Scahill L, Lombroso PJ, et al. Tourette syndrome and tic disorders: A decade of progress. *J Am Acad Child Adolesc Psychiatry*. 2007;46(8):947–968.

Swick SD, Rauch PK. Children facing the death of a parent: The experiences of a parent guidance program at the Massachusetts General Hospital Cancer Center. *Child Adolesc Psychiatr Clin N Am*. 2006;15(3):779–794.

Talmi A, Harmon RJ. Issues in infant psychiatry. In: Sexson SB, ed. *Child and adolescent psychiatry*. Malden: Blackwell Science; 2005:201–224.

Tanguay PE. Pervasive developmental disorders: A 10-year review. *J Am Acad Child Adolesc Psychiatry*. 2000;39(9):1079–1095.

Volkmar FR. Childhood and adolescent psychosis: A review of the past 10 years. *J Am Acad Child Adolesc Psychiatry*. 1996;35(7):843–851.

Waller D. Eating disorders. In: Sexson SB, ed. *Child and adolescent psychiatry*. Malden: Blackwell Science; 2005.

Wazana A, Bresnahan M, Kline J. The autism epidemic: Fact or artifact? *J Am Acad Child Adolesc Psychiatry*. 2007;46(6):721–730.

Zalsman G, Oquendo MA, Greenhill L, et al. Neurobiology of depression in children and adolescents. *Child Adolesc Psychiatr Clin N Am*. 2006;15(4):843–868.

Zametkin AJ, Zoon CK, Klein HW, et al. Psychiatric aspects of child and adolescent obesity: A review of the past 10 years. *J Am Acad Child Adolesc Psychiatry*. 2004;43(2):134–150.

Zucker K. Gender identity development and issues. *Child Adolesc Psychiatr Clin N Am*. 2004;13:551–568.

Dementia, Delirium, and Other Disorders Associated with Cognitive Impairment

Cognition is the information-handling aspect of higher mental functioning. It is a multifaceted activity resulting from the interaction of a number of discrete functions including attention and concentration, memory, language, visuospatial skills, praxis (the ability to carry out learned or skilled movements on command), gnosis (the ability to recognize, or associate meaning with, an object), calculating skills, and executive functions (e.g., planning, organization, proper sequencing, prioritizing, abstraction, and self-monitoring).

A number of neuropsychiatric illnesses are associated with cognitive dysfunction. The *Diagnostic and Statistical Manual of Mental Disorders,* Fourth Edition, Text Revision (DSM-IV-TR) (American Psychiatric Association, 2000), includes a section which focuses on delirium, dementia, and amnestic disorder. These disorders are conceptualized as abnormal deviations from a normal or abnormal cognitive baseline. The cognitive disorders are differentiated from developmental disorders such as mental retardation, which are present from early life onward and associated with an unchanging abnormal cognitive baseline.

It is crucial to recognize that the cognitive disorders feature cognitive impairment, as described in their diagnostic criteria, but are frequently associated with psychopathology as well. Psychiatrists are concerned about the cognitive dysfunction in these illnesses but are perhaps more concerned about anxiety, mood problems, psychosis, personality changes, behavioral problems, and other forms of psychopathology that can accompany cognitive impairment.

Cognitive disorders are very common, especially in the elderly and the medically ill, and place a tremendous economic burden on society. In 2000, an estimated 4.5 million Americans had Alzheimer disease (AD), the most common cause of the syndrome of dementia, and given the rapid growth of the elderly population, an estimated 13.2 million Americans will have AD by 2050. In 2005, it cost over $315 billion to care for the world's 29.3 million people with dementia. Preventing delirium has been shown to significantly decrease health care costs. Diagnosing and treating patients with cognitive disorders are challenging for psychiatrists and other physicians, and alleviating patient suffering and containing health care costs require a good understanding of these disorders.

ASSESSING COGNITION

The cognitive examination is analogous to the physical and general mental status examinations in that it is done to some extent informally, before and during the patient interview. For example, an examiner may note during an interview that a patient with attentional impairment is easily distracted by stimuli in the area. Problems with memory, such as rapidly forgetting things said by the examiner, and problems with language, such as word-finding problems, may also be apparent during an interview. The cognitive examination is also like the physical and general mental status examinations in that informal observations can be supplemented with more formal testing, and the extent of this testing can be tailored to a specific clinical situation. Not all patients need detailed cognitive testing. Cognitive examination should be routine in patients at risk for the cognitive disorders discussed in this chapter. The aged and the medically ill are the groups at highest risk for cognitive dysfunction; therefore, detailed cognitive testing is most often done with these groups.

A number of tests easily administered in the office and at the hospital bedside have been utilized over the years to examine cognition. Normative data established by population testing are not available for many tests, but they can provide a good approximation of a patient's cognitive functioning.

Brief attention can be evaluated by testing a patient's digit span, or ability to repeat a series of numbers. Patients are verbally given a series of numbers at the rate of one per second and asked to repeat the numbers. Testing usually begins with a series of two numbers and progresses upward until the patient fails the task. If a patient cannot repeat more than three digits, this definitely suggests inattention; digit spans of four to five are borderline, and spans of six or greater suggest normal brief attention.

Recent verbal memory can be roughly assessed by asking a patient to remember four unrelated words. Spontaneous recall can be tested at 5, 10, and 30 minutes, and normative data are available for this test. Normal people younger than 60 years remember a mean of approximately three words at 5 minutes, and older than 60 years, about two (Strub and Black, 2000). If a patient cannot remember a word spontaneously, his or her response to cues, or hints, can help differentiate between a memory encoding deficit (i.e., no memory is formed, so cues do not help) and a memory retrieval deficit (i.e., memories are formed but cannot be retrieved without a cue).

Recent nonverbal memory can be assessed by hiding five objects in different locations in a room and then asking the patient for the location of the objects after 5 minutes. Patients younger than 60 years should remember the locations of four to five objects, and older than 60 years, three to four (Strub and Black, 2000).

Language testing examines several subdomains. Verbal comprehension can be assessed by giving patients increasingly difficult commands that they are physically able to carry out (e.g., "touch your nose"; "stick out your tongue, and then point to your stomach"), and reading comprehension can be evaluated by testing patients' abilities to carry out a written command. Language repetition ability should be assessed by giving the patient phrases of increasing length to repeat. Naming abilities can be tested by asking a patient to name objects in the immediate environment or in pictures. Writing can be assessed by asking patients to write a short sentence.

Patients' visuospatial skills can be assessed by asking them to copy increasingly difficult line drawings such as a circle, two overlapping polygons, and a cube. Praxis is tested by giving patients a command to carry out some learned movement (e.g., "show me how you blow out a match"; "show me how you comb your hair").

Executive functioning can be tested in several ways. The Russian neuropsychologist Luria devised tests to assess patients' abilities to perceive and replicate a sequence. When asked to copy an alternating sequence of squares and triangles or a drawing of a double loop, patients with executive dysfunction will often show perseveration, or an inappropriate repetition of elements (e.g., they will continue to draw loops beyond the required two). Luria's "go–no go" test asks patients to tap their finger once on a tabletop after the examiner taps twice but to not tap when the examiner taps once; tapping after one examiner tap suggests perseveration and problems with response inhibition. Luria's hand sequences ask patients to perform a series of two- and three-step hand movements; again, patients with executive dysfunction can fail to perceive the proper sequences or perseverate on one of the movements. Asking patients to draw a standard clock face and place the hands at a specified time can also show problems with planning and organization in patients with executive dysfunction.

Formal, standardized tests of cognition are regularly used in clinical practice. The Mini Mental State Examination (MMSE) is perhaps the most common (Folstein et al., 1975). It is a 30-point test that examines orientation to place and time, immediate and delayed verbal memory, attention and concentration, calculations, language, visuospatial skills, and praxis. The MMSE is useful in patients with delirium and dementia for detecting cognitive dysfunction and following the course of the illness. It should be noted that the MMSE might not detect mild levels of cognitive impairment. It also includes no specific tests of executive functioning and may fail to detect impairment in patients with illnesses characterized by prominent executive dysfunction. Also, in normal individuals there is a positive correlation between years of formal education and MMSE scores; total scores of <30 can therefore be seen in normal individuals who have not pursued postsecondary education.

A few caveats should be mentioned. Before assessing cognition, the examiner should note the patient's level of consciousness, or level of arousal, which can vary from alertness to lethargy, stupor, or coma. Lethargic patients may have false positive findings on cognitive testing because they are unable to remain alert to be tested, and stupor and coma preclude meaningful testing (Strub and Black, 2000). The tests of cognitive functioning discussed earlier are not highly specific, and impairment in one cognitive domain can produce false positive abnormalities when other domains are tested. For example, patients with attentional impairment may perform poorly on all tests of cognitive functioning simply because they cannot attend to the tests.

Specially trained neuropsychologists can perform a wide array of more sophisticated tests that compare a patient's cognitive functioning to well-established normative values, and this information can be helpful with disease diagnosis, monitoring disease progression, and assessing treatment effects. Neuropsychological testing is limited by a need for good patient cooperation (e.g., some patients with advanced dementia and behavioral problems cannot tolerate the several hours of testing commonly done) and the availability of trained neuropsychologists.

DELIRIUM

Defining Delirium

Delirium, an acute neuropsychiatric syndrome, is a manifestation of an underlying medical or surgical condition. It is defined clinically by disturbances in cognition, attention, and level of consciousness (Lipowski, 1990).

Over the years delirium has been known by many synonyms, such as acute brain failure, postoperative psychosis, intensive care unit (ICU) psychosis, and acute confusional state. Although this terminology is quite descriptive, it does not denote the same degree of diagnostic clarity as the term *delirium* and the associated DSM diagnostic criteria. DSM-IV-TR provides diagnostic criteria for delirium. The most important diagnostic signs are an impairment of level of consciousness and change in cognition that develops quickly and may fluctuate throughout the course of the day. In addition to these core symptoms and signs, there must also be evidence that the disturbance in the patient's mental status is due to an underlying medical condition or substance. The determined cause of the altered mental status is then used to further categorize the nature of the delirium from which the patient is suffering. This definition and classification system allows the clinician to effectively differentiate delirium from other important medical and psychiatric disorders and subsequently guide appropriate treatment.

Delirium may be further classified by the patients' motoric presentation. Lipowski (1990) described three subtypes of delirium: hypoactive, hyperactive, and mixed. The hypoactive subtype occurs in patients who appear quiet, lethargic, and withdrawn. Patients having hyperactive subtype may appear restless, psychotic, and/or overtly agitated. In the mixed subtype, the patient's motoric presentation alternates throughout the day with periods of relative hyperactivity and hypoactivity.

Epidemiology

Delirium is a prevalent disorder across clinical populations and health care settings. Studies have shown that between 10% and 24% of elderly patients who present to emergency departments have delirium (Lewis et al., 1995; Naughton et al., 1995). Medically hospitalized patients have rates

---

Clinical Characteristics of Delirium

- Disturbance in awareness with attentional impairment
- Cognitive deficient or perceptional disorder not due to dementia
- Changes have acute onset and fluctuate throughout the day
- Disturbances directly result from general medical condition, substance intoxication, substance withdrawal, or multiple etiologies

of delirium approaching 20%. Delirium may even be more common for specific populations, such as those in the intensive care setting, where rates have been reported as high as 87% (Ely et al., 2001), or the elderly following a hip fracture, where rates more than 60% have been found (Gustafson et al., 1988).

Despite the high prevalence of delirium, its recognition by health care providers is rather poor, with rates of identification as low as 33% (Inouye, 1994). Multiple factors contribute to this poor recognition. Many clinicians expect delirium to present only with agitation and psychosis (the hyperactive form), whereas many patients will present only quietly confused and lethargic (the hypoactive form). Consequently, the hypoactive form often goes unrecognized or misdiagnosed. For example, the hypoactive form of delirium is often mistaken for depression. In addition, the waxing and waning of the patient's mental status may confound the identification of a delirium as different caregivers observe the patient at various times throughout the day. It is also not uncommon for many of the symptoms of delirium (e.g., apathy) to appear primarily psychiatric or "functional" in etiology (e.g., depression) and not organic, thereby distracting the clinician from the correct diagnosis of delirium.

Phenomenology

The presentation of delirium is often quite unpredictable and varied, with a wide range of potential medical, psychiatric, and neurologic signs and symptoms that may vary in quality and quantity throughout the course of the disorder. This variability often leads to significant diagnostic confusion. However, some classic signs and symptoms are associated with this important neuropsychiatric syndrome.

Delirium onset is classically acute and develops rapidly over a period of days or hours. Once present the severity of symptoms often waxes and wanes, with periods of relative clarity alternating with episodes of confusion. Thorough assessment of cognition, however, usually reveals continued attentional impairment even during periods of relative clarity. A disrupted sleep–wake cycle is very common. The term *sundowning* is often used descriptively to illustrate the frequently observed pattern in which the symptoms of delirium become progressively more severe as the day progresses. Another core characteristic is the patient's diffuse cognitive impairment. This is fundamentally a dysfunction of attention, commonly described as a "clouding of consciousness," which may range from an impaired level of arousal to a reduced ability to sustain or shift attention. Impairments of attention will adversely impact other areas of cognition such as memory, orientation, and executive functioning.

Patients with delirium may also experience psychiatric symptoms. The patient may appear quite psychotic with grossly disorganized or illogical thought processes and perceptual disturbances, such as auditory or visual illusions and hallucinations. The illusions and hallucinations may be auditory or visual, but are more commonly visual during an episode of delirium. Therefore, the experience of visual hallucinations by a patient should raise the specter of an organic etiology, such as delirium. Delusions, often paranoid in nature, also occur in delirium but are not as well formed and consistent as the delusions experienced by patients with schizophrenia. Affective lability, or dramatic and inappropriately severe episodes of laughing or crying, may also complicate the course of delirium.

Nonspecific neurologic findings such as language disturbance, tremor, asterixis, and myoclonus also can occur during the course of a delirious episode. Primitive reflexes, such as the snout and grasp reflexes, may be found on careful neurologic examination because frontal lobe inhibition of these reflexes often fails in delirious states.

Etiology

Identifying the etiology of delirium is imperative because management, and ideally reversal, of the insult(s) is the principal goal of delirium treatment. Unfortunately, the etiology is often complex and multifactorial, making the identification and subsequent treatment of an underlying etiology a serious challenge even for the experienced clinician.

Several emergent conditions may lead to the development of delirium (see Table 8-1). These need to be identified acutely because failure to identify and address such critical illnesses may lead to irreversible injury or death. The evaluation of these potentially life-threatening etiologies for delirious states should begin as soon as delirium is suspected.

TABLE 8-1	Emergent Conditions for the Etiology of Delirium
Substance intoxication	
Substance withdrawal	
Infection	
Hypoglycemia	
Hypoxemia	
Central nervous system (CNS) insults	
Trauma	
Ischemic stroke	
Hemorrhagic stroke	
Seizures	
Hypertensive emergency	
Wernicke encephalopathy	

Common precipitants of delirium include medications, infections, end-organ system dysfunction (i.e., cardiopulmonary, renal, or hepatic), electrolyte/metabolic derangement, or central nervous system (CNS) disorders.

Medications are frequently implicated in the development of delirium. Many have the potential to contribute to the development of an altered mental state; however, certain medication classes are more notorious than others for contributing to the onset of delirium. For example, narcotics, sedatives, psychotropics, and medications with anticholinergic properties are common punitive agents. In fact, it has been shown that high anticholinergic drug scores correlate with delirium severity (Han et al., 2001). It is important to note that in vulnerable individuals, medication in therapeutic doses or within therapeutic blood ranges may still cause delirium.

Infections as varied as urinary tract infections, pneumonias, sepsis, meningitis, and human immunodeficiency virus (HIV) infection may cause an individual to suffer an alteration in mental status.

Organ system dysfunction, such as respiratory failure resulting in hypoxia, liver failure leading to hepatic encephalopathy, and renal failure causing uremia, may contribute to delirium in susceptible individuals. Abnormalities of the endocrine system, such as hypoglycemic states and thyroid perturbations, may lead to the development of a delirious state. Metabolic derangements, such as dysregulation of sodium or calcium homeostasis leading to hyponatremia or hypocalcemia, may also contribute to the development of delirium. However, it is often the acuity of the electrolyte imbalance rather than the absolute level that represents the greatest risk. Strokes (ischemic or hemorrhagic), traumatic brain injuries, subdural hematomas, seizures, brain tumors (primary or metastases), and vasculitis are all examples of central nervous system pathology that may lead to a patient presenting clinically with an altered mental status.

Although environmental factors may contribute to the onset of delirium, they are rarely, if ever, the only precipitants. For example, delirious states that occur in the ICU are usually multifactorial in etiology and may be aggravated, but not caused, by the inherent stresses of the ICU environment. This is an important concept, as the descriptive term *ICU psychosis* implies that the ICU environment alone is responsible. This faulty assumption may lead to the dangerous and flawed opinion that no further evaluation for a potential medical cause is required.

Pathophysiology

The pathophysiology of delirium is unclear but is most likely multifactorial and quite complex. Delirium likely requires that a patient with predisposing risk factors suffer a precipitating acute insult that leads to cerebral dysfunction and the subsequent development of delirium.

Various theories of the pathophysiology of delirium exist in the scientific literature. Cerebral dysfunction, both global and regional, has been reported during the course of delirium (Fong et al., 2006; Yokota et al., 2003). Delirium may also be secondary to dysregulation of various neurotransmitters, with acetylcholine and dopamine most often implicated. The predominance of evidence to date supports an underactivity of the cholinergic system and/or an overactivity of the dopaminergic system in the etiology and clinical presentation of delirium (Trzepacz, 2000).

Considerable evidence supports the role of a cholinergic transmission failure in delirium. For example, patients with AD, a disease process with a pronounced reduction in cholinergic activity, are at increased risk for delirium. In addition, disruption of cholinergic transmission has been associated with reduced arousal, attention, and information processing, similar to the deficits seen in delirium. Serum anticholinergic levels have been found to be elevated in patients with delirium, and resolution of these increased levels has been associated with clearing the impaired mental status (Mach et al., 1995). Finally, the adverse cognitive and attentional effects of severe anticholinergic delirium may be reversed by administering the cholinesterase inhibitor physostigmine.

Excess dopamine levels may contribute to the agitation and psychotic symptoms that are often present in delirium. Dopaminergic agonists, such as those used to treat Parkinson disease (PD), are well-known precipitants of delirium. Disease states and medications known to cause delirium, such as hypoxia and opiates, have been associated with excess dopamine states (Broderick and Gibson, 1989; Ota et al., 1991). In addition, dopamine antagonists, particularly the antipsychotics, have been used for years to effectively treat delirium.

Other neurotransmitters, such as γ-aminobutyric acid (GABA), are less commonly implicated in the etiology of delirium, but may contribute in specific disease states such as hepatic encephalopathy and alcohol or sedative/hypnotic withdrawal delirium. Infection or inflammation may cause alterations in mental status through the adverse actions of cytokines. Cytokines may precipitate delirium by mechanisms such as disturbing normal neurotransmitter action or by direct neurotoxic effects.

Evaluation

The evaluation of delirium is based on the patient's clinical presentation and centered on a detailed search for potential causes of the altered mental state. The assessment starts with a careful history of the patient's illness directed toward establishing the onset and subsequent course of the altered mental status. Once the time course is established, events temporally related, and therefore potentially etiologically related, to the onset of delirium become the focus of attention. However, the patient with delirium is often unable to provide the necessary historical details. Therefore, a careful review of the available medical records and discussion with collateral sources of information (the patient's family, friends, or previous caregivers) often provide helpful diagnostic information. Facts about recent trauma, past cognitive decline, and acute and chronic medical conditions, along with a thorough accounting of medications (prescription and over-the-counter) and supplements, should be the focus of these inquiries.

A directed physical examination also needs to be performed. Attention to the patient's vital signs and a pertinent examination of the patient's nervous, cardiac, and pulmonary systems for abnormalities that may reveal the etiology of the patient's delirious presentation is imperative. Observation of the patient's mental status for psychiatric signs and cognitive disturbance consistent with delirium is also important. Evidence of attentional impairment, confusion, and disorientation are often apparent during the initial examination even without formal cognitive testing. Formal testing of the patient's cognitive status may be accomplished through nonspecific tests of cognition such as the MMSE (Folstein et al., 1975). Specific bedside instruments to diagnose delirium and rate the severity of the episode also exist (Breitbart et al., 1997; Inouye et al., 1990; Trzepacz et al., 2001). In addition, numerous informal bedside tests of attention and executive function can be helpful in clarifying the diagnosis of delirium (see the preceding text).

The laboratory evaluation of delirium should be guided by the findings of a careful history and examination and directed toward elucidating potential etiologies of the delirious state (see Table 8-2). Such evaluations usually include a basic metabolic panel, complete blood count, hepatic panel, and a urinalysis with microscopic examination. Tests of thyroid function along with vitamin B_{12} and folate levels should also be obtained. Serum drug levels and a urine drug

TABLE 8-2	Laboratory Evaluation
Potential Laboratory Tests to Consider in the Evaluation of Delirium	
Complete blood count	
Electrolytes	
Renal function tests	
Glucose	
Liver function tests	
Thyroid stimulating hormone	
Vitamin B_{12}	
Folate	
Rapid plasma reagin	
Human immunodeficiency virus	
Urine and serum toxicology screens	
Serum drug levels	
Urinalysis with microscopic examination	
Cardiac enzymes	
Cerebral spinal fluid analysis	
Electrocardiogram	
Structural neuroimaging	
Electroencephalogram	

screen should be performed. Testing for syphilis and HIV may also be considered. An infectious etiology should be suspected if the patient is experiencing a fever or leukocytosis. In these cases, an appropriate evaluation may also include blood cultures, chest radiograph, and a lumbar puncture. If the patient has a history of heart problems or significant risk factors for cardiac disease or if there is suspicion of an acute cardiac event, an electrocardiogram and determination of cardiac enzymes should be performed. Evidence of a pulmonary disease process may lead to ordering a chest radiograph, pulse oximetry, or arterial blood gases.

Computerized tomography (CT) or magnetic resonance imaging (MRI) of the brain is warranted if focal neurologic signs are present on physical examination or in cases of known or suspected head trauma. However, routine use of structural neuroimaging in an unselected population of patients with confusion has been shown to provide little useful clinical information (Hirano et al., 2006). If there is a question of the patient's diagnosis, an electroencephalogram (EEG) can be very helpful in the confirmation of a delirious state. The EEG findings most commonly associated with delirium are diffuse slowing (generalized theta and delta waves) and poor organization of background rhythm along with loss of reactivity to eye opening or closing. Unfortunately, however, the EEG usually provides little specificity to the etiology of delirium; however, some patterns do suggest specific diagnoses.

Treatment

Treating a patient with delirium has two important parts. First, identification and treatment of the underlying medical condition must be initiated. Second, the psychiatric and behavioral symptoms of delirium must be appropriately managed. It must not be forgotten that delirium is a neuropsychiatric manifestation of a medical disorder; therefore, these patients are not routinely admitted to psychiatric units but, rather, are admitted to a medical or surgical unit. Initial treatment should always be directed at reversing the etiology of the delirium. This is essential because the patient's survival may depend on it. All potential factors contributing to the patient's altered mental status need to be aggressively addressed by the treatment team. As a result, medications that may contribute to the onset of the delirium or potentiate an already present delirium need to be discontinued, if possible.

While evaluation and management of potential precipitating and perpetuating causes are underway, the simultaneous management of the adverse and often disruptive behavioral symptoms of delirium is often necessary. This is required in an attempt to ensure the safety of the patient and those around him or her. This important aspect of the treatment of delirium consists of environmental manipulation and pharmacotherapy.

Manipulation of the patient's environment is often helpful in minimizing the behavioral manifestations of delirium. Multiple potentially helpful environmental manipulations have been identified (see Table 8-3). Physically restraining acutely agitated delirium patients is controversial. Physical restraints have been implicated as a precipitating factor in the development of delirium and may iatrogenically contribute to the patient's agitation and risk of injury (Inouye and Charpentier, 1996). Unfortunately, the use of restraints is often necessary when other less restrictive means of managing the patient's agitation have failed and the individual continues to represent a serious risk of harm to self or others. In these rare cases, careful documentation and monitoring of the restrained patient is imperative. The least restrictive manner of restraint required to maintain safety should be utilized for the shortest length of time.

Antipsychotic medications, which exert their action primarily through dopamine antagonism, are the cornerstone of pharmacologic treatment for most cases of delirium. Although they are not approved by the U.S. Food and Drug Administration (FDA) for this indication, antipsychotics have been used for decades for this indication with great success. They help to reduce the adverse behavioral manifestations of delirium. Both the hypoactive and hyperactive motoric subtypes have been shown to benefit from antipsychotics (Platt et al., 1994). Except in cases of delirium secondary to alcohol or sedative-hypnotic withdrawal, antipsychotics have been shown to be more effective than benzodiazepines alone in the management of delirium (Breitbart et al., 1996). Determination of the type and dose of antipsychotic medication along with the route of administration depends on multiple factors, including the patient's age, degree of agitation, clinical setting, and risk of side effects. Monitoring a patient closely after administration is required to determine response and monitor for side effects. The resolution of delirium allows the clinician to gradually taper off the antipsychotic. Delirious patients do not require long-term maintenance pharmacotherapy once the delirium has resolved.

Haloperidol, a high-potency typical antipsychotic, has historically been most often chosen for the symptomatic treatment of delirium and has many properties that make it desirable in this population. Unlike most of the low-potency antipsychotics, it is almost devoid of anticholinergic effects and hypotensive properties. Unlike benzodiazepines, it is not associated with a risk of significant respiratory suppression. Haloperidol also has the benefit of multiple potential routes of administration. It may be administered orally, intramuscularly, and intravenously, although the intravenous route is not approved by the FDA. Despite the increased potency of intravenous

TABLE 8-3	Helpful Environmental Manipulations in Delirium
Maintain the patient's sensory aids (glasses, hearing aids, etc.)	
Minimize noise	
Provide orientation clues (calendars, clocks, familiar pictures)	
Maintain appropriate lighting	
Promote a regular sleep–wake cycle	
Remove potentially dangerous objects	
Encourage family visits	
Provide calming music	

haloperidol compared with oral administration, it is associated with little of the extrapyramidal side effects that often complicate the use of oral or intramuscular haloperidol (Menza et al., 1987). The use of atypical antipsychotics to treat the psychiatric symptoms of delirium is commonplace. Experience to date reveals that the atypical antipsychotics are effective and well tolerated in the treatment of delirium (Rhea et al., 2007).

Whenever antipsychotics are utilized, the clinician must monitor the patient diligently for the development of adverse side effects. Certain side effects require special attention in the medically ill. Extrapyramidal symptoms (EPS), such as dystonias, parkinsonism, and akathisia, are well-recognized side effects of antipsychotic medication and may complicate medical management. In addition, there is increasing appreciation of the association between antipsychotic agents, prolongation of the QTc interval, and the occurrence of *torsades de pointes* (Glassman and Bigger, 2001). Electrolyte abnormalities, such as hypomagnesemia and hypokalemia, and the use of other medications that may prolong the QTc interval are common in the medically ill and should be minimized to reduce the risk of *torsades de pointes*. In addition, certain pharmacodynamic properties of various antipsychotics such as α-adrenergic antagonism and blockade of the cholinergic receptors may induce hypotension and constipation, respectively.

In alcohol and sedative-hypnotic withdrawal delirium, benzodiazepines are considered the first-line pharmacologic agents (Mayo-Smith et al., 2004). Delirious states that are the consequence of seizure activity are also appropriately treated with benzodiazepines. In addition, benzodiazepines may augment high-potency typical antipsychotics in patients with treatment-refractory delirium, potentially reducing the total dose of antipsychotic required and improving the tolerability of the antipsychotic (Menza et al., 1988). Among the benzodiazepines, lorazepam has several advantages, such as a rapid onset of action, short duration of action, and lack of active metabolites. These properties make lorazepam preferred when benzodiazepines are required in the management of delirium.

Prognosis

Delirium has multiple potential adverse effects on patient outcomes. It has been shown to prolong hospitalization (Francis et al., 1990) and increase the cost of health care (Milbrandt et al., 2004). Delirium may also lead to future cognitive decline in some susceptible individuals and increase rates of nursing home placement (Francis and Kapoor, 1992). Medical complications, such as feeding problems and decubitus ulcers, have also been reported to occur more frequently in patients with delirium (Gustafson et al., 1988).

Uncommonly recognized by the treatment team is the psychological toll that delirium takes on the patient as well as the patient's family and caregivers. High stress levels have been found in the patients and nurses, but the spouses of patients experiencing delirium were shown to suffer the highest levels of distress associated with the delirium episode (Breitbart et al., 2002).

In addition to affecting patient morbidity, delirium has also been shown to adversely affect mortality rates (McCusker et al., 2002). This relationship has been shown to remain clinically significant even after controlling for patient age, sex, cognitive function, level of daily living activities, and severity of illness (Inouye et al., 1998). Delirium may therefore herald disability and/or death in afflicted individuals. However, if it is correctly identified and properly treated, patients experience improved outcomes such as decreased length of hospital stays and lower mortality rates (Rockwood et al., 1994).

DEMENTIA

Defining Dementia

Definitions of dementia usually focus on acquired and significant impairment in multiple cognitive domains that is not due to delirium. *Acquired* cognitive dysfunction implies decline from an individual's baseline. *Significant* cognitive dysfunction, or dysfunction that causes impairment in overall functioning, differentiates dementia from conditions such as age-related cognitive decline (ARCD) and mild cognitive impairment (MCI), in which cognitive changes are not associated with any significant loss of functioning (see subsequent text). Impairment in *multiple cognitive domains* differentiates dementia from single-domain disorders such as amnestic disorder

A CASE OF DELIRIUM

An 82-year-old male with a history of probable early AD has been admitted from a nursing home for progressively worsening confusion, wandering, and paranoia compounded by a disruption of his sleep–wake cycle. In the emergency department he was noted to be "seeing things." Collateral information from the patient's family indicates that he has some baseline memory problems, but his current mental state represents an acute change. They also note that his paranoia tends to be worse at night. To address his insomnia, he was recently started on diphenhydramine at bedtime.

The patient cannot provide a coherent history due to an inability to attend to questions posed. He is readily distracted by irrelevant noises and commotion outside his room. When he does attempt to provide an answer, he has trouble finding the right words.

Physical examination reveals normal vital signs and a normal heart, lungs, and abdomen. Mental status examination reveals impaired attention and poor short-term memory with disorientation to time and place. The laboratory evaluation was normal except for a urinalysis that suggested a urinary tract infection.

The patient is given a diagnosis of delirium likely due to multiple etiologies and started on an antibiotic for the presumed urinary tract infection. Diphenhydramine is discontinued due to concerns that its anticholinergic properties may be propagating his impaired mental status. Over the next few days the delirium resolves, and he returns to his prior level of functioning.

(see subsequent text). DSM-IV-TR follows this tradition and defines dementia as a syndrome featuring multiple acquired cognitive deficits including memory impairment *and* a deficit in at least one of the other cognitive realms, such as aphasia, apraxia, agnosia, or executive dysfunction. DSM states that this cognitive dysfunction must represent a decline from a previous higher level of functioning and cause significant impairment in occupational or social functioning and also requires that delirium be ruled out as the cause of the cognitive impairment.

The terms *cortical* and *subcortical* dementia are encountered in the literature. Cortical dementia results when a pathological process that affects mainly the cerebral cortex causes cognitive abnormalities like aphasia, apraxia, and agnosia. AD produces a predominantly cortical dementia. Subcortical dementia (Cummings and Benson, 1984) is caused by pathological processes that affect mainly the basal ganglia, thalamus, and/or white matter and characterized by psychomotor slowing, apathy, depression, and executive dysfunction. Subcortical cerebrovascular disease (CVD) (e.g., lacunar infarcts), PD, and Huntington disease are examples of diseases that cause predominantly subcortical dementias. It should be noted that many diseases said to cause cortical dementia affect subcortical areas as well, and subcortical dementias often include some cortical pathology. The concept of cortical and subcortical dementias is therefore helpful in diagnosing more than a neuropathological reality.

Differentiating delirium from dementia can sometimes be a challenge. Some rules that may help with this are given in Table 8-4.

Causes of Dementia

Numerous neurologic, general medical, and primary psychiatric illnesses can cause the syndrome of dementia. A detailed discussion of all these illnesses is beyond the scope of this chapter. Table 8-5 lists some of the more important causes.

The Dementia Evaluation

Once the syndrome of dementia has been identified in a patient, the search for an etiology begins. It would be inappropriate to give a patient a diagnosis of "dementia" and proceed directly to symptomatic management of memory impairment, agitation, or other problems, just as it would be inappropriate to give a patient a diagnosis of "dyspnea" and proceed directly to a symptomatic treatment like a bronchodilator. Identification of the cause, or causes, of a patient's dementia is important because some etiologies (e.g., depression) produce a dementia that is reversible with treatment, and other etiologies (e.g., chronic vitamin B_{12} deficiency, neurosyphilis) produce a

TABLE 8-4   **Rules to Help Differentiate Delirium from Dementia, and Some Rule Exceptions**

	Delirium	Dementia	Rule Exception
Onset	Hours/days	Months/years	Strategic infarct dementia
Duration	Hours/days	Months/years	Reversible dementia
Course	Waxes/wanes	Progressive	Fluctuation common in dementia with Lewy bodies (DLB)
Night worsening	Common	Less common	REM sleep behavior disorder common in DLB
Level of consciousness	Abnormal/fluctuates	Normal	Often decreased in DLB
Attention	Impaired	Normal until late	Marked impairment with DLB
Hallucinations	Visual common	Less common	Visual common in DLB
Speech	Dysarthria common	Dysarthria uncommon	Dysarthria common in vascular dementia
Tremor	Common	Uncommon	Common in Lewy body diseases
EEG	Prominent generalized slowing	Normal/mild generalized slowing late	Characteristic abnormalities often seen in Creutzfeldt–Jakob disease

EEG, electroencephalography.

TABLE 8-5   **Some Important Causes of Dementia**

Alzheimer disease

Frontotemporal lobar degeneration

Lewy body diseases

Huntington disease

Cerebrovascular disease

Traumatic brain injury

Tumors

Neurosyphilis

HIV infection

Normal pressure hydrocephalus

Vitamin B$_{12}$ deficiency

Creutzfeldt–Jakob disease

Depression

HIV, human immunodeficiency virus.

dementing process that can be arrested with treatment. It is important to identify the remaining nonreversible, nonarrestable diseases (e.g., AD) because disease-specific symptomatic treatments and treatments that may slow the pathological processes of these diseases are now available, and more will undoubtedly be developed. Etiologic diagnosis is the responsibility of all physicians who diagnose dementia, and the expertise of multiple fields may be needed to make a diagnosis in atypical or complex cases.

The neurodegenerative diseases that commonly cause dementia have characteristic natural histories; therefore, obtaining a good history is important in making an etiological diagnosis. Patients can be asked about cognitive dysfunction, neuropsychiatric symptoms, and functional impairment, but usually significant others and medical records must be queried as well to obtain accurate information. As with all medical history taking, it is crucial to ask about the onset of any signs or symptoms manifested because the natural histories of diseases often differ in temporal relationships (e.g., memory impairment is an early manifestation of AD but is a late manifestation of frontotemporal lobar degeneration [FTLD]). General physical (including neurological) and psychiatric (including cognitive) examinations should always be done because they can yield information useful for differential diagnosis. Failure to do a neurologic examination may lead to missing focal neurologic signs, parkinsonism, and other findings that could greatly aid diagnosis.

Medical testing should always be guided by history and examination findings. Inflexible testing protocols may subject patients to unnecessary discomfort and be cost-ineffective. The American Academy of Neurology (Knopman et al., 2001) and the American Psychiatric Association (1997) have published guidelines for appropriate medical testing of patients with dementia.

Structural brain imaging with a CT or MRI scan is required and can identify some reversible and arrestable causes of dementia, such as hematomas, tumors, and hydrocephalus. Structural imaging can also identify infarcts in suspected cases of vascular dementia (VAD) and patterns of atrophy suggestive of specific degenerative diseases (e.g., frontal lobe atrophy suggestive of FTLD).

Functional neuroimaging with a nuclear medicine study such as a single photon emission computed tomography (SPECT) or positron emission tomography (PET) scan may demonstrate areas of altered cerebral blood flow or decreased cerebral metabolism, respectively, consistent with the characteristic spatial distributions of the various neurodegenerative conditions (see subsequent text). The availability of nuclear functional neuroimaging is limited and its cost is significant, though, so this type of imaging is not a required part of the dementia evaluation. Nuclear imaging might be reserved for cases in which diagnostic uncertainty exists, such as cases with symptoms suggestive of AD and FTLD (Small, 2006).

Formal cognitive testing by a trained neuropsychologist can assess patients' cognitive deficits both qualitatively and quantitatively. Neuropsychological testing can identify patterns of impairment characteristic of certain illnesses and be used to monitor patients' progress.

A number of exciting imaging modalities currently in development may revolutionize the diagnosis and treatment of dementia. PET scanning using FDDNP (Shoghi-Jadid et al., 2002), a radiolabeled molecule that binds to amyloid plaques and neurofibrillary tangles, or Pittsburgh compound B (PIB), a radiolabeled molecule that binds to amyloid plaques (Klunk et al., 2004), can demonstrate disease burden *in vivo* and may ultimately aid in the diagnosis and disease course monitoring of illnesses associated with abnormal amyloid and/or τ-protein metabolism. Magnetic resonance spectroscopy (MRS) measures levels of several different naturally occurring metabolites in the brain and by doing so can detect patterns of change suggestive of specific disease processes. Functional magnetic resonance imaging (fMRI), an imaging technique that uses regional blood oxygenation levels as a surrogate marker for regional cortical activation, has demonstrated abnormal activation in patients with AD and may become useful in diagnosis and monitoring treatment effects in patients with dementia (Diamond et al., 2007).

Some Major Causes of Dementia

Alzheimer Disease

Great progress has been made in understanding the pathophysiology of AD and in its diagnosis and treatment since Alzheimer's first case report a century ago. Despite this, AD remains a great cause of suffering and a major contributor to health care costs.

Epidemiology

Many studies have suggested AD is the most common cause of dementia. *The Nun Study* (Snowdon, 2003), a research project in which a group of elderly nuns has been followed longitudinally in an attempt to better understand the risk factors for AD, has suggested that 43% of dementia cases are caused by AD alone and another 34% are caused by AD plus CVD. The prevalence of AD increases with age: it is present in 1% of people aged 60 to 65 years and 40% of people 85 years or older. Some past studies have suggested that women are at greater risk for AD than men, but more recent studies have suggested the risk is probably equal.

Phenomenology

Cognitive dysfunction is prominent in AD. Patients with AD develop memory problems early in their illness. Problems with recent episodic memory are most commonly seen; memories for remote events are usually retained until the later stages of the illness. Patients usually show an encoding memory deficit. In addition to memory problems, dysfunction in other cognitive domains is seen. Executive dysfunction can be seen early in the course of AD but is less prominent than the executive dysfunction accompanying FTLD and subcortical dementias (see subsequent text). Visuospatial dysfunction and problems with calculations are also seen. Language is affected early and significantly. Patients with early- and mid-stage AD show language comprehension problems and "empty speech," or speech lacking in information content. They also make paraphasic errors, or substitute incorrect sounds or words for intended sounds or words. Language testing will reveal problems with object naming. As the disease progresses, patients can develop a posterior (Wernicke's type) aphasia, as might be expected, because the disease process of AD has a predilection for temporoparietal cortical areas. Patients with end-stage AD frequently demonstrate echolalia (repetition of words spoken by an examiner), palilalia (repetition of words spoken by the patient), and eventually mutism.

Psychopathology is noted in almost all cases of AD (Cummings and Victoroff, 1990). Personality changes are common, with apathy, or loss of motivation and interest, being a frequent early sign. With disease progression, patients can become disinhibited and demonstrate socially inappropriate behavior (Mega et al., 1996). Although up to half of patients develop some depressive signs and symptoms such as sadness and crying, only approximately a quarter will develop major depression. Suicide is rare in patients with AD. Psychosis is common, with approximately 50% developing delusions. Fears of spousal infidelity, theft, and a "phantom boarder" (a belief that unwelcome people are living in the home) are common (Cummings and Victoroff, 1990). Psychosis usually occurs in the later stages (Mega et al., 1996) and correlates with a more rapid clinical decline.

Psychiatrists are often asked to treat patients in the middle or later stages of AD who are agitated and/or aggressive. It should be emphasized that agitation and aggression can be caused by many different factors. Agitation in patients with AD commonly indicates a superimposed delirium from an acute medical problem or a new medication. Agitation can also stem from anxiety, a mood disorder, psychosis, personality changes, and physical symptoms such as pain. A request to see an agitated patient with AD should always be followed by an attempt to ascertain the cause(s) of the agitation, and this rule can be generalized to other causes of dementia as well.

Functional impairment becomes more prominent as AD progresses. Patients develop impairment in instrumental activities of daily living (iADLs) such as balancing a checkbook or using a telephone before they develop problems with basic ADLs like dressing or feeding.

The general neurologic examination is usually normal in early AD. Gait abnormalities and seizures can be seen in the later stages of the illness.

Etiology

Age is the most important risk factor for AD. Although it has been reported in patients younger than 24 years, most cases begin after age 65. The incidence of AD doubles with every additional 4 to 5 years of age in the elderly.

Abnormal genes are responsible for most cases with an early onset (younger than 65 years), and genes and other factors likely interact to produce the typical late-onset cases. Gene mutations are thought to account for approximately 10% of all cases of AD. Mutations in the amyloid precursor protein (APP) gene on chromosome 21 can cause dominantly inherited, early-onset AD.

Patients with Down syndrome frequently develop AD by 40 years because they overproduce cerebral amyloid due to the presence of an extra APP gene from their third chromosome 21. The presenilin 1 gene on chromosome 14 and presenilin 2 gene on chromosome 1 code for proteins that form part of the γ-secretase proteolytic enzyme. This enzyme is one of the secretases responsible for cleaving APP, and mutations in these genes may cause an increase in γ-secretase functioning and increase the production of toxic β-amyloid. Presenilin gene mutations have been reported to cause dominantly inherited, early-onset AD, and presenilin 1 mutations account for 50% to 70% of all autosomal dominant AD cases. The apolipoprotein E (apo-E) gene on chromosome 19 codes for a protein that plays a role in cholesterol transport and may aid in neuronal repair. Apo-E genotypes alter the risk of developing late-onset AD, with the E2 allele decreasing AD risk and the E4 allele increasing it. The E4 allele produces an apo-E molecule that is associated with accelerated amyloid aggregation. Almost all E4/4 homozygotes develop AD by 80 years of age.

Risk factors for vascular disease, such as hypertension and diabetes mellitus, are associated with cognitive decline in older individuals. Vascular risk factors may affect the brain in such a way that the amount of AD pathology required to produce the syndrome of dementia is decreased. Vascular risk factors are not correlated with progression of the pathological process of AD, but brain infarcts, which are present in more than one third of patients with AD, worsen cognitive dysfunction in patients with AD pathology.

Genetic abnormalities, and possibly other risk factors, cause AD by increasing the β-amyloid burden in the brain. An abnormal amyloid fragment is produced when APP is cleaved by the β- and γ-secretases (Cummings, 2004). Overproduction of abnormal β-amyloid leads to the formation of senile, or neuritic, plaques, which are aggregations of amyloid, dystrophic neurites, glial elements, apo-E, and a number of other molecules. In AD, plaques are commonly found in the temporoparietal areas important for the association of incoming information from various sensory modalities. Amyloid also accumulates in blood vessels producing cerebral amyloid angiopathy.

Neurofibrillary tangles composed of hyperphosphorylated τ-protein are formed in AD in numerous areas, including the hippocampus, amygdala, basal forebrain (location of the acetylcholine-producing nuclei), and dorsal raphe nucleus (location of serotonin-producing cells). Deposition of β-amyloid precedes cell membrane lipid peroxidation, inflammation, tangle formation, glutamatergic toxicity, and apoptotic cell death (Hardy and Selkoe, 2002).

Evaluation

Despite advances in laboratory testing and neuroimaging, the diagnosis of AD remains largely clinical. Patient histories and examination results are reviewed for patterns of impairment consistent with the known natural history of AD. Standard structural neuroimaging can show patterns of atrophy suggestive of AD (e.g., in the hippocampus), but the lack of specificity of these abnormalities precludes use of structural imaging for definitive diagnosis. Functional neuroimaging using SPECT or PET can show decreased blood flow or hypometabolism in brain areas such as the temporoparietal association areas and medial temporal lobes known to be strongly affected in AD (Silverman et al., 2001). PET imaging using FDDNP or PIB offers the exciting possibility of *in vivo* imaging of plaques and tangles, but is not yet ready for routine clinical use. Tests for some of the genetic abnormalities responsible for autosomal dominant AD are available and should be considered in cases of early-onset AD. Apo-E genotyping is available, but use of this test for the diagnosis of AD is not recommended because knowledge of the genotype only helps understand a patient's risk for developing AD.

Treatment

The acetylcholine-producing neurons in the basal forebrain that project to the hippocampus, neocortex, and other areas are prominently affected by the pathophysiologic process of AD (Whitehouse et al., 1981). Recognition of the cholinergic deficit in AD and the cognitive and neuropsychiatric benefits of increasing cholinergic activity led to the development of several acetylcholinesterase-inhibitor (AChEI) medications. Donepezil is an AChEI that is taken once daily orally. Rivastigmine, a derivative of physostigmine, is given twice daily orally or once daily as a transdermal patch. Galantamine is available in an immediate release form taken twice daily or an extended release form taken orally once daily. Galantamine is believed to improve cholinergic functioning by increasing acetylcholine and allosterically modulating the cholinergic nicotinic receptor. Clinical trials of galantamine for MCI (see subsequent text) suggested an increased risk of death with galantamine treatment, which prompted the FDA to issue an alert in 2005. Previous trials of galantamine in AD did not show an increased risk of death, though, and the drug is still FDA approved for treatment of mild to moderate AD.

AChEIs usually slow the rate of cognitive decline more than they improve cognition in patients with AD (Cummings, 2003a), and patients may benefit from the drugs for several years. In addition, AChEIs can improve neuropsychiatric symptoms such as apathy and hallucinations (Cummings, 2000). It has been suggested that treatment with an AChEI should be deemed ineffective only if it fails to slow a patient's rate of cognitive decline during a trial of 6 months or more (Cummings, 2003a). Discussions are ongoing regarding the overall costs and benefits of treatment with AChEIs.

Overstimulation of N-methyl-D-aspartate (NMDA) receptors by glutamate is thought to produce neuronal excitotoxicity and play a role in the pathogenesis of AD. Memantine, an NMDA antagonist, may be beneficial in all stages of the illness, and patients on AChEIs may benefit when memantine is added (Tariot et al., 2004).

The psychopathology of AD causes significant patient and caregiver suffering and often necessitates treatment with psychological interventions and/or traditional psychotropic medications. An extensive review of the literature on psychological approaches to neuropsychiatric symptoms in dementia found support only for caregiver education and the use of behavior management therapy with patients (Livingston et al., 2005). Few randomized controlled trials of antidepressants in depressed AD patients have been conducted. A recent meta-analysis of some of these studies concluded that the antidepressants studied were superior to placebo in terms of producing a treatment response and achieving remission of depression (Thompson et al., 2007). A case can be made for avoiding tricyclic antidepressants in patients with AD because of the anticholinergic and other serious side effects associated with these medications, but no convincing case can be made for the exclusive use of any other antidepressant at this time. It is common for physicians to begin antidepressant treatment with selective serotonin reuptake inhibitors (SSRIs), and because one controlled study found sertraline to be efficacious in depressed patients with AD (Lyketsos et al., 2003), SSRIs might be reasonable first-line antidepressants.

Antipsychotics have been used for years to treat AD patients with psychosis, agitation, and aggression. In recent years, the atypical antipsychotics have supplanted haloperidol and other typical antipsychotics due to their more favorable side-effect profile. Concerns have arisen, however, about the risks of atypical antipsychotics in patients with dementia. Some studies have suggested an increased risk of stroke in those treated with risperidone or olanzapine. Concerns about an increased mortality rate prompted the FDA in 2005 to add a "black box warning" to the prescribing information of these medications, stating that they are not approved for the treatment of behavioral disorders in patients with dementia. The Clinical Antipsychotic Trials in Intervention Effectiveness—Alzheimer Disease (CATIE-AD) study (Schneider et al., 2006) examined the effectiveness of olanzapine, quetiapine, and risperidone in patients with AD and concluded that the modest efficacy of these medications was offset by their side effects. Despite these concerns, the cautious use of atypical antipsychotics in the AD population can be justified given the fact that psychosis and agitation are common, significant problems and the reality that there are few pharmacologic alternatives. It has been suggested that any AD patient treated with an atypical antipsychotic be monitored closely for side effects and the medication be stopped if no benefit is seen after 2 to 4 weeks of use.

Valproic acid is sometimes used to treat agitation in patients with AD, but recent research has suggested that this drug is not beneficial. There is little research to support the use of other anticonvulsants to treat agitation in AD.

Insomnia is a problem in as many as 25% of patients with AD and can be addressed with nonpharmacological interventions such as exercise, increased daytime light exposure, and improved sleep hygiene (McCurry et al., 2005). There is little research to support the use of any medications in the treatment of insomnia related to AD. Cholinesterase inhibitors may improve rapid eye movement (REM) sleep, but they have also been associated with vivid dreams and insomnia. There is little evidence to support the use of atypical antipsychotics in the treatment of sleep disturbances, and the risks of these medications may outweigh their benefits. Disruption of melatonin secretion has been noted in AD, but it is not clear that supplementing melatonin or using the melatonin receptor agonist ramelteon improves sleep. In clinical practice, patients with AD having insomnia are sometimes given the sedating antidepressants mirtazapine and trazodone or the hypnotics zolpidem, zaleplon, and eszopiclone, despite a lack of support in the literature for using these medications. Benzodiazepine hypnotics and the anticholinergic antihistamines diphenhydramine and hydroxyzine should be avoided because of their possible negative effects on cognition and behavior.

Extensive research is ongoing on treatments that may slow or arrest the pathophysiologic process of AD. A controlled study examining the effects of vitamin E and/or selegiline on the course of AD (Sano et al., 1997) showed that treatment with these antioxidants delayed the onset of severe dementia, placement in a nursing home, and death. Many patients with AD have been treated with a high dose of vitamin E (e.g., 2,000 IU per day) since this finding was reported, but enthusiasm for such treatment has been tempered somewhat by the finding of increased cardiovascular deaths in a meta-analysis of studies of patients taking 400 IU or more of vitamin E per day (Miller et al., 2005). No clear benefit has been shown for treatment with anti-inflammatory medications. Studies of estrogen replacement therapy in postmenopausal women with AD have been disappointing, and one study actually suggested an increased risk of dementia in women treated with estrogen and progesterone (Shumaker et al., 2003). Research is ongoing to investigate ways of decreasing the formation and aggregation of β-amyloid, as well as increasing its clearance. A trial of immunization of patients with AD using β-amyloid was discontinued due to some participants developing subacute meningoencephalitis, but some immunization responders showed a decrease in cognitive decline (Hock, 2003). Passive immunization with intravenous immunoglobulin containing antibodies to β-amyloid may prove to be a safer alternative to active immunization. Statin drugs used to treat hypercholesterolemia may inhibit plaque and tangle formation, but the mechanisms by which this may occur are unclear. Medications that modify the activity of the β- and γ-secretases that generate toxic β-amyloid are avidly being sought (Pissarnitski, 2007).

Prognosis

The rate of progression of AD varies among patients. The time from symptom onset to death varies from 3 to 20 years. In one study, the median time from diagnosis to death was 4.2 years in men and 5.7 years in women (Larson et al., 2004). Patients with end-stage AD become bedridden and die from dehydration, malnutrition, and infections (pneumonia, infected decubitus ulcers, and sepsis).

Frontotemporal Lobar Degeneration

Interest in dementia due to the disease now known as *FTLD* began in the late nineteenth century when Pick first described it. Interest waned in the mid-twentieth century, but in

A CASE OF DEMENTIA DUE TO ALZHEIMER DISEASE

The family of a 77-year-old man relates a 5-year history of gradually worsening cognitive impairment and problems with recent memory and language (e.g., word finding). They say he became unable to pay bills and balance his checkbook about a year ago. The patient's wife becomes tearful when she says that he has no motivation and over the last 6 months he has accused her of having an affair with a man living in their attic.

Office cognitive testing reveals a normal attention span, clearly abnormal recent memory, problems with verbal comprehension and paraphasic errors, and problems with copying complex line figures and calculations. Neuropsychological testing confirms significant deficits in these cognitive domains. Basic laboratory studies are unremarkable. A cranial MRI scan shows only atrophy slightly out of proportion to age, in particular, in the medial temporal lobe.

The patient is given a diagnosis of dementia due to AD.

the 1980s groups working in England and Sweden "rediscovered" the illness and formulated criteria for its diagnosis (Neary et al., 1998). FTLD is of particular interest to psychiatrists because it is often associated with prominent personality changes and other neuropsychiatric symptoms.

Epidemiology

FTLD differs from the other major causes of dementia in that it often manifests before age 65. The mean age of onset is 55 to 62, and in two thirds of cases it is present by age 65. The illness has been reported in patients as young as 21 years. Men and women are at equal risk (Kertesz et al., 2007). FTLD is much less common than AD but is not rare: it may account for 20% of all cases of dementia beginning before age 65.

Phenomenology

Several variants of FTLD have been described, and the clinical manifestations of each are probably determined by particular patterns of brain atrophy.

The behavioral variant of FTLD (bvFTLD) is the most common and may constitute approximately 40% of the FTLD population (Kertesz et al., 2007). Personality changes are a hallmark of bvFTLD. Patients can exhibit apathy, decreased empathy, disinhibition, and loss of social skills (e.g., inappropriate joking, overfamiliarity with other people, and inappropriate sexual comments and behaviors). A lack of concern about hygiene and appearance is common. Patients with bvFTLD can also develop food "faddism" with a marked focus on certain foods or drinks (especially sweets) and hyperoral behaviors, or placing nonnutritive things in the mouth. Aberrant motor behaviors such as pacing can be seen, as can perseverative and compulsive behaviors. Utilization behavior, or the automatic manipulation of objects in the immediate environment, can also be seen. Nonpersecutory delusions are common in bvFTLD, but not depression. Hypochondriasis can be seen. Cognitive testing will reveal significant executive dysfunction in patients with bvFTLD. At autopsy, patients with bvFTLD are usually found to have symmetric, or right slightly greater than left, frontal lobe atrophy.

In patients with the other major variants of FTLD, changes in language are more prominent than changes in behavior. In the semantic dementia (SD) variant, patients lose factual and other real-world knowledge and become unable to grasp the meanings of certain words. Their language output remains fluent. Patients with SD can develop disinhibition and compulsive behaviors like patients with bvFTLD. At autopsy, SD patients are usually found to have left anterior temporal atrophy, but right temporal atrophy can also be seen. These patients constitute approximately 7% of the FTLD population (Kertesz et al., 2007). The other major language variant of FTLD, progressive nonfluent aphasia (PNFA), is characterized by diminished speech output, problems with word finding, and agrammatism (i.e., "telegraphic" speech). Patients with PNFA can also have problems in comprehending complex verbal and written material, but unlike patients with SD, they retain the meanings of individual words. PNFA is associated with atrophy of the left posterior frontal lobe and perisylvian language area.

A memory retrieval deficit can be seen in FTLD in the early stages but is more common in later stages of the illness. Visuospatial skills are usually relatively preserved.

Etiology

Approximately 40% of FTLD cases are genetically determined, and the pattern of inheritance is usually autosomal dominant. Mutations in the τ and progranulin genes on chromosome 17 account for most cases of inherited FTLD. τ gene mutations produce τ-protein-positive inclusions in neurons. Pick disease, with its characteristic intraneuronal Pick bodies, is a "tauopathy." Progranulin is a growth factor that plays a role in cell proliferation and repair. Progranulin gene mutations are a more common cause of FTLD than tau mutations: they account for approximately 25% of familial cases and 5% to 10% of all cases. Progranulin gene mutations produce ubiquitin-only inclusion disease (FTLD-U). The major protein found in FTLD-U is known as *TDP-43*. The profound decrease in empathy and social awareness seen in many patients with FTLD may be related in part to selective loss of von Economo neurons from the orbitofrontal cortex. These specialized neurons have been found in other highly socialized mammals and may play an important role in social functioning.

A CASE OF FRONTOTEMPORAL LOBAR DEGENERATION

The husband of a 60-year-old woman says her personality has changed over the last 2 years. She is no longer interested in her family, friends, or hobbies and stays at home a lot, drinking large amounts of diet soda, smoking, and rummaging through drawers. He is embarrassed to take her to church or social functions because her hygiene has become poor and she makes inappropriate comments about their sex life around strangers.

On interview, the patient denies symptoms of depression. Cognitive examination reveals marked executive dysfunction, including severe perseveration, and essentially normal memory and language. Basic laboratories are unremarkable, as is a cranial CT scan. A brain PET scan shows markedly reduced metabolism in the frontal and anterior temporal lobes.

The patient is given a diagnosis of FTLD.

Evaluation

Cognitive testing of patients with FTLD will reveal prominent executive dysfunction and the language abnormalities discussed earlier. SPECT and PET can be very helpful in the diagnosis of FTLD when they reveal hypoperfusion or hypometabolism in the frontal lobes and/or anterior temporal lobes. Gene testing is available, mainly in the research setting, for some of the mutations that cause the disease.

Treatment

The finding of decreased serotonergic activity in FTLD has led to limited trials of serotonin reuptake inhibitors, but results have been mixed. Because no cholinergic abnormality has been demonstrated in FTLD, cholinesterase inhibitors would be expected to yield no benefit. A study of donepezil noted no cognitive improvement in patients with FTLD, and behavioral worsening occurred in some (Mendez et al., 2007). A recently reported case series found improvement in apathy, agitation, and anxiety in three patients with FTLD treated using memantine (Swanberg, 2007).

Prognosis

Like other degenerative dementias, FTLD usually begins insidiously and progresses slowly. The mean duration of FTLD in general is approximately 6 to 8 years, with a range of 2 to 20 years (Kertesz et al., 2007).

The Lewy Body Dementias

Although PD was described almost two centuries ago and the subcortical Lewy bodies found in PD were identified almost a century ago, it was not until 1961 that a dementing illness associated with cortical Lewy bodies was identified. The concept of dementia with (cortical) Lewy bodies (DLB) was refined in the 1990s and updated in 2005 (McKeith et al., 2005). It has long been recognized that 25% to 30% of patients with PD can develop dementia (Parkinson disease dementia [PDD]), and the similarities and differences between DLB and PDD are currently under study (Lippa et al., 2007).

Epidemiology

DLB usually begins between ages 50 and 80, and a recent study found an average age of 67 years for onset of DLB/PDD. Men are at increased risk for DLB in comparison with women. DLB may account for 20% or more of all dementia cases, making it the second most common neurodegenerative cause of dementia after AD.

Phenomenology

Parkinsonism, particularly bradykinesia, limb rigidity, postural instability, and gait disturbance, is seen in most of the patients with DLB. Postural instability and gait disturbance are more common in DLB and PDD than in PD. Patients with DLB have milder and more symmetric parkinsonism than patients with PD or PDD until the later stages of the illness. In an attempt to differentiate DLB from PDD, a "one year rule" has been proposed wherein patients who develop cognitive and motor impairment within a year of each other are likely to have DLB, and those who develop cognitive and motor impairment more than a year apart are likely to have PDD (McKeith et al., 2005). Other physical symptoms such as syncopal spells and falls are seen in approximately one third of patients with DLB and may be related to dysautonomia. A predominance of motor impairment suggests a diagnosis of PDD over DLB.

Attentional impairment may be prominent in DLB and is more marked in DLB than in PDD. Significant memory impairment appears later in the course of DLB than AD, which can be helpful in differentiating the two illnesses. Patients with DLB frequently appear confused and may be particularly prone to developing delirium with a superimposed acute medical illness. Visuospatial dysfunction can be prominent in DLB. Executive dysfunction is more prominent in DLB than in AD.

Psychopathology can be prominent in DLB as well. Apathy can occur and is first noted in the middle stages. Approximately two thirds of patients with DLB have formed detailed visual hallucinations beginning in the early stages of the illness. Delusions related to the content of hallucinations can be present. Visual hallucinations are correlated with greater cognitive and functional impairment. Psychosis is more severe in DLB than PDD. Approximately 40% of patients with DLB will have depression. Daytime sedation and sleep are often seen in patients with DLB. REM sleep behavior disorder is common in DLB and can precede the onset of the disease by many years. It is also seen in PD. A predominance of cognitive and neuropsychiatric impairment suggests a diagnosis of DLB over PDD.

It is important to mention that symptom fluctuation is noted in most patients with DLB, especially in the middle and later stages. Fluctuation, attentional impairment, and psychosis commonly lead to a misdiagnosis of delirium in patients with DLB.

Etiology

Most cases of DLB arise sporadically, but some are genetically determined. Families with autosomal dominant DLB have been reported. Multiplication of, and mutations in, the α-*synuclein* gene on chromosome 4 can cause PD, PDD, and DLB (Lippa et al., 2007). Abnormal or excess α-synuclein leads to the formation of the abnormal filaments that constitute Lewy bodies. Lewy bodies are found mainly in the substantia nigra and other midbrain structures in PD, but are also widespread in the cortex in DLB and PDD. The severity of dementia in these illnesses correlates with the density of cortical Lewy bodies. Neuronal loss, especially in the cholinergic basal forebrain nuclei, is a downstream effect of Lewy body formation. Coincident AD pathology is common in DLB, and the clinical phenotype of DLB can vary based on the amount of AD pathology present. The apo-E E4 allele is associated with earlier onset of PD and an increased risk of PDD and may increase the risk of developing DLB.

Evaluation

Neuropsychological testing can reveal attentional problems, visuospatial and executive dysfunction, and relative preservation of memory as discussed in the preceding text. Nuclear imaging studies may demonstrate decreased occipital perfusion/metabolism not seen in AD, and this can be helpful in differentiating DLB from AD.

Treatment

Parkinsonism in DLB is less responsive to treatment with levodopa than in PD, and patients with PDD may be less responsive than patients with PD (Lippa et al., 2007). Patients with Lewy body diseases can commonly develop new psychosis or worsening of preexisting psychotic symptoms when treated with dopaminergic drugs.

Patients with DLB have a profound cholinergic deficit and can show marked improvement when treated with a cholinesterase inhibitor. Improvements have been noted in apathy, attentional impairment, psychosis, agitation, sedation, and symptom fluctuation. Patients with PDD can likewise respond to AChEIs. A few case reports and small case series have suggested that patients with DLB can worsen when treated with memantine.

Because psychosis is common in DLB, antipsychotic medications are often considered. In using these medications, physicians should keep in mind the marked neuroleptic sensitivity

A CASE OF DEMENTIA WITH LEWY BODIES

The family of a 69-year-old man says that for several years his sleep has been disturbed by vivid dreams leading to marked agitation. They also say he has vivid visual hallucinations of stray dogs in the house. Over the last 2 years they have noted that he is intermittently "fuzzy" (lethargic and inattentive) during the day and seems to faint on occasion. Over the last year and a half, the family has noted a tremor in both of his arms, slowing of movement, and mild problems with balance. When the patient's primary care physician tried him on olanzapine for the hallucinations, the patient became very sedated and confused and developed severe rigidity.

Cognitive examination shows problems with attention, copying complex figures, and executive functioning. Recent memory is not clearly impaired. Basic laboratories and a cranial MRI are unremarkable. A brain PET scan shows decreased temporoparietal metabolism suggestive of AD but also decreased occipital lobe metabolism not usually seen in AD. This finding, along with the history and examination, leads to a diagnosis of DLB.

characteristic of DLB. Patients with DLB are more neuroleptic sensitive than those with PD. If an antipsychotic is needed, typical antipsychotics should be strictly avoided because of their marked propensity to worsen parkinsonism. Small doses of atypical antipsychotics with low affinity for dopamine D_2 receptors are preferable. Low dose clozapine has been shown to improve psychosis in patients with PD without worsening cognition or motor functioning (Weintraub and Hurtig, 2007). Clozapine side effects, including agranulocytosis, sedation, and orthostasis, limit its use. It is difficult to recommend any other atypical antipsychotic for patients with DLB whose psychosis is not controlled with a cholinesterase inhibitor; some smaller studies have reported effectiveness of quetiapine and olanzapine (Weintraub and Hurtig, 2007).

REM sleep behavior disorder in patients with PD and DLB may respond to melatonin or clonazepam.

There is marked interest currently in developing drugs that may intervene in the pathophysiologic process of the Lewy body dementias. It is hoped that drugs will be developed to interfere with the misfolding and/or toxic aggregation of α-synuclein as well as the toxic effect of α-synuclein on neurons.

Prognosis

The rate of progression of DLB is unclear. A recent study found a median survival of 5 years after symptom onset. In this study, older age at disease onset, fluctuating cognition, hallucinations, and associated AD pathology on autopsy were associated with decreased survival (Jellinger et al., 2007). Patients with end-stage DLB become immobile, develop severe flexion abnormalities, and ultimately die of cardiac or pulmonary disease.

Cerebrovascular Disease

Before the 1970s, "hardening of the arteries" leading to decreased cerebral perfusion was thought to cause plaque and tangle formation and to be the most common cause of dementia. In 1970, Tomlinson et al. showed that plaque and tangle formation did not correlate with arteriosclerotic disease. In 1974, Hachinski showed CVD produced cognitive impairment when it caused destruction of brain tissue and in doing so established the concept of multi-infarct dementia.

Epidemiology

Dementia due solely to CVD may not be as common as once thought. Meta-analyses have suggested that "pure" VAD accounts for approximately 4% to 10% of dementia cases. Mixed dementia (VAD/AD) may in fact be more common than pure VAD and account for approximately 9% to 15% of cases (Jellinger and Attems, 2007). In a recent autopsy study of 1,500 individuals with dementia, pure VAD accounted for 10.8% of cases, mixed dementia 4.6%, and another

5.7% of cases had AD plus significant CVD that did not rise to the level of VAD (Jellinger and Attems, 2007). The prevalence of VAD increases with age and is higher in men than women up to age 85, but in extreme old age this gender pattern may reverse.

Phenomenology

Students have traditionally been taught that VAD begins abruptly and progresses in a "stepwise" fashion, as might be expected in an illness caused by a series of cerebral infarcts. However, some patients with VAD, and especially those with Binswanger disease (see subsequent text), can have an insidious onset and slow progression of their illness that mimics AD and other degenerative dementias.

Cognitive deficits in VAD are determined by the locations of infarcts. Patients with VAD often have more psychomotor slowing and executive dysfunction than patients with AD and a memory retrieval deficit rather than the encoding deficit seen in AD. These findings are consistent with the fact that subcortical ischemic disease, the most common cause of VAD, has a predilection for the "frontal/subcortical circuits." These are composed of areas in the frontal lobe, basal ganglia, and thalamus and the white matter tracts connecting them. CVD involving any of these areas can produce the characteristic cognitive changes mentioned in the preceding text (Mega and Cummings, 1994).

In keeping with the predilection of VAD for the frontal/subcortical circuits, personality changes ranging from lability to apathy are common. Depression is more common, severe, and persistent in VAD than in AD. Hallucinations are more common in VAD than in AD, and delusions are seen in 40% to 50% of patients with VAD. The severity of neuropsychiatric symptoms does not correlate with the severity of cognitive impairment in patients with VAD.

Patients with VAD frequently have focal neurologic signs and symptoms, dysarthria, gait impairment, and urinary incontinence.

Etiology

VAD can result from large-vessel or small-vessel CVD and hemorrhagic or ischemic strokes. Approximately half of all VAD is attributable to small-vessel ischemic disease and approximately 25% to large-vessel infarcts. Small-vessel cases are mostly due to lacunar infarcts (85%), with Binswanger disease, or diffuse white matter ischemic disease, accounting for the remainder. Lacunar infarcts are most often found in the thalamus, basal ganglia, and frontal white matter. In contrast to the older concept of multi-infarct dementia, it has been recognized that single infarcts in certain "strategic" areas can produce cognitive and behavioral changes consistent with dementia. Lacunar infarcts in the anteromedial/dorsomedial thalamus, head of the caudate nucleus, and the genu of the internal capsule can produce dementia (Chui, 2007). Infarction of the angular gyrus can also result in a variety of cognitive abnormalities.

The well-known risk factors for CVD include age, hypertension, diabetes mellitus, hyperlipidemia, cardiac disease (e.g., arrhythmia and congestive heart failure), and smoking. Lesser known factors include obstructive sleep apnea, hypotension (e.g., orthostatic), and elevated fibrinogen and homocysteine levels.

Some genetic abnormalities have also been associated with CVD. The *MTHFR* gene influences plasma homocysteine levels, and variations in this gene have been associated with stroke. Mutations in the *Notch3* gene on chromosome 19 produce the illness known as cerebral autosomal dominant arteriopathy with subcortical infarctions and leukoencephalopathy (CADASIL). Patients with CADASIL develop severe subcortical ischemic disease with lacunes and extensive white matter disease. The apo-E E4 allele may increase the risk for VAD.

Evaluation

Neuropsychological testing can reveal patterns of cognitive impairment consistent with cortical strokes and/or the frontal/dysexecutive syndrome associated with subcortical CVD. Brain imaging will reveal cerebral hemorrhages and infarcts. White matter disease is better assessed with MRI than CT. SPECT and PET scans reveal a patchy distribution of areas of hypoperfusion/hypometabolism in VAD.

Treatment

CVD can be prevented by primary preventive measures such as control of hypertension, diabetes mellitus, and hyperlipidemia and smoking cessation. Hypertension is the most important modifiable risk factor (Chui, 2007). Secondary preventive measures include use of anticoagulant medications such as warfarin and antiplatelet agents. It is unclear at this time if B vitamin supplementation given to lower homocysteine levels results in a decrease in stroke risk.

A recent review of clinical trials of cholinesterase inhibitors and memantine in mild to moderate VAD noted statistically significant cognitive benefits with all drugs but virtually no behavioral or functional benefits (Kavirajan and Schneider, 2007).

Use of traditional psychotropic medications in patients with VAD should follow the guidelines given in the preceding text for other illnesses. Since patients with CVD often have lacunar infarcts in the basal ganglia, they are at increased risk for the development of parkinsonism when treated with dopamine-blocking antipsychotic/mood-stabilizing medications. The possible increase in stroke risk associated with atypical antipsychotics discussed earlier should obviously be given due consideration when treating the VAD population.

Prognosis

VAD usually progresses over 6 to 8 years, and patients usually die of stroke or cardiovascular disease.

AGE-RELATED COGNITIVE DECLINE, MILD COGNITIVE IMPAIRMENT, AMNESTIC DISORDER, AND "PSYCHOGENIC AMNESIA"

Normal, "successful" aging is believed to be associated with subtle cognitive changes. Older studies suggested that a wide range of cognitive changes could be seen in the normal elderly, but they often did not recognize cohort educational effects (e.g., years spent in formal education may be less in an elderly population than a younger one) or adequately control for the effects of illnesses, including dementia, on cognition. More recent research recognizing these potential confounds has suggested that normal aging may have a smaller effect on cognition than previously thought. Declines in speed of information processing have been shown in studies of normal elderly individuals, and this slowing may affect performance on testing of other cognitive skills. Declines in recall memory abilities are seen with normal aging, whereas recognition memory is spared. A slowing of recall memory may account for some of this loss. Normal aging may also be associated with benign language changes such as minor word-finding, comprehension, and naming difficulties. DSM-IV-TR allows elderly people to be given a diagnosis of ARCD if they demonstrate cognitive decline on objective testing that is not attributable to a mental disorder or neurologic condition and does not exceed normal limits given the person's age. Neuropsychological testing may be needed to differentiate between changes in cognition consistent with normal aging and the mild but abnormal changes of early dementia. As people age, there is usually no loss of "crystallized intelligence," or previously acquired knowledge and skills. Patients diagnosed with ARCD develop dementia at the rate of approximately 1% per year.

In recent years, the diagnostic entity MCI has assumed increasing importance. MCI is used to describe people with abnormal declines in cognitive functioning (i.e., declines that exceed the limits set for ARCD) who are not significantly functionally impaired by these declines (i.e., do not meet diagnostic criteria for amnestic disorder or dementia; see subsequent text). Petersen et al. (1997) proposed diagnostic criteria for MCI that require a specific cognitive complaint (corroborated by an informant), objective verification of cognitive impairment, normal overall cognitive functioning, and intact activities of daily living. DSM does not yet include a diagnosis of MCI, and patients with MCI would be given a DSM-IV-TR diagnosis of cognitive disorder not otherwise specified (NOS). Most of the patients with MCI have memory impairment. Patients with memory impairment alone are said to have amnestic MCI, single domain, and those with impairment in memory and one or more additional cognitive functions are diagnosed with amnestic MCI, multiple domain. Patients with cognitive impairment in one or more nonmemory domains can be diagnosed with nonamnestic MCI, single-domain, or nonamnestic MCI, multiple domain (Petersen, 2004). Patients with amnestic MCI are at increased risk for developing dementia due to AD, with a conversion rate of approximately 16% per year (Petersen et al., 2005). Patients with nonamnestic MCI progress to dementia at a lower rate and may develop illnesses other than AD. For example, patients with nonamnestic MCI, single domain, commonly progress to FTLD. Neuropsychiatric symptoms are common in patients with MCI and may be a negative prognostic factor with respect to progression to AD. In a recent study using FDDNP PET, patients with MCI were found to have levels of FDDNP binding intermediate between those of patients with AD and normal controls (Small et al., 2006), as might be expected with an illness conceptualized as lying on a continuum between normal aging and dementia. Given their significant risk of dementia, patients diagnosed with MCI should be followed clinically. Patients should be counseled that not all cases of MCI progress to dementia and some even improve. There is great interest at this time in developing treatments for MCI, both from a symptomatic standpoint and the standpoint of slowing or preventing progression to dementia. Results of studies of cholinesterase inhibitors and vitamin E have been disappointing thus far, and one reported an increase in mortality in patients treated with galantamine (Petersen et al., 2005).

The DSM-IV-TR diagnosis amnestic disorder is used to describe patients who develop significant memory impairment in the absence of other cognitive dysfunction. Patients with amnestic disorder can present with verbal or nonverbal memory difficulties, or both. This impairment must represent a significant decline from the patient's baseline functioning and cause impairment in social or occupational functioning. Patients with delirium or dementia would not qualify for a diagnosis of amnestic disorder because these conditions produce dysfunction in memory as well as nonmemory cognitive domains. Patients with amnestic disorder would not qualify for a diagnosis of ARCD or the non-DSM diagnosis MCI since their memory impairment causes functional impairment. The DSM definition of amnestic disorder requires that the memory impairment may be due to the direct physiological effects of a general medical condition or the persisting effects of a substance of abuse, toxin, or medication. In practice, the diagnosis of amnestic disorder is seldom used because patients with memory loss due to a medical condition or toxin exposure are often found on cognitive testing to have dysfunction in other, nonmemory cognitive domains as well. Some disease processes and toxins can produce isolated memory impairment, though. Alcoholic patients with the isolated and often severe memory impairment associated with Korsakoff syndrome can be given a DSM diagnosis of substance-induced persisting amnestic disorder. Other conditions that can cause amnestic disorder include traumatic brain injury, hypoxic brain injury, and herpes encephalitis. Transient global amnesia (TGA), a non-DSM diagnosis, is a condition characterized by severe anterograde amnesia (i.e., an inability to form new memories) that begins suddenly and resolves within 24 hours. Patients with TGA are usually older (average age 60). During an episode of TGA, patients are disoriented to place and time and repeatedly ask questions about these. Some retrograde amnesia (i.e., an inability to recall previously learned information) is variably present, but patients always remember their personal identities. Patients with TGA are alert and have normal attention and other cognitive functions. Recurrence is rare. Isolated injury of the hippocampus and other medial temporal lobe structures probably underlies the amnestic disorder in these conditions. The cause of TGA has been unclear over the years; it is now believed that venous congestion of the hippocampi following a Valsalva maneuver may be a common cause (Owen et al., 2007).

"Psychogenic amnesia" is called dissociative amnesia and included in the dissociative disorders in DSM-IV-TR. Patients are unable to recall personal information, especially traumatic or stressful information, and usually appear indifferent to this retrograde amnesia. It is usually seen in younger individuals and often correlates with some recent stressor.

CONCLUSION AND FUTURE DIRECTIONS

Delirium, an acute neuropsychiatric disorder of impairment in attention and cognition, is a very common and serious medical problem. The clinician's recognition of delirium is imperative because an alteration in a patient's mental status may be the first clinical sign of a dangerous underlying medical, neurologic, or surgical disorder. Once delirium is recognized, appropriate medical and psychiatric management occur, thereby limiting potentially disastrous consequences.

Most cases of dementia are caused by neurodegenerative diseases that result from abnormal protein metabolism. Neurons differ in their vulnerability to these abnormal proteins, and this produces patterns of neuronal loss unique to each "proteinopathy." Different patterns of neuronal loss lead to different neurophysiological and neurochemical changes, and these specific changes produce characteristic patterns of cognitive dysfunction and psychopathology. We have entered a period of revolutionary change in the way dementia is diagnosed and treated. Advances in the understanding of the pathophysiological processes of the major dementing disorders will allow us to move beyond diagnoses on the basis of clinical phenotypes to more specific diagnoses based on genetic and biochemical abnormalities. With continued advances in biochemical testing and neuroimaging, older phenotypic diagnoses such as AD may give way to pathophysiology-based diagnoses such as "tauopathy" and "synucleinopathy" (Cummings, 2003b). We now understand that even patients with mild clinical dementia have long-standing disease and irreversible neuronal loss. This understanding is leading to a decrease in emphasis on nonspecific, symptomatic treatment of late-stage disease and an increase in emphasis on early identification of disease using new biomarkers. Early identification of dementia will allow treatment with modalities that can arrest or slow disease processes (Dubois et al., 2007).

Clinical Pearls

- A cognitively impaired patient is delirious until proven otherwise.
- Delirium is a neuropsychiatric syndrome with a wide variety of potential presentations and an equally impressive list of possible causes to consider.
- Delirium should always be suspected when a patient suffers an acute deterioration in behavior, function, or cognition.
- The management of delirium involves identifying and reversing the potential causes of the delirium coupled with treating the behavioral manifestations of delirium such as agitation and psychosis.
- Antipsychotics provide the foundation for the psychopharmacological management of the adverse behavior symptoms in most cases of delirium. Benzodiazepines are the mainstay of alcohol or sedative-hypnotic withdrawal delirium.
- Alzheimer disease causes or contributes to over three fourths of dementia cases.
- A number of factors can cause agitation in a dementia patient, and a cause should be sought before treatment is considered.
- Antipsychotics should be used sparingly in dementia patients because studies have shown a significant risk of adverse outcomes.
- A patient who is said to be "depressed" may in fact have a hypoactive delirium or apathy.
- A diagnosis of dementia should always be followed by a search for a cause because some dementias can be reversed or arrested, and disease-specific treatments are available for those that cannot.

Self-Assessment Questions and Answers

8-1. Delirious patients may appear lethargic and apathetic.

A. True
B. False

Patients suffering from delirium may appear withdrawn and fatigued, a motoric subtype of delirium called *hypoactive delirium*. These patients are quietly confused. It is not uncommon for them to be misdiagnosed as suffering from depression.
Answer: A

8-2. Pharmacologic management of delirium depends on the underlying etiology but may include the following:

A. Amitriptyline
B. Haloperidol
C. Zolpidem
D. Diphenhydramine
E. Buspirone

The pharmacotherapy of delirium often depends on the underlying cause of the delirious state.

Antipsychotics, such as haloperidol, are commonly utilized agents. Benzodiazepines may be used in alcohol or sedative-hypnotic withdrawal delirium. Physostigmine, a cholinesterase inhibitor, has been used in severe cases of anticholinergic delirium. Antidepressants (amitriptyline), antihistamines (diphenhydramine), antianxiety agents (buspirone), and hypnotics (zolpidem) have no role in the management of delirium. In fact, amitriptyline and diphenhydramine may worsen the patient's confusion secondary to their potent anticholinergic properties. *Answer: B*

8-3. Which of the following factors *decreases* an individual's risk for developing dementia due to AD?

A. Advanced age
B. Apolipoprotein E E2 allele
C. Apolipoprotein E E4 allele
D. Presenilin gene mutations

E. Risk factors for cerebrovascular disease

All of the factors except apolipoprotein E E2 allele *increase* risk for developing dementia due to AD. *Answer: B*

8-4. A patient with dementia who develops severe parkinsonism after treatment with a small dose of an atypical antipsychotic most likely has:

A. Alzheimer disease
B. Dementia with Lewy bodies
C. Frontotemporal lobar degeneration
D. Vascular dementia

"Neuroleptic sensitivity" is a hallmark of dementia with Lewy bodies. Patients with Alzheimer disease, frontotemporal lobar degeneration, and vascular dementia can also be sensitive to dopamine-blocking antipsychotics but are less sensitive than patients with DLB. *Answer: B*

References

American Psychiatric Association. Practice guideline for the treatment of patients with Alzheimer's disease and other dementias of late life. *Am J Psychiatry*. 1997;154:S1–S39.

American Psychiatric Association. *Diagnostic and statistical manual of mental disorders*, 4th edition, text revision. Washington, DC: American Psychiatric Association; 2000.

Breitbart W, Marotta R, Platt MM, et al. A double blind trial of haloperidol, chlorpromazine, and lorazepam in the treatment of delirium in hospitalized AIDS patients. *Am J Psychiatry*. 1996;153:231–237.

Breitbart W, Gibson C, Tremblay A. The delirium experience: delirium recall and delirium-related distress in hospitalized patients with cancer, their spouses/caregivers, and their nurses. *Psychosomatics*. 2002;43:183–194.

Breitbart W, Rosenfeld B, Roth A, et al. The memorial delirium assessment scale. *J Pain Symptom Manage*. 1997;13:128–137.

Broderick PA, Gibson GE. Dopamine and serotonin in rat striatum during *in vivo* hypoxic-hypoxia. *Metab Brain Dis*. 1989;4:143–153.

Chui HC. Subcortical ischemic vascular dementia. *Neurol Clin*. 2007;25:717–740.

Cummings JL. Cholinesterase inhibitors: A new class of psychotropic compounds. *Am J Psychiatry*. 2000; 157:4–15.

Cummings JL. Use of cholinesterase inhibitors in clinical practice: Evidence-based recommendations. *Am J Geriatr Psychiatry*. 2003a;11:131–145.

Cummings JL. Toward a molecular neuropsychiatry of neurodegenerative diseases. *Ann Neurol*. 2003b;54: 147–154.

Cummings JL. Alzheimer's disease. *N Engl J Med*. 2004;351:56–67.

Cummings JL, Benson DF. Subcortical dementia. Review of an emerging concept. *Arch Neurol*. 1984;41: 874–879.

Cummings JL, Victoroff JI. Noncognitive neuropsychiatric syndromes in Alzheimer's disease. *Neuropsychiatry Neuropsychol Behav Neurol*. 1990;3:140–158.

Diamond EL, Miller S, Dickerson BC, et al. Relationship of fMRI activation to clinical trial memory measures in Alzheimer disease. *Neurology* 2007;69:1331–1341.

Dubois B, Feldman HH, Jacova C, et al. Research criteria for the diagnosis of Alzheimer's disease: Revising the NINCDS-ADRDA criteria. *Lancet Neurol*. 2007;6:734–746.

Ely EW, Margolin R, Francis J, et al. Evaluation of delirium in critically ill patients: Validation of the confusion assessment method for the intensive care unit (CAM-ICU). *Crit Care Med*. 2001;29:1370–1379.

Folstein MF, Folstein SE, McHugh PR. "Mini-mental state." A practical method for grading the cognitive state of patients for the clinician. *J Psychiatr Res*. 1975;12:189–198.

Fong TG, Bogardus ST, Daftary A, et al. Cerebral perfusion changes in older delirious patients using 99mTc HMPAO SPECT. *J Gerontol A Biol Sci Med Sci*. 2006;61A:1294–1299.

Francis J, Kapoor WN. Prognosis after hospital discharge of older medical patients with delirium. *J Am Geriatr Soc*. 1992;40:601–606.

Francis J, Martin D, Kapoor WN. A prospective study of delirium in hospitalized elderly. *JAMA*. 1990;263:1097–1101.

Glassman AH, Bigger JT Jr. Antipsychotic drugs: Prolonged QTc interval, torsade de pointes, and sudden death. *Am J Psychiatry*. 2001;158:1774–1782.

Gustafson Y, Berggren D, Brannstrom B, et al. Acute confusional states in elderly patients treated for femoral neck fracture. *J Am Geriatr Soc*. 1988;36:525–530.

Han L, McCusker J, Cole M, et al. Use of medications with anticholinergic effect predicts clinical severity of delirium symptoms in older medical inpatients. *Arch Intern Med*. 2001;161:1099–1105.

Hardy J, Selkoe DJ. The amyloid hypothesis of Alzheimer's disease: Progress and problems on the road to therapeutics. *Science*. 2002;297:353–356.

Hirano LA, Bogardus ST Jr, Saluja S, et al. Clinical yield of computed tomography brain scans in older general medical patients. *J Am Geriatr Soc*. 2006;54:587–592.

Hock C, Konietzko U, Streffer JR, et al. Antibodies against beta-amyloid slow cognitive decline in Alzheimer's disease. *Neuron*. 2003;38:547–554.

Inouye SK. The dilemma of delirium: Clinical and research controversies regarding diagnosis and evaluation of delirium in hospitalized elderly medical patients. *Am J Med*. 1994;97:278–288.

Inouye SK, Charpentier PA. Precipitating factors for delirium in hospitalized elderly persons. *JAMA*. 1996;275:852–857.

Inouye SK, van Dyke CH, Alessi CA, et al. Clarifying confusion: The Confusion Assessment Method. A new method for detection of delirium. *Ann Intern Med*. 1990;113:941–948.

Inouye SK, Rushing JT, Foreman MD, et al. Does delirium contribute to poor hospital outcomes? *J Gen Intern Med*. 1998;13:234–242.

Jellinger KA, Attems J. Neuropathological evaluation of mixed dementia. *J Neurol Sci*. 2007;257:80–87.

Jellinger KA, Wenning GK, Seppi K. Predictors of survival in dementia with Lewy bodies and Parkinson dementia. *Neurodegener Dis*. 2007;4:428–430.

Kavirajan H, Schneider LS. Efficacy and adverse effects of cholinesterase inhibitors and memantine in vascular dementia: A meta-analysis of randomized controlled trials. *Lancet Neurol*. 2007;6:782–792.

Kertesz A, Blair M, McMonagle P, et al. The diagnosis and course of frontotemporal dementia. *Alzheimer Dis Assoc Disord*. 2007;21:155–163.

Klunk WE, Engler H, Nordberg A, et al. Imaging brain amyloid in Alzheimer's disease with Pittsburgh Compound-B. *Ann Neurol*. 2004;55:306–319.

Knopman DS, DeKosky ST, Cummings JL, et al. Practice parameter: Diagnosis of dementia (an evidence-based review). Report of the Quality Standards Subcommittee of the American Academy of Neurology. *Neurology*. 2001;56:1143–1153.

Larson EB, Shadlen MF, Wang L, et al. Survival after initial diagnosis of Alzheimer disease. *Ann Intern Med*. 2004;140:501–509.

Lewis LM, Miller DK, Morley JE, et al. Unrecognized delirium in ED geriatric patients. *Am J Emerg Med*. 1995;13:142–145.

Lipowski ZJ. *Delirium: Acute confusional states*. New York: Oxford University Press; 1990.

Lippa CF, Duda JE, Grossman M, et al. DLB and PDD boundary issues. Diagnosis, treatment, molecular pathology, and biomarkers. *Neurology*. 2007;68:812–819.

Livingston G, Johnston K, Katona C, et al. Systematic review of psychological approaches to the management of neuropsychiatric symptoms of dementia. *Am J Psychiatry*. 2005;162:1996–2021.

Lyketsos CG, DelCampo L, Steinberg M, et al. Treating depression in Alzheimer disease: Efficacy and safety of sertraline therapy, and the benefits of depression reduction: The DIADS. *Arch Gen Psychiatry*. 2003;60:737–746.

Mach JR, Dysken MW, Kuskowski M, et al. Serum anticholinergic activity in hospitalized older persons with delirium: A preliminary study. *J Am Geriatr Soc*. 1995;43:491–495.

Mayo-Smith MF, Beecher LH, Fischer TL, et al. Management of alcohol withdrawal delirium. An evidence-based practice guideline. *Arch Intern Med*. 2004;164:1405–1412.

McCurry SM, Gibbons LE, Logsdon RG, et al. Nighttime insomnia treatment and education for Alzheimer's disease: A randomized, controlled trial. *J Am Geriatr Soc*. 2005;53:793–802.

McCusker J, Cole M, Abrahamowicz M, et al. Delirium predicts 12-month mortality. *Arch Intern Med*. 2002;162:457–463.

McKeith IG, Dickson DW, Lowe J, et al. Diagnosis and management of dementia with Lewy bodies: Third report of the DLB Consortium. *Neurology*. 2005;65:1863–1872.

Mega MS, Cummings JL. Frontal-subcortical circuits and neuropsychiatric disorders. *J Neuropsychiatry Clin Neurosci*. 1994;6:358–370.

Mega MS, Cummings JL, Fiorello T, et al. The spectrum of behavioral changes in Alzheimer's disease. *Neurology*. 1996;46:130–135.

Mendez MF, Shapira JS, McMurtray A, et al. Preliminary findings: Behavioral worsening on donepezil in patients with frontotemporal dementia. *Am J Geriatr Psychiatry*. 2007;15:84–87.

Menza MA, Murray GB, Holmes VF, et al. Decreased extrapyramidal symptoms with intravenous haloperidol. *J Clin Psychiatry*. 1987;48:278–280.

Menza MA, Murray GB, Holmes VF, et al. Controlled study of extrapyramidal reactions in the management of delirious, medically ill patients: Intravenous haloperidol versus intravenous haloperidol plus benzodiazepines. *Heart Lung*. 1988;17:238–241.

Milbrandt EB, Deppen S, Harrison PL, et al. Costs associated with delirium in mechanically ventilated patients. *Crit Care Med*. 2004;32:955–962.

Miller ER III, Pastor-Barriuso R, Dalal D, et al. Meta-analysis: High-dosage vitamin E supplementation may increase all-cause mortality. *Ann Intern Med*. 2005;142:37–46.

Naughton BJ, Moran MB, Kadah H, et al. Delirium and other cognitive impairment in older adults in an emergency department. *Ann Emerg Med*. 1995;25:751–755.

Neary D, Snowden JS, Gustafson L. Frontotemporal lobar degeneration: A consensus on clinical diagnostic criteria. *Neurology*. 1998;51:1546–1554.

Ota M, Mefford IN, Naoi M, et al. Effects of morphine administration on catecholamine levels in rat brain: Specific reduction of epinephrine concentration in hypothalamus. *Neurosci Lett*. 1991;121:129–132.

Owen D, Paranandi B, Sivakumar R, et al. Classical diseases revisited: Transient global amnesia. *Postgrad Med J*. 2007;83:236–239.

Petersen RC. Mild cognitive impairment as a diagnostic entity. *J Intern Med*. 2004;256:183–194.

Petersen RC, Smith GE, Waring SC, et al. Aging, memory, and mild cognitive impairment. *Int Psychogeriatr*. 1997;9(Suppl 1):65–69.

Petersen RC, Thomas RG, Grundman M, et al. Vitamin E and donepezil for the treatment of mild cognitive impairment. *N Engl J Med*. 2005;352:2379–2388.

Pissarnitski D. Advances in gamma-secretase modulation. *Curr Opin Drug Discov Devel*. 2007;10: 392–402.

Platt MM, Breitbart W, Smith M, et al. Efficacy of neuroleptics for hypoactive delirium. *J Neuropsychiatry Clin Neurosci*. 1994;6:66–67.

Rhea RS, Battistone S, Fong JJ, et al. Atypical antipsychotics versus haloperidol for treatment of delirium in acutely ill patients. *Pharmacotherapy*. 2007;27:588–594.

Rockwood K, Cosway S, Stolee P, et al. Increasing the recognition of delirium in elderly patients. *J Am Geriatr Soc*. 1994;42:252–256.

Sano M, Ernesto C, Thomas RG, et al. The Alzheimer's Disease Cooperative Study. A controlled trial of selegiline, alpha-tocopherol, or both as treatment for Alzheimer's disease. *N Engl J Med*. 1997;336: 1216–1222.

Schneider LS, Tariot PN, Dagerman KS, et al. Effectiveness of atypical antipsychotic drugs in patients with Alzheimer's disease. *N Engl J Med*. 2006;355:1525–1538.

Shoghi-Jadid K, Small GW, Agdeppa ED, et al. Localization of neurofibrillary tangles and beta-amyloid plaques in the brains of living patients with Alzheimer disease. *Am J Geriatr Psychiatry*. 2002;10:24–35.

Shumaker SA, Legault C, Rapp SR, et al. Estrogen plus progestin and the incidence of dementia and mild cognitive impairment in postmenopausal women: The Women's Health Initiative Memory Study: A randomized controlled trial. *JAMA*. 2003;289:2651–2662.

Silverman DH, Small GW, Chang CY, et al. Positron emission tomography in evaluation of dementia: Regional brain metabolism and long-term outcome. *JAMA*. 2001;286:2120–2127.

Small GW. Diagnostic issues in dementia: Neuroimaging as a surrogate marker of disease. *J Geriatr Psychiatry Neurol*. 2006;19:180–185.

Snowdon DA. Nun Study. Healthy aging and dementia: Findings from the Nun Study. *Ann Intern Med*. 2003;139:450–454.

Strub RL, Black FW. *The mental status examination in neurology*, 4th ed. Philadelphia: FA Davis Co; 2000.

Swanberg MM. Memantine for behavioral disturbances in frontotemporal dementia: A case series. *Alzheimer Dis Assoc Disord*. 2007;21:164–166.

Tariot PN, Farlow MR, Grossberg GT, et al. Memantine treatment in patients with moderate to severe Alzheimer disease already receiving donepezil: A randomized controlled trial. *JAMA*. 2004;291:317–324.

Thompson S, Herrmann N, Rapoport MJ, et al. Efficacy and safety of antidepressants for treatment of depression in Alzheimer's disease: A metaanalysis. *Can J Psychiatry*. 2007;52:248–255.

Trzepacz PT. Is there a final common neural pathway in delirium? Focus on acetylcholine and dopamine. *Semin Clin Neuropsychiatry*. 2000;5:132–148.

Trzepacz PT, Mittal D, Torres R, et al. Validation of the delirium rating scale-revised-98: Comparison with the delirium rating scale and the cognitive test for delirium. *J Neuropsychiatry Clin Neurosci*. 2001;13:229–242.

Weintraub D, Hurtig HI. Presentation and management of psychosis in Parkinson's disease and dementia with Lewy bodies. *Am J Psychiatry*. 2007;164:1491–1498.

Whitehouse PJ, Price DL, Clark AW, et al. Alzheimer disease: Evidence for selective loss of cholinergic neurons in the nucleus basalis. *Ann Neurol*. 1981;10:122–126.

Yokota H, Ogawa S, Kurokawa A, et al. Regional cerebral blood flow in delirium patients. *Psychiatry Clin Neurosci*. 2003;57:337–339.

CHAPTER 9

Cynthia M. A. Geppert and Michael P. Bogenschutz

Substance-Related Disorders

Clinicians of every specialty in medicine from pediatrics to pathology will routinely encounter the adverse effects of substance-related disorders during their professional careers. Of all the illnesses and injuries physicians and other health professionals treat, substance abuse and dependence are the most multifaceted; effective assessment and treatment generally must address biological, psychological, social, and even spiritual dimensions of the illness. For decades, there have been effective psychosocial therapies for substance-related disorders, and methadone has been available as an effective treatment for opioid dependence since the 1970s. The last decade has seen great advances in the understanding of the neurobiology of addiction, and new and promising pharmacologic treatments have emerged. At this point in the history of medicine, substance-related disorders can truly for the first time be considered as chronic and relapsing conditions with a recovery rate similar to, if not better than, that of many other common medical diseases such as diabetes and hypertension (McLellan et al., 2000). However, studies have found that many physicians-in-training do not receive adequate education in substance-related disorders and do not feel adequately prepared to treat them in practice despite their prevalence and severity (Miller et al., 2001).

In this chapter, the general epidemiology and etiology of substance-related disorders is first reviewed, and the chapter then provides specific discussions of the phenomenology, diagnosis, and treatment of the major substances of abuse, including alcohol, amphetamine and cocaine, hallucinogens, inhalants, marijuana, opioids, nicotine, phencyclidine (PCP), and sedative-hypnotics. This chapter also outlines future directions in the care of persons with substance-related disorders.

EPIDEMIOLOGY

Drug Use and Treatment in the United States

The most comprehensive annual survey conducted in the United States for substance use and related mental health issues is the National Survey on Drug Use and Health (NSDUH). The 2006 report published by the Substance Abuse and Mental Health Services Administration found that an estimated 20.4 million Americans had used illicit drugs in the month before the survey, with marijuana the most common. More than half of the population consumed alcohol, and 23% endorsed binge drinking, which means they drank five or more alcoholic beverages on a single occasion within the previous 30 days. Approximately 30% of those surveyed were using a tobacco product. Nonmedical use of pain relievers and marijuana were the two illicit drugs most likely to be involved in the initiation of substance use. In 2006, 2.6 million Americans were classified with substance abuse or dependence, and 4 million received some form of help for an alcohol or drug problem. More than half of those who received help did so through a self-help group. Others were treated in emergency departments, rehabilitation facilities, outpatient programs (including intensive outpatient treatment), mental health centers, hospitals, independent practices, or in jails and prisons, which demonstrates the variety and fragmentation of the substance abuse health care delivery system. The number of persons needing treatment at a specialty facility and not obtaining it is far greater than those receiving any kind of treatment, estimated at 21.1 million.

Dual Diagnosis Populations

In recent years, the mental health community has paid increased attention to the high rate of comorbidity between mental health and substance use disorders, called *dual diagnosis* or *co-occurring disorders.* NSDUH indicates that among adults with serious psychological distress, 22.3% were dependent on, or abused, substances, compared with 7.7% among those without a mental health problem. The need for coordinated care for patients with co-occurring disorders is illustrated in the statistic that only 2.8% of persons in this group received both substance use and mental health treatment (Substance Abuse and Mental Health Services Administration, 2006).

Gender, Ethnic, and Age Differences in Substance Use

Complex genetic, cultural, and economic factors underlie epidemiological differences in substance use diagnosis and access to treatment. Rates of substance use disorders are generally about two times higher in men than in women, although the difference seems to be diminishing somewhat in younger age groups. Married adults have higher rates of substance use disorders than those who are single, divorced, or widowed. Poverty and unemployment are also risk factors for substance use disorders. Combined data from the NSDUH from 2002 to 2005 found that the rates of past-year substance use and related disorders were higher among American Indians and Alaskan Natives than among members of other ethnic groups (Substance Abuse and Mental Health Services Administration, 2007). Adolescent substance use is a major public health concern. A hopeful trend identified in the latest survey is that drug use among adolescents has decreased from 11.6% in 2002 to 9.8% in 2006 (Substance Abuse and Mental Health Services Administration, 2003).

PHENOMENOLOGY OF SUBSTANCE DEPENDENCE AND ABUSE

Most of the illnesses covered in this textbook will have disorder-specific criteria in the *Diagnostic and Statistical Manual of Mental Disorders*, Fourth Edition, Text Revision (DSM-IV-TR). Substance-related disorders are an exception in that they share a common category of signs and symptoms which constitute dependence and abuse. To meet the criteria for substance *dependence*, three of the symptoms must be present in a 12-month period and result in impairment of functioning in work, school, or personal life. Substance *abuse* criteria differ in that only one of the symptoms need be found in a 12-month period, but significant impairment still must exist.

Clinical Characteristics of Substance Dependence

- Physical dependence
  - Tolerance
  - Withdrawal
- Loss of control
  - Inability to control duration or amount when using or to stop or control use over time
  - Devoting large amounts of time to finding, using, and recovering from the effects of the substance
- Adverse consequences
  - Decrease in meaningful pursuits in favor of substance use
  - Continued use despite evidence that it causes medical or psychiatric problems

Clinical Characteristics of Substance Abuse

- Repeated failure to meet commitments due to use
- Repeated use in physically dangerous circumstances
- Repeated legal problems due to use
- Recurrent interpersonal conflict due to use

In addition to the substance use disorders (abuse and dependence), DSM-IV-TR also defines substance-related disorders for each class of substance. Most, but not all, substances of abuse cause intoxication and/or withdrawal. Other substances of abuse cause particular substance-related disorders such as delirium, dementia, amnestic, mood, anxiety, sleep, and sexual dysfunction disorders. Often these secondary substance-induced disorders can only be accurately distinguished from primary psychiatric disorders after a period of sobriety is achieved. Factors that have been associated with a relatively good prognosis for recovery from some substances of abuse are absence of family history of substance abuse, social support, high motivation, employment, lack of psychiatric and medical comorbidity, and a shorter duration of illness.

ETIOLOGY AND PATHOGENESIS

Genetics

The genetic contribution to the risk for substance use disorders is well established. In alcohol and nicotine addiction, an estimated 50% to 60% of an individual's risk is due to genetic factors (Tyndale, 2003). For other substances of abuse, the genetic contribution to risk is not as well studied but appears to be comparable (Kendler et al., 2006). No single gene accounts for a large proportion of this risk. Most likely, overlapping sets of genes interact with the environment and predispose to addiction to each of the substances of abuse. Specific polymorphisms of a few genes have been identified that significantly affect addiction liability. In alcohol addiction, the first genes to be established as playing a role in addiction risk were the genes coding for the enzymes responsible for the metabolism of alcohol: alcohol dehydrogenase (ADH) and aldehyde dehydrogenase (ALDH) (Edenberg, 2007). Many of the genes that are candidates for playing a role in addiction code for or affect the expression of receptors for neurotransmitters involved in addiction, affect the release, uptake, or metabolism of neurotransmitters, and/or affect general temperamental characteristics (e.g., impulsivity and novelty seeking) that modulate risk for substance use disorders. It is also likely that genetics can affect response to various pharmacotherapies for addictive disorders.

Psychiatric Comorbidity

Rates of substance use disorders are higher among individuals with most common psychiatric disorders and are particularly elevated among individuals with bipolar disorder, schizophrenia, and antisocial personality disorder. In theory, these high comorbidity rates could be due to substance use disorders causing psychiatric illness, psychiatric illness causing substance use disorders, or a third factor predisposing to both disorders. Each of these models probably plays a role to varying degrees in different cases. Temporally, psychiatric disorders appear to predate the onset of substance use disorders in half or more of dually diagnosed individuals. There is little evidence of any specificity between psychiatric diagnosis and substance of abuse, as would be predicted by the self-medication hypothesis. People with mental illness tend in general to experience more distress and to have fewer coping skills and social supports. They are therefore more likely to resort to substance use in an attempt to cope with unpleasant feelings and situations.

Environmental Risk Factors

Trauma and Stress

Serious trauma histories are ubiquitous among individuals seeking substance abuse treatment, and rates of lifetime posttraumatic stress disorder (PTSD) diagnosis are >50% in some clinical samples (Reynolds et al., 2005). There is now evidence that traumatic experiences have measurable effects on brain development and functioning, which are mediated in part by oxidative stress during overwhelming experiences (Weiss, 2007). These brain changes due to trauma may directly increase risk of addiction (De Bellis, 2002).

Exposure to Drug and Initiation of Drug Use

A person cannot use a drug unless exposed to it and cannot become addicted without using it at least once and usually many times. Exposure is dependent on availability of drugs due to factors such as legal prohibition, prevailing social attitude, price, and drug distribution networks. Initiation of substance use is affected by social networks and, to some extent, by personality/temperament. Because of incomplete brain development, individuals who initiate drug or alcohol use at an earlier age have a greater risk of developing substance use disorders than those who initiate use later.

Social Support for Substance Use versus Abstinence

Substance use behavior is affected by the attitudes of those in the individual's social network. Individuals belonging to religious groups that proscribe substance use are less likely to use those substances and ultimately less likely to become dependent on them. It is well known that peer networks' levels of substance use are a strong predictor of substance use in adolescents. Social support for drinking also has a significant, though smaller, effect on substance use by adults.

Behavioral and Neurobiological Pathogenesis

Brain Reward Mechanism

Decades of research have established that there is a common mechanism of reinforcement or reward for all addictive substances that have been studied. Either directly or indirectly, all of the major classes of addictive drugs cause the release of dopamine in the nucleus accumbens from axons originating in cell bodies in the ventral tegmental area, which is correlated with the pleasurable effects of the drug (Di Chiara et al., 2004). This is a ubiquitous mechanism of reward that is also triggered by natural rewards such as food or sex. However, the amount of dopamine release produced by drugs of abuse is much greater than that produced by natural rewards.

Withdrawal, Tolerance, and Sensitization

Tolerance and withdrawal, discussed earlier, are the defining features of physical dependence. These phenomena occur to varying degrees with the different substances of abuse, and may be understood in a general way using opponent process theory (Koob et al., 1989). The theory states that an organism adapts to counteract the effects of a perturbing stimulus (such as a drug of abuse) in order to maintain homeostasis. In the case of withdrawal, this means that when the substance is removed, the compensatory response of the organism is unopposed and causes effects that are the opposite of the symptoms caused by the drug. Although tolerance to many of the symptoms of intoxication occurs for most drugs, for some effects the opposite occurs: the organism has a greater response with repeated administration of the substance. This is termed *sensitization*. Sensitization has been reported for some of the effects of psychostimulants (Bradberry, 2007).

Motivation and Choice

Although reward and physical dependence are consequences of substance use and play a role in the genesis of addiction, the core features of addiction have to do with alterations in motivation and choice that lead to the seemingly irrational decision to continue using the substance despite obvious devastating consequences (Kalivas and Volkow, 2005). Through repeated cycles of drug use and reward, relatively enduring changes occur in critical brain circuits subsuming motivated behavior, and the addicted individual loses control over his or her use of the substance. Multiple neurotransmitter systems are involved, including dopamine, glutamine, γ-aminobutyric acid (GABA), endogenous opioids, serotonin, endocannabinoids, and cortitropin-releasing factor. Learning mechanisms involving the amygdala, nucleus accumbens, caudate nucleus and putamen, and hippocampus are recruited through the powerful reinforcing effects of substances of abuse, and these mechanisms in turn produce learned responses that contribute to addiction (Volkow et al., 2004).

Motivation is affected through brain areas including the orbitofrontal cortex and anterior cingulate gyrus (Volkow et al., 2004). These areas are hypoactive in addicts at baseline but show an exaggerated response to drug-related cues, and this activation is associated with self-reported craving. Cortical areas including the anterior cingulate, orbitofrontal cortex, and the dorsolateral prefrontal cortex are involved in attention, inhibitory control of behavior, the assignment of value to stimuli in the environment, and other aspects of executive function. Structural and functional changes in these regions lead to impairment in self-monitoring and decision-making.

DIAGNOSIS OF SUBSTANCE USE DISORDERS

As with other medical and psychiatric disorders, diagnosis of substance-related problems relies primarily on a careful and complete history along with a focused physical examination, targeted laboratory tests, and often collateral information. Accuracy, reliability, and rapidity of diagnosis can be improved, especially in primary care settings, through the use of a number of validated instruments, such as the alcohol use disorders identification test (AUDIT), Michigan alcohol screening test (MAST), drug abuse screening test (DAST), and **t**olerance, **w**orried, **e**ye-opener, **a**mnesia, **c**ut-down (TWEAK). The most widely and easily used screening consists of the CAGE (**c**ut-down, **a**nnoyed, **g**uilt, **e**ye-opener) questions (see Table 9-1) (Ewing, 1984).

ALCOHOL-RELATED AND SEDATIVE HYPNOTIC–RELATED DISORDERS

Alcohol is the most widely abused substance in the United States besides nicotine. Alcohol abuse heightens the risk for suicide, homicide, domestic violence, and motor vehicle crashes. Alcohol-induced disorders include intoxication and withdrawal, each with an associated delirium, and the specific disorders of persisting dementia, amnestic, psychotic, mood, anxiety, sexual, and sleep disorders.

Signs and symptoms of alcohol intoxication include slurred speech, lack of coordination, ataxia, nystagmus, and, if severe, stupor or coma. Neurobehavioral changes characteristic of intoxication with alcohol are disinhibition, mood lability and impaired attention, memory, and judgment that causes problems in functioning during or shortly after consumption of alcohol. These symptoms usually have onset within 4 to 12 hours of either stopping or decreasing heavy or sustained alcohol use and generally resolve in 4 to 5 days.

Delirium tremens is a severe form of alcohol withdrawal in patients with chronic alcohol dependence that has a high mortality if untreated. Patients may exhibit agitation and hallucinations, as well as disorientation, confusion, and unstable vital signs. In addition to benzodiazepines, patients require vitamin supplementation and supportive care in a hospital setting.

Alcohol Intoxication and Withdrawal

The differential diagnosis of alcohol intoxication and withdrawal includes use of other central nervous system (CNS) depressants such as benzodiazepines and barbiturates and, in the case of severe withdrawal, other medical and neurologic causes of delirium, seizures, and psychosis. Laboratory tests such as blood alcohol level, urine toxicology screen, liver functions, blood counts and chemistries, and biomarkers, such as carbohydrate deficient transferase (CDT), may assist in making the diagnosis (Montalto and Bean, 2003; Miller and Anton, 2004). Benzodiazepines are the recommended treatment for alcohol withdrawal, and a structured withdrawal scale can assist in determining the most appropriate dose (Mayo-Smith, 1997). Anticonvulsants such as carbamazepine are sometimes utilized to treat withdrawal, and antipsychotics are employed to treat persisting hallucinations and delusions.

Treatment for Alcohol Abuse and Dependence

Psychosocial Therapies

Alcohol abuse and especially dependence are best treated with a combination of pharmacologic and psychosocial therapies. Cognitive behavioral therapy (CBT) aims at correcting the dysfunctional thoughts that lead to maladaptive behaviors and dysphoric emotions that often lead to substance

TABLE 9-1	CAGE Questions

Have you ever:
Felt you should *cut* down on your drinking?
Felt *annoyed* by criticism of your drinking?
Felt bad or *guilty* about your drinking?
Taken a drink first thing in the morning to steady your nerves or get rid of a hang-over? (*eye-opener*)

use. CBT also helps patients improve social skills, relationships, and self-discipline, all of which can prevent relapse. Motivational interviewing (MI) is another effective form of therapy that empathically seeks to increase the patient's awareness and concern about negative consequences of substance use and positive reasons for change and to heighten, and ultimately resolve, associated ambivalence about conflicting life goals. Individual therapy based on the 12-step facilitation model of mutual help and recovery is widely used and has performed favorably in controlled trials when compared with other empirically validated forms of treatment.

Behavioral, group, and family or couples therapies all can be beneficial in treating patients with alcohol disorders. Self-help 12-step programs, of which Alcoholics Anonymous is the original and most widespread, have enabled millions of individuals to achieve and maintain sobriety. Screening and brief interventions in emergency departments and at primary care visits have been shown recently to reduce alcohol use (Hughes and Cook, 1997).

Pharmacologic Treatments

The oldest medication used in the treatment of alcohol dependence is disulfiram. It provides a powerful disincentive to drink for individuals who are taking it, due to the disulfiram-alcohol reaction caused by the inhibition of ALDH (Kristenson, 1995). Consumption of alcohol while taking an adequate dose of this drug leads to the accumulation of acetaldehyde, resulting in unpleasant reactions of flushing, nausea, vomiting, hypotension, and rarely more serious consequences such as seizures or heart attacks. Disulfiram is most successful when used with very motivated patients who are not impulsive and have social support and clinical supervision.

Naltrexone is an opioid antagonist that lessens the reinforcement of alcohol and therefore can reduce both the frequency and amount of drinking. Naltrexone can cause gastrointestinal distress and hepatoxicity and so requires monitoring of liver functions. In 2006, a depot injectable of naltrexone received U.S. Food and Drug Administration (FDA) approval and may improve adherence (Garbutt et al., 2005). The newest medication for the treatment of alcohol dependence is acamprosate (Mason, 2001), which acts through dampening of glutamatergic activity and may reduce craving once a person has achieved abstinence.

Combined Therapy

Clinical trials of all of these medications have generally included some form of psychosocial therapy. A 2006 large randomized controlled trial that combined medications and behavioral therapies found that patients who received naltrexone in a medical management model (up to nine 15-minute sessions) did as well as those who received a more intensive psychosocial treatment in conjunction with medication and medical management (Anton et al., 2006).

AMPHETAMINE- AND COCAINE-RELATED DISORDERS

Amphetamines (including methamphetamine), cocaine, and allied compounds are the major stimulants of abuse. Cocaine interferes with uptake, and amphetamines cause excessive release, of the monoamine neurotransmitters dopamine, norepinephrine, and serotonin in the nucleus accumbens and other parts of the reward system described earlier. These effects initially enhance mood, alertness, and energy but with prolonged and heavy use can be neurotoxic, particularly

A CASE OF WITHDRAWAL

A 66-year-old veteran is admitted to the hospital for treatment of pneumonia. On the second day of hospitalization, he develops tachycardia, fever, elevated blood pressure, and a tremor. Nursing staff report that the man did not sleep the night before and has been agitated and asking to leave the hospital. The psychiatric consultant examines the patient, who describes seeing small animals running over his bed and feels that bugs may be crawling on him. Laboratory studies show elevated liver enzymes and MCV, and the toxicology screen is negative. Review of the chart does not indicate the patient has any psychiatric history.

A CASE OF INTOXICATION

Police bring a 25-year-old construction worker to the hospital emergency department after he tried to attack a convenience store clerk who asked him to pay for his purchases. The psychiatry resident on call is asked to examine the patient. She finds an agitated man pacing around the examination room. When asked why he assaulted the store clerk, the patient states that the clerk was working for the FBI and had been following him for weeks. At times he appears to be responding to internal stimuli. He looks much older than his stated age. On physical examination he appears thin and exhausted with poor dentition and needle marks on both forearms. The resident, with the patient's consent, makes a phone call to his ex-wife, who states that she divorced him because of his drug problem and then hangs up.

in the case of methamphetamine. Stimulants are often consumed in a binge pattern, with amphetamine having longer-lasting effects than cocaine. Addiction can develop rapidly with both drugs, which can be taken orally, snorted, smoked, or injected.

Both substances produce abuse, dependence, intoxication, withdrawal (and delirium during withdrawal), and psychotic, mood, anxiety, sleep, and sexual dysfunction disorders. The symptoms of intoxication with cocaine and amphetamines are similar and include the adverse physical effects of hypertension, tachycardia, dilated pupils, seizures, stereotypical behavior, and, in the case of intranasal use of cocaine, septal necrosis. Deleterious mental effects of these stimulants are insomnia, paranoia, auditory hallucinations, persecutory delusions, anxiety, and aggression. The withdrawal syndrome is the obverse of intoxication as outlined previously and often called a *crash* in which the patient sleeps and eats excessively; feels apathetic, fatigued, depressed, anergic, and anhedonic; and experiences intense cravings to use to relieve this dysphoria (National Institute on Drug Abuse, 1999, 2002). The differential diagnosis of stimulant dependence should consider other drugs, such as PCP and hallucinogens; medical conditions like hyperthyroidism; and primary psychiatric diagnoses, most prominently paranoid schizophrenia and mania.

Although numerous psychotropic medications have been tried in the treatment of cocaine dependence and withdrawal, none has shown consistent benefits in controlled trials, although several promising pharmacotherapies and a vaccine are in development for cocaine (Sofuoglu and Kosten, 2005). Psychosocial therapies are therefore the mainstay of stimulant treatment. Contingency management, a voucher-based system that substitutes positive rewards such as movie tickets or personal items in return for drug-free urine samples and treatment adherence, has yielded consistently positive results (Rawson et al., 2002). CBT can also help patients recognize and avoid relapse triggers and cope with other problematic behaviors surrounding drug use.

CANNABIS-RELATED DISORDERS

Cannabis includes cannabinoid-containing material derived from the plant *Cannabis sativa*. The dried leaves and flowers of the plant are marijuana, and the flowering tops of the female plant contain the highest concentration of cannabinoids. Hashish is a somewhat more potent resin extracted from the plant. Marijuana is the most commonly used illicit drug in the United States. All forms of cannabis exert their psychoactive effects through their agonist effects at the cannabinoid 1 receptor.

Signs and symptoms of cannabis intoxication include euphoria, sedation, sensory distortion and subjective hyperacuity, conjunctival injection, increased pulse and blood pressure, dry mouth, anxiety, and increased appetite. Psychomotor impairment is less marked than with alcohol, but sufficient to impair driving ability significantly. A mild withdrawal syndrome has been described but is not recognized by DSM-IV-TR. Symptoms are similar to, but much less severe than, those of opioid dependence. Other cannabis-induced disorders are cannabis intoxication delirium, cannabis-induced psychotic disorder, and cannabis-induced anxiety disorder. There is considerable evidence that marijuana use increases risk of onset of schizophrenia.

Treatments for cannabis abuse and dependence are not well studied. Psychosocial treatments such as CBT and treatments based on MI that are effective for other addictions are reasonable therapeutic choices for marijuana. There are no known effective pharmacotherapies for cannabis dependence.

HALLUCINOGEN-RELATED DISORDERS

The hallucinogens are a diverse group of serotonergic compounds including lysergic acid diethylamide (LSD), commonly known as *acid*; phenylalkylamines such as mescaline and 3,4-methylenedioxymethamphetamine (MDMA) or "ecstasy"; and tryptamines such as psilocybin and N-dimethyltryptamine (DMT). The term *hallucinogen* is somewhat misleading in that true hallucinations are much less common than the visual illusions and other sensory distortions with this class of drug. Hallucinogenic compounds are widely distributed in nature, and DMT is a naturally occurring compound in the mammalian brain. Subjective effects of hallucinogen intoxication include perceptual changes such as illusions, hallucinations, depersonalization, derealization, and synesthesias, as well as a wide range of unpredictable affective effects, including euphoria, dysphoria, self-transcendence, meaninglessness, anxiety, paranoia, panic, and calm detachment. Physiological effects of hallucinogen intoxication include mydriasis, tachycardia, sweating, palpitations, blurred vision, tremor, and incoordination. When presenting in a medical or psychiatric emergency setting, hallucinogen intoxication may mimic acute psychosis, delirium, or panic. History of recent ingestion of hallucinogens is generally necessary to make the diagnosis, because hallucinogens are not detected with routine urine or serum toxicology.

DSM-IV-TR categorizes the phenomenon of posthallucinogen "flashbacks" as hallucinogen persisting perception disorder. This refers to the clinically significant reexperiencing of any of the perceptual symptoms of hallucinogen intoxication weeks to months after the last use of the drug. Other hallucinogen-induced disorders include hallucinogen intoxication delirium, hallucinogen-induced psychotic disorder, hallucinogen-induced mood disorder, and hallucinogen-induced anxiety disorder.

Although many individuals experiment with hallucinogens, and their use presents significant risks, hallucinogen abuse and dependence do not commonly present for treatment. With the exception of MDMA and related drugs that have stimulant properties, the hallucinogens are not reliably reinforcing and hence very unlikely to produce true addiction. Tolerance to the hallucinogenic effects of most of these drugs is rapid and pronounced, but also rapidly reversible. Withdrawal from hallucinogens is not recognized in DSM-IV-TR, although a period of lethargy and dysphoria lasting up to several days may occur after MDMA use. There are no empirical data on treatment of hallucinogen use disorders, suggesting that relatively nonspecific psychosocial treatments such as MI, CBT, or 12-step approaches would be reasonable choices. Emergent treatment for intoxication generally consists of support, reassurance, and monitoring for safety until the acute effects of the drug wear off. Small doses of antipsychotic medication may be helpful in cases of extreme agitation. As indicated earlier, MDMA and related compounds such as 3,4-methylenedioxyamphetamine (MDA) and N-ethyl-3,4-methylenedioxyamphetamine (MDEA) have somewhat different effects from other hallucinogens, having stimulant properties and more addiction liability. These drugs are sometimes termed *entactogens*, indicating that they promote feelings of empathy and closeness to others. MDMA use is strongly associated with "raves" and, in these contexts, serious medical complications, including severe hyperthermia, rhabdomyolysis, seizures, multiorgan failure, and death. There is also considerable evidence of neurotoxicity in both animal models and humans, although there is uncertainty about how clinically significant these effects are (Gouzoulis-Mayfrank and Daumann, 2006).

INHALANT-RELATED DISORDERS

Inhalants are a diverse and widely available group of breathable chemicals including cleaning fluids, glues, gasoline, spray-paint, and a host of other industrial, household, and office solvents, aerosols, gases, and nitrites. Because of their ubiquity, inexpensiveness, and ready accessibility, they are often the drugs of choice for children and adolescents who sadly do not realize these everyday substances are drugs of abuse or are unaware of the terrible damage they can cause

(Dinwiddie, 1994). "Huffing" is the sustained inhalation of chemicals often from a paper or plastic bag to obtain a feeling of intoxication, mild euphoria, and disinhibition. Chronic use results in brain, liver, bone marrow, nerve, and kidney damage that is often irreversible. Even a single use of inhalants can result in "sudden sniffing death" from cardiac failure. Inhalant abuse is extremely difficult to treat because its young victims often have sustained cognitive impairments that make participation in psychosocial treatments difficult (National Institute on Drug Abuse, 2001). Disorders in addition to intoxication (Gilchrist et al., 1987), abuse, and dependence associated with inhalants include delirium, dementia, psychotic, mood, and anxiety disorders.

NICOTINE-RELATED DISORDERS

Nicotine dependence is the single most common substance use disorder in the United States, with 23% of the population currently dependent. It shares with other substance dependences the DSM-IV-TR defining criteria of physical dependence, loss of control, and adverse consequences. However, the nature of the consequences is very different. Nicotine causes little or no functional impairment or legal or social problems, but the long-term medical consequences make nicotine addiction a leading cause of premature death and disability. Although nicotine causes pleasurable (reinforcing) short-term effects in users, as well as mild increase in heart rate and blood pressure, it does not cause intoxication except in naive users or in overdose. DSM-IV-TR does recognize nicotine withdrawal, with symptoms including dysphoria, insomnia, irritability, anxiety, poor concentration, restlessness, decreased heart rate, and increased appetite.

Unlike all other substance use disorders, nicotine dependence is most often treated in primary care settings. Treatments include effective pharmacotherapies and CBT. The best outcomes are generally found when pharmacotherapy is combined with CBT. Effective treatments include many forms of nicotine replacement therapy (patch, gum, nasal spray, inhaler); bupropion, which is also an effective antidepressant; and varenicline, a partial nicotinic receptor agonist.

OPIOID-RELATED DISORDERS

Opioids are both natural and synthetic compounds and are used medically as analgesics and cough suppressants. Clinically significant effects are due to agonist activity chiefly at the μ opioid receptor. Opioid abuse and dependence, intoxication, and withdrawal are the major disorders, and other opioid-induced disorders are delirium, psychotic, mood, sexual, and sleep disorders. Mild to moderate levels of intoxication with opioids cause drowsiness, pupillary constriction, and slurred speech. Overdose may cause respiratory depression, requiring emergency reversal with naloxone, an opioid antagonist. Stopping opioids once a person has become physically dependent results in the signs and symptoms of opioid withdrawal. Differential diagnosis of opioid disorders encompasses mood disorders such as depression and dysthymia and intoxication with alcohol, sedatives, hypnotics, or anxiolytics. Physical examination, laboratory testing, toxicology screen, and history can help clarify the diagnosis.

The medications methadone and buprenorphine can be used for both opioid withdrawal and maintenance treatment of opioid dependence. Clonidine, an α_2 adrenergic agonist, is used only for the treatment of opioid withdrawal. It suppresses many of the physical symptoms of withdrawal but does little to relieve the psychiatric symptoms.

Chronic opioid use has an exceedingly high relapse rate without opioid substitution, and continued use, especially of intravenous opioids such as heroin, places the individual at risk for medical complications such as endocarditis, shooter's abscesses, and blood-borne infectious diseases (primarily hepatitis B and C and human immunodeficiency virus [HIV]). Death from accidental overdose is frequent (Osher et al., 2003). There are also considerable social and legal consequences of illicit opioid use.

Methadone is a long-acting opioid agonist that, decades of research has shown, reduces opioid and other drug use and criminal activity and improves medical morbidity and psychosocial functioning (Mattick et al., 2002). It can only be administered through licensed and regulated opioid treatment programs where patients receive daily or weekly dosing, counseling, and frequent urine toxicology monitoring. Constipation and sexual problems are the predominant side effects. Methadone maintenance is more effective if combined with psychosocial therapies.

Buprenorphine was FDA approved in 2003 as the first office-based treatment for opioid dependence, with the goal of integrating the treatment of opioid dependence into primary care (Krantz and Mehler, 2004). It is a partial agonist that has a lower risk of respiratory depression and a milder withdrawal syndrome than methadone. It is combined with naloxone in a sublingual form to prevent diversion. To prescribe buprenorphine, practitioners must receive a special certification and waiver from the Center for Substance Abuse Treatment. Buprenorphine has been successfully implemented within a primary care model of medical management.

PHENCYCLIDINE-RELATED DISORDERS

PCP, known as *angel dust*, is a major public health problem most often encountered in the emergency departments of large urban cities such as Washington, DC, or Baltimore (Substance Abuse and Mental Health Services Administration, 2004). PCP was first developed as a human anesthetic but is no longer used in medicine due to its adverse effects, including agitation, delusions, and paranoia (National Institute on Drug Abuse, 2006). By blocking glutamate receptors, PCP causes a profound dissociative effect, which results in distortion of the environment and sense of self. PCP is a white powder that can be snorted, smoked, or ingested. Physiological effects include increased blood pressure and pulse, flushing, and sweating, which can progress to nausea, nystagmus, and ataxia. High doses can lead to seizures and death. The most dangerous aspect of the drug is its propensity to lower the pain threshold while simultaneously increasing aggression, leading to suicidal and homicidal behavior. Management of acute PCP intoxication utilizes supportive care, reduction of stimulation, calming the patient, and, in severe cases, antipsychotics or anxiolytics. PCP-related disorders listed in DSM-IV-TR are abuse, dependence, intoxication (but not withdrawal), and delirium, psychotic, mood, and anxiety disorders.

SEDATIVE-HYPNOTIC–RELATED DISORDERS

The sedative-hypnotic class comprises several different drugs, all of which are similar in facilitating GABA-ergic neurotransmission, either directly or indirectly. Important sedative-hypnotic drugs include the benzodiazepines, barbiturates, meprobamate, chloral hydrate, bromides, and γ-hydroxy butyrate. Most of these drugs have legitimate medical uses, and they are relatively safe if used as prescribed. As a general rule, signs and symptoms of sedative hypnotic–related disorders resemble closely the effects of alcohol. Sedative-hypnotics withdrawal is also similar to alcohol withdrawal, and severe withdrawal can include seizures and delirium, similar to delirium tremens. Intoxication with sedative-hypnotics, particularly when combined with other CNS depressants, can cause severe CNS depression. Treatment rests primarily on stabilization and taper of a cross-tolerant sedative hypnotic. Sedative-hypnotic abuse and dependence commonly co-occur with other substance use disorders. Generally applicable psychosocial treatments are indicated, along with treatment of co-occurring substance use disorders and other psychiatric disorders.

CONCLUSION AND FUTURE DIRECTIONS

Substance-related disorders are among the most prevalent, universal, and deleterious conditions in human experience and for most of history lacked either a known etiology or a treatment. The future directions for substance use research and treatment are promising, with further elucidation of the neurobiological, genetic, and environmental causes and contributors to substance abuse and dependence. It is hoped that these basic science discoveries will be more rapidly translated into efficacious pharmacologic and psychological therapies. The greatest challenges facing substance use clinicians and patients alike in the twenty-first century will be the continuing effort to eliminate the social stigma attached to substance abuse, train adequate numbers of competent professionals, increase access to care, and obtain economic parity in funding for high-quality treatment services.

Clinical Pearls

- Collect information from collateral sources such as family and employers with the patient's consent to improve the assessment of substance use.
- Utilize structured instruments such as the CAGE, AUDIT, and DAST to help diagnose problematic substance use.
- Ask patients *how much* they are drinking or using a drug rather than *if* they are using it. This normalizes substance use and facilitates open communication.
- Ask patients about their longest period of sobriety, how they achieved it, and what triggers led to their relapse.
- Screen intravenous drug users for infectious diseases such as hepatitis C and B and HIV.
- Assess for past or current psychiatric disorders or persistent mood, anxiety, or psychotic symptoms during periods of sobriety that may suggest a primary, rather than substance-induced or secondary, disorder.
- Diagnose and treat insomnia, which is a frequent relapse trigger.

Self-Assessment Questions and Answers

9-1. A 46-year-old teacher has a long history of chronic lower back pain and has become dependent on prescription opioids. When her primary care physician became concerned and reduced the number of pills he prescribed, she began going to other doctors and also making periodic trips to the emergency department to obtain additional medications. She has no prior substance abuse history but is on fluoxetine for major depression. She is married with two teenaged children and is seeking treatment that will allow her to continue working and caring for her family. Which of the following would be the most appropriate treatment approach for this patient?

A. Methadone with no drug counseling
B. Detoxification with clonidine and no follow-up treatment
C. Detoxification with buprenorphine
D. Weekly cognitive behavioral therapy sessions and no medication
E. Buprenorphine maintenance treatment and drug abuse counseling

Patient preferences and contextual factors, such as being a working mother and wife in this case, are important considerations in choosing a treatment. A general principle of substance abuse care is that, when available, combined pharmacologic and psychosocial therapies are most effective; thus answers A and D, which offer single modalities, are less than optimal. A second important principle of substance abuse treatment is that detoxification is only the first step in comprehensive care, and without a more comprehensive treatment plan, patients most often relapse. This

means that answers B and C do not describe treatment approaches that are likely to be successful in the long run. Only answer E, which combines medication treatment with buprenorphine and counseling on a maintenance basis, is an evidence-based treatment that takes into account the patient's particular circumstances. In addition, buprenorphine, as opposed to methadone, is a primarily office-based therapy that is likely to be more convenient and acceptable to this particular patient. *Answer: E*

9-2. A 23-year-old bookstore clerk reports for the evening shift after attending a party. Her supervisor is called midway through the shift by a coworker because the woman is telling customers that she feels as if she is floating outside of her body. The supervisor notices that the clerk's pupils are dilated and she is sweating and tremulous. When asked if she feels ill, the clerk replies, "No. I feel close to God and to everyone." The supervisor wonders what drug the clerk has taken. Which of the following is likely the best answer to the supervisor's question?

A. She is intoxicated with alcohol.
B. She has taken no drug but is experiencing a psychotic break.
C. She has ingested ecstasy.
D. She has used PCP.
E. She has been using amphetamine.

This case presents an experience of methylenedioxymethamphetamine (MDMA) ("ecstasy"). The feeling of "floating outside the body" that describes the phenomenon of depersonalization is often a symptom of MDMA intoxication. Although sweating and tremor could certainly be signs of alcohol withdrawal, the emotional tone of withdrawal is usually anxiety and fear, not intimacy and acceptance, as the clerk expresses. Similarly, phencyclidine (PCP) intoxication often manifests with psychosis, rage, and violence, and amphetamine intoxication with paranoia and hallucinations of a persecutory nature. Although the patient is in the age-range for a first-break psychosis, and this certainly should be considered in the differential, the suddenness of the change in what appears to have been normal behavior and the attendance at a party, often the setting for MDMA use, are highly suspect. *Answer: C*

9-3. The single mother of a 10-year-old who lives in a housing project is worried that her son is becoming involved with drugs. Usually a quiet, obedient, and studious boy, over the last few months he has become sullen and unruly, and his schoolwork has declined. She wonders if he might have allergies because he seems sleepy all the time and has a runny nose. She noticed some office supplies missing from her desk. What drug of abuse is the boy most likely using?

A. Alcohol
B. Inhalants
C. Marijuana
D. PCP
E. Cocaine

Although adolescents unfortunately experiment with all the drugs of abuse listed, the description most closely fits the use of inhalants. Inhalants are common household substances—hence the missing items from the office desk—such as felt-tip markers, correction fluid, and glue. Being somnolent and having runny eyes and nose could be symptoms of marijuana or inhalant use, but given the age of the boy and the setting in an underprivileged area, inhalants are the more likely offender. Similarly, the behavior changes noted, such as irritability and decline in school performance, are somewhat nonspecific, but alcohol intoxication (answer A) would show more marked psychomotor impairment and slurring of speech, and alcohol withdrawal often causes nausea, vomiting, and tremor. Phencyclidine (PCP) intoxication (answer D) would generally cause a more profound psychiatric disturbance, often manifesting with dissociation and aggression. Cocaine intoxication (answer E) presents with insomnia, loss of appetite, hyperactivity, and at times psychotic symptoms. Withdrawal from cocaine could mimic inhalant abuse, because patients are also dysphoric and want to sleep, but it would be harder for this 10-year-old to obtain money sufficient to maintain a cocaine addiction. *Answer: B*

9-4. A 26-year-old college student is working two jobs and also going to school full-time. He begins to use amphetamines so he can get more done. Early in the semester he only uses a small amount of amphetamine before examinations or when he has to work a double shift and finds it very effective to keep him focused and awake. As the semester continues, he starts using every weekend to catch up on assignments he missed during the week. He finds he must use ever-greater dosages of the drug to obtain the same effect. His experience is an example of what neurobiological phenomena?

A. Withdrawal
B. Sensitization
C. Tolerance
D. Dependence
E. Intoxication

If the student was withdrawing from stimulants (answer A), he would likely demonstrate increased need for sleep and food, dysphoria, and craving for the substance, none of which appear to be present. Similarly intoxication (answer E) would show signs and symptoms of increased speech and activity, loss of appetite, insomnia, hypertension, and, often with heavy or prolonged use, psychotic symptoms. Although the young man likely is dependent (answer D) and the case scenario does mention some of the criteria, such as increased use, it does not describe many of the other cardinal symptoms of dependence, such as making the finding and taking of the drug a priority or failed attempts to cut back or stop using. Sensitization (answer B) means that the user obtains an increased effect with the same amount or frequency of substance use, which is the opposite of what is occurring in this situation. This leaves tolerance, the need for higher and higher amounts of a drug to obtain the same psychoactive effects, as the most appropriate answer. *Answer: C*

9-5. A 45-year-old businessman has been prescribed a medication by his primary physician to treat alcohol dependence and is also receiving individual cognitive behaviorally based therapy. His wife is supportive and witnesses him take his medication every morning to improve adherence. One night he is out having dinner with clients, who keep urging him to have a drink. He begins to feel embarrassed and worries that he will lose sales if he does not join in the socializing. Halfway through a glass of bourbon, he begins to feel flushed, dizzy, and nauseated and thinks he may faint. Which of the following medications to treat his alcoholism is he most likely to have been prescribed?

A. Naltrexone
B. Bupropion
C. Acamprosate
D. Disulfiram
E. Clonidine

This man is exhibiting the classic disulfiram reaction, in which patients regularly taking the drug experience hypotension, flushing, nausea, palpitations, and dizziness when they drink alcohol. The mechanism is a build-up of acetaldehyde through the inhibition of acetaldehyde dehydrogenase, which normally metabolizes alcohol in the liver. None of the other agents listed produce these characteristic effects. Naltrexone is an opioid antagonist used to treat both opioid and alcohol dependence but would only produce withdrawal symptoms if the patient used an opioid. Acamprosate is another medication that helps reduce drinking, but it has no adverse effects if alcohol is consumed while taking it. Clonidine is an α-antagonist used to treat opioid withdrawal, which can cause hypotension at higher doses but does not normally result in the flushing and gastrointestinal (GI) disturbance pictured here. Finally, bupropion is an antidepressant medication used in smoking cessation and has no dramatic interaction with alcohol. *Answer: D*

References

American Psychiatric Association. *Diagnostic and statistical manual of mental disorders*, 4th ed., text revision. American Psychiatric Press; 2000.

Anton RF, O'Malley SS, Ciraulo DA, et al. Combined pharmacotherapies and behavioral interventions for alcohol dependence: The COMBINE study: A randomized controlled trial. *JAMA*. 2006;295(17): 2003–2017.

Bradberry CW. Cocaine sensitization and dopamine mediation of cue effects in rodents, monkeys, and humans: Areas of agreement, disagreement, and implications for addiction. *Psychopharmacology (Berl)*. 2007;191(3):705–717.

De Bellis MD. Developmental traumatology: A contributory mechanism for alcohol and substance use disorders. *Psychoneuroendocrinology*. 2002;27(1-2):155–170.

Di Chiara G, Bassareo V, Fenu S, et al. Dopamine and drug addiction: The nucleus accumbens shell connection. *Neuropharmacology*. 2004;47(Suppl 1):227–241.

Dinwiddie SH. Abuse of inhalants: A review. *Addiction*. 1994;89(8):925–939.

Edenberg HJ. The genetics of alcohol metabolism: Role of alcohol dehydrogenase and aldehyde dehydrogenase variants. *Alcohol Res Health*. 2007;30(1):5–13.

Ewing JA. Detecting alcoholism. The CAGE questionnaire. *JAMA*. 1984;252(14):1905–1907.

Garbutt JC, Kranzler HR, O'Malley SS, et al. Efficacy and tolerability of long-acting injectable naltrexone for alcohol dependence: A randomized controlled trial. *JAMA*. 2005;293(13):1617–1625.

Gilchrist LD, Schinke SP, Trimble JE, et al. Skills enhancement to prevent substance abuse among American Indian adolescents. *Int J Addict*. 1987;22(9):869–879.

Gouzoulis-Mayfrank E, Daumann J. Neurotoxicity of methylenedioxyamphetamines (MDMA; ecstasy) in humans: How strong is the evidence for persistent brain damage? *Addiction*. 2006;101(3):348–361.

Hughes JC, Cook CC. The efficacy of disulfiram: A review of outcome studies. *Addiction*. 1997;92(4): 381–395.

Kalivas PW, Volkow ND. The neural basis of addiction: A pathology of motivation and choice. *Am J Psychiatry*. 2005;162(8):1403–1413.

Kendler KS, Aggen SH, Tambs K, et al. Illicit psychoactive substance use, abuse and dependence in a population-based sample of Norwegian twins. *Psychol Med*. 2006;36(7):955–962.

Koob GF, Stinus L, Le Moal M, et al. Opponent process theory of motivation: Neurobiological evidence from studies of opiate dependence. *Neurosci Biobehav Rev*. 1989;13(2-3):135–140.

Krantz MJ, Mehler PS. Treating opioid dependence. Growing implications for primary care. *Arch Intern Med*. 2004;164(3):277–288.

Kristenson H. How to get the best out of Antabuse. *Alcohol Alcohol*. 1995;30(6):775–783.

Mason BJ. Treatment of alcohol-dependent outpatients with acamprosate: A clinical review. *J Clin Psychiatry*. 2001;62(Suppl 20):42–48.

Mattick RP, Breen C, Kimber J, et al. Methadone maintenance therapy versus no opioid replacement therapy for opioid dependence *Cochrane Database Syst Rev*. 2002;(4):CD002209.

Mayo-Smith MF. American Society of Addiction Medicine Working Group on Pharmacological Management of Alcohol Withdrawal. Pharmacological management of alcohol withdrawal. A meta-analysis and evidence-based practice guideline. *JAMA*. 1997;278(2):144–151.

McLellan AT, Lewis DC, O'Brien CP, et al. Drug dependence, a chronic medical illness: implications for treatment, insurance, and outcomes evaluation. *JAMA*. 2000;284(13):1689–1695.

Miller PM, Anton RF. Biochemical alcohol screening in primary health care. *Addict Behav*. 2004;29(7): 1427–1437.

Miller NS, Sheppard LM, Colenda CC, et al. Why physicians are unprepared to treat patients who have alcohol- and drug-related disorders. *Acad Med*. 2001;76(5):410–418.

Montalto NJ, Bean P. Use of contemporary biomarkers in the detection of chronic alcohol use. *Med Sci Monit*. 2003;9(12):RA285–RA290.

National Institute on Drug Abuse *Research report series—cocaine abuse and addiction*. Rockville: U.S. Department of Health and Human Services; 1999.

National Institute on Drug Abuse. *Research report series—methamphetamine abuse and addiction*. Rockville: U.S. Department of Health and Human Services; 2002.

National Institute on Drug Abuse. *InfoFacts inhalants*. 2001, Retrieved April 6, 2002.

National Institute on Drug Abuse. *NIDA InfoFacts: PCP(Phencyclidine)*. 2006.

Osher FC, Goldberg RW, McNary SW, et al. Substance abuse and the transmission of hepatitis C among persons with severe mental illness. *Psychiatr Serv*. 2003;54(6):842–847.

Rawson RA, Huber A, Mccann M, et al. A comparison of contingency management and cognitive-behavioral approaches during methadone maintenance treatment for cocaine dependence. *Arch Gen Psychiatry*. 2002;59(9):817–824.

Reynolds M, Mezey G, Chapman M, et al. Co-morbid post-traumatic stress disorder in a substance misusing clinical population. *Drug Alcohol Depend*. 2005;77(3):251–258.

Sofuoglu M, Kosten TR. Novel approaches to the treatment of cocaine addiction. *CNS Drugs*. 2005;19(1): 13–25.

Substance Abuse and Mental Health Services Administration. *Overview of findings from the 2002 National survey on drug use and health*. Rockville: Department of Health and Human Services; 2003.

Substance Abuse and Mental Health Services Administration. Trends in PCP-related emergency department visits. *Drug abuse warning network report*. Rockville: U.S. Department of Health and Human Services; 2004.

Substance Abuse and Mental Health Services Administration. *Results from the 2005 National survey on drug use and health: National findings*. Rockville: Department of Health and Human Services; 2006.

Substance Abuse and Mental Health Services Administration. *Substance use and substance use disorders among American Indians and Alaska Natives*. The National Survey on Drug Use and Health Report. Rockville; 2007.

Tyndale RF. Genetics of alcohol and tobacco use in humans. *Ann Med*. 2003;35(2):94–121.

Volkow ND, Fowler JS, Wang GJ, et al. The addicted human brain viewed in the light of imaging studies: Brain circuits and treatment strategies. *Neuropharmacology*. 2004;47(Suppl 1):3–13.

Weiss SJ. Neurobiological alterations associated with traumatic stress. *Perspect Psychiatr Care*. 2007;43(3): 114–122.

10

John Lauriello, Tara K. Biehl, Juan R. Bustillo, and Steven M. Jenkusky

Schizophrenia and Other Psychotic Disorders

No other mental illness carries with it the preconceptions, misconceptions, and dread that schizophrenia does. The general public tends to equate schizophrenia with "being crazy," and the clinician is often wary of diagnosing someone with an illness that appears to have such a poor prognosis. In reality, the picture is much different. Schizophrenia is a relatively common illness, with a variety of possible clinical presentations and a range of outcomes. Certainly some patients with schizophrenia are so symptomatic that they are incapacitated and virtually nonfunctioning. However, most of the patients can function at some independent level and have much in common with the average person. Some even function at a very high level, finish school, hold good jobs, and establish families.

In this chapter, what schizophrenia is and what it is not will be explored. The myriad of symptoms that make up the diagnosis of schizophrenia will be looked at and the other psychotic disorders that are commonly considered to be part of the schizophrenia family, including schizophreniform disorder, schizoaffective disorder, brief psychotic disorder, and delusional disorder, will be discussed. The treatment options for schizophrenia, including pharmacologic and psychosocial interventions, as well as the applicability of these treatments to the other related psychotic disorders, will be reviewed.

The Meanings of Psychosis and Schizophrenia

Before going into a formal discussion of schizophrenia, it is helpful to review what is meant by the term *psychosis*. *Psychosis* comes from the Greek words *psykhe* ("mind") and *osis* ("diseased"), meaning "diseased mind." It signifies a loss of reality testing most often accompanied by delusions (false beliefs), paranoia (unwarranted suspicions), and hallucinations (misperceptions of the visual, auditory, or tactile senses). Psychosis is not a diagnosis; rather, it is a cluster of symptoms. It can occur in many conditions, including severe mood states like depression or mania, medical illnesses, or a reaction to a medication or substance.

The psychotic illness later known as *schizophrenia* was first described by Kraepelin (1971) in the late 19th century in an effort to distinguish it from manic depression. He utilized the existing term *dementia praecox* to describe these psychotic patients as having symptoms in common with the dementias but at an unusually early age.

In 1911, Bleuler coined the term *schizophrenia* to better describe the patients Kraepelin had been treating. *Schizophrenia* comes from two Greek words that mean "split mind" and describes the splitting apart of mental functions that Bleuler regarded as the central characteristic of schizophrenia (Kuhn, 2004). Schizophrenia, or "schizophrenic" in lay usage, denotes a split personality or "one who has simultaneously opposing thoughts." Bleuler did intend to emphasize that the "schiz" in schizophrenia was a split, but not one in personality, rather "a split in the meaning and emotion of one's thoughts and behaviors" (Kuhn, 2004). Bleuler also described the "Four As" (autism, attention, affect, and association) as abnormalities that are observed in many patients with schizophrenia. In schizophrenia, Bleuler's autism refers to the inability to develop close interpersonal connections and the tendency to retreat into oneself. Bleuler saw patients with schizophrenia as having difficulties attending to even simple tasks and having a blunted or flat affect or emotional range and jumbled thought processes and associations. Bleuler's Four As are now combined to describe the negative symptoms of schizophrenia. The

TABLE 10-1	Positive and Negative Symptoms of Schizophrenia
Positive Symptoms	**Negative Symptoms**
Delusions	Blunted or flat affect
Hallucinations	Avolition
Disorganization	Alogia
Agitated or bizarre behavior	Attentional problems
Suspiciousness	Anhedonia

positive symptoms mainly describe psychotic symptoms and originally were not a prominent part of either Kraepelin's or Bleuler's descriptions of the illness (see Table 10-1).

Later in the 1950s, the German psychiatrist Schneider (1959) published his "First Rank Symptoms" of schizophrenia, emphasizing "positive" symptoms that he considered pathognomonic for the illness (see Table 10-2). Currently, the evidence that these first rank symptoms are specific for schizophrenia is not very strong, because they can be found in a variety of disorders. However, the influence of the Schneiderian first rank symptoms continues and can be found in the most recently modified *Diagnostic and Statistical Manual of Mental Disorders*, Fourth Edition, Text Revision (DSM-IV-TR) (American Psychiatric Association, 2000) schizophrenia diagnosis section, which will be discussed later in this chapter.

The last 100 years has witnessed a tremendous increase in our understanding of schizophrenia, but its exact etiology is still not fully understood. The signs and symptoms of schizophrenia are now generally accepted as being biological in nature and may be exacerbated or worsened by social factors. Abnormalities in the dopamine system in the brain appear related to the illness, but these changes are not easily detected by imaging or chemical analysis. The best understanding is supported by the effects of potent dopamine receptor blockers (see "Dopamine Hypothesis" discussed later). Schizophrenia clearly runs in families, but these families often have a variety of psychiatric illnesses in their pedigree. There is great excitement in looking at schizophrenia from a genetic perspective, but it is unlikely that a single gene or even a simple set of genes will explain all cases.

EPIDEMIOLOGY

Schizophrenia is a relatively common illness. It affects approximately 1% of the worldwide population at any given time. Owing to the chronic nature of the illness, those afflicted stay afflicted, leading to an ever-growing population. Schizophrenia can theoretically manifest itself at any age, with the most common time of presentation in late adolescence or early adulthood. Men and women are considered to be equally affected, but women tend to be diagnosed at a slightly older age. In general, the earlier the onset of schizophrenia, the more virulent the disease. Children diagnosed at age 5 or 6, although uncommon, face a long struggle with fulfilling

TABLE 10-2	Schneiderian First Rank Symptoms
Hearing one's thoughts out loud
Hearing voices arguing or commenting on one's actions
Feeling one's body is being influenced
Believing one's thoughts are being withdrawn (thought withdrawal) or inserted (thought insertion) by an outside force
Believing one's thoughts are being broadcast for others to hear (thought broadcasting)
Feeling the delusion of being controlled by an external force

developmental milestones necessary for adequate adult functioning. The later the illness presents, the more experience and strengths the person can utilize to cope with the illness.

The Impact of Schizophrenia

Direct and Indirect Economic Costs

The impact of schizophrenia is profound to the individual, his or her family, and society. Economists define the cost of an illness in direct and indirect terms. Direct costs are the upfront costs associated with the treatment of the disease, such as mental health organizations (i.e., community mental health centers, treatment centers), acute hospital stays, clinician costs, nursing homes, medications, and support costs. A 2005 published estimate calculated the direct cost of schizophrenia as $27.7 billion per year in the United States in 2002 alone (Wu et al., 2005). Indirect costs are those "hidden" costs that include the loss of potential wages, in kind support from family, and family burden expenses. In the same 2005 report, the indirect cost of schizophrenia in the United States was estimated to be $32.4 billion per year, which was attributed primarily to lost productivity. Similar high costs were found in other industrialized nations (Fitzgerald et al., 2007).

Life Expectancy and General Health

The life expectancy of a patient diagnosed with schizophrenia is significantly reduced. A recent survey showed a life expectancy more than 30 years shorter than the average person (Auquier et al., 2006; Saha et al., 2007). The leading cause of this shortened life expectancy was cardiac disease due to poor general health maintenance, such as inadequate hygiene practices, poor nutritional habits, limited access to health and dental care, and a high propensity toward smoking. Suicide remains a significant factor for those with schizophrenia and is estimated to be at a much greater rate than for the general population (Bertelsen et al., 2007; Palmer et al., 2005).

Recently an increased rate of metabolic and obesity complications for those with schizophrenia has been brought to the attention of the public. This is in part an inherent aspect of the illness, a byproduct of poor health practices, and due to the use of psychotropic medications, most notably the atypical antipsychotics. A recent analysis of the National Institutes of Mental Health Clinical Antipsychotic Trials of Intervention Effectiveness (CATIE), a large study on antipsychotic use, revealed that a substantial number of enrolled patients with schizophrenia met criteria for metabolic syndrome at baseline (McEvoy et al., 2005; Meyer et al., 2008). Metabolic syndrome is characterized by abdominal obesity, high blood pressure, high cholesterol, and hyperglycemia.

Family Burden

Families are an essential support system for patients with schizophrenia, but historically, families were also "blamed" for malnurturing and causing schizophrenia in their children. Fromm-Reichmann (1948) coined the term *the schizophrenogenic mother* to describe a cold, rigid, and maladaptive parenting style she believed common to families with schizophrenic children. Bateson et al. (1956) described the double bind hypothesis of schizophrenia: a notion that families create a no-win environment for their children which leads to psychosis. Bateson et al. believed that psychosis was an expression of distress and mixed communications experienced early in family life.

In the past, laying responsibility for the illness on the families damned the very people who were obliged to care for their children. Currently, with the acknowledgment of the biological underpinnings of schizophrenia, families are no longer considered the cause of the disorder. Families can, however, improve the outcome of their children if they can reduce stressful interactions in the household. Brown et al. (1966) identified the concept of expressed emotion (EE) to describe conscious or unconscious criticism and blaming of the patient by parents. Numerous studies have shown the advantages of reducing unnecessary and overly punitive criticism, not only in schizophrenia but many other illnesses as well (Wearden et al., 2000).

It should be noted here that sometimes even the best supportive efforts of family and the community are not enough. The very nature and variable course of schizophrenia, along with issues of insight and medication adherence, make this a difficult illness with which to contend for some families. Sometimes the person suffering from the illness or the family providing support may end up alienated, or the family system may become generally fragmented.

THE HEAVY FAMILY BURDEN OF SCHIZOPHRENIA

Mrs. C has cared for her youngest daughter with schizophrenia for more than 35 years. They generally have a good and loving relationship, although at times it is clear Mrs. C is frustrated with her daughter's behavior. Often when her daughter's voices worsen, she screams at the voices, stomps on the floor, and bangs the walls. Mrs. C lives in fear that the landlord will evict them from their apartment. Both mother and daughter are fearful of what will happen if Mrs. C dies. Mrs. C is considering having them move in with her eldest daughter, who would be entrusted to care for the patient if Mrs. C no longer can.

This case illustrates the lifelong responsibility parents assume for their children and the multigenerational aspect of that burden. In the case of Mrs. C, her eldest daughter is prepared to help manage her sister if need be.

Vocational Loss

The ability to work and to be self-sufficient is an important aspect of most people's lives. People with schizophrenia experience a major impairment in their ability to work. Competitive employment (i.e., jobs acquired without the support of government programs or transfer payments) is estimated to be held by <20% of persons with schizophrenia (Lehman et al., 2002). A person's severity of symptoms plays an important role in his or her ability to work, but there are also external disincentives to taking a job, including a reduction or loss of government stipends and associated insurance programs. Great strides have been made to generate some work opportunities for patients that will not jeopardize the financial and supportive safety net they need. The use of supportive employment programs (described in detail under psychosocial treatment later in the chapter) has had some success in connecting people with schizophrenia to work.

Phenomenology

Signs and Symptoms

In the simplest of terms, schizophrenia, which at times can seem like a catchall disorder, is composed of what are called positive and negative symptoms (Table 10-1). Positive symptoms generally refer to symptoms that are present or "added" and can be elicited from the patient through a series of questions. These include auditory or visual hallucinations, delusions, and bizarre behavior. Negative symptoms refer to things that are missing or "subtracted" from the person that one would normally see. These are less likely to be elicited by questioning and must be observed in the patient or determined by history. These include blunted affect, avolition, and alogia. When determining a diagnosis for schizophrenia and other related disorders, it is important to ascertain the level of decline in functioning and the level of perceived stress or impairment for the patient and/or family. This can be done by asking questions such as, Did the person suddenly change or was it more gradual? How many areas of his or her life are affected? Is he or she more socially isolated, able to go to school or work, maintain relationships, and so on?

Diagnosing Schizophrenia

DSM-IV-TR is the diagnostic tool most widely used by clinicians and researchers, especially in the United States. The criteria for diagnosing schizophrenia will be described briefly in this chapter. For more complete diagnostic criteria on each of the described disorders, refer directly to DSM-IV-TR.

The underlying descriptions regarding diagnosing schizophrenia first provided by Kraepelin and Bleuler are still applicable. Reading descriptions of patients with schizophrenia in 1900 would not be remarkably different than reading descriptions of current patients with the disorder. Certainly the context of delusional material might differ, but many themes would be the same. For example, delusions of being controlled by spirits or by God or the devil are still reported today, just as they were many years ago. Beliefs that one is receiving messages from an external source continue. While in 1900 those beliefs might center on a mysterious machine yet to be named, today's patients may describe modern and futuristic satellites and computers.

Approaching a patient with a possible diagnosis of schizophrenia requires an understanding of the criteria for schizophrenia formulated over the last 100 years and a reasonable sense of what is a possibility versus a delusion. For example, it is possible that someone might be investigated by the government or have a cheating spouse, but it is not commonly accepted that aliens are on earth and communicating with people. A person who believes God is speaking to him or her directly may be deeply religious or a member of a church that speaks in tongues, but a person who stays in his or her room, hears God, and believes he or she is the only person in the world with this ability probably has a delusion. DSM-IV-TR provides the framework for a possible diagnosis of schizophrenia, and a diagnosis must satisfy criteria A through E. These criteria are briefly described in the following text. For complete diagnostic criteria, refer directly to DSM-IV-TR.

Criteria for diagnosing schizophrenia

Criterion A states that two (or more) of the following characteristic symptoms must be present for at least 1 month: delusions, hallucinations, disorganization, and/or negative symptoms. With this allowance of either positive or negative symptoms, one could imagine how two patients with the same diagnosis could present very differently and potentially require different treatments.

The remaining criteria for diagnosing schizophrenia include determining the level of disturbance in social and/or work functioning. The symptom presentation and disturbance must be present for a minimum of 6 months and other possible mental illnesses, such as schizoaffective disorder or a mood disorder, must be ruled out.

A subcategory of the illness, late-onset schizophrenia, is reserved for those who present with symptoms for the first time after age 45. An important warning on diagnosing late-onset schizophrenia is that a thorough search for earlier signs and symptoms should be done to definitively diagnose this condition. In many cases, patients who present as late onset have evidence of schizophrenia before age 45, which was either not obvious or unavailable. A good rule of thumb is to focus on occupational and social clues. For example, a man who has graduated from law school but never practiced as an attorney may have decided against pursuing the field for a variety of reasons, including that he may have been too paranoid to work with others.

Treatments

Pharmacologic Treatments of Schizophrenia

During the 19th century more humane treatment of severe mental illness replaced the longstanding religious and moralistic shunning of affected individuals. Humane treatment incorporated many psychosocial concepts utilized now, including vocational and talk therapies. However, even then patients with schizophrenia lived in asylums, and a return to the community was considered unlikely.

The excitement and advances in psychiatry in the first half of the 20th century, notably Freud's psychoanalytic work, provided great insights into the working of the mind and treatments for a variety of "neurotic" conditions (e.g., hysteria). There was similar hope that the success of psychoanalytic therapies for some mental illnesses could also be applied to patients with schizophrenia. Unfortunately, over time, rigorous treatment trials of psychoanalytic therapy did not support its use for schizophrenia (see section on "Psychotherapy"). At the same time, other clinicians attempted to physically change the brain in the hope of remedying some symptoms of schizophrenia. These efforts included psychosurgery (usually frontal lobotomy), insulin coma, and electroconvulsive therapy (ECT). All three certainly changed brain behavior and thinking but were not specific for schizophrenia and could carry lasting untoward effects (da Costa, 1997; Doroshow, 2007; Tharyan and Adams, 2005).

It is now generally accepted that the mainstay treatment of schizophrenia is the appropriate and consistent use of antipsychotic medications. A breakthrough occurred in the early 1950s in France with the discovery of the first antipsychotic, chlorpromazine (also known as *Thorazine*) (Carpenter and Koenig, 2007). Originally intended as a preanesthetic agent, French psychiatrists noticed that it had a calming effect on psychiatrically ill patients. For the first time, a compound could directly counteract psychotic symptoms. Chlorpromazine inspired the development of many agents that shared either biochemical similarities or created similar physical effects in animal models (e.g., catalepsy in rats).

In the early 1960s, Carlsson, winner of the Nobel Prize for Medicine, postulated that these antipsychotic compounds work by counteracting excessive neurotransmitter dopamine activity (specifically the D_2 receptor) in the brain (Toda and Abi-Dargham, 2007). His theory rested on the fact that antipsychotics could mimic a low dopamine condition and induce parkinsonian (or extrapyramidal, also known as *EPS*) side effects in patients. EPS include stiffness, tremor, rigidity, cogwheeling, pill rolling of the fingers, and shuffled gait. Carlsson also theorized that other agents which increase dopamine in the brain, such as amphetamines, could cause psychotic-like syndromes. Therefore, the dopamine hypothesis of schizophrenia was formulated and has remained the predominant biological theory of schizophrenia.

The widespread acceptance of the dopamine hypothesis led pharmacologic development for more than 20 years, producing more and more potent and pure dopamine blockers. Disappointingly, the potency of dopamine blockade did not produce appreciable improvement in outcome and left many patients without adequate relief.

A significant paradigm shift in schizophrenia pharmacotherapeutics occurred with the establishment of the superiority of clozapine for patients with treatment-resistant schizophrenia (Kane et al., 1988). Clozapine was particularly remarkable in that it achieved a greater efficacy in managing the symptoms of schizophrenia without having strong dopamine-blockade properties. It questioned the orthodox view of "the more dopamine blockade, the better." For the first time it was demonstrated that an antipsychotic effect could be separated from the "neuroleptic" or iatrogenic parkinsonian effect. However, clozapine's superiority comes at a great potential price. Clozapine can dangerously lower the white blood cell count of patients. Because of this, it is a second-line antipsychotic, often reserved for patients unresponsive to other medications.

Beginning in the 1980s, the search for other medications that duplicated clozapine's therapeutic effects without its risks gave rise to a new class, or generation, of drugs called the *atypical* or *novel antipsychotics*. The atypicals have in common less reliance on dopamine blockade and more effects on various other neurotransmitters. Currently, they are readily used as first-line agents. The development and use of these atypical antipsychotics have grown rapidly over the last decade. Scientists are still searching for an ideal atypical antipsychotic, one with characteristics thought to include superior efficacy for both positive and negative symptoms, low incidence of EPS and tardive dyskinesia, unchanged prolactin levels, and minimal worrisome metabolic effects.

Medication side effects

All active medications carry some level of side effect burden, and antipsychotics are no exception. The first generation, or typical, antipsychotics are roughly divided into low potency (high mg number) and high potency (low mg number) drugs. The low potency typical antipsychotics tend to have less EPS per mg dose but much more histaminergic and cholinergic effects. Patients taking low potency medication are more likely to become sleepy or orthostatic before getting stiff. High potency typical antipsychotics have a stronger dopamine blockade compared to other neurotransmitters; therefore, patients become stiff before they become sleepy or orthostatic. Either type of typical antipsychotic has a relatively narrow therapeutic window before EPS begin.

Clozapine and the subsequent first-line atypical antipsychotics have a wider therapeutic window. The dose that treats symptoms of schizophrenia is distinctly lower than the dose that causes EPS signs. The scientific rationale for the difference between typicals and atypicals appears to lie in the degree (and possibly the length of time) the medication occupies the dopamine 2 (D_2) receptor. Twelve-hour post–dosing positron emission tomography (PET) studies show that a threshold exists wherein occupation of >60% of the D_2 receptor leads to antipsychotic effect, but >75% D_2 receptor occupation leads to EPS (Kapur and Remington, 2001; Kapur and Seeman, 2001). All typical antipsychotics appear to provide antipsychotic effects at doses that cross the EPS 75% threshold. Atypical antipsychotics vary in terms of how wide the dosing window is to reach the 75% threshold (and both clozapine and quetiapine do not appear to even cross the 60% threshold). However, these medications do occupy >60% of the D_2 receptors at 2 hours post dosing, which may mean that D_2 occupancy can be transient and still effective. Aripiprazole occupies greater than 90% D_2 receptors, but this occupancy is mitigated by its partial agonist effects.

EPS can be unsettling and uncomfortable for patients, a concern in itself, but has also been linked to another side effect called *tardive dyskinesia* (TD). TD is a potentially irreversible hyperkinetic movement disorder that can be both disfiguring and stigmatizing. Various studies estimate the incidence of TD to be between 3% and 7% per year of exposure, with a leveling off after the first 10 years (Kane et al., 1982). It is especially problematic in the elderly, women, and those with comorbid affective disorders. A potential advantage of the atypicals versus the typicals is the lower incidence of TD with atypicals, with incidences <1% per year of exposure (Correll et al., 2004; Kane, 2004; Miller et al., 2007). No cases of TD have been clearly attributed to clozapine. In fact, clozapine has been documented to improve cases of TD. The first-line atypical antipsychotics, although not quite as good as clozapine, all appear to be superior to the typical antipsychotics.

Despite the superior EPS profile of the atypicals, this group has its own side effects. The first of these is an elevation of prolactin. All first-generation typical antipsychotics elevate prolactin, but at least two atypicals (risperidone and paliperidone) do so to an even greater extent. Acute prolactinemia is manifested clinically in women as a loss of menses and in both men and women as galactorrhea and sexual dysfunction. Chronically elevated prolactin has been linked to osteoporosis, most often in women with amenorrhea (Byerly et al., 2007).

Another side effect of the atypicals that concerns clinicians and patients is weight gain. Weight gain and other metabolic changes have been problematic with most antipsychotics since their discovery in the 1950s. However, the weight gain associated with several atypical antipsychotics appears greater than that of the typicals. Clozapine has the greatest associated weight gain, with olanzapine slightly lower, followed by risperidone and quetiapine (Allison et al., 1999). Weight gain is particularly worrisome in patients with schizophrenia because of other risk factors for cardiopulmonary morbidity, including cigarette smoking, poor diets, and sedentary lifestyles. Weight gain must be addressed aggressively with a combination of diet and exercise. If this is unsuccessful, switching to an atypical that has less weight gain association should be considered.

In addition to weight gain, other concerns, such as the emergence of insulin resistance, hyperglycemia, and overt diabetes in patients taking certain atypical antipsychotics, have grown. It is now accepted that many of the atypical antipsychotics (most often those associated with the greatest weight gain) can lead to either type 1 or, more commonly, type 2 diabetes. Regular monitoring of elevated fasting blood glucose is now standard practice for those taking any antipsychotic medication. Likewise, elevations of lipids and triglycerides seem to follow the same general pattern of elevation as blood glucose and require similar monitoring. The treatment of these metabolic problems should include diet, exercise, changing the medication to one of the newer atypical antipsychotics (e.g., ziprasidone, aripiprazole), or initiating hypoglycemics or anticholesterol medications, if necessary (Newcomer and Sernyak, 2007).

Finally, there have been idiosyncratic concerns about specific atypical antipsychotics that have not turned out to be clinically meaningful. An example is the concern about cataracts associated with the atypical antipsychotic quetiapine. Although mainly theoretic in humans, high-dose quetiapine has been shown to cause cataracts in beagle dogs. In practice, cataracts have not appeared to be a problem, with an incidence in the expected normal population range (Whitehorn et al., 2004). Likewise, there had been a concern about the prolongation of the QTc interval with certain antipsychotics, specifically ziprasidone, which has not borne out with greater use (Nemeroff et al., 2005).

Overall, the pharmacologic treatment of schizophrenia has undergone a major change in the last decade. Typical antipsychotics, with a high incidence of neurologic side effects, have been replaced by the atypical antipsychotics, with a far lower rate of these side effects, especially tardive dyskinesia. However, the atypicals have presented new challenges, especially in terms of weight and metabolic elevations. Development of better and safer antipsychotics is still a goal for the future.

Psychotherapies
Psychosocial treatment

Family interventions

One of the most consistent validators of the schizophrenia syndrome is that, like other major psychiatric disorders, it tends to run in families. Although this finding led in the past to premature

A CASE OF TRYING MULTIPLE MEDICATIONS

George is a 42-year-old man who first developed auditory and visual hallucinations at age 20. These symptoms had a profound effect on his ability to function, and he spent a great deal of time revolving in and out of the local psychiatric hospital. Trials of several antipsychotics, including typicals and atypicals, showed limited effect. Finally, at age 30, clozapine was initiated. George disliked the weekly blood draws but accepted them because his voices were greatly improved. George continues on clozapine, supported by disability benefits, but lives independently and has not required a hospitalization in many years.

George clearly suffers from schizophrenia, enduring a rocky decade of treatment. Despite numerous attempts to stabilize him on available first-generation antipsychotics, he eventually required clozapine. Although at age 42 he is chronically disabled, his symptoms have fortunately improved.

speculations regarding the influence of early family environment in the causation of schizophrenia, it is now widely accepted that the familial association is secondary to genetic, not psychosocial, factors. Nevertheless, psychosocial characteristics appear to have a significant impact on the course of the illness.

The concept of "expressed emotion" (EE) was empirically developed by Brown and Rutter (1966) in Britain to explain why some patients with schizophrenia relapsed quickly despite an adequate response to pharmacologic treatment in the hospital. Patients who have extensive face-to-face contact with family members rated high on critical, hostile, or over-involved comments (i.e., high EE families) may have a higher risk of relapse despite adequate medication compliance. It is important to keep in mind that the relationship between high EE and relapse is not specific to schizophrenia and has been found in various other chronic psychiatric and nonpsychiatric illnesses. This relationship is not specific to the family environment but to various social groups and even treatment approaches that are a source of continuous stress for the patient.

The common sense view that persons with a chronic, relapsing illness will tend to manifest exacerbations with continued stress is reaffirmed by the consistent literature on family interventions and outcome in schizophrenia. Most of the controlled trials have documented the effectiveness of various family interventions to reduce relapse, with effect sizes in the same magnitude range as maintenance antipsychotic medication.

Social skills training

Social skills are those specific response capabilities necessary for effective social performance. Most persons with schizophrenia, even those with a favorable response to antipsychotic medications, will have residual symptoms, cognitive impairments, and limited social skills. Because of this, psychosocial interventions aimed at the functional rehabilitation of the patient have been designed and systematically studied since the 1980s (Bellack and Mueser, 1993). Largely following the work on people with physical disabilities, psychiatric rehabilitation uses the principles of learning theory to improve the person's social competence in roles of work, leisure, parenting, marriage, and self-care and help to contribute to more autonomous functioning in the community. Social skills training (SST) should be distinguished from activities in other programs in which the acquisition of skills occurs incidentally. There are three forms of SST: the basic model, the social problem-solving model, and the cognitive remediation model.

Basic social skills model   During SST, dysfunctional, complex social repertoires are identified and broken down into more elementary behaviors, which are learned through repeated performance (Bellack and Mueser, 1993). The elements are then "reassembled" into a whole functional repertoire. Each elementary behavior (e.g., eye contact, speech volume, length of response, questioning) is repeated until learned. The therapist may model the behavior. Next, the patient may role play the integrated social repertoire and finally may practice it in a natural setting.

The literature consistently shows that patients with schizophrenia can be taught various social skills and that learning can persist anywhere between 6 and 12 months (Bellack and Mueser, 1993). The results are mixed on whether the skills learned will lead to an improvement in other important clinical measures, like symptom severity and relapse rate. Even if people with schizophrenia learn social skills, the extent to which these skills generalize in the patients' natural environment and result in improved social competence is a crucial measure of outcome. Generalization has not been clearly demonstrated for the motor skills model. In part to deal with this limitation, problem-solving techniques have been integrated with the more traditional SST model.

Social problem-solving model   The social problem-solving model uses social learning principles and assumes that impairments in information processing underlie the limited social competence present in many patients with schizophrenia. Like traditional SST, complex problem behaviors are identified, and patients are assigned to five distinct modules as targets for improvement: medication management, symptom management, recreation, basic conversation, and self-care. For each of these modules, an emphasis is placed on learning receiving, processing, and sending skills. The hope is that these skills will provide the patient with more flexibility and will result in greater durability and generalization of each module learned. There is some evidence of improvement in measures of social adjustment in the community with this approach (Marder et al., 1996).

Cognitive remediation   That patients with schizophrenia have a multiplicity of cognitive impairments is well established (Braff, 1993). These are most likely not just epiphenomena of symptom severity or medication side effects, because they are present in various subclinical populations (e.g., children at high risk for schizophrenia, nonpsychiatric relatives of patients with schizophrenia, and persons with schizophrenia-spectrum personality disorders). The cognitive impairments are generalized, but some particular functions, such as attention, memory, and planning, may be more impaired than others. Nevertheless, the specificity of cognitive impairments in schizophrenia is still debated. Researchers have reasoned that the limitations on the durability and generalization of SST may be overcome by improving impairments in elementary cognitive functions before teaching social skills. There is some evidence that patients can improve their performance through practice in measures of vigilance and planning, which is the core concept underlying cognitive remediation. However, the transfer of learning to another test has not been documented, even within the same cognitive domain (vigilance or planning), nor has evidence shown any generalization to particular social skills.

Assertive community training

Patients with schizophrenia are often ill prepared to find and maintain proper use of the multiple services they need to function in the community. Providers of these services include psychiatrists, nurses, pharmacists, social workers, and vocational therapists. Traditionally, case managers have functioned as brokers of services. They are contacted by other professionals who identify a need for the patient, and they then work to connect the patient to the provider best able to deliver these services. This approach may be sufficient for patients with physical disabilities and for some patients with mental illness of moderate severity. Unfortunately, many patients with schizophrenia lack the cognitive and social competence to follow through consistently to get their needs met, further increasing their risk of relapsing.

A different approach to case management and service delivery is exemplified by the Assertive Community Treatment (ACT) program (Stein and Test, 1980). Originally developed by researchers in Madison, Wisconsin, in the 1970s, ACT is the most carefully defined, well-documented, and successful program for the delivery of services for persons with chronic mental illness (not just schizophrenia).

Patients are assigned to a multidisciplinary team (case manager, psychiatrist, nurse, general physician, etc.). The team has a fixed caseload of patients and delivers all services when and where needed by the patient, 24 hours a day, 7 days a week. This is a mobile and intensive intervention that provides treatment, rehabilitation, and support activities, including home delivery of medications, monitoring of mental and physical health, *in vivo* social skills training, and frequent contact with family members, among others. There is a high staff to patient ratio.

The original study from Wisconsin followed chronically mentally ill patients assigned to ACT and compared them with a group discharged from the hospital to standard community care (Stein and Test, 1980). After 14 months, the ACT group showed significant advantages in rates of hospitalization, sheltered employment, independent living, and family burden, with essentially no difference in costs. Unfortunately, the advantages were lost after the patients were discharged from the experimental program. In addition, there are no present data on the minimum intensity for the program to maintain gains or which special population of patients may require continuous services.

Because of the comprehensive services provided by ACT and the lack of adequate controls, it is unknown whether the important effect on relapse and hospitalization is due to improved medication adherence, continuity of caregivers, 24-hour coverage, site of service, intensity of services, therapeutic alliance, or a combination of some of these elements.

In summary, when available, ACT-like programs may be particularly effective for relapse prevention in patients with schizophrenia who are frequently hospitalized and may be an especially useful option for patients with a high potential to relapse who do not live with their families or are homeless.

Psychotherapy
Individual therapy

Before the 1960s, individual psychoanalytic-oriented therapy was considered by many to be the optimal treatment for schizophrenia. The first serious challenge to this view came from the landmark study by May et al. (1968) at Camarillo State Hospital.

Hospitalized patients with schizophrenia were randomized to five treatment conditions: antipsychotic medication, individual psychoanalytic-oriented psychotherapy, medication plus psychotherapy, ECT, or "milieu" therapy. The best outcomes were seen in the pharmacotherapy groups, and the worst outcomes were seen in the milieu and psychotherapy-only groups (ECT treatment had intermediate results). Furthermore, the addition of psychotherapy to medication did not result in significant benefits.

These results were criticized because of the relative inexperience of the therapists providing psychoanalytic therapy. Hence, Gunderson (1984) implemented the next major study in Boston during the 1980s and compared individual psychoanalytic-oriented psychotherapy (provided three times a week by experienced psychoanalysts) with supportive therapy (provided once a week by social workers). All patients with schizophrenia were medicated with maintenance antipsychotics, which were by then established as standard treatment, and were then followed for 2 years as outpatients. Again, there were no consistent advantages for the more intensive psychoanalytic treatment.

Following the negative findings in this landmark study, psychoanalytic-oriented individual psychotherapy for most patients with schizophrenia has been practically eliminated in the United States. However, over the last decade, other forms of intensive individual treatment have been examined.

Cognitive behavioral therapy

Cognitive behavioral therapy (CBT) techniques have been developed for patients who continue to experience psychotic symptoms despite optimal pharmacologic treatment. The principal aims of CBT for medication-resistant psychosis are to reduce the intensity of delusions and hallucinations (and the related distress) and to promote active participation of the individual in reducing the risk of relapse and levels of social disability (Tarrier et al., 1993). Interventions focus on rationally exploring the subjective nature of the psychotic symptoms, challenging the evidence for these, and subjecting such beliefs and experiences to reality testing. A handful of well-controlled randomized studies have documented meaningful effects for reducing delusions and hallucinations in cognitively intact, cooperative patients with schizophrenia (Bentall et al., 1994; Chadwick et al., 1994; Tarrier et al., 1993). However, the endurance of these therapeutic effects after discontinuation of therapy is unclear. Although few clinicians have been trained in these techniques, they offer hope and in the future may become widely available, as have similar CBT approaches for depression and anxiety disorders.

Prognostic Factors

In general, the prognosis for patients diagnosed with schizophrenia is improved if they possess insight and understand that they have a mental illness which can benefit from taking medications

A CASE OF SYMPTOMS RETURNING AFTER DISCONTINUING AN ANTIPSYCHOTIC

Carol was a 29-year-old married woman working as an administrative assistant when she began to feel that others were looking at her and commenting on her behind her back. Her husband became concerned and brought her for a psychiatric evaluation. Carol was open to sharing her suspicions and was certain that she was correct about her concerns. She reluctantly agreed to a low dose of an antipsychotic with remarkable results. She was able to return to work, and her husband was quite pleased. However, 15 months later Carol discontinued her medication and again became paranoid. This time she lost her job and was admitted to the psychiatric hospital. She was again restarted on medication and responded well.

consistently, take their medicines regularly as prescribed, have access to adequate health care, and have family or additional support.

How to Approach Treating Patients with Schizophrenia (and Other Related Disorders)

Most patients and their families would like to know immediately what the diagnosis is, and in some cases that is possible, but in others it can require several years. For example, some patients may need to take an antipsychotic for a period of time, after which the patient and clinician may consider trying to change or discontinue the medication. In many cases, the psychosis returns quickly after discontinuation and lends support to a diagnosis of a chronic psychosis, most often schizophrenia. It is imperative to maintain clinical follow-up for several years after a patient discontinues an antipsychotic to monitor for relapse.

OTHER RELATED DISORDERS

Schizophreniform Disorder

Schizophreniform disorder essentially resembles schizophrenia, except for having a shorter duration. This disorder reflects a period of diagnostic uncertainty as to whether the patient will go on to develop schizophrenia. The diagnostic criteria include the Criterion A symptoms of schizophrenia (delusions, hallucinations, disorganized speech or behavior, etc., as described earlier) lasting at least 1 month but <6 months.

Owing to the short duration required for schizophreniform disorder, social and/or occupational impairment is not required but may be seen because this illness sometimes represents the prodromal stage of schizophrenia. The prodrome is composed of what are generally considered "prepsychotic" signs of impairment that could include a decline in academic functioning, an increase in social isolation, and a subtle change in behavior or thought patterns. There is intense worldwide interest in identifying and possibly treating the prodromal symptoms of schizophrenia. There is hope that by intervening early, a full-blown conversion to psychosis can either be delayed or even stopped.

Identifying at-risk individuals is crucial in working with the prodrome. At-risk individuals can include first-degree relatives of patients diagnosed with schizophrenia and/or individuals with mild to moderate signs of impairment. Some studies have shown the use of low dose antipsychotics or CBT techniques to be effective. Clinical hindsight sometimes shows that various soft signs of impairment may have been present for some time before clear psychotic symptoms manifested. Collecting additional information from family members and friends regarding this prodromal time period and the lead-up to manifesting psychotic symptoms can be extremely valuable.

The onset of schizophreniform disorder is similar to that of schizophrenia, often occurring in late adolescence or early adulthood, and the course is variable. As many as one third of patients given this diagnosis provisionally recover within 6 months, while the remaining patients continue to be symptomatic and go on to receive diagnoses of schizophrenia or schizoaffective disorder (American Psychiatric Association, 2000). Other studies found that one third of patients with this disorder went on to receive a diagnosis of an affective disorder, such as major depression or bipolar disorder (Marchesi et al., 2007; Zhang-Wong et al., 1995).

The differential diagnosis of schizophreniform disorder is essentially the same as schizophrenia, with a shorter time frame. As is true when diagnosing any type of psychotic illness, medical or substance-induced causes should be ruled out. If the duration of psychosis is <1 month, brief reactive psychosis may be the appropriate diagnosis.

Modern treatment of schizophreniform disorder is the same as that for schizophrenia, with primary reliance on atypical antipsychotics to control psychosis, as discussed earlier in this chapter. Similar to schizophrenia, patients and families may benefit from additional support and psychosocial treatment while awaiting the resolution of symptoms or further diagnostic clarity over time. Experience working with these patients (sometimes referred to as *first episode* patients) shows that educating both the patient and family during this period is imperative. Both tend to be scared, confused, and concerned and are looking for helpful information that is also realistically hopeful.

Brief Psychotic Disorder

Brief psychotic disorder could be considered on a timeline continuum with schizophreniform disorder and schizophrenia in that it involves similar symptoms but with duration of <1 month. Symptoms can include the presence of hallucinations, delusions, disorganized speech, and/or disorganized or catatonic behavior that lasts from 1 day up to 30 days, with subsequent full recovery. Patients experiencing this disorder can often be frightened, anxious, confused, temporarily quite disabled, and at risk for poor self-care or self-harm. The onset of symptoms is usually sudden and occurs shortly after a traumatic event.

Historically, brief psychotic disorder was called *brief reactive psychosis*, because it was thought to follow a traumatic event, although this is not always the case (Pillmann et al., 2002). The name was later changed to allow for a diagnosis of transient psychosis with no apparent precipitating event. To feel confident in making this diagnosis, other causes of psychosis must be ruled out, including substance-induced psychosis, psychosis related to a medical condition, and other psychiatric illness such as a mood disorder.

When making this diagnosis, it is necessary to choose a specifier from DSM-IV-TR to indicate if the brief psychotic disorder is occurring with or without marked stressors or with a postpartum onset (if occurring within 4 weeks of giving birth).

Brief psychotic disorder is thought to be very rare in the United States and in other developed countries but is more commonly seen in the developing world (American Psychiatric Association, 2000). The average age of onset is in the late 20s to early 30s. The differential diagnosis can be broad and may include ruling out delirium, other medical conditions (such as thyroid illness, Cushing disease, or a brain tumor), substance-induced psychosis (including intoxication), mood disorders, schizophrenia spectrum disorders, and even personality disorders (such as borderline personality disorder). Although challenging to identify, factitious disorder and malingering are part of the differential diagnosis and also must be ruled out.

By definition, patients with brief psychotic disorder will spontaneously remit, but often antipsychotics are utilized and patients may need to be closely followed up or even hospitalized during the psychotic episode. In one study, only 8% of patients with this diagnosis went on to develop schizophrenia, but there is a risk of recurrence of psychosis within 5 years (Marneros et al., 2003).

Schizoaffective Disorder

Schizoaffective disorder describes a somewhat controversial entity, which is defined as the occurrence of continuous psychotic symptoms (Criterion A for schizophrenia) with periods of depression or mania. DSM-IV-TR requires that a patient experience at least 2 weeks of prominent delusions or hallucinations in the absence of prominent mood symptoms. Finally, the mood symptoms must be present for a substantial portion of the total duration of the illness, although the specific duration of the mood symptoms is not defined.

To be considered for a diagnosis of schizoaffective disorder, full criteria for a major depressive episode or manic/mixed episode must be met while the patient is in the mood phase of this illness, and the patient must be experiencing intervening periods of psychosis. To make this diagnosis,

A CASE OF BRIEF PSYCHOTIC DISORDER

Frank is a 42-year-old man with no prior psychiatric history. A year ago, on a drive with his wife, they were involved in a serious motor vehicle crash. Frank was uninjured, but his wife was hospitalized in critical condition. In the intensive care unit, the nurses noticed Frank was talking to himself and appeared easily irritated. He began to insist that only he could sit near his wife's bedside and accused the nurses of trying to kill her. A psychiatric consult was ordered to evaluate him. On interview, Frank was disorganized, guarded, and combative. The psychiatrist admitted him to the psychiatric unit on an involuntary hold. Frank responded quickly to a low dose of an antipsychotic. Fortunately Frank's wife also began to recover and was able to speak to him. After several days in the hospital he no longer had any psychotic symptoms. He was taken off of the antipsychotic a few weeks later and has not had a return of his symptoms.

psychotic symptoms often need to precede the onset of the mood symptoms. Otherwise, a diagnosis of major depressive disorder with psychotic features or bipolar disorder, type I, may be more appropriate, as long as both have incomplete remission that results in lingering psychosis.

Two subtypes of schizoaffective disorder are bipolar and depressive. Bipolar type is diagnosed when symptoms of mania or mixed episodes occur with or without episodes of major depression. Depressive type is diagnosed solely for episodes of major depression. Patients with this disorder sometimes have less severe deficits in psychosocial functioning but often can be severely impaired by poor self-care, lack of insight, prominent negative symptoms, and suicidality.

Little information is available regarding the prevalence of schizoaffective disorder, but the illness is thought to be less common than schizophrenia. Its typical onset is similar to that of schizophrenia, occurring in early adulthood, but can happen anytime from the teens through adulthood. The prognosis for schizoaffective disorder is intermediate between that of schizophrenia and the mood disorders, and there is an increased risk for both schizophrenia and mood disorders in families of patients with schizoaffective disorder (American Psychiatric Association, 2000).

There is some controversy over the validity of this diagnosis, with some authors proposing that schizoaffective disorder is actually a variant of a mood disorder with psychosis (Lake and Hurwitz, 2007). A significant genetic overlap among schizoaffective disorder, schizophrenia, and bipolar disorder contributes to this proposal (Crow, 2007).

In general, pharmacologic treatment for schizoaffective disorder is symptom driven, with most patients requiring an antipsychotic, preferably an atypical, because psychosis is usually a consistent symptom. Many, but not all, atypical antipsychotics theoretically offer the added benefit of treating affective symptoms in addition to psychosis. For the specific subtypes, a mood stabilizer (such as lithium, valproate, lamotrigine, or carbamazepine) may be added for bipolar type or an antidepressant for depressive type. Other nonpharmacologic treatments such as psychosocial rehabilitation or psychotherapy may also be appropriate and helpful.

Delusional Disorder

The key to the diagnosis of delusional disorder is the presence of nonbizarre delusions for at least 1 month, without other psychotic symptoms and features of schizophrenia. In these patients, auditory hallucinations are not present, nor is significant disability in psychosocial functioning except as directly impacted by the false delusional beliefs. To receive this diagnosis, the nonbizarre delusion(s) must not occur in the context of a mood disorder and cannot be induced by substance use or medical illness.

Examples of nonbizarre delusions include descriptions of being followed, poisoned, infected, loved from a distance, or deceived by a spouse or lover. The key is to evaluate if the delusion is possible, which may be difficult because it is possible for a spouse to be unfaithful or the patient to be ill or infected with something. Some individuals with delusional disorder may show little impairment in functioning, while others may be significantly impaired, expending excessive time focusing on the delusion, even being unable to work or maintain relationships. The onset of delusional disorder can occur almost anytime from the teens to old age and may or may not occur in response to a severe stressor.

DSM-IV-TR identifies several subtypes of the disorder based on the theme of the delusion: erotomanic, grandiose, jealous, persecutory, somatic, mixed, or unspecified.

Erotomanic type includes feeling that another individual, often of a higher status, is in love with the patient or the other way around. The object of the delusion may be an acquaintance or a stranger, and the patient may make efforts to contact the person ranging from sending letters and making phone calls to stalking. Patients may get involved with law enforcement due to their efforts to contact, possess, or even rescue the object of their delusion.

Grandiose type involves patients feeling that they have a special talent, ability, or insight, or that they have a special relationship with someone of importance. Their perception of these talents or abilities should be evaluated in comparison to their level of functioning.

Jealous type is applied when the patient is convinced of infidelity by his or her lover or spouse, based on a persistent misreading of clues and subsequent efforts by the patient to confront his or her partner and control the partner's behavior.

Persecutory type, the most common, involves the fixed belief that one is being spied on, followed, poisoned, maligned, or manipulated. Often these patients become engaged in the legal system to try to right some perceived wrong and may become violent.

Somatic type includes delusional beliefs about bodily sensations or functions, including feeling malodorous, infested by parasites, dysmorphic, or that certain organs are no longer functioning.

Mixed type is used when multiple themes exist and one is not considered to be predominant. Unspecified type is used when no clear theme is identifiable but the presence of delusions and an impact on functioning are clear.

For patients with delusional disorder, significant psychosocial consequences can ensue secondary to these fixed delusions. Patients may become irritable and dysphoric. Anger and violence may occur with the persecutory type, resulting in injury and arrest. Patients with somatic delusion may undergo the risks and expense of extensive medical testing. The differential diagnosis is wide and includes ruling out other psychotic disorders, medical illnesses such as dementia, the use of substances, and mood disorders. Patients who abuse stimulants can develop persecutory delusions. Hypochondriasis and body dysmorphic, obsessive-compulsive, and paranoid personality disorders may all present with similar symptoms and should be carefully ruled out.

The treatment of delusional disorder is very difficult because these patients almost always lack insight into their delusions and often are firmly convinced of their accuracy. Patients rarely come to treatment of their own accord with the delusions, although they may pursue medical treatment for reasons connected to their belief system. Establishing a therapeutic relationship is a very delicate matter, because the patient may be quick to interpret the therapist's behavior as manipulative. For some patients it can be almost impossible to rationally engage them around the content of their delusions. Therefore, the approach often involves engaging the patient in treatment of secondary symptoms, such as anxiety. Antipsychotics are the medication of choice, with efficacy of perhaps 50% for compliant patients (Manschreck and Khan, 2006). Some evidence also suggests that when medications are given involuntarily, up to 75% of delusional patients may see a response (Herbel and Stelmach, 2007). Occasionally the violent, delusional patient may need psychiatric hospitalization or incarceration. CBT can sometimes be helpful in reducing the strength of the beliefs or delusions for the patient and their associated affect (O'Connor et al., 2007). A therapist may also be able to build a relationship with this kind of patient and help him or her entertain other less-threatening views or cognitions that may help in coping with the world.

CONCLUSION AND FUTURE DIRECTIONS

In this chapter schizophrenia and its related psychotic disorders have been described. Schizophrenia is a hallmark psychiatric illness, due to the magnitude of the symptoms and the effect on the person's overall functioning. The medical diagnosis of schizophrenia first appeared in the late 19th century and, despite changes in diagnostic criteria, it remains essentially the same illness as first described. Psychosis, disorganized thinking and behavior, along with reduced social interactions, remain its cardinal symptoms. What has changed is a better understanding of its pathophysiology and treatment.

Most experts believe that some common abnormality is in the dopamine system in the brain and may be corrected by blocking dopamine receptors. However, the root causes of schizophrenia remain unclear. Schizophrenia runs in families but is not entirely explained by genes. Identical twins are only 50% concordant for schizophrenia despite sharing the same genes. Environmental factors probably play some role, and certainly chemicals that release dopamine (e.g., marijuana, amphetamines) are related to many who present with the illness. In the future, it is expected that these important threads of information will be connected and a more accurate etiology will be discovered. Likewise, treatments continue to advance and should be able to provide patients with safer and more effective means to control the illness.

Clinical Pearls

- Psychosis is a group of symptoms that occurs in a variety of diagnosed illnesses.
- Schizophrenia affects 1% of the population and has high direct and indirect costs.
- Schizophrenia can be diagnosed with a combination of positive and negative symptoms and must affect functioning.
- Before diagnosing late-onset schizophrenia, make sure that an earlier presentation has not been missed—especially look at occupational functioning before age 45.
- Antipsychotic medication is the only class of medication indicated for schizophrenia.
- All current antipsychotics block the dopamine-2 receptor in some manner.
- The second-generation antipsychotics, or "atypical antipsychotics," appear to have fewer neurologic side effects than the first-generation or "typical antipsychotics."
- Patients with schizoaffective disorder manifest a mood disorder during a significant portion of their illness, but they always have a period of psychotic symptoms without diagnosable affect problems.
- The psychosocial treatments of schizophrenia have been proved to enhance outcome for the illness in combination with antipsychotic treatment.
- The key to the diagnosis of delusional disorder is the presence of nonbizarre delusions without other psychotic symptoms and features of schizophrenia.

Self-Assessment Questions and Answers

10-1. A 19-year-old man presents at the psychiatric emergency department with his mother. He is very guarded and unwilling to talk to the nurse or psychiatrist. His mother informs the evaluation team that he was well until a month ago. At that time, he was playing in a local rock band, staying up late, and, according to his friends, smoking marijuana daily. He began to suspect that his bandmates were going to take the band on the road without him. He seemed to talk to himself and get very angry at the slightest provocation. He admitted to his bandmates that he was hearing the voice of God. He isolated himself, and finally his mother convinced him to come to the emergency department. Which of the following is true?

A. This 19-year-old has schizophrenia.
B. A substance-induced psychotic disorder must be ruled out.
C. His mother is to blame for allowing him to play in a rock band.
D. He will most likely not require treatment with an antipsychotic.

This is a classic case of a potential first episode of psychosis. It is possible that he is having a substance-induced psychosis, and confirming the extent of his current use (by toxicology screen and collaborative history) is important. It is possible that with abstinence from illegal substances his psychosis will resolve. However, in the meantime he most likely will require antipsychotic treatment for some period. He cannot be diagnosed with schizophrenia at this time. First, the substance use must be ruled out; if that is negative, he might meet the diagnosis of schizophreniform disorder since the symptoms are only 1 month in duration. If after 6 months with these symptoms he remains symptomatic, the most likely diagnosis becomes schizophrenia. *Answer: B*

10-2. Jill is a 30-year-old woman with a diagnosis of schizophrenia for the last 10 years. She has taken a variety of antipsychotics with some partial improvement in her condition. It appears she has faithfully taken her medications. Recently, Jill's symptoms have worsened, and she has been admitted to the hospital several times despite three documented trials of first-line antipsychotics. Which is the most likely next choice for Jill?

A. Consider clozapine.
B. Consider electroconvulsive therapy.
C. Reconsider the diagnosis because the antipsychotics are not working.
D. Switch to a depot antipsychotic.

Jill appears to be treatment resistant to the first-line antipsychotic medications. The first thing to consider is whether she is taking her medication. According to the history, the psychiatrist is confident she is. If the psychiatrist had some doubts, Jill could be started on a depot antipsychotic to ensure that she is receiving it. Electroconvulsive therapy is a potential treatment for treatment-resistant schizophrenia, but the data are mixed on its benefits so it would be used if the patient had a contraindication to or a failed trial of clozapine. Data support clozapine as the only proven medication for treatment-resistant schizophrenia. *Answer: A*

10-3. Pat is a 32-year-old unmarried administrative assistant in a large Wall Street brokerage house. She is an excellent worker and prides herself in meeting all of her boss' requests. Pat lives by herself and has never married. Two weeks ago Pat found out her boss was divorcing his wife. Her reaction was ecstatic because she believed that now she and her boss could be together romantically. When she told her boss, he was surprised and tried to let her down gently. She became distraught. Which is the most likely diagnosis for Pat?

A. Adjustment disorder with depressed mood

B. Delusional disorder, erotomanic subtype
C. Schizophrenia
D. No diagnosis; it was just a misunderstanding

Pat presents with the classic description of delusional disorder, erotomanic type. She has secretly believed that she had a more personal and significant relationship with her boss that was far beyond a work relationship. Despite zero evidence to support this, her boss' upcoming divorce is proof that they will be together. When confronted with the reality from her boss, she decompensates. *Answer: B*

10-4. Which best states the use of cognitive behavioral therapy (CBT) in treating schizophrenia?

A. CBT should be used instead of pharmacologic treatment of schizophrenia.
B. CBT should be used when pharmacologic treatment of schizophrenia is not effective.
C. CBT can reduce the intensity of delusions and hallucinations.
D. CBT cannot work with patients with psychosis due to impaired reality testing.

CBT for schizophrenia has the potential to reduce the intensity of delusions and hallucinations and promote better social functioning and lower relapse. It should not be used in place of antipsychotic medications, but as a complement to them. It can be successful in patients with impaired reality testing if the patient is open to questioning the delusions or hallucinations. *Answer: C*

10-5. All effective antipsychotics have been shown to:

A. Block the dopamine 2 receptor
B. Have the same side effect profile
C. Be available in long-acting preparations
D. Be free of tardive dyskinesia

To date, all effective antipsychotics block the D_2 receptor, even clozapine, which is a weak D_2 blocker. Antipsychotics can have very different side effect profiles, and only a few are available as long-acting injections. None are free of tardive dyskinesia, although the atypicals have been reported to have a lower rate than typical antipsychotics. *Answer: A*

References

Allison DB, Mentore JL, Heo M, et al. Antipsychotic-induced weight gain: A comprehensive research synthesis. *Am J Psychiatry*. 1999;156(11):1686–1696.

American Psychiatric Association. *Diagnostic and statistical manual of mental disorders*, 4th ed, text revision. Washington, DC: American Psychiatric Association; 2000.

Auquier P, Lançon C, Rouillon F, et al. Mortality in schizophrenia. *Pharmacoepidemiol Drug Saf*. 2006;15(12):873–879.

Bateson G, Jackson D, Haley J, et al. Toward a theory of schizophrenia. *Behav Sci*. 1956;1:251–264.

Bellack A, Mueser K. Psychosocial treatment of schizophrenia. *Schizophr Bull*. 1993;19:317–336.

Bentall RP, Haddock G, Slade PD. Cognitive therapy for persistent auditory hallucinations: From theory to therapy. *Behav Ther*. 1994;25:51–66.

Bertelsen M, Jeppesen P, Petersen L, et al. Suicidal behaviour and mortality in first-episode psychosis: The OPUS trial. *Br J Psychiatry Suppl*. 2007;51:s140–s146.

Braff D. Information processing and attention dysfunctions in schizophrenia. *Schizophr Bull*. 1993;19:233–254.

Brown GW, Bone M, Palison B, et al. *Schizophrenia and social care*. London: OUP; 1966.

Brown GW, Rutter M. The measurement of family activities and relationships: A methodological study. *Hum Relat*. 1966;19:241–263.

Byerly M, Suppes T, Tran QV, et al. Clinical implications of antipsychotic-induced hyperprolactinemia in patients with schizophrenia spectrum or bipolar spectrum disorders: Recent developments and current perspectives. *J Clin Psychopharmacol*. 2007;27(6):639–661.

Carpenter WT, Koenig JI. The evolution of drug development in schizophrenia: Past issues and future opportunities. *Neuropsychopharmacology*. 2008;33(9):2061–2079.

Chadwick P, Lowe C, Horne P, et al. Modifying delusions: The role of empirical testing. *Behav Ther*. 1994;25:35–49.

Correll CU, Leucht S, Kane JM. Lower risk for tardive dyskinesia associated with second-generation antipsychotics: A systematic review of 1-year studies. *Am J Psychiatry*. 2004;161:414–425.

Crow TJ. How and why genetic linkage has not solved the problem of psychosis: Review and hypothesis. *Am J Psychiatry*. 2007;164(1):13–21.

da Costa DA. The role of psychosurgery in the treatment of selected cases of refractory schizophrenia: A reappraisal. *Schizophr Res*. 1997;28(2–3):223–230.

Doroshow DB. Performing a cure for schizophrenia: Insulin coma therapy on the wards. *J Hist Med Allied Sci*. 2007;62(2):213–243.

Fitzgerald PB, Montgomery W, de Castella AR, et al. Australian Schizophrenia Care and Assessment Programme: Real-world schizophrenia: Economics. *Aust N Z J Psychiatry*. 2007;41(10):819–829.

Fromm-Reichmann F. Notes on the development of treatment of schizophrenics by psychoanalysis and psychotherapy. *Psychiatry*. 1948;11:263–273.

Gunderson JG, Frank AF, Katz HM, et al. Effects of psychotherapy in schizophrenia: II. Comparative outcome of two forms of treatment. *Schizophr Bull*. 1984;10:564–598.

Herbel BL, Stelmach H. Involuntary medication treatment for competency restoration of 22 defendants with delusional disorder. *J Am Acad Psychiatry Law*. 2007;35(1):47–59.

Kane J, Honigfeld G, Singer J, et al. Clozapine for the treatment-resistant schizophrenic. A double-blind comparison with chlorpromazine. *Arch Gen Psychiatry*. 1988;45:789–796.

Kane JM, Woerner M, Weinhold P, et al. A prospective study of tardive dyskinesia development: Preliminary results. *J Clin Psychopharmacol*. 1982;2:345–349.

Kane JM. Tardive dyskinesia rates with atypical antipsychotics in adults: Prevalence and incidence. *J Clin Psychiatry*. 2004;65(Suppl 9):16–20.

Kapur S, Remington G. Dopamine D(2) receptors and their role in atypical antipsychotic action: Still necessary and may even be sufficient. *Biol Psychiatry*. 2001;50(11):873–883.

Kapur S, Seeman P. Does fast dissociation from the dopamine D(2) receptor explain the action of atypical antipsychotics? A new hypothesis. *Am J Psychiatry*. 2001;158(3):360–369.

Kraepelin E. In: Barclay RM, Edinburgh E, Livingstone S, eds. *Dementia praecox and paraphrenia. Facsimile Edition*. Chapter II. Huntington, NY: Robert E. Krieger Publishing Company, Inc; 1971.

Kuhn R. Eugen Bleuler's concepts of psychopathology. *Hist Psychiatry*. 2004;15(3):361–366.

Lake RL, Hurwitz N. Schizoaffective disorder merges schizophrenia and bipolar disorders as one disease—there is no schizoaffective disorder. *Curr Opin Psychiatry*. 2007;20:365–379.

Lehman AF, Goldberg R, Dixon LB, et al. Improving employment outcomes for persons with severe mental illnesses. *Arch Gen Psychiatry*. 2002;59:165–172.

Manschreck TC, Khan NL. Recent advances in the treatment of delusional disorder. *Can J Psychiatry*. 2006;51(2):114–119.

Marchesi C, Paini M, Ruju L, et al. Predictors of the evolution towards schizophrenia or mood disorder in patients with schizophreniform disorder. *Schizophr Res.* 2007;97(1–3):1–5.

Marder SR, Wirshing W, Mintz J, et al. Two-year outcome of social skills training and group psychotherapy for outpatients with schizophrenia. *Am J Psychiatry.* 1996;153:1585–1592.

Marneros A, Pillmann F, Haring A, et al. Features of acute and transient psychotic disorders. *Eur Arch Psychiatry Clin Neurosci.* 2003;253(4):167–174.

May PRA, Tuma AH, Dixon WH. Schizophrenia: A follow-up study of the results of five forms of treatment. *Arch Gen Psychiatry.* 1968;38:776–784.

McEvoy JP, Meyer JM, Goff DC, et al. Prevalence of the metabolic syndrome in patients with schizophrenia: Baseline results from the Clinical Antipsychotic Trials of Intervention Effectiveness (CATIE) schizophrenia trial and comparison with national estimates from NHANES III. *Schizophr Res.* 2005;80(1):19–32.

Meyer JM, Davis VG, Goff DC, et al. Change in metabolic syndrome parameters with antipsychotic treatment in the CATIE Schizophrenia Trial: Prospective data from phase 1. *Schizophr Res.* 2008; 101(1-3):273–286.

Miller D, Eudicone JM, Pikalov A, et al. Comparative assessment of the incidence and severity of tardive dyskinesia in patients receiving aripiprazole or haloperidol for the treatment of schizophrenia: A post hoc analysis. *J Clin Psychiatry.* 2007;68(12):1901–1906.

Nemeroff CB, Lieberman JA, Weiden PJ, et al. From clinical research to clinical practice: A 4-year review of ziprasidone. *CNS Spectr.* 2005;10(11):s1–s20.

Newcomer JW, Sernyak MJ. Identifying metabolic risks with antipsychotics and monitoring and management strategies. *J Clin Psychiatry.* 2007;68(7):e17.

O'Connor K, Stip E, Pélissier MC, et al. Treating delusional disorder: A comparison of cognitive-behavioural therapy and attention placebo control. *Can J Psychiatry.* 2007;52(3):182–190.

Palmer BA, Pankratz VS, Bostwick JM. The lifetime risk of suicide in schizophrenia: A reexamination. *Arch Gen Psychiatry.* 2005;62(3):247–253.

Pillmann F, Haring A, Balzawiet S, et al. The concordance of ICD-9 acute and transient psychosis and DSM-IV brief reactive psychosis. *Psychol Med.* 2002;32(8):1483–1484.

Saha S, Chant D, McGrath J. A systematic review of mortality in schizophrenia: Is the differential mortality gap worsening over time? *Arch Gen Psychiatry.* 2007;64(10):1123–1131.

Schneider K. *Clinical psychopathology.* New York: Grune & Stratton; 1959.

Stein L, Test MA. An alternative to mental hospital treatment: I. Conceptual model, treatment program and clinical evaluation. *Arch Gen Psychiatry.* 1980;37:392–399.

Tarrier N, Beckett R, Harwood S, et al. A trial of two cognitive-behavioral methods of treating drug-resistant psychotic symptoms in schizophrenic patients, I: Outcome. *Br J Psychiatry.* 1993;162:524–532.

Tharyan P, Adams CE. Electroconvulsive therapy for schizophrenia. *Cochrane Database Syst Rev.* 2005;(2):CD000076.

Toda M, Abi-Dargham A. Dopamine hypothesis of schizophrenia: Making sense of it all. *Curr Psychiatry Rep.* 2007;9(4):329–336.

Wearden AJ, Tarrier N, Barrowclough C, et al. A review of expressed emotion research in health care. *Clin Psychol Rev.* 2000;20(5):633–666.

Whitehorn D, Gallant J, Woodley H, et al. Quetiapine treatment in early psychosis: No evidence of cataracts. *Schizophr Res.* 2004;71(2-3):511–512.

Wu EQ, Birnbaum HG, Shi L, et al. The economic burden of schizophrenia in the United States in 2002. *J Clin Psychiatry.* 2005;66(9):1122–1129.

Zhang-Wong J, Beiser M, Bean G, et al. Five-year course of schizophreniform disorder. *Psychiatry Res.* 1995;59(1-2):109–117.

CHAPTER

11

Christopher H. Warner and William V. Bobo

Mood Disorders

The mood disorders are a large, heterogeneous group of clinical syndromes defined in the *Diagnostic and Statistical Manual of Mental Disorders*, Fourth Edition, Text Revision (DSM-IV-TR) (American Psychiatric Association, 2000a). Their predominant feature is a disturbance in mood state so severe that it interferes with functioning and well-being. Dysfunctions in mood range from severe depression to uncontrollable elation or irritability. Two general classes are among the currently defined mood disorders: unipolar depressive disorders, which are characterized by severe depression and/or loss of capacity for experiencing pleasure (e.g., anhedonia) without hypomanic or manic mood episodes (defined in subsequent text), and bipolar disorders, which are characterized by both episodic depression (and/or anhedonia) and hypomania or mania. This chapter begins with a discussion of the epidemiology of mood disorders as a broad class of illnesses and then describes the clinical and defining features of the individual mood episodes and syndromes. The chapter closes with a synopsis of proposed etiologies for the individual mood disorders, followed by guidelines to their diagnosis and treatment and illustrative case material.

EPIDEMIOLOGY OF MOOD DISORDERS

Mood disorders, along with anxiety disorders, are the most common psychiatric problems, presenting in approximately one quarter of all primary care patients. In general, both mood and anxiety disorders are associated with varying risk of disease chronicity, leading in many cases to long-term problems functioning in social, domestic, and occupational roles, and economic burden. The adverse impact of mood disorders on general health indicators in the United States is either equal to or, in most cases, greater in magnitude than most other chronic diseases, including cardiovascular disorders. As such, mood disorders are a global public health concern.

Depressive Disorders

It is estimated that more than one in five Americans will be affected by a depressive disorder in their lifetimes (Kessler et al., 1994). The National Comorbidity Survey (Kessler et al., 1994) and the Epidemiologic Catchment Area Study (Regier et al., 1993) noted that each year a little more than one out of every ten individuals will suffer from a depressive disorder. The lifetime prevalence and 1-year prevalence for each of the specific depressive disorders are listed in Table 11-1. Psychosocial and role functioning are impaired in a great majority of cases, and the degree of impairment is directly attributed to the depressive symptoms themselves (Kessler et al., 2003).

In spite of considerable advances, our understanding of the pathogenesis and risk factors for developing depressive illnesses is still evolving. Most depressive disorders present before age 45, with the average age of onset between ages 30 and 35, and most commonly occur in the spring and fall. Family history is a clear risk factor for onset of depressive disorders, and those with a family history of depressive disorders are more likely to have earlier episodes. Gender is another known risk factor: depressive disorders are twice as common in women as they are in men. Rates do not vary significantly based on race or ethnicity.

Socioeconomically, lower status and higher risk of depression are weakly correlated, but depression appears to have a notably higher prevalence (3:1) in those who are unemployed. Geographically, the prevalence of depression in rural locations is believed to be lower than in

TABLE 11-1 Prevalence of Mood Disorders		
Disorder	**1-Year Prevalence (%)**	**Lifetime Prevalence (%)**
All depressive disorders	10–15	20–25
Major depressive disorder	3–10	5–17
Dysthymic disorder	3	3–6
All manic disorders	0.5–1.4	1.3–6.4
Bipolar I disorder	0.5–1.3	0.8–1.6
Bipolar II disorder		0.5–4.8
Cyclothymia		0.5–1

(Howland and Thase, 1993; Narrow, 1999; Kessler et al., 1994, 2003; Regier et al., 1993.)

urban locations. Some studies have documented a lower risk of developing depressive disorders in the lower latitudes (e.g., closer to the equator) than in more temperate regions in the higher latitudes.

The onset, course, and outcome associated with individual depressive disorders will be summarized in the appropriate sections mentioned in subsequent text. One aspect is worth special mention. Depressive disorders are associated with increased early mortality compared with the general population, even when only subsyndromal depressive symptoms not satisfying criteria for major depression are present (Cuijpers and Smit, 2002). Much of this risk is attributable to suicide, with a 6% lifetime risk (Inskip et al., 1998).

Bipolar Disorders

Manic episodes are not as common as the depressive episodes, even during the long-term course of bipolar disorder; however, prevalence rates have been increasing over the last 10 years, leading to an increase in the diagnosis of bipolar disorder and recognition of bipolar syndromes in younger cohorts. The lifetime and 1-year prevalence rates for each of the currently recognized bipolar syndromes (excluding bipolar disorder, not otherwise specified [NOS]) are listed in Table 11-1. Worldwide lifetime prevalence rates show remarkable consistency and also appear to indicate that bipolar illnesses go undiagnosed for 6 years before treatment is sought. An even greater delay in the institution of proper treatment may be encountered if the first mood episode or episodes are depressive rather than manic, because the first treatment sought may be for a presumed unipolar depression. Frequency estimates for bipolar disorders are limited somewhat by problems of definition, because many forms of bipolar disorder at varying levels of severity are believed to exist. We will focus our discussion on the currently defined bipolar syndromes—bipolar I disorder, bipolar II disorder, and cyclothymic disorder.

The peak age of onset for most bipolar disorders occurs in a range between ages 15 and 19 years, although the disorders may present at any age. First onset of illness after age 30 is uncommon (16% or fewer of all cases) and even rarer after age 45. Those with a family history of bipolar disorder may have their first mood episode at an even younger age than 15. Bipolar II disorders have a slight tendency to present at a later age. Unlike depression, bipolar disorders as a whole appear to be gender neutral, although more recent reports suggest that bipolar II disorder is more common in women than in men. Rates do not vary significantly based on race or ethnicity, although historically, bipolar I disorder among African Americans was underdiagnosed in favor of schizophrenia. Mixed results for investigations of socioeconomic risk for bipolar disorder suggest that the extreme low and high ends of the strata confer added risk, although the relationship appears to be somewhat weak.

The evidence for genetic influence in developing bipolar disorder is much stronger. Family studies indicate that over 65% of patients with a bipolar illness have a family history of an affective disorder, and the level of risk increases with the presence of a major affective disorder in a primary relative. Twin studies provide even stronger evidence of a genetic association. The lifetime risk of bipolar disorder in monozygotic twins is estimated at 40% to 70%, while the risk of bipolar disorder in first-degree relatives is 5% to 10%. Monozygotic versus dizygotic concordance rates for bipolar disorder are 62% versus 8%, with a 59% estimate of heritability. Although this concordance rate is strong, it is <100%. As such, environmental and other nongenetic factors are still of critical importance. The exact mode of risk inheritance is unknown, and an active search continues for specific susceptibility genes for bipolar disorders.

MOOD EPISODES

DSM-IV-TR provides operationalized diagnostic criteria for four different types of mood episodes: depression, manic, hypomanic, and mixed. These episodes are not separate disorders by themselves. However, they form the basis for the syndromal mood disorder diagnoses described in subsequent text.

Major Depressive Episode

Depression has many connotations and can be used to describe feelings such as demoralization or disappointment and transient reactions to grief and loss. In contrast, major depressive episodes are distinct mood episodes hallmarked by a depressed mood (usually described as morbid sadness) or a loss of interest or pleasure (anhedonia) plus additional characteristic symptoms.

During depressive episodes, patients often feel discouraged, defeated, helpless, hopeless, and unable to cope with the stresses of everyday life. Individuals with severe depression may find it impossible to motivate themselves to carry out even the most common daily tasks. Depressed patients may begin to think of themselves in negative terms and feel like failures or feel that their families and/or friends would be better off without them. The thought processes of some people with severe depression may become so distorted that their thinking becomes delusional. Others may experience auditory hallucinations. In any case, considerable dysfunction in everyday living stems directly from the symptoms themselves.

It is important to recognize that patients with depression will not always present complaining of a depressed mood. Rather, they may present with complaints of fatigue, weakness, anxiety, and irritability or with somatic complaints such as recurrent headaches or gastrointestinal problems. If depression is suspected, a thorough evaluation should be conducted. The comprehensive interview should include a thorough history of present illness that is reviewed for the symptoms of a major depressive episode. Simply inquiring about whether the patient has been feeling "sad" or "blue" or experiencing depression that is "difficult to shake" can be enough to start this process. A simple mnemonic commonly used to help remember the diagnostic criteria is SIGECAPS

Clinical Characteristics of a Major Depressive Disorder

- At least a 2-week period of maladaptive functioning clearly changed from previous functioning
- Marked distress and/or significant impairment in social or occupational functioning
- No evidence of a physical or substance-induced etiology for symptoms or another major mental disorder
- At least five of the following, one of which must be either depressed mood or loss of interest or pleasure:
  - Depressed mood
  - Loss of interest or pleasure
  - Appetite disturbances with weight change >5% of body weight within 1 month
  - Sleep disturbance
  - Psychomotor disturbance
  - Fatigue or loss of energy
  - Feelings of worthlessness or excessive or inappropriate guilt
  - Diminished ability to concentrate or indecisiveness
  - Recurrent thoughts of death or suicidal ideation

TABLE 11-2	**Differential Diagnosis for Depression**			
Psychiatric	**Medical**	**Nutrition**	**Substance**	**Medications**
Major depressive disorder	Inflammatory conditions: systemic lupus erythematosus	Vitamin deficiencies (B_{12}, folate, niacin, thiamine)	Alcohol	Corticosteroids
Dysthymic disorder	Infectious: syphilis, Lyme disease, HIV encephalopathy,		Cocaine	β-Blockers
Adjustment disorder with depressed mood	mononucleosis		Amphetamines	Calcium channel blockers
Schizoaffective disorder	Endocrine: Addison disease, Cushing disease, hyperthyroidism, hypothyroidism,		Marijuana	H2 blockers
Bipolar disorder	prolactinomas, hyperparathyroidism		Sedatives/ Hypnotics	Sedatives
Attention-deficit/ hyperactivity disorder	Neoplasm: pancreatic cancer, disseminated carcinomatosis		Narcotics	Muscle relaxants
Bereavement				Hormones (estrogen, progesterone, testosterone)
Substance-induced mood disorder				Chemotherapy agents
Mood disorder due to a general medical condition				

(**s**leep, **i**nterest, **g**uilt, **e**nergy, **c**oncentration, **a**ppetite, **p**sychomotor agitation/retardation, **s**uicidal thoughts). Additionally, a review of medical symptoms, family history, and social history, including substance use history, should be conducted to assess for the potential of other possible causes. Suicidal ideation and behavior should always be specifically assessed, as reviewed in the subsequent text.

Several screening tools exist to supplement the above investigations and help determine the presence and severity of depression. One of the most common is the Patient Health Questionnaire, which has a nine-item and a two-item version. These questionnaires are self-administered versions of the Primary Care Evaluation of Mental Disorders depression module. They assess the diagnostic criteria for depression on a scale of 0 ("not at all") to 3 ("nearly every day") and can be easily scored by the administering provider.

The differential diagnosis for depression is rather large, and to make a final diagnosis of major depressive episode, a full physical and laboratory evaluation should be conducted. Table 11-2 outlines the differential diagnosis for depression. No diagnostic laboratory evaluation is pathognomonic for depression. However, a number of studies are indicated for clarification of the differential, including complete blood count (CBC), thyroid stimulating hormone (TSH), rapid plasma reagin (RPR), serum electrolytes, liver function tests, human immunodeficiency virus (HIV), vitamin B_{12}, erythrocyte sedimentation rate, and a toxicology screen. Additionally, consideration should be given to a computerized tomography (CT) of the head. Although the dexamethasone suppression test was once touted as a potentially effective biological screening tool for major depression, it lacks sufficient sensitivity for everyday practice and is therefore not utilized in routine settings.

Manic Episode

Mania is a mood disturbance characterized by a distinct period of abnormally elevated, expansive, or irritable mood. For the diagnosis of a manic episode, the patient must have both the mood disturbance and three of the characteristic symptoms if the primary mood disturbance is characterized by euphoria or four or more of the characteristics if the primary mood disturbance is irritability. Collectively, these changes must have persisted for 7 or more consecutive days or

Clinical Characteristics of a Manic Episode

- A distinct period of abnormally and persistently elevated, expansive, or irritable mood, lasting at least 1 week, of sufficient severity to cause marked impairment in social or occupational functioning
- No evidence of a physical or substance-induced etiology for symptoms or another major mental disorder
- At least three of the following (four if the mood is primarily irritable):
  - Grandiosity
  - Decreased need for sleep
  - Hyperverbal or pressured speech
  - Flight of ideas or racing thoughts
  - Distractibility
  - Increase in goal-directed activity or psychomotor agitation
  - Excessive involvement in pleasurable activities with high potential for painful consequences

have been severe enough to result in hospitalization. The manic patient is, therefore, typically euphoric or expansive, evidencing limitless enthusiasm; however, the mood and affect of manic patients may also be irritable, argumentative, irrational, angry, or labile. As such, hostile or even assaultive behavior may occur during a manic episode. Regardless of primary mood state (euphoric or irritable), patients are in an abnormally activated state characterized by little need for sleep, increased energy in spite of lacking sleep, and increased levels of arousal leading to marked decreases in concentration, increased "thrill or pleasure seeking" behaviors, impulsivity, and impaired judgment. Their speech is usually loud and/or rapid with circumstantial or tangential associations. One particular speech pattern observed in many manic patients has been termed *pressured* speech, which, in addition to being rapid, is also difficult to interrupt. When severe, manic patients may develop psychotic symptoms such as delusions and hallucinations, and many times may be paranoid. Psychotic features are common, occurring in well over half of manic patients.

One of the most common and disabling features of mania is patients' significantly impaired insight into the true nature of their situation. Patients may not realize that their mood changes and behavior are the result of a mental disorder. Excessive involvement in pleasurable activities during a manic state can lead to increased spending to the point of bankruptcy or marriage-ending sexual misadventures without patients having an insight into the consequences of their actions until after the manic episode ends. With or without psychotic features, manic episodes can pose significant danger to the safety of patients and those around them and should therefore be treated as psychiatric emergencies. Unfortunately, due to patients' limited insight and their entertaining and adventurous nature, their presentation to treatment may sometimes be delayed. In some instances, such dramatic changes in mood and behavioral state may be blamed on the abuse of substances when, in fact, manic mood changes can lead to experimentation with drugs. Many times family or friends may force manic patients into treatment, or involuntary hospitalization may be required.

As with major depressive episodes, if a manic episode is suspected, a thorough evaluation should be conducted. The comprehensive interview should include a thorough history of present illness that is reviewed for the symptoms of a manic episode. The DIG FAST mnemonic is commonly used to help remember the diagnostic criteria (**d**istractibility, **i**njudiciousness, **g**randiosity, **f**light of ideas, **a**ctivities [increase in goal-directed activities], **s**leep [decreased need for], and **t**alkativeness). Other instruments, such as the Mood Disorder Questionnaire, may be used to screen for past manic (or hypomanic) episodes in depressed patients. As with other conditions, a thorough review of medical symptoms, family history, and social history, including substance use history, is indicated. Furthermore, a collateral history from family, friends, or other

TABLE 11-3	Differential Diagnosis for Manic Episodes		
Psychiatric	**Medical**	**Substance**	**Medications**
Bipolar I disorder	Neurologic conditions: multiple sclerosis, stroke, head trauma, temporal lobe epilepsy, frontal lobe syndrome, Huntington disease, subcortical dementia Endocrine: hyperthyroidism, Cushing syndrome Autoimmune: systemic lupus erythematosus (SLE) Infections: human immunodeficiency virus (HIV) encephalitis, herpes simplex virus	Cocaine Amphetamines Caffeine Alcohol	Antidepressants Steroids Amphetamines Levodopa (L-dopa) Adrenocorticotropin

medical providers is essential because many manic patients lack insight into their condition and may be unreliable in their responses to an interview.

A full physical and laboratory evaluation should be conducted to evaluate the complete differential diagnosis for manic episodes (see Table 11-3). As with depression, no laboratory evaluation is diagnostic for mania. However, the same laboratory tests recommended for depression should be performed. Additionally, consideration should be given to performing a head CT and, if indicated, serum levels for prescribed medications.

Hypomanic Episode

Hypomanic episodes are similar to manic episodes but less severe. The two key features that distinguish a hypomanic from a manic episode are shorter duration of the episode (4 consecutive days of symptoms in hypomania versus 7 or more days for mania) and lack of social or occupational dysfunction in a hypomanic episode. In addition, hypomanic episodes are not associated with psychotic symptoms such as hallucinations or delusions and are not severe enough to necessitate hospitalization. Patients with a suspected hypomanic episode should receive the same evaluation as those with suspected manic episodes. The mnemonic DIG FAST also applies for hypomanic episodes, with consideration of the aforementioned distinguishing features.

Mixed Episode

At times, patients may present with the symptoms of both a major depressive episode and manic episode at the same time for 7 or more consecutive days, termed *mixed episodes*. Operational criteria for a mixed episode call for satisfying the full criteria for both a manic and major depressive episode but duration is 1 week. Mixed episodes tend to be more difficult to treat, and irritability is usually the predominant mood state. Similar to manic episodes, this condition will likely require hospitalization for treatment due to the impaired judgment, lack of insight, and, in particular, increased risk for self-injurious behavior. Bipolar patients with mixed episodes are at high risk, especially for suicidal thinking and behavior.

DEPRESSIVE DISORDERS

The current psychiatric diagnostic system recognizes three basic depressive mood disorders: major depressive disorder, dysthymic disorder, and depressive disorder NOS. Table 11-4 highlights the key characteristics and differences among these disorders. All are characterized by the occurrence of prolonged depressive mood states that are severe enough to result in psychosocial dysfunction. Depressive disorder NOS is reserved for clinically significant depression of undetermined etiology (e.g., the current depressive episode cannot be determined or attributed to a general medical illness or a substance) or episodes of idiopathic depression that do not satisfy diagnostic criteria for major depression or dysthymia. Some well-recognized depressive syndromes, such as premenstrual dysphoric disorder (PMDD) and postpsychotic depression, are currently classified under depressive disorder NOS.

Clinical Characteristics of a Hypomanic Episode

- A distinct period of sustained elevated, expansive, or irritable mood, lasting for at least 4 days, clearly different from nondepressed mood, yet does not cause marked impairment in social or occupational functioning such as in acute mania
- No evidence of a physical or substance-induced etiology for symptoms or another major mental disorder
- At least three of the following also present to a significant degree:
  - Inflated self-esteem or grandiosity
  - Decreased need for sleep
  - More talkative than usual
  - Flight of ideas or racing thoughts
  - Distractibility
  - Increase in goal-directed activity or psychomotor agitation
  - Excessive involvement in pleasurable activities with high potential for painful consequences

---

The etiopathophysiology of mood disorders has not been determined but is believed to reflect abnormalities at multiple physiologic levels. At the molecular level, there is robust evidence for a crucial role played by genetic factors, especially for major depression. The heritability of major depression has been estimated from twin studies as ranging from 31% to 42% (Sullivan et al., 2000). In spite of the large influence of genetic factors, the mode of inheritance for depressive disorders has not been precisely determined.

Abnormalities at the brain systems level have received the greatest amount of attention in the last several decades and have to this point contributed the most to the development of effective antidepressant drug therapies. They involve hypothesized deficiencies in the biogenic monoamines serotonin (5-HT), norepinephrine (NE), and dopamine (DA). These monoaminergic systems

TABLE 11-4   Mood Disorders

Disorder	Characteristic Episode	Required Time Course	Key Absence Findings
Major depressive disorder	Major depressive episode	2 wk	No manic or hypomanic episode
Dysthymic disorder	Depressed mood more often than not but does not meet criteria for major depressive episode	2 yr	No manic, hypomanic episode, or major depressive episode
Bipolar I disorder	Manic episode	N/A	N/A
Bipolar II disorder	Hypomanic episode and major depressive episode	N/A	No manic episode
Cyclothymic disorder	Recurrent hypomanic episodes and depressive episodes that do not meet the criteria for major depressive episode	2 yr	No manic or major depressive episodes

N/A, not applicable.

are distributed extensively in limbic and prefrontal cortical circuits, structures that are critical to the regulation of mood, motivation and drive, and neurovegetative functioning. Most of the available antidepressants, which will be discussed later, have as their general mode of activity increasing synaptic availability of these monoamines by inhibiting their degradation (in the case of monoamine oxidase inhibitors [MAOIs]) or presynaptic reuptake (in the case of tricyclic antidepressants [TCAs], selective serotonin reuptake inhibitors [SSRIs], and serotonin and norepinephrine reuptake inhibitors [SNRIs]). Although these molecular mechanisms have been the dominant model for informed antidepressant drug development, they cannot explain the delayed onset of therapeutic effect of these medications. As such, a major focus of preclinical and clinical research has been identification of long-term changes in brain systems resulting from chronic treatment with antidepressants.

Major life stressors often precede major depressive episodes and are believed to be important in maintaining them. It is hypothesized that interactions with these and other molecular targets result in the signs and symptoms of depression (Shelton, 2007). Specifically, interactions between molecular targets and stress may alter neuronal size, reduce synaptic connectivity, and interfere with neuronal repair in major depression. Several studies have suggested that stress can cause structural alterations in limbic brain regions that may result from neuronal atrophy and loss. Early biochemical hypotheses implicated abnormal stress-induced elevations in cortisol levels, which were found in a proportion of moderate to severely depressed patients. Cortisol elevation has been associated with neuronal loss in limbic structures, particularly the hippocampus, in many disorders in addition to depression. Therefore, the interactions of environmental stressors and genetic or molecular targets may cause abnormal activity in the hypothalamic-pituitary-adrenal (HPA) axis, causing downstream structural alterations in key brain regions and signs and symptoms of clinical depression. Stress can cause downregulation of brain-derived neurotrophic factor (BDNF), the most abundant and widely distributed neurotrophic factor in these locations. Chronic treatment with antidepressants appears to increase BDNF expression, leading to enhancement of neuronal survival and synaptic functioning.

Neuroimaging technologies have helped to uncover many of the aforementioned alterations in morphology of limbic and other important brain structures in depression, especially reduction in hippocampal size (Videbech and Ravnkilde, 2004). These technologies have also identified depression-associated abnormalities in the activity of other limbic structures and other brain regions responsible for regulation of emotional, cognitive, and neurovegetative functioning and response to environmental stress. For example, many functional magnetic resonance imaging (fMRI) studies of individuals with depression have shown relative overactivity in brain regions associated with emotion and relative underactivity in areas associated with cognition. These findings are in accord with neuropsychologic studies that document depression-associated bias toward processing negative, emotionally laden information (Leppanen, 2006). Positron emission tomography (PET) neuroimaging studies have documented reduced concentrations of serotonin transporters (5-HTTs) and abnormal postsynaptic binding activity of serotonin in depression. PET and single photon emission computed tomography (SPECT) neuroimaging studies have also uncovered depression-related abnormalities in the hypothalamus, which may help explain alterations in neurovegetative functions, such as sleep, appetite, and sexual drive, and in the basal ganglia, which may help explain the psychomotor slowing and, in tandem with limbic abnormalities, the concentration problems and cognitive dulling that often accompany severe depressive states.

Major Depressive Disorder

Phenomenology

Major depressive disorder (MDD) is the most common of the mood disorders. It is characterized by one or more major depressive episodes without a history of mania or hypomania. The hallmark symptoms include a depressed mood and/or a loss of interest in things formerly enjoyed or capacity for experiencing pleasure for a period of 2 or more weeks. At its most severe, it can lead to psychosis and suicide.

MDD is generally described in terms of its frequency and severity. It can occur as either a single episode or as a recurrent illness with multiple episodes. Recurrent MDD is diagnosed when the individual has two or more major depressive episodes with at least 2 months of normal mood symptoms between them.

Severity is generally described as mild, moderate, severe without psychotic features, or severe with psychotic features. Mild refers to cases where only the minimum diagnostic requirements are met and the symptoms only result in minor social or occupational dysfunction. Moderate severity implies a higher degree of dysfunction, while severe refers to the presence of several symptoms in excess of those required to make the diagnosis and marked impairment. The addition of the qualifier "with psychotic features" refers to the presence of delusions or hallucinations in addition to the core mood symptoms. Additionally, there are several subtype specifiers for MDD including atypical, melancholic, or catatonic features.

The *atypical features* specifier is applied when a patient's mood brightens in response to actual or potential positive events during the course of a major depressive episode, a phenomenon termed *mood reactivity*. Two of the following additional features are required for the diagnosis of MDD with atypical features: significant weight gain and/or increase in appetite; hypersomnia; leaden paralysis or a heavy feeling in the arms or legs; or a long-standing pattern of interpersonal rejection sensitivity that results in social and occupational dysfunction.

The *melancholic features* subtype is characterized by loss of pleasure in all or almost all activities and/or the lack of reactivity to usually pleasurable stimuli. Additionally, three or more of the following are required: a depressed mood that is experienced as qualitatively different from the feeling experienced after a loss; depression that is regularly worse in the morning, with the patient awakening at least 2 hours earlier than usual; marked psychomotor retardation or agitation; significant anorexia or weight loss; and excessive or inappropriate guilt.

The *catatonic features* specifier is applied when a major depressive episode is dominated by at least two of the following: motor immobility, including waxy flexibility or stupor; apparently purposeless excessive motor activity that is not responsive to external stimuli; extreme negativism, manifested by maintenance of a rigid posture or resistance to commands; unusual voluntary movements (including maintaining inappropriate or bizarre postures, stereotyped movement, prominent mannerisms, or prominent grimacing); or echolalia or echopraxia (purposeless mimicking of words or behaviors).

Treatment

There are numerous biological and nonbiological treatments for depression. Biological treatments include antidepressant medications, electroconvulsive therapy (ECT), naturopathic treatments (such as St. John's Wort), newer modalities such as repeated transcranial magnetic stimulation (rTMS), luminotherapy (i.e., "bright light therapy"), vagal nerve stimulation (VNS), and experimental treatments such as deep brain stimulation (see also Chapter 24). Nonbiological treatments include various psychotherapeutic approaches, three of which will be discussed in detail due to established efficacy in the setting of mild-to-moderate depression (see also Chapter 23). Specific pharmacologic properties of individual antidepressant medications will be discussed in Chapter 22. The clinical use of biological and nonbiological treatments for depression will be discussed in this chapter.

Biological treatments

Selection of specific treatments for depression depends on several factors. In general, psychotherapy is recommended for mild depression, while antidepressant medications are indicated for moderate to severe depression, but the combination of medication and psychotherapy may be the most potent approach of all (American Psychiatric Association, 2000b; Feldman, 2007; National Institute for Clinical Excellence, 2004). If psychotic features are present, the combination of an antidepressant and antipsychotic medication is indicated. This severe form of depression may also respond preferentially to ECT; other indications for ECT include melancholic features, catatonic features, suicidal ideation, severe treatment resistance, or any instance where a more rapid treatment response than medications can offer is needed. ECT also may be the safest option to treat depression in the setting of pregnancy. While depression with melancholic features responds favorably to treatment with TCAs, major depression with atypical features responds more favorably to treatment with SSRIs and MAOIs. When choosing among the antidepressant therapies, other factors to consider include past treatment responses and patient preference. Major depression with seasonal onset (typically during fall and winter months) may respond favorably to luminotherapy.

Luminotherapy is an effective treatment for major depression with seasonal onset. Patients are exposed to a 2500 to 10,000 lux light source for 30 to 120 minutes, usually first thing in the morning (Winkler et al., 2006). Complications from this procedure are rarely encountered, although relapse rates are high once treatment is stopped.

ECT is one of the most rapidly effective treatments for depression, especially for patients whose depression is complicated by psychotic or catatonic features, suicidal ideation, and refractoriness or intolerable/dangerous side effects due to pharmacologic treatment. There are no absolute contraindications to ECT. Relative contraindications include space occupying intracranial lesions, increased intracranial pressure, recent cerebrovascular accident, recent myocardial infarction, and unstable cardiopulmonary disease. Most of the risks of ECT are related to the use of anesthesia rather than the controlled seizure. Common adverse effects include headache, typically reversible deficits in short-term memory, postictal confusion, and, rarely, longer lasting amnestic effects. Although bilateral lead placement is considered to be more clinically efficacious, it is also associated with more adverse cognitive effects than nondominant unilateral lead placement. Despite considerable improvements in the safety of the ECT procedure through the use of anesthesia and being perhaps the most clinically effective antidepressant treatment available (UK ECT Review Group, 2003), ECT is still underutilized, likely a result of the negative stigma associated with it.

Alternative treatments are less well studied. Of these, the best studied is St. John's Wort, which has been shown to be effective in the treatment of mild-to-moderate depression. Although the exact mechanism of action is uncertain, at least one of the ingredients is an inhibitor of monoamine oxidase. As such, the same precautions as called for the MAOIs may also apply here, especially if St. John's Wort is combined with other psychotropic drugs. S-adenosylmethionine (SAM-e), like St. John's Wort, is another natural product available without a prescription. The antidepressant effects are less well studied, and the pharmacologic mechanism of action is unknown; however, there is evidence of serotonin, norepinephrine, and dopamine potentiation. The efficacy and tolerability, as well as the potential for drug–drug interactions, of these agents are areas of active investigation. As such, the place of these remedies in the overall antidepressant armamentarium is uncertain.

VNS is a relatively new approach that is indicated for refractory depression that has been unresponsive to antidepressant drugs or ECT (Groves and Brown, 2005). Because it is a relatively new treatment, the effectiveness of VNS in comparison with other approaches still requires systematic investigation. Repeated transcranial magnetic stimulation (rTMS) is an experimental therapy that has been proposed as an alternative to ECT and may result in fewer cognitive effects and greater overall tolerability; however, the effectiveness of this approach has not been firmly established (Loo et al., 2008).

Psychosocial interventions

Cognitive behavioral therapy (CBT) and interpersonal psychotherapy (IPT) have established clinical efficacy for the treatment of major depression and, in the context of mild-to-moderate illness, are believed to be as effective as antidepressant medications (Wampold et al., 2002). Both are time-limited, manualized approaches that focus on current patterns of thinking, behaving, and interacting, which are believed to precipitate and sustain depressive symptoms. In CBT, specific styles of habits of thinking and behaving are identified and systematically challenged using a variety of techniques. In IPT, a similar approach is used, though with a focus on interpersonal problems and challenges in the patient's life. Both CBT and IPT can be delivered in an individual (i.e., one-to-one) or a group format. Although these two approaches are generally recommended as first line among the psychotherapies, other less well-studied approaches have also been shown to be helpful, including psychodynamic psychotherapy, behavioral therapy, marital therapy, and supportive therapy.

General therapeutic strategy

Successful treatment of major depression and related syndromes requires an integrated biopsychosocial approach. In many cases, combined treatment using medication and psychotherapy, typically CBT or IPT, is indicated, though not necessarily for milder cases of depression (Jindal and Thase, 2003). Persistent monitoring of safety issues such as treatment tolerability and suicidal ideation is required at every treatment stage. In general, there are three such stages: the acute stage, continuation treatment, and maintenance treatment.

The goal of acute phase treatment is stabilization of severe depression. Antidepressants should be offered for moderate to severe depression, while psychotherapy without medication may be considered for milder cases (Jindal and Thase, 2003). First-line medication treatment options include SSRIs, SNRIs, or bupropion according to most practice guidelines. Choice of initial agent depends on several factors, including prior response to antidepressants (including that of family members with depression), adverse event profile, medical comorbidity, substance use history, history of nonadherence (in which case medications that require only once daily dosing would be given higher consideration), cost of medications, and type of depression. Major depression with psychotic features warrants combining an antipsychotic and antidepressant and/or ECT. Atypical depression may respond more favorably to SSRIs or MAOIs, while melancholic depression may respond best to an SSRI, TCA, or SNRI. Because of the delayed onset of therapeutic action of these drugs, an adequate treatment trial, assuming correct dosage, is 4 to 6 weeks.

Absence of any meaningful clinical response calls for consideration of switching to another antidepressant. Switching within the same pharmacologic class may achieve better clinical results—for instance, switching from one SSRI to another after failure to respond to the first medication has a 40% to 70% chance of achieving a therapeutic response. It is not certain how successful switching to a third antidepressant from the same class is, and most recommend switching to an antidepressant from another class at this stage.

Several options may be considered for partial responses, including increasing the dose of the medication, switching medications if the dose cannot be raised, augmenting with a second non-antidepressant drug, or combining antidepressants. Switching to a different antidepressant drug hazards losing the partial therapeutic effect already achieved. Watchful waiting at partially effective doses hazards further progress, although some patients may require longer than 6 weeks to respond to a given medication at a given dose. As such, combining medications is a commonly employed strategy. Common augmenting agents include lithium, thyroid hormone, buspirone, stimulants, and atypical antipsychotic drugs, even in the absence of psychotic features. Antidepressants that are combined are generally members of different pharmacologic classes (e.g., SSRI and bupropion). As of this writing, no evidence suggests that one combination or augmentation strategy is superior to another or to switching antidepressants. Great care should be taken when combining other antidepressants with TCAs, particularly SSRIs, due to potential drug–drug interactions that may raise the blood concentration of TCAs. Psychotherapy is also considered a first-line augmenting treatment for antidepressant partial response and should not be overlooked.

If successful, acute phase treatment lasts for up to 10 weeks, while continuation phase treatment lasts 6 to 9 months. This stage focuses on the elimination of residual depressive symptoms and prevention of relapse. In general, the same medication treatment that achieved symptom remission is continued. Elimination of any residual depressive symptoms is an important goal, because their presence is a predictor of eventual full depressive relapse and can result in significant morbidity. As such, adjustments in the medication regimen to meet this goal are often required. Patients should be cautioned about premature discontinuation of drug treatment, as early relapse can occur.

Some patients are able to discontinue medication treatment after completing the continuation phase treatment, whereas others require ongoing treatment in the maintenance phase. The goal of maintenance phase treatment, which lasts up to 3 years or longer, is prevention of disease recurrence. It is indicated for patients with recurrent episodes of depression, residual depressive symptoms, "double depression" (i.e., a major depressive episode occurring against the backdrop of dysthymic disorder), or history of severe depressive episodes with high psychosocial morbidity or suicide risk (American Psychiatric Association, 2000b). Many patients who recover during maintenance phase treatment consent to lifelong antidepressant treatment.

Treatment-resistant depression

Approximately 30% to 40% of patients treated in usual care settings will not achieve significant symptom relief after two drug trials of adequate design and duration, and fewer still achieve remission. This assumes that nonadherence, the most important determinant of treatment nonresponse, has been ruled out, along with occult medical illness and psychiatric comorbidities, active substance misuse, and effects of concomitant medications or drug interactions. Before being considered treatment resistant, patients should receive at least two adequate treatment trials with medicines from two different classes, ideally for at least 6 to 8 weeks at the highest tolerable dose. Many patients are treated with serial trials of antidepressant monotherapy among the first-line options discussed earlier. Failure of multiple first-line options typically results in a trial of TCAs, the optimal dosing of which may be monitored by plasma concentrations. For some patients, use of TCAs at the high end of the dosing range may still yield only low therapeutic drug concentrations. MAOIs are usually reserved for third- or fourth-line consideration. Assuming a partial response has occurred to optimization of antidepressant dose, the augmenting or combination treatment options discussed earlier may be considered. If the augmenting options are unsuccessful, other options that have less evidential support include dopamine agonists, modafinil, lamotrigine, pindolol, and various nutraceuticals (Gotto and Rapaport, 2005). Combinations of antidepressants have long been studied and are effective for many. All medication combinations should be closely monitored for potential drug interactions or increased adverse effects, especially for any combination involving MAOIs. All patients should be offered a trial of psychotherapy (Jindal and Thase, 2003). Some may ultimately require ECT.

Prognosis

Major depression is a recurring disorder for a majority of patients, many of whom respond only partially to treatment. For many, depressive symptoms persist unremittingly as a chronic disease. Approximately one in seven patients will commit suicide (Nierenberg et al., 2001). Response to treatment is highly variable. In most studies, 70% to 80% of individuals achieve a significant reduction in symptoms, though as many as half may not respond to an initial treatment trial. Finding valid predictors of treatment response continues to receive intensive study. Naturalistic studies have shown a direct relationship between both the length and number of depressive episodes and risk of poor recovery, as does incomplete treatment of the current depressive episode (Keller and Boland, 1998). The presence of comorbid substance abuse and anxiety disorders portends worse prognosis for the depressive disorder and also increases suicide risk. Major depression with psychotic features has a poorer long-term outlook compared with nonpsychotic depression (Keller and Boland, 1998). The presence of certain types of personality disorder pathology is associated with poorer outcome. Comorbid dysthymic disorder with major depression also has a worse long-term prognosis as compared to major depression alone (Keller and Boland, 1998). Finally, lack of psychosocial support and access to care predicts poor outcome.

Dysthymic Disorder

Phenomenology

The essential feature of dysthymic disorder is a chronically depressed mood present for most of the day and occurring on more days than not for at least 2 years. Additionally, the severity of the mood disorder cannot meet the criteria for a major depressive episode. Patients will often present with a chronic, low-grade depression and complain of being depressed for as long as they can remember. Brief periods of normal mood may be present within the 2-year period but can never last for >2 months. Beyond depressed mood, the criteria for dysthymic disorder (two of which are required for the diagnosis) are slightly different than those of major depression, including chronic appetite disturbance, sleep difficulties, fatigue or subjective sense of low energy, poor self-esteem, concentration problems, difficulty in decision making, and sense of hopelessness.

Dysthymic disorder has a lifetime prevalence of about 3% and affects females twice as often as males (Weissman et al., 1988). Typical dysthymic disorder presents during adolescence (early-onset type); however, the disorder may present after age 21 (late-onset type). Early onset may be associated with greater risk of lifetime comorbidity with major depression, substance abuse, and personality disorders relative to the late-onset type (Klein et al., 1999). The course of dysthymic disorder is highly variable, with some patients experiencing clinically significant symptoms every day, and some having a highly fluctuant course.

The differentiation of dysthymia from chronic major depression can therefore be difficult. In general, dysthymia is more chronic, and the mood symptoms are more persistent and only mild to moderate in severity. Dysthymia is usually without a clear onset, although patients with the late-onset type are more likely to experience the onset of illness in the context of identifiable psychosocial stressors. This is in contrast to major depressive episodes, which may be mild to moderate but generally have an identifiable onset and are often episodic in nature. Although it rarely warrants psychiatric hospitalization and is generally not associated with psychosis, the sheer chronicity of the depressed mood in patients with dysthymia can result in considerable psychosocial morbidity and dysfunction and renders patients at especially high risk for developing recurrent, superimposed episodes of major depression.

Treatment

In comparison with major depression, dysthymic disorder has less severe neurovegetative symptomatology. In addition, early conceptualizations of what is now defined as dysthymic disorder emphasized character and temperamental pathology. As such, early treatment recommendations emphasized the use of psychoanalytic and related forms of psychotherapy. More recent research has shown that CBT and IPT are effective treatments for dysthymic disorder. Aggressive treatment of dysthymic disorder is warranted because of the aforementioned considerable morbidity and risk of developing superimposed major depressive episodes. Contemporary approaches to treatment call for combined psychotherapy and medication treatment. There is robust evidence for the efficacy of SSRIs and TCAs in dysthymic patients (de Lima and Hotopf, 2003). MAOIs have also been shown to be effective; however, they are not considered first-line treatments for dysthymic disorder. There is some open label evidence for the use of other antidepressant treatments, including bupropion, venlafaxine, mirtazapine, and duloxetine.

Prognosis

The clinical presentation, course, and treatment response for dysthymic disorder are highly variable. Remission rates after successful treatment are reported as ranging from 46% to 71% for up to 6 years (Hermens et al., 2004). Recovery rates may be even higher, especially if medication and psychotherapy are combined (Klein et al., 2000). Similar to major depression, prognostic markers include duration of depressive illness, psychiatric and substance-related comorbidity, burden of general medical illness, and past responses to treatment. The age of onset may also be a prognostic marker. Early-onset dysthymic disorder is associated typically with greater psychiatric comorbidity related to axis II pathology and substance abuse, and greater incidence of progression to major depression. Although the global depressive symptom burden is believed to be less than that of major depression, the functional disability and psychosocial morbidity associated with dysthymic disorder, especially over the long term, is often profound. As such, aggressive treatment is as indicated in the setting of dysthymic disorder as it is in major depression to prevent these poor long-term outcomes.

Depressive Disorders Not Otherwise Specified

Conditions in which the physician has concluded that clinically significant depression is present but cannot determine if it meets the criteria for MDD, dysthymic disorder, adjustment disorder with depressed mood, or depressive disorder due to another condition (secondary depression) are

A CASE OF DYSTHYMIC DISORDER

A 28-year-old married woman presents for evaluation of "always feeling down." She notes that she has felt this way for several years and that more days than not she is waking up earlier than intended, finds she has little appetite, and has minimal motivation. She denies any clear event that she can tie to her starting to feel like this and notes that her friends and husband are getting very frustrated with her because she is "just blah." She saw her primary care physician about this 1 to 2 years ago, and he prescribed fluoxetine, which she took for 2 months but discontinued when she did not feel any improvement and never sought follow-up. During the interview she denies any history of problems with being able to focus, wanting to harm herself, or her symptoms being more severe. She cannot report having a "good week" in >3 years. Additionally, she denied any history of being very energetic, not requiring sleep, and being very active and productive. She denies any problems at work, other than not interacting with her coworkers when they want to go out. She denied feeling anxious or edgy when around people or feelings of embarrassment. She came today because her mother told her that she used to "feel like Eeyore all the time too" until she got some help.

classified as depressive disorder NOS. Several special types of depressive disorders are classified under the depressive disorder NOS heading, including premenstrual dysphoric disorder (PMDD), minor depressive disorder, and recurrent brief depressive episodes.

Premenstrual Dysphoric Disorder

PMDD is a condition marked by depressed mood, anxiety, mood lability, and decreased interest in activities that is associated with most menstrual cycles for the preceding year. Although nearly 80% of women will have some physical symptoms during their menstrual cycles and about 20% to 40% have premenstrual syndrome, only about 2% to 10% of women meet the diagnostic criteria for PMDD (American College of Obstetricians and Gynecologists, 1995). The symptoms tend to appear during the last week of the luteal phase of the estrous cycle and remit within a few days after the onset of menses. Additionally, there is at least a 1-week period of no symptoms during the typical 28-day cycle. When present, the depressive mood symptoms must cause social and occupational dysfunction. Multiple treatments have proved effective for this condition, including lifestyle and dietary changes, nutritional supplementation, psychotherapy, and pharmacotherapy. Lifestyle changes include regular exercise, maintaining a healthy and balanced diet, getting regular sleep, and smoking cessation. Nutritional supplementation includes vitamins B6 and E, calcium, and magnesium. Together, these treatment approaches can exert a noticeable ameliorating effect; however, the size of their effect is usually quite modest. By contrast, psychotherapeutic interventions including cognitive therapy, relaxation therapy, and light therapy achieve greater overall symptom relief. SSRIs, various hormonal treatments (such as gonadotropin releasing hormone agonists and oral contraceptives), benzodiazepines (usually as adjunctive treatment), and vasoactive medications (including spironolactone) have also proven to be effective treatments.

Minor Depressive Disorder and Recurrent Brief Depressive Episodes

Minor depressive disorder is a condition in which the patient has depressive symptoms for a period of at least 2 weeks; however, insufficient symptom criteria are satisfied in order to meet the criteria for a major depressive episode or dysthymic disorder. Recurrent brief depressive episodes are major depressive episodes that last for >2 days but <2 weeks and occur at least once a month for a year. These forms of depressive illness have not been as extensively studied as the depressive syndromes reviewed earlier. A thorough history to rule out past episodes of mania or hypomania should be undertaken in patients who experience recurrent brief depressive episodes to rule out a bipolar spectrum illness.

BIPOLAR DISORDERS

The bipolar disorders are sometimes referred to as *manic depression*. This group of disorders involves various combinations of manic, hypomanic, mixed, and major depressive episodes.

Table 11-4 highlights the key characteristics and differences among these disorders. The bipolar disorders include bipolar I disorder, bipolar II disorder, cyclothymic disorder, and bipolar disorder NOS.

Without treatment, people afflicted with bipolar disorders may demonstrate extreme emotional fluctuations throughout their lives. Yet some of the most well-respected leaders and creative minds have been thought to have these conditions, including Vincent van Gogh (1853–1890), Isaac Newton (1642–1727), and Abraham Lincoln (1809–1865).

As with depressive disorders, the pathophysiology of bipolar disorders is unknown but thought to involve a confluence of pathological processes at multiple physiological levels. Genetic factors are believed to play a key role in the molecular pathophysiology of bipolar disorder. Estimates of heritability based on twin studies range from 65% to 80% (Berrettini, 2004), making bipolar disorders among the most heritable of all mental illnesses. The exact mode of genetic inheritance is unknown. In addition, because the heritability of the disorder is far short of 100%, environmental contributors are assumed to play a key role in the etiology.

At the neurochemical level, there is evidence for disruption of biogenic amine neurotransmitter function, similar to that of major depression. In addition to the monoamine neurotransmitters, disruptions in glutamanergic neurotransmission have also been implicated in the pathophysiology of bipolar disorder. Alterations in neurotransmitter levels are not consistently replicated enough to formulate a biogenic amine hypothesis for bipolar disorder. Neuroendocrine studies have implicated HPA axis abnormalities with a bit more consistency. For instance, the depressive phase of bipolar disorders appears to be associated with relative hypercortisolemia, while the manic state is associated with lower cortisol levels. How this relates to clinical symptoms of severe depression and mania, hypomania, or mixed mood episodes remains to be determined.

Although neurochemical abnormalities appear to be widespread in bipolar disorder, pathological processes in specific brain regions are also implicated. In particular, there is evidence of deficits in frontal cortex functioning in bipolar manic patients, coupled with relative hyperactivity in limbic structures such as the amygdala and ventral striatum (Strakowski et al., 2005). These are key regions of interest in bipolar disorder and other psychiatric illnesses, because the frontal cortex is responsible for exerting top-down executive control over more primitive brain structures, and the amygdala and ventral striatum are key mediators of modulation of emotions, psychomotor activity, and the sensation of reward. There is also evidence of disruption of functional connectivity between the frontal lobe and other areas of the brain in bipolar patients, suggesting dysregulation of the communication pathways between key brain regions. Thus, poorly coordinated patterns of cross talk between neurobiological systems and neuroanatomic regions may be responsible for the chaotic symptom presentation and course of bipolar spectrum disorders and the profound neurocognitive deficits that are manifest in bipolar patients, even in euthymic states.

Some of the more recent findings in the neurobiology of bipolar disorder involve structural abnormalities and their possible links with changes in gene expression. Volumetric brain imaging studies using structural magnetic resonance imaging (MRI) have shown reduced prefrontal gray matter volumes among bipolar patients, as well as an increase in the number of white matter hyperintensities—all of which suggest that the clinical manifestations of bipolar disorder may stem in part from cellular breakdown in key brain regions (Brambilla et al., 2005). The mood stabilizer medication lithium has been found to increase neuronal cell survival, which may relate to its potentiation of cell survival factors (Bcl-2 and BDNF) and inhibition of the proapoptotic factors Bax and p53 (Chuang, 2005). Lithium has also been associated with increases in markers of neuronal integrity on proton magnetic resonance spectroscopy (1H-MRS) imaging and increases in cortical gray matter volume on structural MRI. Valproate, another mood stabilizer medication, has also been shown to increase Bcl-2. These changes may relate to the cognitive dysfunction observed in bipolar patients, which may predict much of the functional incapacity associated with bipolar disorders.

Finally, increasingly consistent findings in bipolar disorder point to an etiopathological role of disrupted neuronal signal transduction/secondary messenger pathways. Most investigations have centered on disease-associated alterations in cyclic adenosine monophosphate (cAMP), cyclic guanosine monophosphate (cGMP), phosphoinositol and calcium signaling, as well as alterations in the cAMP/protein kinase A (cAMP/PKA) and protein kinase C (PKC) transduction pathways.

These are compelling molecular targets, because they are involved in the physiological functioning of many neurotransmitter systems.

Furthermore, changes in gene expression resulting from altered intracellular signaling may take several weeks, coincident with the delayed onset of therapeutic activity of biological treatments for bipolar disorder. Lithium exposure results in the modulation of several of these secondary messenger systems. As is the case for major depression, effective treatments for bipolar disorder, including lithium and ECT, result in increased BDNF expression over long-term exposure, thus promoting neuronal and synaptic viability and survival. The role of these intracellular processes in the pathophysiology of bipolar disorder and the mechanism of action of effective bipolar treatments are rapidly advancing fields of study.

Bipolar I Disorder

Phenomenology

A diagnosis of bipolar I disorder is assigned if there is a history of at least one episode of mania or at least one mixed episode, and all secondary causes have been ruled out. Even though these two types of mood episodes are most important in defining the disorder, the predominant mood state during the course of bipolar I disorder is depression. During these depressive periods, the greatest functional disability occurs, though severe devastation may be wrought in a relatively shorter period of time during manic episodes, as reviewed earlier. Because bipolar disorders typically involve depressive mood states, misdiagnosis and delays in treatment are frequently encountered. This is a significant public health concern, because the treatments for bipolar depressive states and major depression are different, and use of antidepressant medications without mood stabilizers in the setting of bipolar depression may result in sudden mood state switching into the manic range and increase the frequency of mood cycling over time.

When classifying bipolar I disorder, it is important to specify the most recent episode. For example, if the patient presents with acute mania with no prior history of a mood-related problem, the diagnosis is qualified as "Bipolar I Disorder, Single Manic Episode," but if someone with a history of bipolar I disorder presents with a severe depressive episode, the diagnosis is qualified as "Bipolar I Disorder, Most Recent Episode Depressed." In the latter case, such a patient would have had a past history of confirmed mania or mixed mood state.

Many patients with bipolar I disorder who present with acute manic, mixed, or depressive mood episodes also experience psychotic features. In most cases, the psychotic features are mood congruent—that is, the psychotic themes are consistent with the presenting mood state. For instance, patients who present in an acute manic state with psychotic features tend to experience grandiose delusions, sometimes with auditory hallucinations that reflect grandiose themes. Patients who are depressed, by contrast, may express nihilistic delusional beliefs. When the content or theme of the psychotic features reflects the nature of the mood state with which they are associated, the psychotic features are termed *mood congruent*. Those that do not relate in any meaningful way to the associated mood state are termed *mood incongruent* and are believed to portend a worse prognosis compared with mood-congruent psychotic features.

Treatments

The pharmacologic properties of individual mood stabilizers and other medicines used in the treatment of bipolar disorder will be covered in Chapter 22. In this section, pharmacologic treatments will be discussed in the broader context of acute and long-term treatment of bipolar disorders.

The cornerstone of treatment of bipolar disorder, regardless of polar mood state, is pharmacologic treatment with mood stabilizers. The term *mood stabilizer* refers to medications that are effective for acute stabilization and longer-term maintenance treatment of bipolar disorders. There are three traditional mood stabilizer medications: lithium, valproate, and carbamazepine. Other medications that could be classified as mood stabilizers under this definition include atypical antipsychotics and lamotrigine. Many of these medications are used in combination over long-term treatment, because many appear more effective for some phases of bipolar disorder and less effective for others. As such, different pharmacologic approaches may be utilized depending on which phase of bipolar illness and/or its treatment (e.g., acute mania/hypomania, acute depression, mixed episodes, long-term maintenance treatment) is being addressed.

Acute mania

Acute mania often presents dramatically with severe agitation and/or grandiosity, impulsivity, sleeplessness, cognitive dysfunction, and overactivation that may progress to psychotic symptoms, overt aggression, and other forms of dangerous and disinhibited behaviors. As such, acute episodes of mania are treated as medical emergencies and require rapid institution of treatment.

Selection of particular medications, or combinations of them, is based on several factors, including severity of the current episode, presence of psychotic symptoms, past treatment responses, adverse effect profile of individual drugs, comorbid psychiatric or medical conditions (including concomitant substance abuse), and clinical subtype.

Often, a mood stabilizer with established effectiveness for acute mania is chosen, such as lithium, valproic acid, or carbamazepine. Under ideal circumstances, treatment with a single mood stabilizer may be all that is required; however, the lag time to therapeutic benefit with these medications (up to 3–4 weeks) can be considerable in some patients, and therapeutic response is not always complete with one medicine. As such, mood stabilizer medications are often combined with one another (e.g., adding valproic acid to lithium) or with antipsychotic drugs acutely in order to achieve a more rapid or complete therapeutic effect. The combination of valproic acid and carbamazepine is typically best avoided in order to limit drug–drug interactions between the two that may result in increased concentrations of toxic metabolites of both drugs. If a patient presents in an acute manic state with psychotic features, treatment with an antipsychotic medication is warranted.

Older typical neuroleptic drugs (e.g., haloperidol, chlorpromazine) are also effective for treating acute mania, but their long-term use is limited by increased risk of extrapyramidal adverse effects (EPS) and tardive dyskinesia. Additionally, long-term use of typical neuroleptics may induce depressive symptoms. Newer atypical antipsychotic drugs are more commonly used based on the lower risk of EPS and tardive dyskinesia, and they do not appear to be associated with increased risk of depression during long-term use.

Other biological treatments, most having less support from clinical evidence than the options mentioned earlier, with the exception of ECT, are discussed in a separate section later in the chapter. ECT may be a preferred option for patients who are pregnant, as several of the mood stabilizers have teratogenic potential. Psychotherapy and other intensive psychosocial treatments are not typically initiated during an acute manic episode but are instead introduced as the patient begins to improve.

Acute bipolar depression

Acute bipolar depression presents with the same clinical features as acute episodes of major depression. Although antidepressants are effective in reducing depressive symptoms in both bipolar and unipolar depressive disorders, they may increase risk of mood switching from depression to mania or hypomania in patients with bipolar disorder. The preferred first-line option for treating acute bipolar depression is the use of a mood stabilizer or other medications with evidence of efficacy in this phase of illness.

Even though traditional mood stabilizers such as lithium, valproate, and carbamazepine may be effective for some, they are far more effective in the setting of acute mania rather than depression in bipolar disorder. The anticonvulsant medication lamotrigine has established efficacy in the treatment of acute bipolar depression when used as a single agent; however, lamotrigine has not been shown to be effective for mania. As such, patients with a history of frequent or severe manic episodes prior to becoming depressed who are being considered for lamotrigine treatment often receive concomitant therapy with more established antimanic agents such as lithium or atypical antipsychotic drugs.

Lamotrigine may be added to existing mood stabilizer treatment during depressive episodes. It must be titrated slowly to its target dose of 200 to 400 mg daily to limit the risk of potentially fatal drug rashes. Although lamotrigine is generally well tolerated, caution must be exercised when combining it with certain other medications. Because valproic acid inhibits the metabolism of lamotrigine, its starting dose in the presence of valproate is half of the usual starting dose, and the titration schedule is approximately twice as slow. By contrast, because carbamazepine accelerates the metabolism of lamotrigine, starting doses are higher and the titration schedule more aggressive.

A CASE OF MIXED MOOD EPISODE

A 23-year-old single woman is brought to the emergency department by her fiancé. Four weeks before, she developed depressed mood, inability to enjoy hobbies, unprovoked tearfulness, and insomnia with fatigue during the day. These symptoms persisted unremittingly and progressively worsened. She became increasingly irritable and angry. During the evaluation, she reported feeling depressed, worthless, and suicidal and repeatedly discussed feelings of guilt over her perceived shortcomings and failures. She also complained of not being able to "slow down" her mind and body and that her thoughts were overcrowded. She was talking very fast and seemed to jump from topic to topic. She acknowledged having recurrent thoughts about taking her life over the last few days and had considered multiple methods. Her fiancé reported that she had been psychiatrically hospitalized recently and had discontinued her medication 3 months ago to lose weight for their wedding. The emergency department physician reported that her screening laboratories were normal, including a negative urine drug and β-HCG assessments.

The presence of psychotic depressive episodes warrants use of an antipsychotic medication. The same considerations in terms of choice of agent for manic episodes also apply to the treatment of psychotic depression. The atypical antipsychotics quetiapine and olanzapine (in combination with fluoxetine) have established efficacy for the treatment of bipolar depression, with or without psychotic features, as single interventions. Both have established efficacy for the treatment of acute mania.

Poor or partial symptomatic responses may be managed by combining medication treatments or ECT, particularly in severe cases. ECT may be a preferred option for patients who are pregnant, actively suicidal, or refusing food or drink or other situations where a rapid treatment response is urgently needed. The practice of combining antidepressants with mood stabilizer medications is controversial and risks precipitating an acute manic episode or increasing mood cycle frequency. Antidepressant monotherapy should be avoided. Psychosocial interventions are best initiated when acute symptoms subside.

Mixed episodes

Although DSM-IV-TR characterizes mixed mood episodes as those that satisfy the criteria for both major depressive and manic episodes, mixed mood episodes have a variable presentation in the clinical environment (e.g., a major depressive episode with subsyndromal manic or hypomanic features). As with acute mania, first-line options for mixed episodes include antimanic mood stabilizers (lithium, valproic acid, and carbamazepine). Although mixed episodes have been classically described as being less responsive to lithium than valproic acid or carbamazepine, evidence for this relationship is not strong. Thus, lithium remains a reasonable choice as a mood stabilizer for mixed episodes. Antipsychotic drugs, particularly atypical agents, have also been shown to be effective for mixed episodes, as single agents or in combination with antimanic mood stabilizers. Although lamotrigine does not appear to be effective for treating acute mania, it may be useful for treating acute mixed episodes, particularly if depressive symptoms predominate.

Mixed mood episodes may occur independently or mark the transition point between mania/hypomania and depression, or *vice versa*. As such, antidepressants are best avoided or discontinued during mixed episodes, if possible, in order to prevent induction of "pure" manic episodes or increasing mood lability. In general, if patients transition into "pure" manic episodes or mixed symptomatology persists during the course of acute treatment for mixed episodes, the general guidelines provided earlier for acute mania may be followed. If the patient transitions into a bipolar depressive episode, the general guidelines for bipolar depression may be followed. Regardless of mood phase transitioning, refractory cases may ultimately respond to ECT.

Maintenance treatment

Once the acute phase symptoms are successfully treated, most patients will require ongoing pharmacologic treatment. The goals are to prevent future occurrences of acute mood episodes and to prevent subsyndromal recurrences of depressive or manic symptoms, which are associated with marked dysfunction and increased risk of acute illness recurrence, especially in patients who have had two or more manic episodes or one severe manic episode.

Although combinations of medications may be needed during acute phase treatment, the ideal circumstance is to treat with one medication during the maintenance phase if at all possible. For maintenance treatment following an acute manic or mixed episode, there is considerable support for the use of lithium. There is also evidence to support valproic acid and lamotrigine as single agents in this role. Atypical antipsychotic drugs may also be effective as single agents.

Many factors determine the choice of maintenance medication. An important consideration is the nature of the acute episode preceding maintenance treatment. Following acute depressive episodes, maintenance treatment with lamotrigine is a reasonable first choice as a single agent in patients with no history of severe or recurrent manias or in combination with an antimanic medication if such a history is present. Lithium has also been shown to be effective in this role; however, it appears to be more effective in preventing recurrences of mania than depression. Additionally, there is some evidence of a less favorable response to lithium during long-term treatment among patients with rapid cycling, a high number of prior mood episodes, and comorbid substance use disorders. Less evidence supports single agent valproic acid and carbamazepine in preventing recurrences of depression compared with preventing manic episodes. Emerging evidence supports the long-term use of atypical antipsychotic drugs, especially olanzapine. Clinicians must consider the long-term adverse effect profiles and their interaction with the patient's general medical status (discussed in further in Chapter 22). Therapeutic monitoring recommendations for specific drugs should be followed closely.

Because breakthrough symptoms are so frequently encountered during long-term therapy, combinations of medications are often required. In general, combining medications should be done after ensuring that the dosage and, when applicable, serum drug concentrations have been confirmed as adequate. If dosages are low or serum drug levels are subtherapeutic, the next step before adding a second agent may be optimizing the dose of the first medication. Particularly effective combinations may include lithium and lamotrigine, lithium and either valproic acid or carbamazepine, or a traditional mood stabilizer and an atypical antipsychotic drug. Psychosocial treatments are also important adjuncts to medication for the prevention of bipolar relapse.

Rapid cycling

Rapid cycling bipolar disorder, defined as a long-term course characterized by four or more mood episodes over a 12-month period, is associated with poorer response to pharmacotherapy, greater dysfunction, and higher suicide risk compared with nonrapid cycling bipolar illness. In some studies, use of antidepressants has been associated with greater risk of rapid cycling and higher frequency of mood episodes among patients with a known rapid cycling course. Other medications/compounds have also been associated with potential mood cycling effects, including stimulants, sympathomimetics, other drugs of abuse, and corticosteroids. If unnecessary, these medications should be avoided, and if possible, antidepressants should be tapered and discontinued as an initial step in treating patients with a current or past rapid cycling course. Substance use disorders should be treated. Mood stabilizer medications that are effective during maintenance treatment should be selected and optimized. The combinations of medications discussed in the preceding text for maintenance phase treatment may be used if rapid cycling persists in spite of the above maneuvers.

Other biological treatments

Other anticonvulsant medications have less evidence to support their use in bipolar disorder. Benzodiazepines are often used as pharmacologic adjuncts to mood stabilizer and/or antipsychotic drugs in acute manic or mixed states due to their rapid sedating properties and beneficial effects on sleep. Typical neuroleptic drugs such as haloperidol are also effective antimanic agents and often used also for adjunctive treatment due to their rapid sedating properties. Their use is typically restricted to short-term treatment due to their motor adverse effects and the increased risk of causing tardive dyskinesia during long-term treatment.

One advantage of typical neuroleptics is extensive clinical experience in the setting of pregnancy. They may be safer alternatives than many of the above mood stabilizers for the treatment of mania during pregnancy. Finally, ECT is a highly effective treatment for both polar phases of bipolar disorder, especially when psychotic features are present. ECT may also be the safest bipolar treatment during pregnancy.

The use of antidepressant medications for bipolar depression, both acutely and during maintenance phase treatment, is controversial because of concern about increased risk of antidepressant-associated conversion to mania and increase in mood cyclicity. The relative liabilities of the antidepressant classes for causing such effects have not been precisely determined; however, TCAs are believed to confer the greatest risk, while less risk is associated with SSRIs, MAOIs, and bupropion. The risk associated with SNRIs is also believed to be relatively low, even though they, like TCAs, feature blockade of multiple amine reuptake pumps in their pharmacodynamic profile. Regardless, antidepressants are generally not used in the absence of a known concomitant mood-stabilizing medicine to guard against mood switching and the development of rapid cycling. Antidepressants are generally discontinued after recovery from acute bipolar depression after several weeks to several months of clinical stability. Some patients, however, appear to respond better to prolonged combination therapy with an antidepressant and mood stabilizer rather than a mood stabilizer alone.

Psychosocial interventions

The benefits of psychotherapy and psychosocial interventions should not be overlooked. Effective modalities include psychoeducational interventions for patients and their support systems, illness management training, establishing a structured daily routine, problem solving skills training, and couples/marital therapy (Scott and Colom, 2005). Many of the most severely impaired patients will require case management, housing assistance, and legal services. Specific psychotherapeutic interventions that enhance adherence to treatment, recognition of symptoms indicative of early relapse, and symptom management, including cognitive behavioral approaches, have also shown promise in remedying residual symptoms and preventing relapse (Vieta et al., 2005). Family-focused treatment, which aims to improve communication, problem solving, and general illness awareness within the family context, has also been shown to reduce relapse rates in bipolar patients (Vieta et al., 2005). In general, psychotherapeutic strategies are believed to be more effective for depressive episodes. Their benefit in the setting of manic or mixed episodes, particularly in the presence of psychotic features, is not nearly as well established.

Prognosis

Early comparative studies suggested that the long-term outlook in bipolar disorders was much more favorable than that of schizophrenia; however, research in the last two decades has suggested that this may have been overly optimistic. Between 20% and 40% of bipolar patients have a poor overall response to mood stabilizer treatment, and between 35% and 60% of patients have chronic mood symptomatology in spite of treatment and a poor overall outcome.

In terms of disease-specific outcome, depressive mood states are responsible for most of the long-term morbidity associated with bipolar disorder. The presence of psychotic features (especially if they are mood incongruent), rapid cycling, and mixed episodes predicts worse outcome. As with major depression, subsyndromal affective symptoms are frequently present and portend a poorer long-term prognosis, requiring aggressive treatment, particularly of depressive episodes, with the goal of achieving symptom remission.

Emphasis on treatment adherence is another important prognostic marker. The single biggest predictor of relapse and rehospitalization is poor adherence to treatment. Between 20% and 55% of patients are believed to be poorly adherent.

Finally, 8% to 22% of patients with bipolar disorders exhibit suicidal behavior. Risk of suicide is increased for patients with rapid cycling, mixed episodes, psychotic features, comorbid substance abuse, and greater medical and psychiatric comorbidity. Better outcomes are observed among patients who remain adherent to their treatment regimen, retain insight into the nature of their illness, are substance free, and have adequate psychosocial support. The degree of cognitive impairment, even during periods of euthymia, will likely emerge as another major determinant of functional capacity in bipolar illness.

A CASE OF BIPOLAR I DISORDER

A 20-year-old single male college student is brought in by his parents due to concerns over his recent behaviors while home on break. He has been "very odd" in that he cannot seem to stay on task, appears hyperactive, and is not sleeping at night. What finally prompted them to bring him in for evaluation was when he awoke them at 1 AM requesting his father's physics books and then reawakened them at 4 AM citing that he had solved the next step in proving Einstein's theory of relativity. They became concerned that he was using drugs, although he had no prior history, and searched his room. They found no evidence of any substances but did note multiple religious items throughout the room and an open journal with an entry that was written in very small print entitled "the writings of the messiah." They contacted his college roommate, who noted that he had been doing fine until a week ago, when he began studying for finals. The roommate cited a distinct change with an increase in energy and very limited sleep. During the interview, he talked very rapidly and seemed to jump from topic to topic. He denied that there was anything wrong and expressed confusion as to why he needed to be seen.

Bipolar II Disorder

Phenomenology

In contrast to bipolar I disorder, bipolar II disorder requires the history of at least one major depressive episode and at least one hypomanic episode. A diagnosis of bipolar I disorder would supersede the diagnosis of bipolar II disorder if there is a history of a manic episode. Table 11-4 helps to distinguish bipolar II from bipolar I and cyclothymic disorders.

Treatment and Prognosis

Recommendations for the treatment of bipolar II disorder have generally echoed those for bipolar I disorder in spite of the lack of treatment studies focused on bipolar II patients. Bipolar II disorder is believed by many to be a less severe form of illness than bipolar I disorder; however, functional outcome studies comparing both forms of bipolar illness indicated that the degrees of functional impairment in work, social, domestic, and recreational domains are equal.

In addition, measures of life satisfaction and overall social maladjustment indicate little, if any, difference between bipolar I and bipolar II disorders over the long term. The comparable degrees of dysfunction between these disorders in spite of differences in frequency and severity of manic mood states may be explained by more frequent and severe depressive episodes, higher burden of substance-related and psychiatric comorbidity, and risk of suicidal behavior associated with bipolar II disorder compared with bipolar I disorder. Whether this translates to clear differences in responsiveness to standard treatments for bipolar I disorder is unclear.

Cyclothymic Disorder

Phenomenology

Cyclothymic disorder, or cyclothymia, is a chronic mood disorder characterized by numerous hypomanic and dysthymic episodes over a 2-year period or longer. During this time period (≥1 year for children or adolescents), patients do not experience a symptom-free period lasting longer than 2 months. The mood episodes are not due to a medical condition, the effects of substances or medication, or other mental health condition. History of a major depressive, manic, or mixed episode would result in a superseding diagnosis of bipolar I or II, as appropriate. Additionally, the mood symptoms must result in clinically significant distress or impairment in social, occupational, or other important domains of functioning.

In general, cyclothymia has an insidious onset in adolescence or early adult life and persists unremittingly with prolonged periods of cyclical, often unpredictable, mood changes. Many times, people close to patients will describe them as moody, unpredictable, inconsistent, or unreliable. This can result in patterns of unstable relationships and recurrent occupational problems. In addition to these problems in life functioning, rates of comorbid substance abuse are high.

Treatment and Prognosis

Like bipolar II disorder, the same modalities used to treat bipolar I disorder are used to treat cyclothymia. However, these treatments are generally not empirically supported for use in cyclothymia. Studies focusing on course and outcome of cyclothymia are also relatively few, and differences in response to standard treatments have not been extensively investigated. This may be related in part to the sheer clinical heterogeneity among patients who are diagnosed with cyclothymia. Depression is believed to be the predominant mood state, which may predict significant functional burden. Treatment response may depend to a great degree on the extent of substance-related and psychiatric comorbidity. Many of the prognostic markers reviewed for bipolar I disorder are similar for cyclothymic disorder. Studies of clinical outcome for cyclothymic disorder and bipolar II disorder are clearly warranted.

SECONDARY MOOD DISORDERS

When a medical or drug-induced condition can be pinpointed as the etiology for the mood disorder, then a secondary mood disorder is diagnosed. The differential diagnosis list for mood disorders is very broad (Tables 11-2 and 11-3). A thorough history and physical, including laboratory evaluation, is necessary. Laboratory, electrophysiologic, and radiographic studies may also be indicated. Possible clues to an organic cause for mood symptoms include onset of symptoms after age 40, rapid onset and evolution of symptoms, altered sensorium, atypical psychotic symptoms (e.g., extra-auditory hallucinations, including fully formed visual and tactile hallucinations), dense cognitive impairments greater than what is typical of the psychiatric syndrome in question, presence of abnormal vital signs, history of known medical illnesses that can present with psychiatric symptoms, known substance use problems, advanced age, extensive polypharmacy, multiple medical problems, and recent change in medical status and/or medications.

Mood Disorder Secondary to a General Medical Condition

The characteristic feature of a mood disorder secondary to a general medical condition is that the mood disturbance is determined to be a result of the effects of a medical illness. For example, if patients have a hypothyroid condition, they may initially present with a depressed mood and the symptoms of a major depressive episode but should appropriately be diagnosed as having a secondary mood disorder.

Unlike the primary mood disorders, the secondary mood disorders do not require that full criteria be met for the mood episodes. All that is required is for the patient to develop clinically significant mood symptoms. The physician should qualify the diagnosis as with depressive features, manic features, or mixed features. Clinical management depends on the identification and successful treatment of the underlying cause. Improvement in psychiatric symptoms may lag slightly behind normalization of illness-specific biomarkers. Thus, absence of immediate improvement with normalization of laboratory indices does not exclude the diagnosis of a secondary mood disorder.

Substance-Induced Mood Disorder

When a mood disorder is determined to be due to the physiologic effects of a substance, a substance-induced mood disorder is diagnosed. Like mood disorders that are due to general medical conditions, all the criteria for a major mood disorder do not have to be met to make the diagnosis of substance-induced mood disorder. Only the development of clinically significant mood symptoms is required. The physician should qualify the diagnosis as with depressive features, manic features, or mixed features. Clinical management relies on identifying the offending substance and discontinuing its use. Normalization of mood state may not occur immediately, but may lag behind substance discontinuation.

CONCLUSIONS AND FUTURE DIRECTIONS

The mood disorders represent a large, clinically heterogeneous group of disorders characterized primarily by clinically significant changes in mood and regulation of emotional and neurovegetative functioning. Collectively, they are frequently encountered in primary care and psychiatric and nonpsychiatric subspecialty settings and are associated with a significant degree of illness-related burden, functional disability, and comorbidity. Even though the etiology and pathophysiology of affective disorders are not fully understood, there has been laudable progress in the last few decades toward a greater understanding of the neurobiological underpinnings of mood disorders and, importantly, how environmental stressors and early life trauma may interact with neurobiological systems to produce the signs and symptoms of unipolar depressive and bipolar illnesses. The successful management of mood disorders depends most heavily on accurate diagnosis and aggressive treatment, particularly for bipolar disorders, which are often undiagnosed or mistakenly diagnosed as unipolar depression. Although there are numerous effective treatment modalities for both major depression and bipolar I disorder, there is a relative lack of evidence for the treatment of other mood disorders. Because all mood disorders appear to be associated with significant residual symptomatology, aggressive treatment is required regardless of the diagnosis. Psychosocial interventions are crucial for amelioration of residual symptoms and improving functional outcome for many patients, especially when combined with pharmacotherapy. Future outcome studies will shed light on which treatment modalities, delivered singly or in combination with one another, are most effective for particular types of patients or symptom profiles. Even now, molecular neurobiological approaches are yielding a diverse array of promising targets for future drug development for mood disorders that may be exploited for clinical use in the near future.

Clinical Pearls

- The essential features of a major depressive episode are depressed mood or loss of interest or pleasure for 2 or more weeks plus four or more physiologic symptoms.
- Dysthymic disorder requires that mild depressive symptoms be present most of the day, more days than not, for 2 years, with <2 months free of symptoms.
- Major depressive disorder is a recurrent illness with an increasing likelihood of future episodes after each recurrence.
- The factors most likely to affect recurrence of major depressive episodes are inadequate treatment, history of prior episodes, comorbid conditions, and premature discontinuation of treatment.
- Psychotherapy and pharmacotherapy are equally effective options for treatment of mild-to-moderate depression.
- After achieving successful control of acute depressive symptoms with pharmacotherapy, the same medication should be continued for at least 6 to 9 months to prevent recurrence of symptoms.
- A history of depression is not required to make a diagnosis of bipolar I disorder, only a manic episode.
- Patients with bipolar disorder spend more time depressed than manic; it is important to ask about their history of mania.
- The key differences between a hypomanic and manic episode are the level of severity, the degree of social/occupational dysfunction, and the need for hospitalization.
- There are no specific laboratory or radiologic findings for mood disorders; however, laboratory evaluations should be performed and radiologic studies should be considered in new-onset mood symptoms to rule out general medical conditions and substance abuse.
- ECT may be a preferred option for pregnant patients in manic episodes due to the teratogenic potential of mood stabilizers.
- The use of antidepressants should be avoided in the treatment of acute bipolar depression due to the increased risk of mood switching; mood stabilizers are the preferred first-line option.
- Indications for hospitalization in mood disorders include acute mania, acute risk of suicide, psychosis, or impaired ability for self-care.
- Always consider comorbid personality issues or substance use disorders in patients with mood disorders that do not respond to appropriate treatments, because these are commonly associated with mood disorders and may need to be major areas of therapeutic focus.

Self-Assessment Questions and Answers

11-1. Which of the following is the most common mood disorder?

A. Bipolar I disorder
B. Bipolar II disorder
C. Cyclothymic disorder
D. Dysthymic disorder
E. Major depressive disorder

Depressive episodes are far more common than the manic and hypomanic episodes required for bipolar disorder. It is estimated that nearly one in five Americans will have a depressive episode in their lifetimes and approximately one in ten will be depressed at some point during the year. Major depressive disorder is twice as likely to occur in women and most likely to occur in spring and fall. *Answer: E*

11-2. A patient is recently diagnosed with major depressive disorder after his first episode of depression and started on treatment with a selective serotonin reuptake inhibitor. He has never had to take a chronic medication and is concerned about whether he will be on this "for life." How long can he expect to be on the medication?

A. 6 weeks
B. 2–3 months
C. 4–6 months
D. 9–12 months
E. 2 years

Because this is his first episode of depression, acute phase management with an antidepressant lasts up to 10 weeks and then should be followed by a 6- to 9-month maintenance phase of continued treatment to prevent recurrence of symptoms. This is assuming that the patient responds to the first medication. After completion of the maintenance phase, the patient can be counseled about the risks and benefits of discontinuing treatment. If the patient has a history of recurrent episodes after completing courses of treatment, consideration should be given to continuous pharmacotherapy. *Answer: D*

11-3. Which of the following is the best treatment option for a patient presenting with depressed mood who has a prior history of manic episodes?

A. Carbamazepine
B. Lamotrigine
C. Lithium
D. Sertraline
E. Venlafaxine

This patient has acute bipolar depression. Lamotrigine has established efficacy as a single agent in this condition. Even though traditional mood stabilizers such as lithium, valproate,

and carbamazepine may be effective for some, they are far more effective in the setting of acute mania rather than depression in bipolar disorder. Antidepressants may increase risk of mood switching from depression to mania or hypomania in patients with bipolar disorder, so sertraline and venlafaxine should be avoided without the concurrent initiation of a mood-stabilizing agent. *Answer: B*

11-4. A 27-year-old man with no prior mental health history comes for an initial visit with the psychiatrist. Two months ago he started a new job where he works in marketing. He does not like his boss and feels that he is constantly being berated. Since that time he notes increasingly depressed mood, early morning waking, decreased energy and concentration at work, and increased irritability. He denies any thoughts of wanting to harm himself or others and notes that he is "not motivated to get things done at work." At home he gets irritable with his spouse on weeknights because he is "dreading having to go to work the next day" but feels much better and is more relaxed on weekends. He denies any prior history of depression or mental health care and any periods of decreased need for sleep, elevated mood, feelings of being anxious more often than not, or recurring fears of embarrassment in certain situations. What is the most likely diagnosis?

A. Adjustment disorder with depressed mood
B. Bipolar II disorder
C. Dysthymic disorder
D. Major depressive disorder
E. Secondary mood disorder

In this case, the patient has no prior history of elevated mood symptoms and no previously identified medical or substance use concerns, which make a secondary mood disorder or bipolar II disorder unlikely. Additionally, his symptoms have been present for only the last 6 weeks, which does not meet the necessary criteria of 2 years for dysthymic disorder. The differentiation between major depressive disorder and adjustment disorder becomes a little more difficult. This gentleman does have five of the criteria, including a depressed mood for more than the last 2 weeks resulting in occupational dysfunction; however, his symptoms do not appear to be global, because he reports not having the same level of symptoms on the weekends. In this case, with an abrupt onset and one clear identifiable stressor, an adjustment disorder should be considered.

Although not formally classified as a mood disorder in DSM-IV-TR, an adjustment disorder with depressed mood is a frequent clinical depressive syndrome. An adjustment disorder is a psychiatric disorder that occurs following an identifiable psychosocial stressor (such as divorce, job loss, physical illness). The individual's response to that stressor is considered to be extreme or in excess of what would normally be expected or results in significant impairment in the individual's social, occupational, or interpersonal functioning. In general, the symptoms will remit in time or when the stressor is removed, and removal of the stressor is the primary treatment. However, if that is not possible, the individual should be treated similar to major depressive disorder. *Answer: A*

11-5. A 25-year-old woman with a history of worsening depressive symptoms presents to a psychiatrist for the first time for treatment of her depression. She reports no prior history of depressive symptoms and has never been seen previously by a mental health provider. She denies any medical problems and is not taking any medications, over-the-counter medications, herbal supplements, or illicit substances at this time. She reports that her symptoms began 2 to 3 months ago and includes a decreased desire to do anything, decreased energy, difficulty concentrating, decreased appetite coupled with an 11 lb weight loss, and insomnia. She reports daily thoughts that she would be better off dead and notes that she has contemplated taking all of the acetaminophen

that she has in her house. Her husband is with her and reports that she has ongoing thoughts that their child is possessed by an evil spirit and that she has been making phone calls to several local churches, requesting an exorcism. She last saw her medical provider 4 months ago and was noted to have a normal examination and laboratory work. Which of the following is the best first course of management for this condition?

A. Admit for inpatient treatment.
B. Start cognitive behavioral therapy.
C. Start electroconvulsive therapy.
D. Start treatment with a mood stabilizer.
E. Start treatment with a selective serotonin reuptake inhibitor.

Mild-to-moderate major depressive disorder can be treated equally effectively with either psychotherapy or medications (selective serotonin reuptake inhibitors are generally considered first-line treatment). The most effective method is a combination of psychotherapy and pharmacotherapy. More severe cases may require augmentation with additional medications or the use of electroconvulsive therapy (ECT) for those who are unable to tolerate medications or who have conditions that make ECT the safest option, such as multiple medical problems or pregnancy. However, this example outlines a case of major depressive disorder, severe with psychotic features. In view of her delusions about her child, infanticide is a serious concern and this patient should be hospitalized immediately for a full evaluation and immediate initiation of treatment under close observation. *Answer: A*

References

American College of Obstetricians and Gynecologists. ACOG Committee Opinion No. 155: Premenstrual syndrome. *Int J Gynaecol Obstet*. 1995;50:80–84.

American Psychiatric Association. *Diagnostic and statistic manual of mental disorders*, 4th ed., text revision. Washington, DC: American Psychiatric Association; 2000a.

American Psychiatric Association. Practice guideline for the treatment of patients with major depressive disorder (revision). *Am J Psychiatry*. 2000b;157(Suppl 4):1–45.

Berrettini W. Linkage and association studies of bipolar disorders. In: Charney DS, Nestler EJ, eds. *Neurobiology of mental illness*, 2nd ed. New York: Oxford University Press; 2004:369–379.

Brambilla P, Glahn DC, Balestrieri M, et al. Magnetic resonance findings in bipolar disorder. *Psychiatr Clin North Am*. 2005;28:443–467.

Chuang DM. The antiapoptotic actions of mood stabilizers: Molecular mechanisms and therapeutic potentials. *Ann N Y Acad Sci*. 2005;1053:195–204.

Cuijpers P, Smit F. Excess mortality in depression: A meta-analysis of community studies. *J Affect Disord*. 2002;72:227–236.

de Lima MS, Hotopf M. A comparison of active drugs for the treatment of dysthymia. *Cochrane Database Syst Rev*. 2003;(3):CD004047.

Feldman G. Cognitive and behavioral therapies for depression: Overview, new directions, and practical recommendations for dissemination. *Psychiatr Clin North Am*. 2007;30:39–50.

Gotto J, Rapaport MH. Treatment options in treatment-resistant depression. *Prim Psychiatr*. 2005;12: 42–50.

Groves DA, Brown VJ. Vagal nerve stimulation: A review of its applications and potential mechanisms that mediate its clinical effects. *Neurosci Behav Physiol*. 2005;29:493–500.

Hermens ML, van Hout HP, Terluin B, et al. The prognosis of minor depression in the general population: A systematic review. *Gen Hosp Psychiatry*. 2004;26:453–462.

Howland RH, Thase ME. A comprehensive review of cyclothymic disorder. *J Nerv Ment Dis*. 1993;54: 229–234.

Inskip HM, Harris EC, Barracough B. Lifetime risk of suicide for affective disorder, alcoholism, and schizophrenia. *Br J Psychiatry Suppl*. 1998;172:35–37.

Jindal RD, Thase ME. Integrating psychotherapy and pharmacotherapy to improve outcomes among patients with mood disorders. *Psychiatr Serv*. 2003;54:1484–1490.

Keller MB, Boland RJ. Implications of failing to achieve successful long-term maintenance treatment of recurrent unipolar depression. *Biol Psychiatry*. 1998;44:348–360.

Kessler RC, McGonagle KA, Zhoa S, et al. Lifetime and 12-month prevalence of DSM-III-R psychiatric disorders in the United Sates: Results from the National Comorbidity Survey. *Arch Gen Psychiatry*. 1994;51:9–19.

Kessler RC, Berglund P, Demler O, et al. Epidemiology of major depressive disorder: Results from the co-morbidity survey replication. *JAMA*. 2003;289:3095–3105.

Klein DN, Schatzberg AF, McCullough JP, et al. Early- versus late-onset dysthymic disorder: Comparison in out-patients with superimposed major depressive episodes. *J Affect Disord*. 1999;52:187–196.

Klein DN, Schwartz JE, Rose S. Five-year course and outcome of dysthymic disorder: A prospective, naturalistic follow-up study. *Am J Psychiatry*. 2000;157:931–939.

Leppanen JM. Emotional information processing in mood disorders: A review of behavioral and neuroimaging findings. *Curr Opin Psychiatry*. 2006;19:34–39.

Loo CK, McFarquhar TF, Mitchell PB. A review of the safety of repetitive transcranial magnetic stimulation as a clinical treatment for depression. *Int J Neuropsychopharmacol*. 2008;11(1):131–147.

Narrow WE. *One-year prevalence of depressive disorders among adults 18 and over in the US: NIMH ECA prospective data*. Rockville: National Institute of Mental Health; 1999.

National Institute for Clinical Excellence. *Depression: Management of depression in primary and secondary care. Clinical Guideline 23*. London: National Institute for Clinical Excellence (NICE); 2004.

Nierenberg AA, Gray SM, Grandin LD. Mood disorders and suicide. *J Clin Psychiatry*. 2001;62 (Suppl 25):27–30.

Regier DA, Narrow WE, Rae DS, et al. The de facto mental and addictive disorders service system. Epidemiologic Catchment Area prospective 1-year prevalence rates of disorders and services. *Arch Gen Psychiatry*. 1993;50:85–94.

Scott J, Colom F. Psychosocial treatments for bipolar disorders. *Psychiatr Clin North Am*. 2005;28: 371–384.

Shelton RC. The molecular neurobiology of depression. *Psychiatr Clin North Am*. 2007;30:1–11.

Strakowski SM, Delbello MP, Adler CM. The functional neuroanatomy of bipolar disorder: A review of neuroimaging findings. *Mol Psychiatry*. 2005;10:105–116.

Sullivan PF, Neale MC, Kendler KS. Genetic epidemiology of major depression: Review and meta-analysis. *Am J Psychiatry*. 2000;157:1552–1562.

UK ECT Review Group. Efficacy and safety of electroconvulsive therapy in depressive disorders: A systematic review and meta-analysis. *Lancet*. 2003;361:799–808.

Videbech P, Ravnkilde B. Hippocampal volume and depression: A meta-analysis of MRI studies. *Am J Psychiatry*. 2004;161:1957–1966.

Vieta E, Pacchiarotti I, Scott J, et al. Evidence-based research on the efficacy of psychologic interventions in bipolar disorders: A critical review. *Curr Psychiatry Rep*. 2005;7:449–455.

Wampold BE, Minami T, Baskin TW, et al. A meta-(re)analysis of the effect of cognitive therapy versus "other therapies" for depression. *J Affect Disord*. 2002;68:159–165.

Weissman MM, Leaf PJ, Bruce ML, et al. The epidemiology of dysthymia in five communities: Rates, risks, comorbidity and treatment. *Am J Psychiatry*. 1988;145:815–819.

Winkler D, Pjrek E, Iwaki R, et al. Treatment of seasonal affective disorder. *Expert Rev Neurother*. 2006;6:1039–1048.

CHAPTER 12

James W. Murrough, Sanjay J. Mathew, and Dennis S. Charney

Anxiety Disorders

Anxiety disorders are among the most common psychiatric illnesses in the United States and lead to considerable morbidity and public health costs. Anxiety and fear are universal human experiences with both psychological and physical aspects. These emotions serve an essential role in shaping adaptive behavior. Although short-term increases in anxiety may be adaptive, long-term increased anxiety may lead to suffering and disability. An anxiety disorder is considered to be present when the level or duration of anxiety in an individual leads to significant distress or functional impairment. The anxiety disorders currently recognized in the *Diagnostic and Statistical Manual of Mental Disorders,* Fourth Edition, Text Revision (DSM-IV-TR) (American Psychiatric Association, 2000), are a group of related but distinct entities that share potentially debilitating anxiety as a core symptom: panic disorder, agoraphobia, social phobia, specific phobia, obsessive-compulsive disorder (OCD), posttraumatic stress disorder (PTSD), generalized anxiety disorder (GAD), and acute stress disorder.

DSM-IV-TR also recognizes that anxiety disorders may be caused by specific substances, either prescribed medications or illicit drugs, or by general medical conditions; these disorders are labeled substance-induced anxiety disorder or anxiety disorder due to a general medical condition, respectively (see Chapters 9 and 28 for a complete discussion of these disorders). DSM-IV-TR also has a residual category for disorders of anxiety that do not fit into any of the defined syndromes: anxiety disorder not otherwise specified (NOS).

This chapter begins with a brief overview of the epidemiology and etiology of anxiety disorders. Subsequent sections focus on each of the anxiety disorders and discuss signs and symptoms, differential diagnosis, and treatment.

EPIDEMIOLOGY

Findings from the National Comorbidity Survey (NCS) and other national and international community surveys suggest that anxiety disorders are very common in the general population. Approximately 1 in 4 adults will have an anxiety disorder at some point in his or her life. Anxiety disorders are also the most common psychiatric illnesses in children and adolescents. However, different anxiety disorders have different peak ages of onset, which may reflect a trajectory of brain development. Separation anxiety and specific phobia tend to occur in middle childhood, social phobia and panic disorder in adolescence, and GAD and OCD in early adulthood.

The approximate prevalence of specific anxiety disorders in US adults is as follows: panic disorder, 3.5% (5.1% in women, 1.9% in men); specific phobia, 12.5%; social phobia, 12%; OCD, 2% to 3%; PTSD, 5% to 6% in men, 10% to 14% in women; GAD, 5% to 6% (Kessler et al.,1994, 1995, 2005). Risk factors for developing anxiety disorders include female gender, lower socioeconomic status and fewer years of education, a family history of anxiety disorders, and certain early patterns of temperament and personality. Gender differences in the prevalence of anxiety disorders begin to emerge at approximately age 6 years. Women have approximately a twofold increase in lifetime rates of panic disorder, agoraphobia, simple phobia, and GAD. Notably, there is no reported gender difference in OCD or social phobia. Although the reason for this is not known, relevant factors likely include differential reporting of symptoms (underreporting in men), as well as gender-specific social, psychological, and biological factors.

The major anxiety disorders have all been shown to aggregate in families, and numerous twin studies confirm both genetic and nongenetic modes of familial transmission. Among the anxiety disorders, panic disorder has demonstrated the highest rates of familial aggregation and genetic heritability. Individuals who have a first-degree biological relative with panic disorder are eight times more likely to develop the disorder compared to the general population (Katon, 2006). If the onset of panic disorder occurs before age 20, the risk in first-degree relatives is increased up to 20 times.

Aspects of temperament and personality that emerge early in development have been shown to predict the onset of anxiety disorders, including panic disorder, later in life. A well-studied early predictor of anxiety disorders is behavioral inhibition, a trait marker of vulnerability in children characterized by increased withdrawal or physiological reactivity to novel stimuli. In one study, the risk of developing social phobia in adolescence was increased twofold for an individual with a personal history of inhibition as a toddler. Early environmental influences, such as a parenting style characterized by overprotection or rejection, have also been shown to be risk factors for developing social phobia later in life.

ETIOLOGY

The cause of a specific anxiety disorder in a given individual is usually difficult to determine, although it likely represents a complex interaction between vulnerability factors, both inherited and stemming from early experience, and ongoing psychosocial stress. The last two decades have witnessed considerable advances in understanding the neural basis of fear and anxiety, which has enabled the development of testable biological models of human anxiety disorders. Although the role of life experiences in the etiology of anxiety disorders has been widely studied, the retrospective nature of the data limits the conclusions that can be drawn. On one hand, the risk of developing an anxiety disorder is elevated in an individual who has been exposed to early physical, sexual, or emotional trauma or other forms of extreme stress. On the other hand, most cases of anxiety disorders arise in the absence of an identifiable, specific causal factor.

Although the concept of stress as related to psychological and biological systems is difficult to define, it is essential to the conceptualization of psychiatric illnesses, including anxiety disorders. Humans and animals regularly demonstrate a relatively predictable set of immediate physiological and behavioral responses to a highly stressful event, for example, a life-threatening situation. These include the so-called fight-or-flight response mediated by epinephrine, norepinephrine (NE), and the sympathetic nervous system and alterations in endocrine, growth, vascular, and digestive physiology mediated by cortisol and the hypothalamic-pituitary-adrenal (HPA) axis. These responses likely represent the evolution of adaptive functions in the face of danger and threat and remain highly valuable today in the immediate response to danger. However, prolonged or dysregulated activation of these systems likely contributes importantly to several types of psychiatric morbidity, including PTSD and major depression. DSM-IV-TR recognizes two mental disorders that specifically result from exposure to extreme stress or threat: PTSD and acute stress disorder. Of great interest in current psychiatric research is the identification of vulnerability or protective factors, such as behavioral traits, psychological coping styles, early life events, or genetic or other biological factors, that mediate the transition from acute response to prolonged disability following exposure to a traumatic event (Charney, 2004).

Neurobiology of Fear and Anxiety

Animal studies have identified a network of brain regions that subserve behaviors related to fear and anxiety, for example, in paradigms utilizing classical conditioning or fear-potentiated startle. The amygdala is a set of nuclei within the medial temporal lobe that has emerged as the key brain structure in the acquisition and expression of fear-related behaviors. A network of interconnected structures, including the amygdala, the hippocampus, the orbitofrontal cortex (OFC) and medial prefrontal cortex (mPFC), the anterior insula, and related parts of the thalamus, sensory cortices, and brain stem nuclei, participates in the evaluation of sensory information (appetitive vs. aversive) and the organization of appropriate responses related to fear or threat (Drevets and Charney, 2005). An important principle of this neuroanatomical organization is that "higher" prefrontal regions, including OFC and mPFC, send dense *inhibitory* projections to "lower" limbic regions, including the amygdala, and serve to modulate the neural activity therein.

On the basis of anatomical knowledge from animal studies, neuroimaging studies using positron emission tomography (PET) and functional magnetic resonance imaging (fMRI) have investigated homologous neural structures in humans. These studies have begun to identify specific brain regions that play a role in fear and anxiety in humans and that may act as substrates for anxiety disorders (Rauch et al., 2006).

In addition to the emerging neuroanatomical correlates of anxiety disorders, specific neurochemical systems are implicated in stress-related and anxiety-related disorders. NE is increased by stressful or novel environmental stimuli, and several symptoms experienced by patients with anxiety disorders, such as panic attacks, are characteristic of increased NE function. The HPA axis and corticotropin-releasing hormone (CRH) are activated by stress and demonstrate abnormalities in several anxiety disorders. Preclinical investigations of γ-aminobutyric acid (GABA) have demonstrated anxiolytic properties of enhanced GABA function and anxiogenic properties of impaired GABA function. Benzodiazepines are thought to exert their anxiolytic effects by binding to the GABA channel and potentiating GABA-ergic transmission. Other neurochemical systems implicated in the stress response and anxiety disorders include serotonin (5-HT), dopamine, glutamate, and several neuropeptides including arginine vasopressin, neuropeptide Y, galanin, and cholesystokinin (CCK) (Neumeister et al., 2005).

PANIC DISORDER AND AGORAPHOBIA
Phenomenology and Differential Diagnosis

Panic disorder is characterized by recurrent discrete attacks of anxiety accompanied by several somatic symptoms, such as palpitations, paresthesias, hyperventilation, diaphoresis, chest pain, dizziness, trembling, and dyspnea. Often the condition is accompanied by agoraphobia that consists of excessive fear (and often avoidance) of situations in which escape or obtaining help would be difficult, such as driving, crowded places, stores, or being alone. Current DSM-IV-TR classifications include panic disorder without agoraphobia, panic disorder with agoraphobia, and agoraphobia without history of panic disorder (American Psychiatric Association, 2000).

Panic disorder usually begins with a spontaneous panic attack that often leads the individual to seek medical treatment, such as presenting to an emergency department believing that he or she is having a heart attack, stroke, "going crazy," or experiencing some other serious medical event. Some time may pass before subsequent attacks or the patient may continue to get frequent attacks. Patients may feel constantly fearful and anxious after the first attack, wondering what is wrong and fearing it will happen again. Some patients experience nocturnal attacks that awaken them from sleep.

The differential diagnosis of panic disorder and agoraphobia includes anxiety disorders due to general medical conditions; anxiety due to substances such as caffeine, cocaine, or amphetamines; withdrawal from alcohol, sedative-hypnotics, or benzodiazepines; other phobic conditions; GAD; or psychosis. Medical illness that may produce symptoms similar to panic attacks must be excluded. Endocrine disturbances (e.g., pheochromocytoma, thyroid disorder, or hypoglycemia) may produce similar symptoms and can be excluded with appropriate clinical history and

Clinical Characteristics of a Panic Attack

Rapid onset and relatively short duration of some of the following:
- Heart palpitations
- Difficulty breathing
- Diaphoresis
- Chest pain
- Gastrointestinal discomfort or nausea
- Dizziness or lightheadedness
- Feelings of dissociation
- Belief that one is dying or seriously ill
- Paresthesias

Clinical Characteristics of Panic Disorder

- Recurrent, unexpected panic attacks
- Persistent worry for at least 1 month about having additional panic attacks or significant behavioral change related to panic attacks
- May include agoraphobia

laboratory evaluations. When gastrointestinal symptoms are prominent, the clinician may need to exclude the diagnosis of colitis. Symptoms of tachycardia, palpitations, chest pain or pressure, and dyspnea may be confused with cardiac or respiratory conditions. Lightheadedness, faintness, dizziness, derealization, shaking, numbness, and tingling may suggest a neurologic condition.

Panic disorder differs from GAD in that the panic attacks are distinguished by recurrent discrete, intense episodes of panic symptoms, although in both disorders anticipatory anxiety and generalized feelings of anxiety may be present. Although some of the same situations may be feared, agoraphobia differs from social and simple phobias in that the fear is related to feeling trapped or being unable to escape and often becomes generalized.

Panic disorder is frequently associated with major depression, other anxiety disorders, and alcohol and substance abuse. In clinical samples as many as two thirds of patients with panic disorder report experiencing a major depressive episode at some time in their lives. Similarly, studies of patients seeking treatment for major depression report high rates of panic in these patients and their relatives. Once symptoms begin, patients often describe becoming demoralized as a result of fear related to the symptoms and imagined causes, as well as impairment when their activities are restricted by their agoraphobia. Unlike patients with depression, those with panic disorder usually lack vegetative symptoms and have a normal desire to engage in activities but avoid them because of their phobias.

Treatment

Treatment of panic disorder and other anxiety disorders begins with patient education. Symptoms of panic are experienced as highly unpleasant and fear provoking; patients often believe that they have a life-threatening medical illness. It is important for clinicians to educate patients as to the nature of panic attacks and panic disorder and to provide reassurance that, although their condition is associated with significant distress, they do not have a life-threatening medical illness. Clinical experience suggests that patients respond well to education and experience significant relief of distress. Several resources are available to aid in patient education, including the Anxiety Disorders Association of America (www.adaa.org).

Pharmacotherapy

Evidence-based pharmacologic treatment of panic disorder includes the use of selective serotonin reuptake inhibitors (SSRIs), serotonin-norepinephrine reuptake inhibitors (SNRIs), tricyclic antidepressants (TCAs), benzodiazepines, and monoamine oxidase inhibitors (MAOIs) (see Table 12-1). Short-term efficacy does not differ among SSRIs, TCAs, and benzodiazepines; each demonstrates a treatment response rate between 50% and 80% (Mitte, 2005).

SSRIs should be considered first-line pharmacologic treatment for panic disorder given their demonstrated efficacy, safety, and low side-effect profile. The clinician should be aware of potential early activating or anxiety-potentiating effects of the SSRIs, sometimes described by the patient as *jitteriness*. Strategies to help avoid these effects, which may interfere with treatment and adherence, include beginning at a low dose with a slow titration schedule.

Although benzodiazepines are rapidly acting and highly anxiolytic, there are concerns regarding dependence and abuse potential, as well as potentially significant withdrawal symptoms and reemergence of anxiety symptoms with discontinuation of the medication. Up to 80% of patients treated with benzodiazepines for longer than 4 months develop a discontinuation syndrome including anxiety, irritability, insomnia, headache, and disturbances in concentration.

TABLE 12-1	[a]Pharmacotherapy for Anxiety Disorders		
Medication	**Class**	**Indications**	**Daily Dosing Range (mg)**
Sertraline	SSRI	PD, SAD, PTSD, OCD	50–200
Paroxetine	SSRI	PD, SAD, PTSD, GAD, OCD	10–60
Fluoxetine	SSRI	PD, OCD	20–60
Escitalopram	SSRI	GAD	10–20
Fluvoxamine	SSRI	OCD	50–300
Venlafaxine XR	SNRI	PD, SAD, GAD	37.5–225
Duloxetine	SNRI	GAD	30–120
Buspirone	Azaspirone	Anxiety disorders	5–30
Alprazolam	Benzodiazepine	PD, anxiety disorders	0.75–4
Clonazepam	Benzodiazepine	PD	0.5–4
Clomipramine	TCA	OCD	75–300

[a]SSRI, selective serotonin reuptake inhibitor; SNRI, serotonin-norepinephrine reuptake inhibitor; TCA, tricyclic antidepressant; PD, panic disorder; SAD, social anxiety disorder (also social phobia); PTSD, posttraumatic stress disorder; GAD, generalized anxiety disorder; OCD, obsessive-compulsive disorder.
Disorders listed under Indications have received U.S. Food and Drug Administration (FDA) approval; the term *anxiety disorders* refers to an FDA-approved indication for anxiety that is not more specifically defined.

A very slow taper over several months may be required to minimize the patient's discomfort during benzodiazepine discontinuation.

One clinically useful application of benzodiazepines in the treatment of panic disorder, as well as other anxiety disorders, may be their use as an adjuvant when beginning therapy with an SSRI or SNRI. A recent trial found that the addition of clonazepam 0.5 mg three times daily to sertraline treatment of panic disorder resulted in more rapid early reduction of anxiety symptoms compared to treatment with sertraline alone. However, this group difference did not persist at later points in the study, indicating an early, but not maintained, benefit of benzodiazepine adjunctive treatment. This early use of benzodiazepines may help counteract the potential activating side effects of the SSRIs or SNRIs.

There is a paucity of data to direct the clinician to the next step in treatment if a patient fails an initial trial of an SSRI. The first step should be optimization, which involves maximizing adherence to treatment and dose escalation as tolerated. If the initial treatment trial continues to be inadequate, potential strategies include short-term augmentation with a benzodiazepine or switching to a different medication within the same class (another SSRI) or to a different class of medication (SNRI, TCA, MAOI).

Psychotherapy

Cognitive behavioral therapy (CBT) has been demonstrated to be highly effective in the treatment of several anxiety disorders, including panic disorder. CBT is generally conducted over 12 to 16 sessions and focuses on techniques of exposure therapy and cognitive restructuring (see Chapter 23). Clinical studies generally demonstrate comparable response rates to pharmacotherapy or CBT for panic disorder. Some data suggest that the combination of an antidepressant plus CBT is superior to either treatment alone, although this difference does not appear to be maintained at long-term follow-up. The decision to initiate treatment with medication versus CBT in a given patient will depend on several factors, including the patient's preference for a pharmacologic or nonpharmacologic approach and motivation to participate in psychotherapy. A recent study of a psychodynamic intervention in patients with panic disorder demonstrated efficacy, but further studies are needed.

A CASE OF A PANIC ATTACK

A 23-year-old single woman in good physical health presented to the emergency department at a local hospital with a chief complaint of chest pain. She was walking down the street when she experienced the sudden onset of palpitations, chest tightness, shortness of breath, and lightheadedness. She reported that these symptoms came out of the blue and caused her great alarm. Nothing like this has ever happened to her before, and she is fearful that there is something wrong with her heart. Blood work, ECG, and CXR findings are normal.

SOCIAL PHOBIA

Phenomenology and Differential Diagnosis

Social phobia, also known as *social anxiety disorder*, is a common psychiatric disorder that can lead to significant suffering and disability. Healthy individuals commonly experience social fears, especially in public-speaking situations. For some people, fear of social or performance situations becomes persistent and overwhelming and limits their social or occupational functioning because of intense anxiety and, often, avoidance.

Two clinically recognized variants of social phobia are a generalized type, in which the individual experiences significant and functionally limiting anxiety in nearly all social situations, and a more circumscribed type limited to performance in a particular social situation, such as public speaking. The latter type is also referred to as *nongeneralized* or *performance-related social phobia*. Onset is typically in adolescence, and the course of the illness tends to be chronic. The mean length of illness is 10 years before the individual presents to medical attention.

Social phobia is characterized by a persistent and exaggerated fear of humiliation or embarrassment in social or performance situations, leading to high levels of distress and possibly avoidance of those situations. Patients may become fearful that their anxiety will be evident to others, which can intensify their symptoms or even produce a situational panic attack. The fear may be of meeting people or speaking, eating, or writing in public and relates to the fear of appearing nervous or foolish, making mistakes, being criticized, or being laughed at. Often physical symptoms of anxiety such as blushing, trembling, sweating, and tachycardia are triggered when the patient feels that he or she is under evaluation or scrutiny. The diagnosis requires interference with one's normal routine or academic, occupational, or social functioning or marked distress about the phobia. In children, a 6-month duration is required.

Probably the most difficult diagnostic distinctions are between social phobia and normal performance anxiety, or social phobia and panic disorder. Normal fear of public speaking usually diminishes as the individual is speaking or with additional experience, whereas in social phobia the anxiety may worsen or fail to attenuate with rehearsal. The degree of impairment or distress distinguishes a clinically significant disorder. Individuals with social phobia may experience situational panic attacks resulting from anticipation of or exposure to the feared social

Clinical Characteristics of Social Phobia

- Persistent fear or anxiety related to embarrassment in social situations or feeling scrutinized by others
- Avoidance of the feared situation
- Feared situation almost always provokes phobic responses
- The individual recognizes the fear or related phobic reactions as excessive/out of proportion
- Significant distress and impairment

activity. Some patients with panic disorder/agoraphobia avoid social situations due to fear of embarrassment if a panic attack should occur, but usually their initial panic attack is unexpected (e.g., occurs in a situation they previously did not fear), and the subsequent development of phobias is generalized beyond social situations. Social phobia and panic disorder may coexist. In major depression, social avoidance may develop from apathy rather than fear and resolve with remission of the depressive episode. Patients with PTSD might appear to have social avoidance, but careful exploration of their symptoms more likely will reveal avoidance of trauma-related cues, loss of interest, or hypervigilance.

Social phobia is more common in women than men, although equal rates of men and women present for medical care. Social phobia is associated with lower socioeconomic status and education. Comorbidity with other phobic disorders is common (>50%). Major depression and alcohol use disorders are comorbid in 15% to 20% of cases.

Treatment

Pharmacotherapy

Most studies of the efficacy of pharmacotherapy for social phobia have focused on the generalized type, in which functionally limiting anxiety occurs in most social situations. Medications that have demonstrated benefit in randomized, placebo-controlled trials include the SSRIs, SNRIs, and MAOIs, as well as other medications including mirtazapine, clonazepam, gabapentin, and pregabalin (Table 12-1).

The SSRIs and the SNRI venlafaxine are considered first-line treatment for social phobia, and more than 20 controlled trials have demonstrated efficacy for these medications. The response rates are generally between 50% and 80% after 12 weeks of treatment. There is little evidence for the superiority of one of these medications over another, and the choice of medication should be guided with consideration of tolerability and side effects. To minimize side effects, the initial dose should be low, and the clinician should slowly titrate to the target dose. Although some patients experience significant symptom reduction in the first 2 to 4 weeks, other patients may require up to 12 weeks of treatment for a clinically significant benefit to be observed. It is therefore important to maintain treatment for an adequate amount of time before determining that a treatment trial has failed.

Although benzodiazepines are commonly used to treat social phobia, the data regarding the efficacy of this class of medication are more limited than those for the SSRIs and SNRIs. Benzodiazepines carry significant risks of abuse, dependence, and withdrawal, and the clinician should be judicious in their use. Several open trials have demonstrated the efficacy of clonazepam given three times daily for the treatment of social phobia. To minimize the potential for withdrawal symptoms, the patient should be gradually tapered from clonazepam (e.g., at a rate of 0.25 mg every 2 weeks).

Relapse rates are up to 60% when pharmacotherapy is discontinued before 12 months of maintenance therapy. A reasonable strategy would be to continue pharmacotherapy for at least 12 months, followed by a slow taper and close monitoring for relapse with early reinitiation of therapy.

Medication on an as-needed basis may be appropriate for treatment of the nongeneralized, or performance-related, type of social phobia. For example, musicians and public speakers have used β-blockers such as propranolol for performance anxiety. Short-acting benzodiazepines such as alprazolam may also be of benefit when taken 30 minutes before a performance event such as public speaking. Again, the clinician is urged to use caution when prescribing benzodiazepines, given their high abuse potential.

Psychotherapy

CBT is first-line treatment for social phobia, and clinical trials suggest that there is generally equal efficacy between CBT and pharmacologic treatments (see Chapter 23 for a complete discussion of the theory and clinical application of CBT). Briefly, CBT for social phobia usually focuses on negative, so-called automatic, thoughts that precede engagement in a social event, such as "The audience will think that I do not know what I am talking about." The therapist challenges these automatic thoughts through a process known as *cognitive restructuring*. Another important component to the application of CBT to social phobia is exposure therapy. The patient is asked

A CASE OF SOCIAL PHOBIA

A 29-year-old single businessman stated that at age 12 his voice cracked during an audition and people laughed at him. A few years later he became very anxious when he had to speak in class. He gradually became more anxious or avoided any situation in which he might be called on or observed, even to answer a roll call. His avoidance of professional meetings was interfering with his work.

to generate a hierarchical list of anxiety-provoking situations, and then, with the help of the therapist, the patient is exposed to these situations, beginning with the least anxiety-provoking and proceeding to more anxiety-provoking situations. This type of CBT includes role-playing and homework assignments. Of all the anxiety disorders, social phobia may be the most amenable to group CBT, along with social skills training.

In clinical trials, improvement is usually observed after 6 to 12 weeks and up to two thirds of patients will be considered to have a response at 12 weeks. In one study, 89% of patients who completed a course of CBT were found to have maintained a clinical improvement at 5-year follow-up compared with a group of patients who were treated with psychoeducation alone. Indeed, compared to pharmacotherapy, there are data to suggest that the treatment benefits of CBT are more durable. This is balanced by data suggesting that there is a more rapid onset of benefit with pharmacotherapy compared to CBT. Studies do not generally support superior efficacy of combination treatment compared to pharmacotherapy or CBT alone, although this treatment strategy may be of benefit for some patients.

SPECIFIC PHOBIA

Phenomenology and Differential Diagnosis

Specific phobia can be diagnosed when impairment or subjective distress results from excessive fear and avoidance of a specific object or situation. As for other phobias, the patient has a marked and persistent fear that he or she recognizes is excessive or unreasonable. Exposure to the phobic stimulus almost always produces an anxiety response, and the situation is either avoided or endured with intense distress. The previous name for this disorder, *simple phobia*, was changed to *specific phobia* in DSM-IV, and differentiation from other anxiety disorders was emphasized in that the anxiety or avoidance is not better accounted for by OCD, PTSD, panic disorder with agoraphobia, agoraphobia without history of panic disorder, or social phobia. DSM-IV-TR recognizes four subtypes of specific phobia: animal, natural environment (e.g., storms, water, heights), blood-injection-injury, situational (e.g., airplanes, elevators, enclosed places), and an "other" category for phobias that do not fit into any of the subtypes.

The onset of animal phobia is usually in childhood. Blood-injection-injury phobia usually begins in adolescence or early adulthood and can be associated with vasovagal fainting on exposure to the phobic stimulus. Age of onset may be more variable for other specific phobias. Many childhood-onset phobias remit spontaneously. Impairment depends on the extent to which the

Clinical Characteristics of Specific Phobia

- Significant and excessive fear or anxiety evoked by a specific object or situation
- Avoidance of the feared situation
- Feared situation almost always provokes phobic response
- The individual recognizes the fear or related phobic reactions as excessive/out of proportion
- Significant distress and impairment

phobic object or situation is routinely encountered in the individual's life. If the phobic object or situation is unpredictable, as in weather, or an internal sensation, such as fear of vomiting, the illness can be particularly debilitating.

Unlike common minor fears, the avoidance, anticipatory anxiety, or distress when exposed to the phobic situation results in marked distress or some degree of impairment in activities or relationships. Unlike social phobia, the fear does not involve scrutiny or embarrassment, and unlike agoraphobia, the fear is not of being trapped or having a panic attack. The nature of the fear is specific to the phobia, such as a fear of falling or loss of visual support in height phobia or fear of crashing in a flying phobia. Unlike the avoidance characteristic of PTSD, the fear in a specific phobia is not related to a traumatic event.

Treatment

Pharmacotherapy

Psychopharmacology has generally been considered to be only minimally effective in the treatment of specific phobia. In a study of alprazolam, a benzodiazepine with a short half-life, patients with flying phobia did experience an acute reduction in subjective anxiety during a flight compared to those given placebo; however, the alprazolam group fared worse and experienced more anxiety compared to the placebo group on a subsequent flight a week later. Other studies of medications, either alone or in combination with psychotherapy, have generally yielded negative results.

In contrast, a landmark study by Ressler et al. (2004) demonstrated that administration of D-cycloserine, a partial agonist at the N-methyl-D-aspartate (NMDA) receptor, accelerated the effects of virtual reality–based exposure for height phobia. The use of agents designed to enhance learning, in combination with behavioral or cognitive therapy, may hold significant promise for the treatment of anxiety disorders and is an active area of research (Anderson and Insel, 2006).

Psychotherapy

The standard treatment for specific phobias is exposure, to achieve habituation to (or extinction of) the fear response. Exposure is conducted in a graded manner, proceeding from the least to the most anxiety-producing aspect of the stimulus. The exposure can be *in vivo*, in which the patient is actually exposed to the feared object or situation, or the exposure can take place in the office through the use of imagery and, more recently, through virtual reality techniques. Although *in vivo* exposure therapy has a history of documented success, two recent studies comparing *in vivo* to virtual reality–based exposure found that the two methods were equally effective (Choy et al., 2007). Applied muscle tension has been used to treat specific phobia as well, with most data being obtained for the blood-injection-injury type.

CBT for specific phobia has been used less frequently but has demonstrated effectiveness in certain types of phobia (see Chapter 23). Patients have shown significant improvement in four out of five studies examining the effectiveness of CBT in specific phobia. CBT works to restructure distorted or irrational thoughts that contribute to pathological fear or anxiety in response to the phobic object. For fear of flying, CBT might focus on questioning the chances of an actual crash occurring.

OBSESSIVE-COMPULSIVE DISORDER

Phenomenology and Differential Diagnosis

DSM-IV-TR classifies OCD as an anxiety disorder, although current thinking suggests that it may be etiologically less related to other anxiety disorders, such as PTSD or panic disorder, and more related to a group of so-called obsessive-compulsive (OC) spectrum disorders or obsessive-compulsive related disorders (OCRD) (Bartz and Hollander, 2006).

OCD is underdiagnosed and undertreated. One reason is that patients often harbor significant embarrassment and shame regarding their symptoms. Patients with OCD may see their symptoms as strange, odd, or alien and may be reluctant to discuss them with others, including health care providers. It is essential that clinicians have a high index of suspicion and are able to recognize the signs and symptoms of OCD. Patients on average see three to four physicians and spend 9 years seeking treatment before the illness is recognized (Jenike, 2004).

Clinical Characteristics of OCD

- Recurrent obsessions (intrusive thoughts or ideas) or compulsions (repetitive behaviors or mental acts designed to reduce anxiety resulting from the obsessions)
- The individual recognizes the obsessions or compulsions as excessive/abnormal
- Significant distress and impairment

OCD is defined by the presence of obsessions or compulsions that produce discomfort or impairment. Obsessions are thoughts, impulses, or images that are recurrent, persistent, intrusive, and recognized as senseless (at least initially). Compulsions are behaviors (rituals) or mental acts (counting, praying) that are repetitive, purposeful, and intentional; are in response to an obsession; are performed in a stereotyped manner or according to certain rules to prevent discomfort or a dreaded event; and are initially recognized as excessive or unreasonable. Obsessions and compulsions are not in themselves pleasurable, and patients usually attempt to ignore, suppress, or neutralize obsessions. In clinical samples, both obsessions and compulsions are almost always present, and multiple obsessions and/or compulsions are common.

The most common obsessional thoughts involve contamination (e.g., exaggerated fear or avoidance of germs), so-called pathological doubt (e.g., preoccupation or fear of making the wrong decision or completing routine daily tasks), and order or symmetry. Obsessions may also involve violent, aggressive, or sexual thoughts or images. Common compulsions (depending on the related obsession) include cleaning, checking, arranging, counting, hoarding, and repeating. Compulsive cleaners may spend hours meticulously dusting and vacuuming. Compulsive hoarders are unable to discard useless objects, resulting in a home cluttered with mail, bags of used containers, dust balls, and so on. Some patients need to repeat tasks over and over to "get it right" or repeatedly rearrange objects so that they assume an exact pattern. Fear of contamination can result in avoidance of any contact with dirt or any object that might have come in contact with the feared contaminant or was sold in the same store as the contaminant. Examples of obsessions and compulsions are listed in Table 12-2.

The differential diagnosis of OCD may include schizophrenia, major depression, phobias, Tourette syndrome, and obsessive-compulsive personality disorder (OCPD). In OCD, behavior can be bizarre and have an impact on social and occupational functioning similar to that of schizophrenia. However, the behaviors are limited to the execution of compulsive rituals. When reality testing is lost, the loss is limited to convictions regarding obsessive ideas and does not extend to other areas of thinking. Occasionally, the depressive ruminations seen in major depressive episodes may be mistaken for obsessions, but depressive ruminations have a brooding, depressive, or guilty quality and resolve with recovery from the episode. Avoidance of contaminants or

TABLE 12-2	**Common Obsessions and Compulsions**
Obsessions	**Compulsions**
Contamination/illness	Checking
Violent images	Cleaning/washing
Fear of harming others/self	Counting
Perverse/forbidden sexual thoughts, images, or impulses	Hoarding/collecting
Symmetry/exactness	Ordering/arranging
Somatic	Repeating
Religious	

other objects and situations may resemble the avoidance seen in phobic disorders, but the fear is not of being trapped, as in agoraphobia, or social embarrassment, as in social phobia, but is directly related to the obsessional thought. The repetitive, irresistible movement or utterances of Tourette syndrome may be difficult to differentiate from OCD, and the disorders may coexist.

Comorbidity with OCD is common; 50% to 60% of patients meet criteria for major depression at some point in their lives. Comorbidity with other anxiety disorders is also common, with lifetime prevalence ranging from 15% to 25% for panic disorder, social phobia, and GAD. With relevance to the concept of the OC spectrum of disorders, higher rates of disorders with obsessional or compulsive elements are found in patients with a primary diagnosis of OCD, including hypochondriasis, body dysmorphic disorder, anorexia nervosa, several of the impulse control disorders, and Tourette syndrome and other tic disorders.

Treatment

Pharmacotherapy

Clomipramine was the first medication discovered to have a specific effect on OCD symptoms, likely due to its serotonin reuptake–inhibiting properties. More recently, multiple randomized, controlled trials of SSRIs have demonstrated their efficacy in OCD, and SSRIs are considered first-line pharmacotherapy given their tolerability and safety (Table 12-1). The response rates for OCD are lower than those seen for other illnesses treated with SSRIs, such as major depression. Approximately 40% to 60% of patients with OCD will demonstrate a response to SSRIs. Symptomatic reductions in OCD are also relatively low, typically in the range of 20% to 40%, compared to major depression, in which reductions of at least 50% are expected. Return of symptoms is common when effective medication is decreased or discontinued. In one double-blind discontinuation study, 90% of patients relapsed after their medication was switched to placebo.

No single SSRI has demonstrated superior efficacy over another; however, individual patients may respond to one member of the class of SSRIs and not another. The reason for this phenomenon is not known. If a patient fails to respond to a specific agent, serial trials of other SSRIs are required. For nonresponders, the first step in management should always be to optimize the initial medication trial. Begin with low doses so that side effects are tolerated, adjust doses slowly to allow time to respond, increase the dose to the maximum recommended or higher, and continue medication trials to 12 weeks (additional improvements have been reported for up to 28 weeks). Higher doses and longer trials may be required to treat OCD compared to other SSRI-responsive disorders such as major depression.

There are few controlled trials to evaluate the efficacy of augmentation therapy when response to an initial treatment is incomplete. However, several studies suggest benefit from adding a dopamine antagonist to an SSRI, typically an atypical antipsychotic. A single placebo-controlled study demonstrated efficacy of the benzodiazepine clonazepam in reducing the symptoms of OCD. Other agents that have been used for augmentation and for which the efficacy data are limited include buspirone, trazodone, clonidine, pindolol, and tryptophan. A reasonable treatment algorithm proposed by Dell'Osso et al. (2007) suggests starting with a combination of an SSRI and CBT; if there is no response, switch to another SSRI; if there is still no response, augment with clomipramine, a benzodiazepine, buspirone, an antipsychotic, or a mood stabilizer; if there is still further no response, consider an MAOI; and finally consider deep brain stimulation or other neurosurgical techniques for treatment-refractory cases, as discussed in the following text.

Psychotherapy

A type of CBT known as *exposure and response prevention* is an important component in the treatment of OCD. Multiple open and controlled trials have repeatedly demonstrated the efficacy of behavioral therapy in the treatment of OCD, with up to 85% of patients reporting at least some improvement in symptom severity and 50% reporting very much improvement.

Treatment for OCD focuses on exposing the patient to stimuli that produce anxiety and obsessional thoughts (e.g., a dirty object thought to be contaminated with germs) and then preventing the compulsion or ritual that would typically follow the obsession (e.g., compulsive hand washing). The patient is instructed to make a hierarchical list of anxiety-producing stimuli or situations, and then exposure is begun in therapy, starting with the least distressing and progressing incrementally to more distressing stimuli. A process of habituation is conducted such that the stimuli become less anxiety-provoking with subsequent exposures. Therapists may also include CBT, in which false beliefs are challenged. Data suggest that improvement in symptom severity is correlated with longer duration of exposure to anxiety-provoking stimuli. Given the cost and other practical constraints, group CBT has been developed for exposure and response prevention, and initial results suggest efficacy comparable to individual therapy.

Other Somatic Treatments

In severe, debilitating cases that have failed all attempts at more conservative treatment, neurosurgical techniques such as cingulotomy, subcaudate tractotomy, stereotactic limbic leukotomy, or anterior capsulotomy can be beneficial. The effectiveness of these procedures is likely based on the disruption of connections among the frontal cortex, basal ganglia, thalamus, and limbic structures. The more recent surgical technique of DBS, used in the treatment of Parkinson disease, is currently being developed and studied for the treatment of OCD (Dell'Osso et al., 2005). Electrodes are surgically implanted in the patient's brain and can be turned on or off, without making pertinent lesions, to activate or disrupt function in putative neural circuits, mediating the symptoms of OCD. Although current data are limited by small sample sizes, the application of DBS holds significant promise for the treatment of otherwise refractory OCD.

POSTTRAUMATIC STRESS DISORDER AND ACUTE STRESS DISORDER

Phenomenology and Differential Diagnosis

PTSD is a syndrome that develops in some individuals who are exposed to an extremely stressful event that provokes fear, horror, or helplessness. The syndrome is characterized by three clusters of symptoms: reexperiencing the trauma, avoiding reminders of the trauma, and increased physiologic arousal and startle. Exposure to extreme stress also increases the risk of other psychiatric disorders, including major depression, GAD, panic disorder, and substance abuse. Acute stress disorder was only recognized as a unique mental disorder in DSM-IV and describes a similar disorder to PTSD that occurs earlier (within 4 weeks) and remits within 4 weeks.

Reexperiencing phenomena include intrusive memories, flashbacks, nightmares, and psychological or physiological distress in response to reminders of the trauma. Intrusive memories are spontaneous, unwanted, distressing recollections of the traumatic event. Repeated nightmares contain themes of the trauma or a highly accurate and detailed recreation of the actual event(s). Flashbacks are dissociative states in which the person feels as if he or she were actually reliving the event and loses contact with the current environment, usually for a few seconds or minutes. Reactivity to trauma-related stimuli can involve intense emotional distress or physical symptoms similar to those of a panic attack when exposed to sights, sounds, smells, or events that were present during the traumatic event. Avoidance can include thoughts, feelings, situations, or activities that are reminders of the trauma. Numbing might occur through amnesia for parts

---

Clinical Characteristics of PTSD

- Exposure to an extremely stressful event that provokes fear, horror, helplessness
- For at least 1 month:
  - Reexperiencing the trauma through intrusive memories, nightmares, flashbacks
  - Actively avoiding reminders of the trauma
- Increased physiologic arousal (insomnia, irritability, increased vigilance, exaggerated startle)
- Significant distress and impairment

of the event, emotional detachment, restricted affect, or loss of interest in activities. Increased arousal can include insomnia, irritability, hypervigilance (exaggerated watchfulness, feeling on guard, checking for danger), increased startle response (jumpiness), or impaired concentration.

The immediate response to fear or threat is nearly universal, but a minority of people exposed to a potentially traumatic event develops prolonged stress-related psychopathology such as PTSD. In some individuals exposed to a traumatic event, the initial fear response, which is adaptive in the short term, may become prolonged, leading to a relatively sustained heightened state of fear. The identification of individual factors that mediate resilience or vulnerability to trauma is an active area of research. The current conceptualization is that inherited factors and early life experiences make up a background of risk or protection that modulates the impact of subsequent stressful life events on the individual.

Although the initial response to fear is biologically mediated, the subjective interpretation of the event can have an important influence on how the trauma is experienced and the risk of developing PTSD. Factors that influence how a traumatic event is perceived include the degree of controllability of the event, the perceived threat, actual personal loss, and predictability. The experience of trauma or exposure to extreme stress can result in feelings of vulnerability and helplessness. Resilience in the face of trauma may be related to the individual's ability to contain the initial fear response and relatively quickly reestablish normal emotional tone. Avoidance may develop in the face of a heightened fearful state. Avoiding stimuli that remind the patient of the trauma actually perpetuates the fear state by reducing opportunities to habituate to the stimuli and increasing social isolation (Yehuda, 2002).

Events that lead to PTSD usually involve interpersonal violence such as rape or assault, exposure to life-threatening situations such as combat or crashes, or natural disasters. The National Vietnam Veterans Readjustment Study (NVVRS) (Kulka et al., 1990) examined PTSD in Vietnam veterans and matched civilian controls. The lifetime rate of PTSD in male Vietnam veterans was 31%, and 15% had current PTSD. Rates in women were 27% and 9% respectively. Victims of sexual assault are at especially high risk for subsequent mental health problems and suicide. In a survey of 20- to 30-year-olds, 39% experienced a traumatic event, and the lifetime rate of PTSD in those exposed to trauma was 24% (the lifetime population prevalence is 9%). Risk factors for exposure to traumatic events included family history of any psychiatric disorder, history of conduct disorder symptoms, male gender, extroversion, and neuroticism. Risk factors for PTSD following exposure to trauma included separation from parents during childhood, family history of anxiety, preexisting anxiety or depression, family history of antisocial behavior, female gender, and neuroticism.

Although female gender has consistently demonstrated itself to be a risk factor for the development of PTSD, the reason remains uncertain. Even when adjusting for the type and severity of trauma, the risk of developing PTSD is twice as high in women compared with men. Although it is possible that biological sex differences account for the increased relative risk, few data suggest this. There is evidence that gender differences in social support after a trauma may be an important mediating factor. Women report lower levels of support after being the victim of a violent crime than men. Therefore, it is important to remember that women's experience of a trauma may be different than men's, even if the nature of the trauma is similar (Nemeroff et al., 2006).

In adjustment disorder, the stressor is usually less severe, and the characteristic symptoms of PTSD, such as reexperiencing and avoiding, are not present. Avoidance of trauma-associated stimuli may resemble a phobia; however, in PTSD the avoidance is limited to reminders of the trauma. The physiological response to events symbolizing the trauma may resemble panic attacks, but in pure PTSD no spontaneous attacks occur, nor do attacks occur apart from trauma-related stimuli. Many of the symptoms resemble those of major depression. If a full depressive syndrome also exists, both diagnoses should be made; the same is true of coexisting anxiety disorders. Note that comorbidity with substance dependence, especially alcohol, is common.

Treatment

Pharmacotherapy

It is important for primary care physicians and other clinicians to ask about and recognize the symptoms of PTSD so that therapy can be initiated as soon as possible after the traumatic event. Rapid assessment and treatment are hoped to prevent many of the complications and disability associated with prolonged PTSD. Patients with PTSD are often reluctant to discuss their symptoms, given the propensity toward avoidance of thoughts and feelings related to the event inherent in the disorder. Patients may feel ashamed or assume that their illness represents a character flaw or personal weakness.

Few medications have been shown to be effective at targeting the core symptoms of PTSD, such as intrusive memories, avoidance, or hyperarousal. Instead, several medications that have demonstrated efficacy in other mood and anxiety disorders have been shown to be of some benefit to patients with PTSD (Table 12-1). SSRIs are considered first-line treatment for PTSD, given their favorable safety and tolerability profile. Two SSRIs, sertraline and paroxetine, have U.S. Food and Drug Administration (FDA) approval for use in PTSD. Although there are no well-controlled clinical studies to guide treatment decisions, current consensus treatment guidelines recommend at least an 8-week trial of an SSRI and then a switch to another class of antidepressant (e.g., venlafaxine) if there is no response. If there is only a partial response, the addition of a mood stabilizer such as valproic acid may be of some benefit.

The use of benzodiazepines in the treatment of PTSD should be avoided, given the potential of abuse and dependence and the lack of demonstrated efficacy. A randomized, controlled trial of alprazolam did not show efficacy greater than placebo, and neither alprazolam nor clonazepam is superior to placebo in the immediate aftermath of a traumatic event.

Psychotherapy

Specific techniques of CBT, namely exposure therapy and cognitive restructuring, have demonstrated efficacy in the treatment of PTSD (see Chapter 23). In exposure therapy, the patient is exposed to thoughts, feelings, or other reminders of the trauma, and the resulting anxiety and physiological responses are modulated with the help of the therapist, leading to habituation over time. Cognitive restructuring is designed to help patients confront false beliefs, or so-called automatic thoughts, that are generated in the aftermath of the trauma and may contribute to avoidance behavior and other maladaptive sequelae (e.g., the patient may have the automatic thought "I am in danger" or "My environment is not safe").

GENERALIZED ANXIETY DISORDER

Phenomenology and Differential Diagnosis

Pathologic forms of anxiety characterized by diffuse "apprehensive expectation" have long been recognized in psychiatry and were referred to as *anxiety neurosis* by Freud and his followers in the early 1900s. However, GAD was not recognized as a mental disorder, separate from other forms of anxiety, until DSM-III-R (American Psychiatric Association, 1987).

GAD is characterized by chronic excessive anxiety about life circumstances accompanied by symptoms of motor tension, vigilance, and scanning of the environment. The individual often awakens with apprehension and unrealistic concern about future misfortune. One patient described experiencing the anxiety of a final examination with every task he was assigned at work. The current diagnostic criteria require a 6-month duration of symptoms to differentiate the disorder from more transient forms of anxiety such as adjustment disorder with anxious mood. DSM-IV-TR criteria emphasize that the worry is out of proportion to the likelihood or impact of the feared events, pervasive (focused on many life circumstances), difficult to control, not related to hypochondriacal concerns or PTSD, and not secondary to substances or medical etiologies. Tension or nervousness may be manifested by three of the following: restlessness, easily fatigued, feeling keyed up or on edge, difficulty concentrating or mind going blank, and irritability. In addition, significant functional impairment or marked distress is required for the diagnosis.

Patients with anxiety disorders, including GAD, often present to general practitioners with somatic complaints such as fatigue, chronic musculoskeletal symptoms, chest discomfort, or shortness of breath. A thorough medical assessment is necessary to rule out a medical illness before making the diagnosis of GAD or another psychiatric disorder. Common medical problems that must be considered include cardiac, pulmonary, neurologic, and endocrine disturbances, particularly hyperthyroidism. Substance use (e.g., stimulants, caffeine, cocaine), withdrawal (e.g., from sedative-hypnotics, alcohol, benzodiazepines, opioids), or prescribed medications (e.g., sympathomimetics, steroids) must also be considered. Factors that suggest an underlying

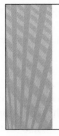

Clinical Characteristics of GAD

- Excessive, difficult-to-control, daily worry about several different situations or events for at least 6 months
- Associated somatic symptoms such as restlessness, fatigue, difficulty concentrating, irritability, muscle tension, sleep disturbance
- Significant distress and impairment

medical cause of anxiety include onset after age 35, no personal or family history of an anxiety disorder, and no apparent increase in current psychosocial stress in the patient's life.

High rates of GAD have been reported in general medical populations, and GAD is the most common anxiety disorder to present to primary care clinics. It has a variable age of onset with a mean age of 35 years. The illness is more common in women, people who are single compared with those married, individuals in lower socioeconomic levels, and disadvantaged ethnic groups. GAD may begin as childhood overanxious disorder. In clinical samples, the prevalence in men and women appears to be equal, and the course tends to be chronic.

Risk factors for developing GAD include a family history of anxiety disorders and increased exposure to psychosocial stress during development and adulthood. A history of exposure to physical, sexual, or emotional trauma is a well-documented risk factor. GAD is also more common in individuals who smoke tobacco and have general medical illnesses. Comorbidity is common. Major depression is the most prevalent comorbid psychiatric disorder, affecting up to two thirds of patients with GAD. Panic disorder affects one in four patients with GAD, and alcohol abuse is present in more than one third of patients.

Persistent anxiety may develop between attacks in panic disorder, but usually it is apprehensive anxiety related to panic and phobias. GAD is not diagnosed if it is limited to episodes of depression; however, as discussed in the following text, it may share etiological elements with depression. In patients with somatization disorder, the focus of worry is about health concerns and physical symptoms, rather than apprehensive worry about life circumstances.

Treatment

Pharmacotherapy

SSRIs are considered first-line treatment for GAD given their demonstrated efficacy and favorable side-effect profile and safety. Two SSRIs (paroxetine, escitalopram) and extended-release venlafaxine (venlafaxine XR) are FDA approved to treat GAD (Table 12-1). An 8-week placebo-controlled trial of paroxetine showed reduced anxiety symptoms in 72% of patients on active medication compared with 56% of patients taking placebo. In a 24-week relapse prevention study, the relapse rate for patients taking paroxetine was 11%, compared with 41% in patients switched to placebo. As in depression, the SSRIs and SNRIs may take several weeks and up to several months to exert their full effects. In patients who respond, therapy should be continued for at least 6 months to prevent relapse. On the basis of the clinical picture and weighing the risks and benefits of medication therapy, the clinician and patient may elect to continue maintenance therapy or attempt a slow taper while monitoring for recurrence of symptoms. Common side effects when beginning treatment include restlessness or sedation and jitteriness.

The judicious use of benzodiazepines, such as clonazepam or lorazepam, can be highly effective for short-term treatment of anxiety symptoms. Long-term use is not recommended, given the risks of tolerance, dependence, and withdrawal. In a randomized trial comparing two antidepressants, paroxetine and imipramine, to a benzodiazepine in patients with GAD, the benzodiazepine was more effective than either antidepressant at 2 weeks, but less effective than either at 8 weeks. The most effective use of a benzodiazepine may be adjunctive use when starting an SSRI or SNRI to offer patients early rapid anxiety relief before the anxiolytic properties of the antidepressants take effect. Short-term use may also counteract the possible early activating properties of the SSRIs or SNRIs. If the clinician elects to use a benzodiazepine, it is important to slowly taper the medication before discontinuation to prevent withdrawal symptoms, which may include tremor, diaphoresis, worsening anxiety, agitation, and seizure.

Buspirone is a nonbenzodiazepine anxiolytic that acts as a partial agonist at the 5-HT1A receptor and has demonstrated some benefit in patients with GAD.

Psychotherapy

CBT has been demonstrated to be highly efficacious for GAD. Patients learn to identify anxiety-provoking thoughts and relapse them with more adaptive ways of thinking through a process known as *cognitive restructuring*. Patients may be instructed to keep a thought log at home to record specific thoughts that precede the anxious worry. Behavioral therapy helps patients assess the validity of negative thoughts by exposure to real-life experiences. For a complete discussion of the theory and practice of CBT, please see Chapter 23.

CONCLUSION AND FUTURE DIRECTIONS

Anxiety disorders are very common and likely to be encountered with significant frequency in the general medical clinic, as well as in psychiatric practice. A familiarity with the phenomenology, differential diagnosis, and treatment of the various anxiety disorders will be an important skill for most clinicians.

There has been a burgeoning of research in the neural mechanisms and etiology of mental illness across the diagnostic categories. For anxiety disorders in particular, emerging mechanistic and explanatory models have grown out of collaboration and translational research among neural, behavioral, and clinical domains. Animal studies performed by Joseph LeDoux, Michael Davis, and others on the neuroanatomy of fear and fear-related learning have provided a foundation to generate testable hypotheses regarding the biology of human anxiety disorders. This work will begin to inform nosologic categories such that disorders will be grouped by shared etiology rather than clinical phenomenology. One example is the conceptualization of a subset of anxiety disorders, including PTSD and panic disorder, that may be characterized as disorders of fear-related circuitry. These disorders would be viewed as fundamentally reflecting aberrant functioning in brain regions mediating fear, including the amygdala, hippocampus, and regions of the prefrontal cortex. Similarly, OCD may harbor neurobiological underpinning more closely related to other illnesses conceptualized on the OC-related spectrum and less related to other anxiety disorders. These considerations and others are currently under investigation in the development of DSM-V.

Clinical Pearls

- Suspect panic attacks in patients without physical pathology who present with somatic symptoms suggestive of cardiac, endocrine, and neurologic disorders.
- When prescribing antidepressants, be sure to warn patients about a possible initial "activation syndrome" and use small doses to begin treatment.
- SSRIs should be considered first-line treatment for most anxiety disorders. Minimize use of benzodiazepines due to the significant potential for dependence, abuse, and withdrawal.
- The combination of pharmacotherapy and behavioral therapy is optimal for the treatment of OCD. SSRIs are specifically effective for OCD, whereas most other agents are ineffective. Behavioral therapy consisting of exposure to ritual-eliciting stimuli and prevention of the compulsive response is beneficial in most cases.
- Exposure therapy is a specific type of CBT that has demonstrated efficacy in relieving symptoms of PTSD. First-line pharmacotherapy is with an SSRI; adjunctive therapy with a mood stabilizer may be of some benefit.
- The essential feature of GAD is excessive daily worry that is out of proportion to what the patient would expect, in addition to somatic symptoms (muscle tension, restlessness), for at least 6 months.

Self-Assessment Questions and Answers

12-1. Which of the following early environmental influences has been associated with the development of an anxiety disorder later in life?

A. Delay in standard vaccinations such as measles, mumps, rubella
B. Parenting style characterized by overprotection or rejection
C. Presence of older siblings
D. Presence of younger siblings
E. Prolonged or complicated delivery at birth

Early environmental factors that have been associated with the development of an anxiety disorder later in life include a parenting style characterized by overprotection or rejection, as well as other factors that might disrupt the mother-child relationship. *Answer: B*

12-2. Individuals who have a first-degree relative with panic disorder have an increased relative risk of developing panic disorder of:

A. 2 times
B. 4 times
C. 6 times
D. 8 times
E. 20 times

Individuals who have a first-degree relative with panic disorder are eight times more likely to develop panic disorder compared with individuals in the general population. *Answer: D*

12-3. Brain regions thought to be important in suppressing or modulating activity in the amygdala and underactive in patients with posttraumatic stress disorder or other fear-based anxiety disorders include the:

A. Brain stem
B. Cerebellum
C. Medial prefrontal cortex
D. Primary sensory cortex
E. Thalamus

Preclinical and human neuroimaging studies implicate ventral and medial regions of the prefrontal cortex as important in suppressing and containing fear and anxiety-related neural activity in the amygdala, and evidence exists for dysfunction of these areas in posttraumatic stress disorder and other anxiety disorders. *Answer: C*

12-4. A patient who presents with anxiety related to hand washing and housecleaning many times per day would be most appropriately diagnosed with which disorder?

A. Generalized anxiety disorder
B. Obsessive-compulsive disorder
C. Panic disorder
D. Posttraumatic stress disorder
E. Specific phobia

Obsessive-compulsive disorder is most appropriately diagnosed when a patient presents with intrusive thoughts related to fear of germs and associated behaviors (such as cleaning or hand washing). For a diagnosis, the patient should experience clinically significant distress and/or impairment resulting from the intrusive thoughts and behaviors. *Answer: B*

12-5. When a patient is prescribed an SSRI for treatment of symptoms related to generalized anxiety disorder, in what time frame can clinical improvement be expected?

A. 1 to 2 days
B. 1 week
C. 2 weeks
D. 4 to 8 weeks
E. 6 months

Most patients will experience clinically significant improvement in anxiety symptoms in 4 to 8 weeks after beginning treatment with an SSRI. *Answer: D*

References

American Psychiatric Association. *Diagnostic and statistical manual of mental disorders*, 3rd ed, revised. Washington, DC: American Psychiatric Association; 1987.

American Psychiatric Association. *Diagnostic and statistical manual of mental disorders*, 4th ed, text revision. Washington, DC: American Psychiatric Association; 2000.

Anderson KC, Insel TR. The promise of extinction research for the prevention and treatment of anxiety disorders. *Biol Psychiatry*. 2006;60:319–321.

Bartz JA, Hollander E. Is obsessive-compulsive disorder an anxiety disorder? *Prog Neuropsychopharmacol Biol Psychiatry*. 2006;30:338–352.

Charney DS. Psychobiological mechanisms of resilience and vulnerability: Implications for successful adaptation to extreme stress. *Am J Psychiatry*. 2004;161:195–216.

Choy Y, Flyer AJ, Lipsitz JD. Treatment of specific phobia in adults. *Clin Psychol Rev*. 2007;27:266–286.

Dell'Osso B, Altamura AC, Allen A, et al. Brain stimulation techniques in the treatment of obsessive-compulsive disorder: Current and future directions. *CNS Spectr*. 2005;10:966–983.

Dell'Osso B, Altamura AC, Mundo E, et al. Diagnosis and treatment of obsessive-compulsive disorder and related disorders. *Int J Clin Pract*. 2007;61:98–104.

Drevets WC, Charney DS. Anxiety disorders: Neuroimaging. In: Sadock BJ, Sadock VA, eds. *Kaplan and Sadock's comprehensive textbook of psychiatry*, 8th ed. Philadelphia: Lippincott Williams & Wilkins; 2005.

Jenike MA. Obsessive-compulsive disorder. *N Engl J Med*. 2004;350:259–265.

Katon WJ. Panic disorder. *N Engl J Med*. 2006;354:2360–2367.

Kessler RC, Berglund P, Demler O, et al. Lifetime prevalence and age-of-onset distributions of DSM-IV disorders in the National Comorbidity Survey Replication. *Arch Gen Psychiatry*. 2005;62:593–602.

Kessler RC, McGonagle KA, Zhoa S, et al. Lifetime and 12-month prevalence of DSM-III-R psychiatric disorders in the United States: Results from the National Comorbidity Survey. *Arch Gen Psychiatry*. 1994;51:8–19.

Kessler RC, Sonnega A, Bromet E, et al. Posttraumatic stress disorder in the National Comorbidity Survey. *Arch Gen Psychiatry*. 1995;52(12):1048–1060.

Kulka RA, Schlenger WE, Fairbank JA, et al. *Trauma and the Vietnam war generation*. New York: Brunner/Mazel Publishers; 1990.

Mitte K. A meta-analysis of the efficacy of psycho- and pharmacotherapy in panic disorder with and without agoraphobia. *J Affect Disord*. 2005;88:27–45.

Nemeroff CB, Bremner JD, Foa EB, et al. Posttraumatic stress disorder: A state-of-the-science review. *J Psychiatr Res*. 2006;40:1–21.

Neumeister A, Bonne O, Charney DS. Anxiety disorders: Neurochemical aspects. In: Sadock BJ, Sadock VA, eds. *Kaplan and Sadock's comprehensive textbook of psychiatry*, 8th ed. Philadelphia: Lippincott Williams & Wilkins; 2005.

Rauch SL, Shin LM, Phelps EA. Neurocircuitry models of posttraumatic stress disorder and extinction: Human neuroimaging research—past, present and future. *Biol Psychiatry*. 2006;60:376–382.

Ressler KJ, Rothbaum BO, Tannenbaum L, et al. Cognitive enhancers as adjuncts to psychotherapy: Use of D-cycloserine in phobic individuals to facilitate extinction of fear. *Arch Gen Psychiatry*. 2004;61:1136–1144.

Yehuda R. Post-traumatic stress disorder. *N Engl J Med*. 2002;346:108–112.

Somatoform Disorders

Somatoform disorders are conditions in which patients present with prominent physical complaints or concerns in the absence of any obvious illness. These concerns often lead to frequent medical consultation and numerous tests and interventions. Because of the apparent medical nature of their complaints, patients usually present to primary care physicians or emergency departments. In general, these disorders are underrecognized and patients tend to be symptomatic for years or even decades before diagnosis. Even after recognition of a somatoform disorder, treatment is difficult without a multimodal approach that includes primary care physicians, mental health professionals, and an integrated health system. New evidence-based treatments are emerging that provide guidance for clinicians and, it is hoped, improved outcomes for patients.

Somatoform disorders are believed to have psychological underpinnings. When people are under psychosocial stress, they may express their symptoms physically rather than verbally or emotionally. Certain patients may be more prone to this than others. The concept of *alexithymia*, which comes from the Greek for "lack of words for feelings," has been introduced to identify these patients. It is common in those who have many medical and psychiatric disorders, including eating disorders, acquired immunodeficiency syndrome (AIDS), and substance abuse (Sifneos, 1996). When asked about mood, these patients often lack the words needed to describe their internal experiences. They are also noted to generally lack fantasies and to have literal or concrete thought processes (Sifneos, 1996). These factors contribute to their inability to recognize the psychological factors that are helping to produce their symptoms and lead to their preference for medical care rather than psychiatric care.

Somatoform disorders bring to the fore the differences between disease and illness. *Disease* describes the physical process by which people enter the sick role, while *illness* describes the social role people enter while sick. Patients enter a state of illness once they are defined as sick by themselves and others, and this role can come to dominate their lives (Eisenberg, 1977). In patients with somatoform disorders, the subjective experience of being sick becomes salient enough that patients begin to misinterpret or misrepresent the bodily signals of disease they are receiving. Once this process goes on long enough, patients can develop relatively fixed images of themselves as sick people that cannot be easily changed. Because of this, somatoform disorders are often chronic and difficult to treat.

Various somatoform disorders, each with a different focus on expression, interpretation, and meaning of symptoms, have been described. The origin is controversial, but a number of theories have been proposed. The physical symptoms patients experience may represent unconscious emotions and thoughts that have no other outlet. If patients were reared by parents who responded to somatic complaints more rapidly than emotional concerns, they may have learned to express distress physically rather than verbally. One factor they share is that the symptoms are not intentionally produced (as in factitious disorder or malingering, which are described later) but develop out of unconscious processes. The symptoms are probably best understood as communicating material that the patient cannot consciously describe or understand but needs expression anyway.

Somatization Disorder

Epidemiology

In general, somatoform disorders are more common in women, and somatization disorder is five times more common, with overall prevalence estimates ranging from 0.2% to 2% in women and approximately 0.2% among men (Sadock and Sadock, 2007). It is also more common in first-degree relatives of patients with the disorder. Male relatives of patients with somatization disorder are more likely to have antisocial personality disorder and alcoholism compared with the general population. The prevalence of the disorder varies across cultures; among Greek and Puerto Rican men, for example, the disorder is equally as common as in women. In general, the prevalence is higher in those who are less educated and belong to lower socioeconomic classes.

Etiology

Somatization disorder appears to have a genetic component. Monozygotic twins share the disease at three times the rate of dizygotic twins (Sadock and Sadock, 2007). Patients with somatization disorder have higher rates of alcoholism and antisocial personality disorder among male relatives, a finding that suggests these disorders share a common genetic trait with somatization disorder, which has variable expression modulated, in part, by gender. Another theory is that patients with somatization disorder are experiencing difficulty with maturation and the assumption of adult roles. In order to avoid responsibility, they unconsciously adopt the sick role and remain in a dependent state.

Phenomenology

Somatization disorder is the prototype somatoform disorder. Originally called hysteria or Briquet syndrome, it is characterized by symptoms in multiple physical domains that continue for many years and lead to significant impairment in functioning. Investigation reveals no underlying physical cause. The disorder must include at least four pain complaints, at least two types of gastrointestinal disturbance, a pseudoneurologic feature, and a sexual symptom. These concerns may not all be present at once, and in order to make the diagnosis, a careful history must be taken. Reviewing past medical and psychiatric records is often essential to uncover a somatization diagnosis. Patients are not intentionally creating or lying about their symptoms, as in factitious disorder or malingering; patients with somatization disorder believe that their symptoms are real and have not done anything to produce them.

Patients present for medical care before age 30. Common presenting complaints include back pain, headaches, abdominal pain, pelvic pain, nausea, vomiting, dizziness, fainting, seizures, weakness, paralysis, and painful sexual intercourse. Presentations can be dramatic, and histories are often vague and impressionistic. Patients are less concerned with details than with communicating their distress. By the time the diagnosis is made, patients have often had many unnecessary tests and procedures that are usually unrevealing. They frequently express frustration with their physicians when tests are negative or further evaluation is deemed inappropriate. Often in the course of medical evaluation, incidental findings lead to more invasive tests and produce iatrogenic morbidity (e.g., spinal surgery for disk compression leading to paralysis).

Patients often have comorbid psychiatric illness, most commonly, mood, anxiety, personality, and substance use disorders (Sadock and Sadock, 2007). Patients often report a history of childhood abuse or neglect (Mai, 2004). Medical physicians often refer patients to psychiatry for comorbidities rather than somatization disorder itself and frame it as part of an overall plan to help the patient feel as well as possible in spite of physical problems.

Differential Diagnosis

The most important item in the differential diagnosis of somatization disorder is undiagnosed physical illness. Even in patients with established somatization disorder, careful evaluation of new complaints is essential. The primary ways that somatization symptoms can be differentiated from real illness are the involvement of multiple organ systems in ways that are not biologically plausible and consistently normal findings on physical examination and laboratory evaluation (Sadock and Sadock, 2007). Illnesses that have multiple effects, such as multiple sclerosis, systemic lupus erythematosus, and thyroid disease, may appear to be somatization disorder and should be considered when the diagnosis is proposed.

Other psychiatric disorders can have physical symptoms as part of their presentation. Major depressive disorder and anxiety disorders can have physical pain and fatigue as prominent symptoms. However, these symptoms tend to have temporal relationships to the onset of the other signs of depression or anxiety and resolve with psychiatric treatment. Patients with schizophrenia or other psychotic disorders may express somatic concerns or delusions, but these are typically bizarre and in the context of other false beliefs.

Treatment

The standard of care for patients with somatization disorder is the psychiatrist's referral letter to the primary care physician. This letter describes the illness to the physician and outlines a treatment plan (see Table 13-1). Regularly scheduled visits; appropriate, evidence-based examinations and evaluations; and the avoidance of invasive tests are all recommended in the letter (Smith et al., 1986). Perhaps most importantly, physicians are encouraged not to suggest to patients that the illness is all in their heads. This statement often leads patients to terminate their relationships with their physicians and start the whole process over again with someone new. The letter has been shown to decrease the patient's utilization of health care resources (Smith et al., 1986). Because patients may resist psychiatric treatment, often primary care physicians must manage somatization disorder.

Psychotropic medication appears to be of limited utility in somatization disorder. Because patients have high rates of comorbid psychiatric disorders, any pharmacotherapy should be targeted toward other psychiatric symptoms.

Psychotherapy has been shown to be helpful in somatization disorder. Patients randomized to cognitive behavioral therapy (CBT) were shown to have a decrease in health concerns and lower rates of service utilization when compared to patients who received treatment as usual (Allen et al., 2006). Group psychotherapy has also been used with some apparent benefits. Patients with somatization disorder often struggle to remain in psychotherapy long enough to receive benefit.

Prognosis

Somatization disorder tends to be waxing and waning and chronic. Patients rarely achieve full remission but can have a decrease in symptom frequency and medical visits. The greatest risks come from iatrogenic harm, which can be reduced by recognition of the condition and avoidance of unnecessary medical procedures.

TABLE 13-1	**Common Recommendations to Primary Care Physicians for Patients with Somatoform Disorders**
Disorder	**Recommendations to Primary Care Physicians**
Somatization disorder	• Avoid unnecessary tests • Have appointments at regular intervals • Support patient's suffering without feeling the need to repair it • Refer to mental health for comorbid conditions
Conversion disorder	• Explain diagnosis and reassure patient • Offer psychiatric referral
Hypochondriasis	• Offer psychiatric referral • Treat with antidepressants • Provide support and empathy to patient
Pain disorder	• Avoid iatrogenic drug dependence • Referral to specialty pain clinic
Body dysmorphic disorder	• Avoid unnecessary cosmetic procedures • Psychiatric referral in all cases

Conversion Disorder

Epidemiology

Conversion disorder has a prevalence rate of approximately 0.1% but is far more common in psychiatric and neurologic populations (Sadock and Sadock, 2007) and more common in women with a male-to-female ratio of at least 2:1 (Barsky et al., 2004). Unlike other somatoform disorders, it is common in children and adolescents, where the gender ratio is equal. Like somatization disorder, conversion disorder is seen more commonly in patients with lower levels of education. Those from rural areas develop conversion disorder more commonly; even more striking is the increased prevalence among people from the developing world.

Etiology

When patients present with conversion disorder, they may be trying to resolve or express an unconscious conflict. For example, if patients present with the inability to speak, it may represent their fear of saying something they know might cause harm to themselves or someone else. Psychogenic seizures, a common form of conversion disorder, may result from unconscious aggression that needs discharge but cannot be safely expressed. Neuroimaging research has contributed valuable information about disrupted frontal lobe function during conversion reactions that suggests a biological component as well (Stonnington et al., 2006).

Phenomenology

Patients with conversion disorder present with symptoms that appear neurologic or medical in origin. However, investigations reveal no underlying physical disease. Psychological factors are thought to be important in the development of symptoms; patients often present during or immediately after a crisis, such as the death of a loved one. Symptoms may relate to the underlying psychological stress. For example, if patients feel overburdened by family or work responsibilities, they may be unable to walk ("stand on their own feet") or if they see something forbidden, they may develop blindness. The patients are unaware that their symptoms are not caused medically and not motivated by any gain. Classically, patients are described as indifferent to their symptoms *(la belle indifférence)* but frequently are concerned about what is happening to them and demand explanation.

Common conversion symptoms often have a sudden onset in the setting of psychological stress and include psychogenic, nonepileptiform seizures (pseudoseizures), blindness, deafness, paralysis, mutism, falling, and psychogenic vomiting. Gait problems are common; *astasia-abasia* is a term that describes a dramatically unbalanced gait that could not result from weakness or loss of balance without falls. Patients do not fall but continue to walk in an unbalanced manner with writhing of the torso and thrusting of the limbs.

Differential Diagnosis

As with somatization disorder, underlying medical illness is the most common possibility for patients with conversion disorder. A thorough evaluation to rule out a physical cause is essential before making a diagnosis. For example, in psychogenic, nonepileptiform seizures, video electroencephalography (EEG) monitoring is the standard of care, with the diagnosis only made after observed motor activity in the absence of EEG changes. Symptoms that wax and wane, inconsistent findings between different examinations and examiners, and the presence of a known psychological stressor all increase the likelihood of conversion disorder (Sadock and Sadock, 2007).

Treatment

Patients with conversion disorder will often have spontaneous resolution with only limited interventions (Table 13-1). Suggestion while under hypnosis or amobarbital interviews can be tried to alleviate the symptoms (Stonnington et al., 2006). Improvement in the psychological stressor can lead to symptom relief in the absence of other interventions. There is some debate about telling patients the diagnosis, but most experts now recommend informing patients that they do not have an underlying physical illness and that stress may be the cause of their symptoms (Stonnington et al., 2006). If this message is delivered in an empathic and positive manner, patients can often accept the diagnosis and may benefit from the knowledge.

A CASE OF NONEPILEPTIFORM SEIZURES

A 37-year-old woman presents to a tertiary care hospital for further evaluation of intractable seizures. For 3 months, she has had two or three seizures every day, which are routinely witnessed by her husband and children. They report that they last for a few minutes, involve the movement of all four limbs in a rhythmic manner, and then she is able to resume what she was doing. She says she does not know why she is having seizures. On examination, she is pleasant, cooperative, and without obvious neurologic deficits. Forty-eight-hour video EEG monitoring reveals no abnormalities in spite of five seizure-like events.

After the acute episode, psychotherapy can assist patients by improving their insight into their response to stress and provide them with tools to manage stress more effectively. CBT has been used with some success in patients with conversion disorder to assist with recognizing the first signs of conversion and aborting a full episode. Relaxation training, muscle relaxation, and visualization exercises can all be used in the context of CBT to assist patients with their symptoms. Treatment with medication is often unhelpful unless the patient has comorbid anxiety or depression; then treatment for the comorbidities is indicated.

Prognosis

Conversion disorder has a high rate of spontaneous resolution but 25% to 50% of patients suffer relapses within the first year. When patients have multiple episodes of conversion symptoms, the disorder can become chronic and debilitating. In general, those with psychogenic, nonepileptiform seizures have a worse prognosis and require ongoing treatment after the episode resolves.

Hypochondriasis

Epidemiology

Hypochondriasis differs from other somatoform disorders in that it is equally prevalent among men and women. Education, ethnic background, and socioeconomic status do not appear to affect prevalence. The rate in the general population is likely approximately 2%, but in primary care settings the disorder is more common, with estimates ranging from 3% to 10% (Escobar et al., 1998).

Etiology

In hypochondriasis, patients may have altered processing of physical signals that leads to assigning exaggerated importance to trivial physical sensations. This overemphasis leads the patient to engage in abnormal health-related behaviors, such as frequent physician visits and constant anxiety about health. Similar to somatization disorder, patients with hypochondriasis may be seeking relief from burdening responsibilities without being conscious of their conflict.

Phenomenology

Patients with hypochondriasis believe they have a medical illness and their health is at risk. They spend significant amounts of time worrying about their illness and frequently seek medical care to obtain confirmation of their fears. Normal exams and physician reassurance do not assuage patients' fears but, rather, cause them to become angry and frustrated with their physicians or seek another opinion. A key component of the condition is anxiety over health. Bodily symptoms are often misinterpreted. Normal sensations are thought to be signs of illness and lead to anxiety and abnormal health-related behaviors, such as repeated visits to physicians. These worries are not delusional in quality because, although their beliefs are false, they are not fixed and can usually be swayed by a normal examination or test result. However, this effect does not last; soon their fear returns, they begin worrying, they think they have a serious illness, and the cycle begins again.

Differential Diagnosis

Hypochondriasis differs from somatization disorder in that the patient's focus is on having a serious illness rather than physical symptoms (Noyes et al., 2006). Patients with hypochondriasis experience far more anxiety than those with somatization disorder and can be differentiated from those with conversion disorder by the acute onset of symptoms and the relative lack of anxiety patients with conversion disorder experience. Body dysmorphic disorder leads to anxiety about appearance but not about a serious underlying illness. Patients with pain disorder are focused on pain rather than being anxious about an underlying illness. Unlike patients with factitious disorder, patients with hypochondriasis do not intentionally produce their symptoms.

As with other somatoform disorders, patients with hypochondriasis must be carefully evaluated to ensure they do not have a real underlying medical illness. Diseases with vague symptoms, such as myasthenia gravis, multiple sclerosis, or connective tissue diseases, may account for physical sensations. Even in patients who have an established history of hypochondriacal behavior, evidence-based evaluations are appropriate to rule out an undiagnosed illness.

Treatment

Treatment with paroxetine, a selective serotonin reuptake inhibitor (SSRI), may be helpful (Greeven et al., 2007). If patients have comorbid depression or anxiety, those symptoms can be treated with psychotropics as well. Physicians often notice hypochondriacal anxiety more readily than patients, but if patients can acknowledge that they are in distress, they might be amenable to anxiolytics. Patients may benefit from CBT that focuses on the triggers for hypochondriacal concerns and provides tools other than visiting physicians for relief (Greeven et al., 2007). Group therapy may also help by enhancing their support systems. If patients are not open to psychiatric treatment, regular doctor appointments for reassurance and support are recommended to decrease their anxiety and sense of hopelessness (Table 13-1). This may also help decrease the amount of unnecessary evaluation these patients undergo. They are more likely to benefit from physicians who assist them with coping rather than focus on complete elimination of symptoms.

Prognosis

Hypochondriasis tends to be chronic, with periods of improvement followed by relapse. Patients have better prognoses if they have treatable anxiety or depression and are open to psychiatric care for these conditions. Avoiding iatrogenic harm is essential to maintaining a favorable prognosis.

Pain Disorder

Epidemiology

Pain disorder is likely the most common of all the somatoform disorders. Lifetime prevalence has been estimated as high as 12% (Sadock and Sadock, 2007). Because the disorder is common and not often formally diagnosed, data are lacking on gender ratio, education, and socioeconomic status.

Etiology

Pain disorder often develops in the context of chronic pain from traumatic, musculoskeletal, or orthopedic injury. Genetic factors may play a role, but the mechanism is likely polygenetic and difficult to elucidate. Psychological factors may also play a role. Guilt transformed into physical discomfort and the belief that suffering is an appropriate punishment may propagate or potentiate pain. Other factors are unknown.

Phenomenology

Patients with pain disorder present with predominant complaints about pain, which can be in any anatomic location but commonly include headaches and neck, back, abdominal, and pelvic pain. Psychological factors are thought to be important in the development or maintenance of the pain. Patients often have underlying medical conditions. They repeatedly visit physicians and describe in detail the frequency, character, and intensity of the pain. They often have great impairment in their social or professional lives because of pain. Depression is a common comorbidity.

Differential Diagnosis

Deciding which patients with chronic pain have pain disorder is difficult. Patients must have some obvious psychological contribution to the pain; however, there is evidence that patients with chronic pain from documented medical causes have changes in their personality profiles that may be caused by the pain (Tyrer, 2006) and make them seem to have psychological factors contributing to their pain when in fact their pain is causing psychological changes.

Pain disorder differs from the other somatoform disorders in that patients tend to focus on pain above other factors. Other symptoms tend to be absent. Patients with conversion disorder have nonpainful presentations. Other psychiatric disorders can have physical discomfort or increased pain as a feature, but in pain disorder the pain is the central or only symptom.

Treatment

Patients are best served in multidisciplinary pain clinics that have specialty programs designed to treat patients suffering with chronic pain (Table 13-1). Analgesics are of limited benefit, and narcotic medications carry the risk of abuse and dependence. Dual action (serotonin and norepinephrine) antidepressants such as venlafaxine and duloxetine can benefit patients with pain disorder (Kroenke et al., 2006). Tricyclic antidepressants also have established effectiveness, but patients must be monitored closely for side effects. Adjunctive supportive psychotherapy aimed at improving functioning is also of benefit, as is relaxation training and physical therapy aimed at regaining function.

Prognosis

Patients with pain disorder tend to have chronic courses and significant disability. Those who retain function and have a shorter duration of pain tend to have better long-term outcomes.

Body Dysmorphic Disorder

Epidemiology

Body dysmorphic disorder is rare in psychiatric settings but probably has a prevalence rate as high as 15% in plastic surgery clinics (Jakubietz et al., 2007) and has higher prevalence among women. Age of onset is usually during adolescence, but patients do not typically present for treatment until the disorder has been present for at least a few years.

Etiology

Patients share a number of features with those who have obsessive-compulsive disorder (OCD), and body dysmorphic disorder may be a subtype of OCD. If it is, serotonin dysfunction may underlie the excessive focus on appearance typical in body dysmorphic disorder (Grant and Phillips, 2005).

Phenomenology

Patients have undue concern about deficits in appearance even in the absence of obvious abnormalities. They spend excessive time examining the defective area, including their hair, skin, eyes, ears, nose, breasts, stomachs, and genitals, and ruminating about the perceived imperfection. Frequently, others cannot even notice that something is amiss. Patients often seek medical care for their concerns, particularly from dermatologists and plastic surgeons. If they receive treatment for one area of concern, they often shift their focus to another perceived abnormality. They have high rates of comorbid depression, and as many as 25% attempt suicide (Phillips and Menard, 2006). Obsessive-compulsive traits are common.

Differential Diagnosis

Body dysmorphic disorder must be differentiated from anorexia nervosa. Patients with anorexia also have excessive concern about their body image, but this is focused on weight and shape rather than a perceived bodily imperfection. Patients with gender identity disorder are uncomfortable with their gender rather than preoccupied with the appearance of their genitals. OCD may be a premorbid condition, but patients with body dysmorphic disorder alone do not have the discomfort with the condition typical in OCD. If patients have unshakable and irrational beliefs about their appearance even after direct confrontation, delusional disorder, somatic subtype, can be diagnosed as well.

Treatment

Patients with body dysmorphic disorder do not benefit from plastic surgery and should not be considered good surgical candidates. They likely benefit from the treatment of comorbid psychiatric diagnoses such as depression and OCD, especially when the high suicide rate is considered (Table 13-1). Medications that have been used in delusional disorder, such as pimozide, clomipramine, and olanzapine, may also be of use if patients have both conditions as comorbidities. CBT focusing on the excessive concerns and alleviating the resulting anxiety can decrease symptoms and may increase the rate of remission (Phillips et al., 2006).

Prognosis

Patients often have long courses that begin in adolescence. Concerns can shift from one body part to another, and those who receive surgery do not appear to derive any benefit compared with those who do not. If anything, morbidity and mortality from surgery produce far more harm than the potential benefit from cosmetic procedures.

Undifferentiated Somatoform Disorder

Undifferentiated somatoform disorder is much more common than somatization disorder (Escobar et al., 1987; Abbey, 2005). In fact, the prevalence may be as high as 10% for broadly defined somatoform disorders. Patients present with numerous chronic complaints that may be as debilitating as those found in full somatization disorder while not meeting the restrictive criteria (see subsequent text). The patients are similar in demographics to those who have somatization disorder.

The diagnosis is reserved for patients who have at least one unexplained physical symptom that persists for at least 6 months. Often, patients have more than one symptom but do not meet full criteria for somatization disorder. There is good evidence that patients with at least three unexplained symptoms are similar to patients with full somatization disorder in presentation, course, and prognosis (Escobar et al., 1987). They also share similar family histories, comorbid psychiatric illnesses, and levels of service utilization. In the future the diagnosis of somatization disorder may become less strict to include these patients.

Somatoform Disorder Not Otherwise Specified

The category Somatoform Disorder Not Otherwise Specified is for patients who have had unexplained somatic symptoms or hypochondriacal health concerns for <6 months. The *Diagnostic and Statistical Manual of Mental Disorders,* Fourth Edition, Text Revision (DSM-IV-TR) (American Psychiatric Association, 2000), makes special note of patients with pseudocyesis or the false belief that one is pregnant. Patients are not pregnant and have negative pregnancy tests but may have enlargement of the abdomen and the hormonal changes associated with pregnancy. They often have a change in menstrual frequency or even frank amenorrhea. Symptoms may resolve when patients become convinced that they are not pregnant, but in some cases patients continue to hold the delusional belief even when the expected outcome (delivery) does not occur.

FACTITIOUS DISORDER

People with factitious disorder fake having medical or psychological illness to gain access to the sick role. The essence of the diagnosis is the deception the patient is utilizing as part of the presentation. Physical or psychological symptoms are intentionally produced, and patients retain awareness at all times that they are misleading those caring for them.

Epidemiology

In the general medical hospital, factitious disorder is fairly rare. Most estimates find that approximately 1% of patients referred for psychiatric consultation have factitious disorder. Given that approximately 5% of hospital patients typically receive a psychiatric consultation, this would suggest that about 0.05% of patients in the general hospital have factitious disorder. Patients who work in health care fields, including nurses, medical technicians, and physicians, have elevated rates. Women present with physical signs and symptoms three times as often as men, but men present with psychological signs and symptoms twice as often as women (Sadock and Sadock, 2007). Patients frequently have comorbid personality, substance use, and mood disorders.

Etiology

Patients with factitious disorder wish to gain access to the sick role. On an unconscious level they are likely trying to re-create the dynamic that exists between parent and child, with their role as the child. Patients receive certain basic needs no matter the setting in which they are hospitalized. Food, shelter, and the time and attention of caregivers are all essentially guaranteed when patients assume the sick role. Those who have a history of childhood neglect or abuse may use the sick role to re-create and then master through alteration the past mistreatment they suffered. Unfortunately, the usual outcome is that they receive the same type of disapproval their parents offered. This time, though, it comes from hospital staff who become frustrated and angry with patients for deceiving them.

Phenomenology

Patients intentionally feign symptoms and are only able to give limited history. Collateral information must be obtained from family, friends, and past medical records. Patients with primarily psychological features may present with false reports of hallucinations, delusions, or other psychotic phenomena and may feign bizarre behavior such as mutism, posturing, and catatonia. Reports of suicidal ideation or attempts are common. Alongside these features, patients often report fantastic, grandiose personal histories, a phenomenon known as *psuedologica fantastica*. They may report that they are famous or remarkable for little known but glorious past achievements. They often begin their tales with an element of the truth but then expand on it in exciting and improbable ways. Their stories nearly make sense but often fall apart with further questioning or attempts at external verification.

Patients with physical symptoms are more commonly encountered in the general hospital. They create physical signs and symptoms through a variety of means, such as injecting bacteria or feces into intravenous lines to produce fever and sepsis, taking high doses of thyroid hormone to appear hyperthyroid, injecting insulin to produce hypoglycemic crisis, and using anticoagulants to produce serious bleeding complications. Patients often have a history of numerous surgeries and present asking for further operations to assist with intra-abdominal adhesions. Because these patients often have a medical background, they may be familiar with signs and symptoms of illness as well as the most effective means to spur physician action.

Factitious disorder by proxy is a rare condition in which parents induce illness in their children so that their children may assume the sick role. Although there are undoubtedly psychological motivations for such actions, factitious disorder by proxy is child abuse and, once identified, must be reported to the proper authorities.

Differential Diagnosis

Patients with factitious disorder must be differentiated from those with genuine psychological or medical illness. Exogenous use of medication to produce a medical illness can often be detected with laboratory evaluation. For example, the measurement of C peptide, produced in amounts roughly equal to that of insulin by the pancreas, in patients with suspected factitious hypoglycemia can help to distinguish endogenous excess of insulin from surreptitious insulin injection (Barsky et al., 2004). Although factitious disorder with psychological features can be harder to detect, patients should have their stories confirmed as best as possible. Factitious disorder must be distinguished from conversion disorder and malingering. In conversion disorder, the production of symptoms is unconscious and usually related to a psychological factor. In factitious disorder, patients are aware that they are producing symptoms even if they are unaware of the factors motivating them to do so. In contrast, patients who are malingering are aware of their motivation, typically secondary gain from being ill (benefits, housing, etc.).

Treatment

Patients with factitious disorder do not respond to any known psychological treatments. While in the hospital, efforts should first be targeted to recognition and diagnosis. The main morbidity is iatrogenic. Following diagnosis, the likelihood of further surgery or testing decreases dramatically. Providing patients with the diagnosis in the presence of primary care physicians and nursing staff can help decrease the patients' negative reaction. The diagnosis can be framed in terms of the patients' suffering or as a psychiatric illness to assist patients with saving face and being more honest with their physicians. Patients are sometimes amenable to psychiatric treatment and should be offered the option of inpatient care or outpatient follow-up. Providing clear information to hospital staff is often necessary because patients with factitious disorder often anger their care providers. By explaining that it is a behavioral disorder and that the patient likely has serious psychological disturbance, the hospital staff are more likely to treat the patient with dignity.

Prognosis

Factitious disorder tends to be chronic, although good quality long-term data are largely lacking. After discovery in one hospital, patients typically move to another hospital and repeat the cycle. Patients tend to have extended periods in the hospital or other care settings and therefore have limited interpersonal or professional success. If they are able to accept ongoing psychiatric care, it may improve their prognosis.

MALINGERING

Malingering is the intentional production of symptoms in order to obtain both the sick role and some further secondary gain. Patients are typically interested in the material goods associated with illness, including disability benefits and housing. Patients in prison may be interested in obtaining special treatment. Malingering may help patients avoid military or work duties, and patients frequently produce symptoms in order to obtain drugs with high liability for dependence, such as sedatives and opiates. Patients encountered in medicolegal settings, including prisoners and those involved in litigation, are more likely to be malingering than those seen in a general psychiatric clinic (Ford, 2005). Detecting malingering can be difficult but, in spite of the covert nature of the disorder, must be attempted to optimize care for the patient.

Epidemiology

Malingering is rare in the general population but increases in prevalence in psychiatric settings. In the military, it is estimated to have a prevalence up to 5%. Among patients with criminal history, the prevalence may be as high as 25% (Sadock and Sadock, 2007). Common comorbid diagnoses include antisocial and borderline personality disorders in adults and conduct disorder in children and adolescents.

Phenomenology

Patients may present with malingering in order to avoid responsibility, gain material goods, obtain favorable judgments in criminal and civil proceedings, and access drugs of abuse. Patients may present with specific complaints and requests and become quickly frustrated with delays in care or proposed alternatives. They may have rapid escalation in their behavior if their demands are not met and must be monitored for impulsive destructive behavior and suicide attempts.

Differential Diagnosis

Malingering must be distinguished from conversion disorder and factitious disorder, as outlined in the section on factitious disorder. Genuine medical or psychiatric illness must be ruled out. In general, patients with malingering are less cooperative with their care than patients with conversion, but their oppositional style can be found in factitious disorder. As with factitious disorder, malingering does not rule out comorbid psychiatric disorders.

Treatment

There is no specific treatment for malingering. Once the diagnosis has been made, the entire treatment team involved with the patient should be made aware so that they can respond appropriately to requests and set limits when needed. Patients often leave treatment once their deception has been discovered. Disregarding the behavior can sometimes lead to its extinction through behavioral mechanisms. Because patients often have comorbid psychiatric disorders, they may benefit from ongoing treatment and decrease their malingering behaviors over time.

Prognosis

Patients with a history of malingering are at risk of repeated episodes. Long-term follow-up can be difficult to obtain but, in general, the behaviors decrease when the potential to gain is lost.

FUTURE DIRECTIONS

Recently, research into somatoform disorders has strengthened the evidence base for psychiatric treatment. Structured psychotherapies like CBT have been shown to be effective at decreasing problematic health care–related behaviors. Group therapy has also been shown to improve short-term outcomes. Psychotropic medications such as SSRIs and venlafaxine have been shown in trials to improve symptoms and functioning in patients with somatoform disorders. New techniques such as functional neuroimaging are providing better insight into the biologic factors that promote the somatoform disorders. Greater appreciation of the high prevalence of these disorders in primary care is helping to increase knowledge of the disorders among nonpsychiatrists. Somatoform disorders can be challenging to treat, but when there is successful detection and treatment, both patients and health care professionals benefit. For every surgery that is prevented or procedure that is avoided, patients have lower risk of iatrogenic harm and further complications.

Clinical Pearls

- Patients with somatization disorder have high rates of iatrogenic morbidity and mortality and should have as few procedures and surgeries as possible.
- For many patients, the best treatment for somatization disorder is a stable relationship with one primary care physician who provides them with consistent and reasonable care.
- Conversion disorder may respond well to suggestions of improvement during hypnosis.
- Hypochondriasis is the only somatoform disorder that is as common in men as in women.
- Body dysmorphic disorder has high rates of comorbid depression and suicide attempts.
- Patients who do not meet full criteria for somatization disorder are still at high risk for the complications of somatization disorder and likely to benefit from the same interventions.
- Once the diagnosis of factitious disorder is presented to patients, they often become angry and leave the hospital against medical advice only to seek admission to another nearby hospital soon afterwards.
- Malingering is more common in patients who have pending medicolegal action.
- For many somatoform disorders, CBT has been shown to be effective in decreasing health-related behaviors.

Self-Assessment Questions and Answers

13-1. A 45-year-old man presents to the emergency department with complaints of blindness in one eye that began suddenly 2 hours earlier. He has an afferent reflex in the other eye and appears to blink to threat when his functioning eye is closed. Computed tomography of the head was interpreted to be within normal limits. Ocular pressure is normal. His symptoms continued after admission to the hospital. Visual evoked potentials, magnetic resonance imaging of the brain, and lumbar puncture results for multiple sclerosis were all normal. What is the next step?

A. Cerebral arteriogram to evaluate for retinal artery occlusion
B. Discharge from the hospital
C. Psychiatric consultation

D. Functional neuroimaging
E. Transfer to a psychiatric hospital

This patient likely has conversion disorder. He has a sensory deficit of sudden onset without evidence of underlying medical illness. Few details about his life circumstances have been collected. Psychiatric consultation will help obtain a history of his psychiatric disorders, development, and recent stressors. The psychiatrist will be able to advise his physicians about the likelihood of conversion as well as suggest to him that recovery may come soon. If necessary, the psychiatrist could hypnotize him or use an amobarbital interview to facilitate the suggestion process. *Answer: C*

13-2. A 24-year-old woman presents to her dermatologist with concerns about her skin. She states that it is discolored and asks for an expensive and experimental bleaching procedure. She has a history of rhinoplasty, breast augmentation, and liposuction. She reports that she has spent 2 hours a day for the last 2 months figuring out exactly where the discoloration begins and can assist with pointing it out. Which of the following questions is necessary when obtaining her history?

A. "Are you having any thoughts of suicide?"
B. "Will you promise not to have any more surgeries after this?"
C. "Do you ever feel like people are following you?"
D. "Will you be able to pay cash for this procedure?"
E. "Have you spent a lot of time in the sun?"

13-3. Which of the following medications would you consider for her?

A. Buspirone
B. Bupropion
C. Clomipramine
D. Haloperidol
E. Venlafaxine

This patient likely suffers from body dysmorphic disorder because she has excessive concern about minor defects in appearance and spends a significant amount of time preoccupied with this concern. Patients with body dysmorphic disorder have been shown to be at elevated risk for suicide and should be evaluated psychiatrically before any procedures or surgeries. Medications for obsessive-compulsive disorder (OCD), such as clomipramine, have been demonstrated to be of some utility in these patients. *Answers: A, C*

13-4. A 43-year-old man presents to the hospital with complaints of recurrent fainting. He says when he is home alone, he will fall while walking to the bathroom. He was found on the floor by his roommate after hitting his head on the bathroom basin. He does not reveal it upon presentation but is aware of why the fainting occurs (hypoglycemia). He wants to be admitted to the hospital but does not have any further motive. Given these facts, the correct diagnosis is:

A. Somatization disorder
B. Conversion disorder
C. Factitious disorder
D. Malingering
E. Hypochondriasis

The patient is producing hypoglycemia by injecting insulin. He wishes to gain access to the sick role but is unaware of why. This is a factitious disorder. Conversion disorder is not intentionally produced; symptoms start in the unconscious. Malingering is done with some gain in mind, other than entering the sick role, such as avoiding legal problems or financial gain. Somatization disorder presents with many diffuse complaints in the absence of obvious illness; this man has an isolated complaint. Hypochondriasis is the fear of a serious medical illness in the context of the misinterpretation of minor bodily symptoms, and those with it rarely have presentations as dramatic as fainting. *Answer: C*

13-5. A 53-year-old woman presents to a primary care physician with complaints of nausea, vomiting, loss of appetite, headache, back pain, chest pain, difficulty walking, neck pain, vaginal dryness, and periods of blindness. She says most of these symptoms have been present in one form or another for >20 years. She has a history of hypertension, a hysterectomy, and is a smoker. She denies the use of other drugs. Following a normal physical examination, the next appropriate step would be to:

A. Assure the patient that she is fine and that it is all in her head.
B. Recommend psychiatric care.
C. Refuse to see the patient again.
D. Obtain blood tests and an ECG.
E. Admit to the hospital for further testing.

Although the patient may have somatization disorder, her risk factors and clinical history are concerning for coronary artery disease. Patients with somatization disorder develop medical illness at the same rate as other people and require evidence-based evaluation. Blood tests to evaluate myocardial damage and metabolic profile along with an ECG are minimally invasive and will provide useful information immediately. If the tests are normal, the patient should continue to receive care from the same physician and, if possible, receive an outpatient psychiatric referral for evaluation. *Answer: D*

References

Abbey SE. Somatization and somatoform disorders. In Levenson JL, ed. *Textbook of psychosomatic medicine*. Arlington, VA: American Psychiatric Publishing, Inc.; 2005.

Allen LA, Woolfolk RL, Escobar JI, et al. Cognitive-behavioral therapy for somatization disorder. *Arch Intern Med*. 2006;166:1512–1518.

American Psychiatric Association: *Diagnostic and Statistical Manual of Mental Disorders*, 4th Edition, Text Revision, Washington DC, American Psychiatric Association;2000.

Barsky AJ, Stern TA, Greenberg DB, et al. Functional somatic symptoms and somatoform disorder. In: Stern TA, Fricchione GL, Cassem NH, et al., eds. *Massachusetts general hospital handbook of general hospital psychiatry*. 5th ed. Philadelphia: Mosby;2004.

Eisenberg L. Psychiatry and society: A sociobiologic synthesis. *N Engl J Med*. 1977;296:903–910.

Escobar JI, Burnam A, Karno M, et al. Somatization in the community. *Arch Gen Psychiatry*. 1987;44: 713–718.

Escobar JI, Gara M, Waitzkin H, et al. DSM-IV hypochondriasis in primary care. *Gen Hosp Psychiatry*. 1998; 20:155–159.

Ford CV. Deception syndromes: Factitious disorders and malingering. In: Levenson JL, ed. *Textbook of psychosomatic medicine*. Arlington, VA: American Psychiatric Publishing, Inc.;2005.

Grant JE, Phillips KA. Recognizing and treating body dysmorphic disorder. *Ann Clin Psychiatry*. 2005;17(4): 205–210.

Greeven A, van Balkom AJLM, Visswe S, et al. Cognitive behavior therapy and paroxetine in the treatment of hypochondriasis: A randomized controlled trial. *Am J Psychiatry*. 2007;164:91–99.

Jakubietz M, Jakubietz RJ, Kloss DF, et al. Body dysmorphic disorder: Diagnosis and approach. *Plast Reconstr Surg*. 2007;119:1924–1930.

Kroenke K, Messina 3rd N, Benattia I, et al. Venlafaxine extended release in the short-term treatment of depressed and anxious primary care patients with multisomatoform disorder. *J Clin Psychiatry*. 2006;67(1):72–80.

Mai F. Somatization disorder: A practical review. *Can J Psychiatry*. 2004;49:652–662.

Noyes Jr R, Stuart S, Watson DB, et al. Distinguishing between hypochondriasis and somatization disorder: A review of the existing literature. *Psychother Psychosom*. 2006;75:270–281.

Phillips KA, Menard W. Suicidality in body dysmorphic disorder: A prospective study. *Am J Psychiatry*. 2006;163:1280–1282.

Phillips KA, Pagano ME, Menard W, et al. A 12-month follow-up study of the course of body dysmorphic disorder. *Am J Psychiatry*. 2006;163:907–912.

Sadock BJ, Sadock VA. *Kaplan & Sadock's synopsis of psychiatry*, 10th ed. Philadelphia: Lippincott Williams & Wilkins, 2007.

Sifneos PE. Alexithymia: Past and present. *Am J Psychiatry*. 1996;153(7 Suppl):137–142.

Smith GR, Monson RA, Ray DC. Psychiatric consultation in somatization disorder. *N Engl J Med*. 1986;314: 1407–1413.

Stonnington CM, Barry JJ, Fisher RS. Conversion disorder. *Am J Psychiatry*. 2006;163(9):1510–1517.

Tyrer S. Psychosomatic pain. *Br J Psychiatry*. 2006;188:91–93.

Dissociative Disorders

According to the *Diagnostic and Statistical Manual of Mental Disorders* Fourth Edition, Text Revision (DSM-IV-TR) (American Psychiatric Association, 2000), "the essential feature of the dissociative disorders is a disruption in the usually integrated functions of consciousness, memory, identity, or perception of the environment." This disturbance can be sudden or gradual, transient or chronic. The DSM-IV-TR dissociative disorders are dissociative identity disorder, depersonalization disorder, dissociative amnesia, dissociative fugue, and dissociative disorder not otherwise specified (NOS). The study of the dissociative disorders began at the end of the 18th century. However, the modern notion that these conditions are a distinct group of disorders, with systematic research about them, did not really begin until the advent of DSM-III in 1980. At that time, conditions that developed from the 19th century construct of *hysteria* were distributed among different diagnostic categories: dissociative disorders (the subject of this chapter), somatoform disorders (such as conversion disorder and somatization disorder, Chapter 13), posttraumatic stress disorder (PTSD, Chapter 12), and even borderline personality disorder (Chapter 20).

Janet (1901) is the founder of modern approaches to dissociation and dissociative disorders. He developed theories of hysteria and dissociation, suggesting that many cases of hysteria are based on covert, dissociated aspects of the personality that were engendered by traumatic experiences in susceptible individuals. Freud and Breuer's (1895) revered *Studies in Hysteria* referenced Janet's work, used similar notions of fixed ideas and traumatic etiology, and introduced the cathartic method of cure for hysteria, for example, in the famous case of Anna O. Freud posited that the dynamic unconscious, intrapsychic conflict, and intrapsychic defenses surrounding unacceptable thoughts, wishes, and memories gave rise to hysteria, thereby underemphasizing and even disregarding the role of real traumatic experiences in the genesis of dissociation. Modern conceptualization of dissociative disorders often involves a synthesis of Janetian ideas and Freudian ones, validating external experiences while at the same time attending to their intrapsychic elaborations.

The scientific investigation of dissociation dates to Prince's (1908) experiments using a crude polygraph to measure galvanic skin resistance (GSR) across the alter states of a patient with dissociative identity disorder—a physiological measure of arousal that remains of interest today. Prince reported seeing differential GSR reactivity to words that were emotionally laden for various alter states. The advent of reliable and valid measures of dissociation over the last two decades has opened up new avenues of experimental investigation (Bernstein and Putnam, 1986; Steinberg, 1995). A variety of physiological, neuroendocrine, cognitive, and brain imaging studies are increasingly informing clinicians about the biological underpinnings of dissociation and the impact of dissociation on physical and mental functioning.

Systematic research has consistently found a robust relationship between dissociation and traumatic experiences (Vermetten et al., 2007). The role of trauma in Western culture crosses into historically taboo subjects, such as rape, incest, child abuse, and domestic violence, and their actual prevalence in our society. In addition, the study of trauma leads to larger legal and social questions (Dalenberg, 2006). Studies now document unusually high rates of trauma in patients with dissociative disorder (although this linkage is notably weaker for depersonalization disorder). In addition, numerous studies have found significantly higher levels of dissociative symptoms in traumatized, compared with nontraumatized, clinical and general population samples (van Ijzendoorn and Schuengel, 1996). Although these findings significantly link dissociation with antecedent trauma, they are not sufficient to demonstrate that the trauma actually "causes" the

TABLE 14-1	Prevalence of Dissociative Disorders from Two Population Studies	
Diagnosis	Ross 1997 (%)	Johnson et al., 2006 (%)
Dissociative amnesia	6.0	1.8
Dissociative fugue	0.0	0.0
Dissociative identity disorder	1.3	1.5
Depersonalization disorder	2.8	0.8
Dissociative disorder NOS	0.2	4.4
All dissociative disorders	10.3	8.5

NOS, not otherwise specified.

dissociation. Vulnerabilities and diatheses toward dissociation presumably also play a role and have not been well elucidated so far. Dissociation also appears to serve as a major mediating process between traumatic experiences and subsequent psychopathology, such as PTSD, and therefore is an important target for prevention and early intervention efforts. Stress-resistant, or resilient, individuals are characterized, in part, by their lack of dissociative responses to major stressors (Morgan et al., 2001).

There are only two systematic general population studies of the prevalence of dissociative disorders (see Table 14-1) (Johnson et al., 2006; Ross, 1997). The data from the earlier study were later reanalyzed, yielding a more conservative 3% to 5% prevalence for all pathological dissociation (Waller and Ross, 1997).

DISSOCIATIVE AMNESIA

Clinical Presentation and Diagnosis

In DSM-IV-TR the essential feature of dissociative amnesia is "inability to recall important personal information, usually of a traumatic or stressful nature, that is too extensive to be explained by normal forgetfulness." To be diagnosed as dissociative amnesia, the memory disturbance should not occur exclusively during the course of dissociative identity disorder, dissociative fugue, PTSD, acute stress disorder, or somatization disorder or should be more pronounced than the particular disorder would dictate. It should also not be due to the effects of substances or neurologic or other medical conditions.

Dissociative amnesia has two basic presentations. One is a dramatic and sudden disturbance in which extensive aspects of memory for personal information are not available to conscious verbal recall. These patients are often seen in emergency departments or general medical or neurologic services, because the sudden development of memory loss requires medical assessment. A more prevalent form of dissociative amnesia is a deletion from conscious memory of significant aspects of one's personal history. Patients do not ordinarily complain of this, and it is usually only discovered in taking a careful life history. Dissociative amnesia typically has a clear-cut onset and offset; for example, a patient may report that she does not remember being in fifth grade, although she has a clear memory for other school years.

Epidemiology

Dissociative amnesia has been reported in approximately 6% of the general population. Some factors associated with dissociative amnesia after traumatic experiences are trauma caused by human assault rather than natural disaster, repeated trauma as opposed to single traumatic events, longer duration of trauma, fear of death or significant harm during trauma, trauma caused by multiple perpetrators, close relationship between the perpetrator and victim, betrayal by a caretaker as part of abuse, threats of death or significant harm by the perpetrator if the victim discloses his or her identity or information regarding the traumatic experience, violence of the trauma, and earlier age at onset of trauma (Loewenstein, 2001).

Etiology

Different theories have been developed to explain dissociative amnesia. In the behavioral states and information processing model (Putnam, 1998), dissociation is conceptualized as a basic part of the psychobiology of the human response to life-threatening danger: a protective activation of altered states of consciousness that change perception, pain sensation, time sense, and sense of self. Alternatively, extreme psychological conflict can precipitate dissociative amnesia. In many cases of acute dissociative amnesia, the psychosocial environment out of which the amnesia develops is not traumatic *per se* but, rather, massively conflictual, with the patient experiencing intolerable emotions of shame, guilt, despair, rage, and desperation, from which simply fight or flight seems impossible or psychologically unacceptable. Another explanatory model emphasizes developmental attachment theory (Lyons-Ruth et al., 2006) and betrayal trauma (Freyd, 1996). Betrayal by a trusted and needed other, such as a parent, is thought to influence the way in which a traumatic event is processed and remembered. In this scenario, the amnesia is protective of the child's developmentally mediated need for attachment, allowing for the preservation of overall emotional and cognitive growth despite the maltreatment.

Differential Diagnosis

In considering the diagnosis the clinician must first determine that the phenomenon is beyond "normalcy" in its extent. In patients with dementia, organic amnestic disorders, and delirium, the memory loss for personal information is embedded in a far more extensive set of cognitive, language, attentional, behavioral, and memory problems. Causes of organic amnestic disorders include Korsakoff psychosis, cerebral vascular accidents, postoperative amnesia, postinfectious amnesia, anoxic amnesia, and transient global amnesia. Electroconvulsive therapy may also cause a marked, usually temporary, amnesia. In posttraumatic amnesia due to brain injury, there is usually a clear history of physical trauma, a period of unconsciousness or amnesia or both, and objective clinical evidence of brain injury. In most epilepsy cases, the clinical presentation is quite different from that of dissociative amnesia, with clear ictal events and sequelae. Patients with nonepileptic seizures (also known as *pseudoseizures*) may also have dissociative symptoms such as amnesia and a history of psychological trauma. The diagnosis can ultimately be clarified by telemetry or ambulatory electroencephalogram (EEG) monitoring.

A variety of substances can cause amnesia, commonly including alcohol, sedative-hypnotics, anticholinergics, steroids, narcotics, psychedelics, marijuana, and phencyclidine. Transient global amnesia may be mistaken for a dissociative amnesia, especially because stressful life events may precede either disorder. However, transient global amnesia has a sudden onset of complete anterograde amnesia and learning abilities, pronounced retrograde amnesia, preservation of memory for personal identity, and anxious awareness of memory loss. Patients usually are older than 50 years and have risk factors for cerebrovascular disease.

Patients with dissociative identity disorder often present with amnestic episodes but are also characterized by a plethora of additional symptoms. Amnesia is a criterion symptom for both acute stress disorder and PTSD. Clinical judgment needs to be exercised to determine whether the extent of the amnesia warrants a separate dissociative disorder diagnosis. Feigned amnesia is more common in patients presenting with the acute, classic forms of dissociative amnesia. There is no absolute way to differentiate dissociative amnesia from factitious or malingered amnesia.

Course and Prognosis

Acute dissociative amnesia frequently spontaneously resolves once the person is removed to safety from traumatic or overwhelming circumstances. The amnesia may resolve in hours, weeks, or months. If it does not spontaneously resolve, psychotherapy, hypnotherapy, pharmacologically facilitated interviews, or combinations of these modalities can be helpful. In unusual cases, a chronic course can develop, with the patient seemingly unable to tolerate recall of the events that surrounded the onset of the amnesia.

Treatment

Phase-oriented treatment is the current standard of care for trauma disorders, including dissociative amnesia (Loewenstein, 2001). Three basic phases are recognized. The initial stabilization phase focuses on safety, symptom control, containment of affects and impulses, and education about

A CASE OF DISSOCIATIVE AMNESIA

Mrs. Jones was a 35-year-old working mother of three children who lived at home with her husband. She had been having an affair with a coworker for 3 years, and one day her husband inadvertently found out about the affair. Despite all her pleadings, he was unwilling to discuss the situation in any way and in a rage left her and the children, stating that he would never come back. Mrs. Jones' mother almost immediately moved in to help. Mrs. Jones' mother brought her to a psychiatrist 3 days after the incident because Mrs. Jones was acting very strangely at home. She was found to have developed an acute amnesia, whereby she had selectively forgotten her workplace, her profession, and the man with whom she was having an affair. She could remember all other aspects of her life, including her personal identity and her family life. Further probing revealed no evidence of any organic insult that could have prompted her mental state or suggestion of malingering. Over the next 2 days, Mrs. Jones began to recover a considerable portion of her lost memories. She continued individual psychotherapy with the psychiatrist to better understand the factors that had precipitated such an overwhelming psychic response and to explore ways to work through her recent traumatic experience.

trauma treatment. The focus of the second phase is on integrating traumatic material in greater depth. Finally, the third phase is one of resolution, in which the traumatized person is reconnected to ordinary life. Classic free-association suggestions are often the most helpful in understanding factors that interfere with recall and for allowing recall to occur at a pace that the patient can tolerate. Memory accuracy is improved if the clinician asks the patient nonleading questions. Cognitive therapy can also be beneficial. As a patient is more able to correct cognitive distortions, particularly about the meanings of prior trauma, more detailed recall of traumatic events may occur.

There is no known pharmacotherapy for dissociative amnesia other than pharmacologically facilitated interviews. A variety of agents have been used for this purpose, including sodium amobarbital, thiopental (Pentothal), oral benzodiazepines, and amphetamines. Currently, no adequately controlled studies have been conducted that assess the efficacy of any of these agents compared with other treatment methods.

DEPERSONALIZATION DISORDER
Clinical Presentation and Diagnosis

For many years, the ubiquity of depersonalization as a psychiatric symptom obscured its broader recognition as a disorder. Recent research has identified clinical features and neurobiological correlates that distinguish it from other psychiatric disorders with symptoms of depersonalization and validate its standing as a unique disorder. The essential feature is the subjective sense of detachment or estrangement from oneself. An individual may report feeling like an automaton, having little sense of agency, as if in a dream or fog, watching oneself like in a movie, or not being able to feel one's feelings. Patients experiencing depersonalization often have great difficulty expressing what they are feeling and use banal phrases, such as "I feel dead," "nothing seems real," or "I am standing outside of myself." Therefore, depersonalized patients may not adequately convey to the examiner the distress they experience, and accordingly, clinicians may not take the severity of this disorder as seriously as they should. Often depersonalization is accompanied by *derealization*, coined by William Mapother, the sense that the surrounding world appears strange, foreign, or dream-like. It is conceptualized as a dissociative alteration in the perception of the environment. Objects may appear as if viewed from a great distance and two dimensional, without depth or substance. Sounds come from a distance, muffled and distorted. Colors dim and lose their vitality or appear two dimensional.

First described by Maurice Krishnaber in 1872, depersonalization was formally named in 1898 by Ludovic Dugas, who sought to convey "the feeling of loss of ego." When such experiences become persistent or recurrent, depersonalization disorder may be diagnosed. Individuals must have intact reality testing (i.e., know that their sense of unreality is not real), and the depersonalization must not occur exclusively in the context of another psychiatric disorder, a neurologic or other medical disorder, or ongoing substance use. Although in DSM-IV-TR derealization in the absence of depersonalization (which is quite uncommon) is diagnosed as a separate miscellaneous disorder under dissociative disorders NOS, leading experts in the field agree that depersonalization and derealization are not likely to be distinct disorders.

Epidemiology

Transient experiences of depersonalization and derealization are very common in normal and clinical populations. They are the third most commonly reported psychiatric symptoms, after depression and anxiety, with an estimated 1-year prevalence of approximately 20%. Depersonalization can occur transiently in settings of severe stress, trauma, conflict, sleep deprivation, travel to unknown places, or intoxication. Substances most associated with inducing depersonalization are marijuana, hallucinogens, the dissociative anesthetic ketamine, and 3-4 methylenedioxymethamphetamine (Ecstasy). In rare cases, such drug ingestions, even sporadic, can trigger a devastating, chronic depersonalization syndrome. Depersonalization as a disorder is notably rarer than as a symptom, with an estimated lifetime prevalence of 2% to 3%.

Etiology

Traditional psychodynamic formulations have emphasized the disintegration of the ego or cohesive sense of self that occurs with depersonalization. The split between an observing and a participating self can be likened to the division of the intellectual and the emotional self. These explanations stress the role of overwhelmingly painful experiences and conflicts as triggering events. The high rates in normal adolescents and in patients who are conceptualized as having borderline or narcissistic personality organizations are cited as evidence that ego immaturity or ego deficits are predisposing factors. Attention has been drawn to the similarities between depersonalization and obsessive-compulsive symptoms. Similarly, it has long been noted that patients with acute or chronic overwhelming anxiety, panic, or depression can sometimes evolve a clinical picture of chronic depersonalization even when the original condition subsides.

Clinical studies in depersonalization disorder have found elevated childhood interpersonal trauma, especially emotional abuse and emotional neglect, as well as traumatic loss of significant others (Simeon et al., 2001). In some, growing up with a very unstable and traumatizing parent with a severe mental illness has been implicated. In general, the traumas reported by patients with depersonalization disorder tend to be less severe than those typically reported by patients with other dissociative disorders. A substantial number of individuals with depersonalization disorder cannot identify any traumatic or stressful antecedents. Stressors typically viewed as nontraumatic in nature, such as interpersonal, financial, or occupational losses, can also be associated with the onset, as well as with exacerbations, of depersonalization disorder. In addition, chemical stressors, such as marijuana, hallucinogens, and stimulants, have been known to precipitate chronic depersonalization in some people; these individuals may be conceptualized as having a neurobiological or genetic vulnerability.

The epilepsy literature shows a longstanding clinical association between symptoms of depersonalization and derealization and temporal lobe and limbic system dysfunction. In the 1950s, Penfield reported depersonalization symptoms elicited during neurosurgery by stimulation of the superior and middle temporal gyri. In healthy volunteers, elegant experiments have suggested that the out-of-body experience may be subsumed by the inferior parietal lobule. Brain imaging studies in depersonalization disorder itself have suggested altered brain activation patterns in posterior cortical sensory association areas, which may relate to the perceptual alterations and sense of unfamiliarity (Simeon et al., 2000), and prefrontal cortical hyperactivity that overly inhibits limbic activation, which may relate to the hypoemotionality of depersonalization (Lemche et al., 2007).

Differential Diagnosis

The variety of conditions associated with depersonalization as a symptom complicate the differential diagnosis of depersonalization disorder. Therefore, a thorough psychiatric and medical evaluation is essential, including standard laboratory studies, drug screening, an EEG, and brain imaging if there is any suspicion of a lesion. A range of neurologic conditions have been reported as causes and need to be ruled out, including seizure disorders, brain tumors, postconcussive syndrome, metabolic abnormalities, vertigo, Ménière's disease, and sleep apnea. Depersonalization is also common after head injury.

Depersonalization can also be a symptom occurring in the context of panic attacks, social anxiety, depression, and even schizophrenia. A thorough longitudinal history must therefore be obtained because depersonalization disorder is only diagnosed if its duration, course, and extent are clearly independent of these other disorders. Patients with borderline personality disorder may experience transient stress-related dissociation that can primarily take the form of depersonalization and derealization. In this case depersonalization disorder should be diagnosed if the symptoms are too persistent and recurrent, in the judgment of the clinician, to be accounted for by the personality disorder. Finally, depersonalization disorder should not be diagnosed if the symptoms occur in the context of another dissociative disorder with additional dissociative symptoms such as dissociative identity disorder.

Course and Prognosis

Depersonalization after stressful or traumatic experiences or intoxications commonly remits spontaneously after removal from the traumatic circumstances or the end of the episode of intoxication. Depersonalization accompanying mood, psychotic, or anxiety disorders commonly remits with definitive treatment of these conditions. However, sometimes depersonalization does not resolve after resolution of these proximal antecedents; at other times, it can occur without any apparent proximal precipitant and continue, leading to the diagnosis of depersonalization disorder.

Depersonalization disorder can have an episodic, relapsing and remitting, or chronic course. The latter is most common, occurring in two thirds of patients (Simeon et al., 2003). Sometimes the disorder is episodic initially but later becomes chronic. Many patients with chronic depersonalization may have a course characterized by severe impairment in occupational, social, and personal functioning. Average age of onset is in adolescence or young adulthood. Many patients with depersonalization disorder are initially treated for anxiety or mood symptoms, and the primary nature of the depersonalization disorder becomes apparent to the clinician later on, once the anxiety or mood symptoms improve or remit. Over the lifetime, traumatic or stressful events, unfamiliar situations, and high levels of sensory input may exacerbate the disorder.

Treatment

Clinicians caring for patients with depersonalization disorder often find them to be a clinically refractory group. Medication treatment trials to date, which have primarily examined serotonin reuptake inhibitors and lamotrigine, have not found efficacy. Clinical experience suggests that a portion of these patients may respond partially to various groups of psychiatric medications, singly or in combination, such as antidepressants, mood stabilizers, benzodiazepines, stimulants, cognitive enhancers, and opioid inhibitors.

Many different types of psychotherapy, such as psychodynamic, cognitive, cognitive-behavioral, hypnotherapeutic, and supportive, have been used to treat patients with depersonalization disorder. No systematic data exist comparing these modalities. Clinical experience suggests that patients with depersonalization who have the most robust responses to these specific types of standard psychotherapy are those with shorter duration of the disorder, more fluctuant symptoms in duration and intensity, as well as symptoms that can be understood and modulated according to the contexts in which they occur and their internal elaboration. Stress management strategies, distraction techniques, reduction of sensory stimulation, and relaxation training may also be somewhat helpful.

A cognitive behavioral model of the disorder was recently put forth that emphasizes journaling, distraction techniques, reduction of avoidance behaviors, and breaking the vicious cycle of mounting anxiety, fear, and depersonalization (Hunter et al., 2003). In a small study, 30% of patients no longer met criteria for the disorder after such a course of treatment. Some severely impaired patients with depersonalization disorder may require long-term supportive treatment, with the clinician being acutely aware of the patient's interpersonal sensitivity, distress, and sense of hopelessness about the condition.

A CASE OF DEPERSONALIZATION DISORDER

Alisa, a 17-year-old teenager, grew up as an only child in a dysfunctional home. Her father was an alcoholic of whom she was terrified, and her mother was loving but depressed and withdrawn. Alisa had one very close friend, Amanda, to whom she confided all her troubles. When Alisa was 16, her mother was diagnosed with advanced cancer and given little time to live; Alisa did everything she could to care for her. Four months later, Alisa was devastated by the news that Amanda was accidentally hit and killed by a drunk driver. One month later her mother died. During the funeral, Alisa started to feel increasingly unreal and foggy, outside of her body, watching the service like a detached observer. She imagined that she was having a terrible day and that she would wake up the next morning feeling better. Alisa's depersonalization did not lessen by the next day, however, but persisted for several months, at which point she decided to approach her school counselor.

DISSOCIATIVE FUGUE

Clinical Presentation and Diagnosis

Dissociative fugue is the least studied and rarest of the dissociative disorders. The symptoms are reminiscent of both dissociative amnesia and dissociative identity disorder. The essential feature is sudden travel away from one's home and inability to recall some or all of one's past life, accompanied by a confusion about who one is or even assumption of a new identity. In the United States, James described one paradigmatic case of fugue with change of personal identity. Ansel Bourne, an itinerant preacher, disappeared from his home in Providence, Rhode Island, in January 1887, after withdrawing $500 from his bank account to pay some bills. Two months later, he "awoke," finding himself in Norristown, Pennsylvania, where he had been living quietly under the name of A. J. Brown and working as a shopkeeper. He had no memory for the time between his disappearance and his return to the Bourne identity. During the fugue, Bourne apparently behaved "normally."

Etiology

Traumatic circumstances leading to an altered state of consciousness dominated by a wish to flee are thought to be the underlying cause of most fugue episodes. These can include combat, rape, recurrent childhood sexual abuse, massive social dislocations, and natural disasters. They can also include more ordinary life circumstances that are overwhelmingly conflictual, unbearable, and inescapable. In such cases, patients are usually struggling with extreme emotions and impulses, such as overwhelming fear, guilt, or shame, intense incestuous, sexual, suicidal, or violent urges, or a combination of these, that are in conflict with the patient's conscience or ego ideals. Conceptually, dissociation allows people to flee without consciously knowing that they are doing so.

Course and Prognosis

Dissociative fugues have been described to last from days to months. Approximately half of patients report more than one fugue during their lifetime. Although most patients recover most of their autobiographical memory before the onset of fugue, in rare cases amnesia can be refractory.

Differential Diagnosis

In dissociative fugue, there is *purposeful* and considerable travel away from one's home or customary place of daily activities, which differs from the confused or aimless wandering during an episode of dissociative amnesia. Patients with dissociative identity disorder may have symptoms of dissociative fugue, usually recurrently throughout their lives, but they have additional dissociative symptoms as well. In complex partial seizures, patients have been noted to exhibit wandering, semipurposeful behavior, or both during the ictal or postictal state, for which there is subsequent amnesia. Serial, telemetric, or both EEGs usually show abnormalities associated with behavioral pathology. Wandering behavior during a variety of general medical conditions, toxin-related and substance-related disorders, delirium, dementia, and organic amnestic syndromes could

A CASE OF DISSOCIATIVE FUGUE

Mr. Allen was a 48-year-old respected lawyer who lived with his wife and four children. After disappearing one day, he was found 2 months later in a distant city, living under a different name. He was living in a local church residence and had no memory of his past or who he was. He was returned home and started treatment; it was gradually uncovered that he had been feeling intensely unhappy with his marriage, children, and job over the past several years. Mr. Allen's earlier life was notable for an isolated and cold upbringing, as well as horrific combat experiences that he had never before shared. His dissociative fugue episode may be conceptualized as the only escape, short of suicide, for a man who could no longer bear his life as it was but was prevented by complex dynamics of guilt, shame, and rage from actively changing it.

theoretically be confused with dissociative fugue. A full medical and neurologic evaluation is indicated in these patients, including physical examination, laboratory tests, and toxicologic screening. Serial or telemetric EEGs should also be conducted to exclude a seizure disorder. Malingering of dissociative fugue may occur in individuals who are attempting to flee a situation involving legal, financial, or personal difficulties, as well as in soldiers who are attempting to avoid combat or unpleasant military duties.

Treatment

Dissociative fugue is usually treated with an eclectic, psychodynamically informed psychotherapy that focuses on helping the patient recover memory for identity and recent experiences (Loewenstein, 2001). Hypnotherapy and pharmacologically facilitated interviews are frequently necessary adjunctive techniques to assist with memory recovery. Therapy should be carefully paced, following the three-phase approach discussed previously. Once initial stabilization is achieved, subsequent therapy is focused on helping the patient regain memory for identity, life circumstances, and personal history. During this process, extreme emotions related to trauma, severe psychological conflict, or both may emerge that need to be addressed. Clinicians should be prepared for the emergence of suicidal ideation or self-destructive ideas and impulses as the traumatic or stressful prefugue circumstances are revealed.

DISSOCIATIVE IDENTITY DISORDER

According to DSM-IV-TR, dissociative identity disorder, previously known as *multiple personality disorder*, is characterized by the presence of two or more distinct identities or personality states. These recurrently take control of the person's behavior, resulting in large memory gaps that cannot be explained by ordinary forgetfulness. Each of these identity states (also referred to as *alters, self-states, alter identities*, or *parts*) has its own relatively distinct and enduring way of perceiving, relating to, and thinking about the self and the world.

Clinical Presentation

Patients with dissociative identity disorder often present in highly complex as well as covert ways that can make early diagnosis challenging and often result in years of misdiagnosis, especially by less well-informed clinicians. Hallmark symptoms at presentation are summarized in the following text (Kluft, 2005; Loewenstein, 1991).

Amnesia Symptoms

As part of the general mental status examination, clinicians should routinely inquire about experiences of losing time or major gaps in the continuity of recall for personal information. Patients rarely spontaneously report these experiences; therefore, they require active inquiry by the interviewer to be uncovered. In some instances, patients report coming to or waking up in the midst of some activity with little or no recall of how they came to be involved in that activity. In other instances, patients find evidence of having done or acquired things for which they have no recall. Dissociative time loss experiences are too extensive to be explained by normal forgetting and typically have sharply demarcated onsets and offsets. Patients often report significant gaps in autobiographical memory, especially for childhood events, that do not fit the normal expected decline in autobiographical recall for younger ages.

Process Symptoms

Dissociative process symptoms include depersonalization and derealization, dissociative hallucinations, passive influence and interference experiences, and dissociative cognitions. Patients frequently report feeling spaced out or disconnected from themselves and others and may report profound out-of-body experiences. Dissociative auditory hallucinations commonly take the form of voices heard as originating from within the person (pseudohallucinations), not from outside. Individual hallucinated voices typically have distinctive age and gender attributes. Patients generally recognize that the voices are hallucinations and may be reluctant to reveal their existence for fear of being considered psychotic. Hallucinated voices often come to be identified with specific alter personality states. Visual hallucinations typically take the form of detailed images with traumatic or frightening content. Tactile, gustatory, and olfactory hallucinations may also occur, as well as intrusive posttraumatic flashbacks. Analgesia (i.e., not feeling pain) is also common.

Passive influence and interference symptoms include many first-rank Schneiderian symptoms such as audible thoughts, voices arguing with each other, influences playing on the body, thought withdrawal and insertion, and made feelings, impulses, and actions. These symptoms were once considered to be pathognomonic of schizophrenia, but they can also be found in patients with affective, organic, and dissociative disorders. In dissociative identity disorder, the agents of the passive influence symptoms are usually experienced as internal, not external as in psychotic disorders. Patients with dissociative identity disorder generally do not have delusional explanations for these experiences.

The recognition that dissociative patients frequently manifest subtle, but often clinically significant, cognitive impairments emerges from clinical research with psychological and cognitive test batteries (Brand et al., 2006; Dorahy, 2001).

Dissociative Alterations in Identity

Clinically, dissociative alterations in identity may first be manifested by odd first-person plural or third-person singular or plural self-references. In addition, patients may refer to themselves using their own first names or make depersonalized self-references. Patients often describe a profound sense of concretized internal division or personified internal conflicts between parts of themselves. In some instances, these parts may have proper names or may be designated by their predominate affect or function, for example, "the angry one" or "the protector."

A set of behaviors, collectively referred to as *switching behaviors*, may be manifest during evaluation or therapy sessions, including intrainterview amnesias, in which the patient does not recall or is confused about the session. A variety of physical signs, including pronounced upward eye rolls or bursts of rapid blinking and eyelid fluttering, may also occur. The patient's tone of voice and manner of speaking, posture, and demeanor may show marked alteration. These cognitive, behavioral, and physical shifts are manifestations of alter personality switching, overlap and interference between alter states, or both. These alters can best be conceptualized as distinct self-states, each organized around a prevailing affect, sense of self, body image, state-dependent autobiographical memories, and limited behavioral repertoires. The set of alter personality states, usually referred to as the *personality system*, constitutes the personality of the individual.

Epidemiology

A conservative analysis of epidemiologic data suggests a prevalence of approximately 1.3%, and dissociative identity disorder is five to nine times more commonly diagnosed in women. Reasons may include gender-related differences in types of maltreatment, differences in clinical presentations, and the possibility that more men with dissociative alterations in identity end up in the criminal justice system.

Etiology

Dissociative identity disorder is attributed to the interaction of overwhelming stress (typically extreme childhood mistreatment), insufficient nurturing and compassion in response to overwhelmingly hurtful experiences during childhood, and dissociative capacity (ability to uncouple one's memories, perceptions, or identity from conscious awareness). Children are not born with a sense of a unified identity—it develops from many sources and experiences. In overwhelmed children, many parts of what should have blended together remain separate (Putnam, 1998). In contrast to most children who achieve cohesive, complex appreciation of themselves and others, severely mistreated children may go through phases in which different perceptions and emotions are kept segregated. Such children may develop an ability to escape the mistreatment by "going away" or "retreating" into their own minds. Each developmental phase may be used to generate different selves (Kluft, 2007).

Chronic and severe abuse (physical, sexual, or emotional) during childhood is almost always reported in patients with dissociative identity disorder, ranging from 85% to 97% of cases in various studies (Ross, 1997). Early life experiences resulting in severe disturbances of attachment with the primary caregiver, such as disorganized attachment, have also been strongly implicated (Lyons-Ruth et al., 2006). A minority of patients were not abused but experienced important early losses (such as the death of a parent), serious medical illnesses with repeated painful surgical procedures, or other overwhelmingly stressful events.

The few neurobiological studies in dissociative identity disorder have documented brain alterations related to the disorder, such as widely different brain circuits activated in the "apparently normal" versus "traumatic" identity states by traumatic memories (Reinders et al., 2006), as well as smaller hippocampal and amygdalar volumes (Vermetten et al., 2006). Therefore the neurobiology of the "diunity" of the mind, body, and brain has begun to be elucidated (Frewen and Lanius, 2006).

Differential Diagnosis

On average, more than 6 years pass between first psychiatric contact and the diagnosis of dissociative identity disorder. Although often misportrayed as flamboyant and overt, only a small minority of patients present this way. Most are reticent about revealing their dissociative symptoms, especially hallucinations, amnesia, and identity divisions, and initially present as relatively inhibited and obsessional, with many affective and somatic complaints. A subgroup of patients with dissociative identity disorder shows interpersonal dynamics consistent with borderline personality disorder. Very frequently PTSD comprises a secondary diagnosis. The presence of auditory hallucinations, disturbed thinking and behavior, confusion due to amnesic gaps, and Schneiderian first-rank symptoms contribute to the misdiagnosis of schizophrenia in approximately half of patients with dissociative identity disorder at some point in their psychiatric histories. Rapid changes in affect associated with alter personality switching often lead to a misdiagnosis of rapid-cycling bipolar disorder or schizoaffective disorder. Concerns about factitious and malingered dissociative identity disorder are common. A mixture of factors can lead to this presentation, including misdiagnosis, actual factitiousness, and assumption of a social role of an abuse victim or a patient with dissociative identity disorder. Indicators of falsified or imitative dissociative identity disorder include those typical of other factitious or malingering presentations such as symptom exaggeration, lies, use of symptoms to excuse antisocial behavior (e.g., amnesia only for bad behavior), amplification of symptoms when under observation, refusal to allow collateral contacts, and legal problems. Patients with genuine dissociative identity disorder are usually confused, conflicted, ashamed, and distressed by their symptoms and trauma history. Patients with nongenuine dissociative identity disorder frequently show little dysphoria about their disorder.

Course and Prognosis

Little is known about the natural history of untreated dissociative identity disorder. Limited evidence suggests that the disorder becomes less overt over time, although severe symptoms can persist into older age. A relapsing and remitting course is common, and patients can more or less successfully mask or suppress symptoms for periods of time. Individuals with untreated dissociative identity disorder often continue involvement in abusive relationships or violent subcultures, which can result in repeated trauma for themselves as well as trauma for their children, leading to intergenerational transmission of the disorder. Some patients with dissociative identity disorder die by suicide or as a result of their intentional or accidental high-risk

A CASE OF DISSOCIATIVE IDENTITY DISORDER

Mrs. Hirsch, a 37-year-old married woman, was employed as a local librarian in the small town where she lived. She discovered her 5-year-old daughter "playing doctor" with several neighborhood children, and although this event was of little consequence, Mrs. Hirsch became fearful that her daughter would be molested and therefore was increasingly depressed, panicky, and somatic. She withdrew from her husband, found it harder to take care of her children, and deteriorated at work. Finally she met with a psychiatrist and described dense amnesia for the first 13 years of her life. For as long as she could remember, she had had an imaginary protector companion. She also heard voices in her head of several women and children as well as her father's derogatory voice. She reported that since age 13 her life was punctuated by repeated episodes of amnesia for work, her marriage, the birth of her children, and her sex life with her husband. Her husband noted that sometimes she spoke like a child and at other times would adopt a Southern accent. Questioned more closely about her early life, the patient appeared to enter a trance and stated in a childlike voice, "I just do not want to be locked in the closet." Over the course of long-term psychotherapy, the patient, in the alter identities, described chronic physical abuse, sexual abuse, and emotional torment by her father.

behaviors. Patients range widely in their level of functioning. Prognosis is poorer in patients with comorbid psychotic disorders, borderline personality disorder, severe medical illnesses, refractory substance abuse and eating disorders, significant antisocial personality features, criminal activity, and ongoing perpetration of abuse and repeated victimization.

Treatment

Current treatment approaches have evolved considerably with the conceptualization of dissociative identity disorder as a complex developmental trauma disorder and are well delineated (Chu et al., 2005; Kluft, 2001; Loewenstein, 2006; Putnam, 1989). Appropriate treatment follows a phasic model that is the current standard of care for many trauma-spectrum disorders. The phases include symptom stabilization; optional focused, in-depth attention to traumatic material; and integration or reintegration, in which the patient with dissociative identity disorder moves more completely away from a life based on chronic trauma and victimization.

Intensive psychotherapy, twice or thrice weekly, is the golden standard for treating these patients. Integration of the identity states is the most desirable outcome. For patients who cannot or will not strive for integration, treatment aims to facilitate cooperation and collaboration among the identities and to reduce symptoms. The first priority of psychotherapy is to stabilize the patient and ensure safety before evaluating traumatic experiences and exploring problematic identities. Some patients benefit from hospitalization during various phases of treatment, in which dangerous symptoms or comorbidities can more effectively be stabilized or continuous support and monitoring can be provided as painful memories are addressed. Hypnosis is often used to explore traumatic memories and diffuse their effect. It may also help with accessing the identities, facilitating communication between them, and stabilizing and interpreting them. As the reasons for the dissociations are addressed, therapy can move to the point at which the patient's selves, relationships, and social functioning can be reconnected, integrated, and rehabilitated. Some integration occurs spontaneously over the course of treatment, as the psychological need to hold on to the dissociated states lessens.

Although no medications to date are known to have a direct antidissociative effect, they are widely used to help manage symptoms of depression, anxiety, impulsivity, and substance abuse (Loewenstein, 2005). Some medications most commonly used as adjuvants during psychotherapy of these patients are antidepressants to assist mood, anxiety, and obsessive-compulsive disorders and PTSD; mood stabilizers for more pronounced mood swings; benzodiazepines for sleep and overwhelming anxiety; atypical antipsychotics for disorganizing anxiety and quasi-psychotic thinking; clonidine or prazocin for symptoms of hyperarousal; and opioid antagonists for numbing symptoms and addictions.

DISSOCIATIVE DISORDER NOT OTHERWISE SPECIFIED

The DSM-IV-TR category of dissociative disorder NOS covers all the conditions characterized by a primary dissociative response that do not meet diagnostic criteria for one of the other dissociative disorders described previously. Therefore, dissociative disorder NOS is a heterogeneous collection of dissociative reactions, some of which are common expressions of distress in other cultures but relatively rare in Western societies.

One major subgroup in this category, often clinically diagnosed in the West as much or more than dissociative identity disorder, might be viewed as a "milder" variant of the latter disorder. These patients are similar in clinical presentation, life history, clinical course, and treatment response to those with dissociative identity disorder but their sense of subjective self-fragmentation does not meet full DSM-IV-TR criteria for alter identities, or they do not present with prominent amnesia for their alter identities.

Also included within dissociative disorder NOS are the many cultural variants of dissociative trance. Anthropologists have identified forms of dissociation in every culture examined. In some instances, it takes the form of specific trance state disorders; in others, it is manifest in religious rites and rituals; and, in still others, it is manifest in traditional healing practices. All of these forms of dissociation are common in many non-Western societies.

Furthermore, DSM-IV-TR includes under dissociative disorder NOS those dissociative reactions elicited by extremely coercive, persuasive practices such as torture, brainwashing, thought reform, mind control, and indoctrination intended to induce an individual to relinquish basic political, social, or religious beliefs in exchange for antithetical ideas and beliefs. Finally, Ganser syndrome, a rare and poorly understood condition characterized by giving approximate answers, is also included in this category.

CONTROVERSIES ABOUT DISSOCIATIVE DISORDERS

Confusion and controversy surround the dissociative disorders. Current controversies have their origins in 19th century disagreements about the nature of "hysteria." In modern U.S. psychiatric nosology, the classical hysteria concept has given rise to a number of DSM disorders: somatoform disorders, dissociative disorders, PTSD, anorexia nervosa, and histrionic and borderline personality disorders.

When viewed within a larger sociopolitical perspective, dissociation theory intersects with many of the most controversial social issues of modern times. Even in the 19th century, contention centered on whether hysteria was related to traumatic experiences or was caused by suggestive influences, among other explanations. Recent systematic research consistently has found a robust relationship between dissociation and traumatic experiences. The role of trauma in Western culture, particularly intergenerational violence and sexual abuse, crosses into historically taboo subjects such as rape, incest, child abuse, and domestic violence and their actual prevalence in society. In addition, the study of trauma leads to larger legal, social, and cultural questions related to peace and war, the meaning of violence in society, and even varying religious views about the relationship among men, women, and children and the nature of the family.

In modern psychiatry and psychology, these disorders are the focus of controversies that include the longstanding debates between mentalists and behaviorists, "psychodynamically oriented" and "biologically oriented" clinicians, various researchers in cognitive psychology, cognitive researchers and clinical researchers and practitioners, and different theoretical schools at odds over the nature of hypnosis. Some fundamentalist Christian clinicians even have viewed demonic possession as part of the differential diagnosis of dissociative disorders.

Issues here include the significance of early trauma for human psychopathology, the existence of "unconscious" mental life and "intrapsychic defenses" such as "repression," the nature of memory, and the nature of hypnosis and whether it involves altered states of consciousness. Further, dissociative amnesias and delayed recall of traumatic events raise difficult-to-answer questions about the reliability of traumatic memory. The latter issue has been a significant controversy in the psychiatric community that has spilled over into the courts and the popular media, arenas where dispassionate scientific inquiry is unlikely to be the central concern of the participants.

From the middle of the 19th century to the present, the popular media has nurtured public fascination with various forms of dissociation, especially multiple personality. Robert Lewis Stevenson's *The Strange Case of Dr. Jekyll and Mr. Hyde* is the most well known. Other popular 19th century novels and plays focused on fugue, amnesia, and crimes committed under the influence of hypnosis or in somnambulistic states. From at least the 1930s onward, sensational reports of patients with generalized dissociative amnesia and/or fugue were featured in the daily newspapers. Similar cases still periodically appear in the news when amnestic patients are found and cannot be identified.

In the late 20th century, popular accounts of multiple personality such as *The Three Faces of Eve, Sybil*, and a recent spate of similar first-person accounts continued in this vein. The widespread use of multiple personality as a fictional plot device—generally to give a bizarre twist to a story—has contributed to the public and professional confusion that surrounds this disorder. Similarly, amnesia for life circumstances and for trauma is also a recurrent story mechanism in contemporary novels, films, and television—and almost never portrayed accurately. Media stereotyping occurs for many forms of mental illness, but the distortions typical in most fictional depictions of dissociative disorders are particularly misleading.

Highly publicized criminal and civil cases such as the "Hillside Strangler," the Franklin murder case, and the Ramona case have brought additional media attention to claims of multiple personality, amnesia, and "recovered memory." These contentious cases, with their warring academic experts and sensationalized media depictions, have also fueled popular stereotyping of dissociative disorders. Media "spin" about these cases has often been inaccurate and misleading.

For example, dissociative identity disorder, formally known as *multiple personality disorder*, is often confused with schizophrenia in the popular media and culture. Although some symptoms of dissociative identity disorder superficially resemble those of schizophrenia (e.g., hearing voices), dissociative identity disorder and schizophrenia are unrelated conditions. People with schizophrenia do not develop "split personalities," and they have a different symptom picture and clinical presentation from patients with dissociative identity disorder.

Because of all this, one commentator ruefully observed that most clinicians get the bulk of their training about dissociation and dissociative disorders from the media. For the foreseeable future, because of the complexity of the social, cultural, philosophical, and political issues these conditions evoke, it is unlikely that debates about them will remain purely in the academic arena.

CONTROVERSIES ABOUT TRAUMA AND MEMORY

A major recent controversy, played out primarily in the media and the courts, involves the question of whether traumatized individuals can, at one time, fail to recall some or all of a traumatic experience and then recall it later. This idea was not controversial when soldiers with posttraumatic disorders frequently reported amnesia for wartime trauma (Sargent and Slater, 1941). However, controversy flared with court cases involving claims of childhood sexual abuse with alleged perpetrators sued or prosecuted on the basis of reported delayed recall of these traumas. In the alternative form, "accused" parents and/or "recanting" former victims have sued mental health providers, alleging malpractice and/or alienation of affections based on the notion that there is no such thing as dissociation, amnesia, "repression" of memory, and dissociative disorders. These cases have been the subjects of considerable media attention.

There appears to be professional consensus currently that individuals can show delayed recall for traumatic experiences. However, controversy surrounds the purported mechanism for this phenomenon. Some ascribe this to specific posttraumatic memory difficulties such as dissociation. Others do not support the notion of a "special" mechanism for amnesia, ascribing it to "normal forgetting," deliberate attempts to suppress recall of the memories, and/or refusal to disclose memories that are accessible (Brown et al., 1998, 1999b; Dalenberg, 2006). In general, memories of trauma with delayed recall have not been shown to be more or less accurate than memories that have been reportedly "continuous"; each can be shown by independent corroboration to be essentially accurate, partially accurate, or confabulated.

Most research shows a relationship between dissociative disorders and traumatic experiences. An alternative etiological model for dissociative identity disorder posits that dissociative identity disorder is not an authentic condition but one created through "iatrogenic" factors. "Iatrogenic" defines disorders or symptoms that arise due to actions of a practitioner, such as a physician, psychologist, or therapist. In the iatrogenesis or sociocognitive model of the etiology of dissociative identity disorder (Lilienfeld et al., 1999; Spanos, 1996), suggestive influences by therapists who strongly believe in dissociative identity disorder and "repressed memories" for trauma are posited to be the iatrogenic factors. This model posits that dissociative identity disorder develops as a learned social role in patients who are suggestible, "fantasy prone," or highly hypnotizable and who may show features of borderline personality disorder. According to the sociocognitive model, naive therapists induce dissociative identity disorder behavior in susceptible patients by overtly or covertly cueing the patient to act like someone with multiple personalities. This model is an analog of the sociocognitive model for hypnosis, which hypothesizes that hypnosis is not caused by an altered state of consciousness but only by a learned social role (Spanos, 1996).

A major controversy exists among professionals about the validity of these two models. This controversy has spilled into the media and has been an issue in legal cases in which plaintiffs have sued practitioners, alleging "implantation" of false memories of childhood maltreatment and/or iatrogenic creation of dissociative identity disorder (Brown et al., 1998).

Despite this controversy, only limited research data support the sociocognitive model for dissociative identity disorder (Brown et al., 1999a; Loewenstein, 2007), and no research study of a clinical population has attempted to test this model. Proponents of the sociocognitive model have raised questions about the validity of the self-reports of childhood trauma from patients with dissociative identity disorder. However, recent studies including large samples of maltreated children with dissociative disorders as well as intensively validated case studies provide independent corroboration of patients' reports of maltreatment (Hornstein and Putnam, 1992; Lewis et al., 1997).

Clinical Pearls

- In the first psychiatric interview with a new patient, the clinician must always ask about traumatic stress history.
- Two nonleading, broad questions can help to elicit trauma history:
  - "Did anything terrible, overwhelming, or traumatic ever happen to you as a child or adult?"
  - "What is the worst, most traumatic thing that ever happened to you?"
- Dissociation symptoms should be asked about in a first interview even in the absence of a known trauma history.
- A question to inquire about depersonalization/derealization is "Do you ever feel detached from yourself, unreal, like in a fog or dream?"
- A question to inquire about dissociative amnesia is "Do you ever lose time, or find yourself in a different place without knowing why or how?"
- A question to inquire about identity states is "Do you ever feel as if you are somehow more than one person, or have others told you that you act like a totally different person?"
- In patients presenting with combinations of mood disorders, anxiety disorders, questionable psychotic symptoms, eating disorders, substance use disorders, impulsivity, and interpersonal difficulties, the clinician must consider early life trauma and dissociative disorders in the differential.
- There is no antidissociative drug to date. All dissociative disorders are treated primarily with psychotherapy.

Self-Assessment Questions and Answers

14-1. Mr. Jones is a 40-year-old man who was taken to the emergency room by his wife. He appeared confused and distraught and could not remember anything that had taken place over the past day. His wife reported that the day before he had found out that his brother had terminal cancer. Which of the following would need to be ruled out before making a diagnosis of dissociative amnesia?

A. Alcohol intoxication

B. Alcohol intoxication, delirium, and stroke

C. Delirium

D. Depersonalization

E. Stroke

Before an individual's amnesia can be attributed to psychogenic causes (e.g., dissociative amnesia), all medical causes must be excluded, and in Mr. Jones' case, alcohol intoxication, delirium, and stroke are such medical etiologies. *Answer: B*

14-2. Ann had seen her new psychiatrist over several sessions when she started revealing curious symptoms such as feeling foggy or dead in her body, finding new shoes and clothes in her closet, and losing several hours of time once a week or more. Which of the following dissociative symptoms was Ann describing or inferring?

A. Amnesia

B. Depersonalization

C. Identity alteration

D. Amnesia and depersonalization

E. Amnesia, depersonalization, and identity alteration

14-3. Ann's most likely diagnosis, given the information above, is:

A. Depersonalization disorder

B. Dissociative amnesia

C. Dissociative fugue

D. Dissociative identity disorder

E. Schizophrenia

Patients with dissociative identity disorder experience the entire constellation of dissociative symptoms, although they may not report all of them to their doctor concurrently or over such a brief time period as Ann, especially if the right questions are not asked by the clinician. *Answers: E, D*

14-4. Which of the following is true?

A. Depersonalization cannot be triggered by ingesting drugs.

B. Dissociative amnesia must be precipitated by multiple overwhelming traumatic events.

C. Dissociative fugue is the most common of the dissociative disorders.

D. Dissociative identities can be viewed as a developmental failure to develop a cohesive self.

E. Only fluoxetine has proven efficacy for treating dissociative symptoms.

Children are not born with a sense of a unified identity. Compared with most children, who achieve cohesive, complex appreciation of themselves and others, severely mistreated children may keep different perceptions and emotions segregated and develop an ability to escape mistreatment by "retreating" into their own minds. Each developmental phase may be used to generate different selves. Depersonalization can be triggered by ingesting drugs such as marijuana and hallucinogens. Dissociative amnesia can be precipitated by a single, overwhelming traumatic event. Dissociative fugue is by far the rarest of dissociative disorders. Although solid epidemiological data do not exist, it is estimated approximately at 1/10,000. No medication has proven efficacy for treating dissociative symptoms. *Answer: D*

14-5. Which of the following is true of depersonalization symptoms?

A. Depersonalization symptoms are most often transient in the general population.

B. Depersonalization symptoms are not typically accompanied by derealization symptoms.

C. Individuals commonly have impaired reality testing about their depersonalization symptoms.

D. Depersonalization disorder does not relapse or remit.

E. Average age of onset is in middle age.

Depersonalization symptoms typically are accompanied by derealization symptoms. By definition, if individuals do not have the knowledge that their depersonalization symptoms are not "real" but rather are "as if" experiences, the condition would fall in the psychotic spectrum, such as a person who did not just have the feeling that she was living a dream but who truly believed her life to be a dream. Depersonalization disorder can have an episodic, relapsing and remitting, or chronic course; the latter is most common. Average age of onset is in adolescence or young adulthood. *Answer: A*

References

American Psychiatric Association. *Diagnostic and statistical manual of mental disorders*, 4th ed, text revision. Washington, DC: American Psychiatric Association; 2000.

Bernstein EM, Putnam FW. Development, reliability, and validity of a dissociation scale. *J Nerv Ment Dis*. 1986;174:727–735.

Brand B, Armstrong JA, Loewenstein RJ. Psychological assessment of patients with dissociative identity disorder. *Psychiatr Clin North Am.* 2006;29:145–168.

Brown D, Scheflin AW, Hammond DC. *Memory, trauma, treatment, and the law.* New York: Norton; 1998.

Brown DW, Frischholz EJ, Scheflin AW. Iatrogenic dissociative identity disorder: An evaluation of the scientific evidence. *J Am Acad Psychiatry Law.* 1999a;27:549–638.

Brown DW, Scheflin AW, Whitfield CL. Recovered memories: The current weight of the evidence in science and in the courts. *J Am Acad Psychiatry Law.* 1999b;27:5–156.

Chu JA, Loewenstein RJ, Dell PF, et al. Guidelines for treating dissociative identity disorder in adults. *J Trauma Diss.* 2005;6:69–149.

Dalenberg CJ. Recovered memory and the Daubert criteria: Recovered memory as professionally tested, peer reviewed, and accepted in the relevant scientific community. *Trauma Violence Abuse.* 2006;7:274–311.

Dorahy M. Dissociative identity disorder and memory dysfunction: The current state of experimental research and its future directions. *Clin Psychol Rev.* 2001;5:771–795.

Freud S, Breuer J. *Studien über Hysterie.* 1895.

Frewen PA, Lanius RA. Neurobiology of dissociation: Unity and disunity in mind-body-brain. *Psychiatr Clin North Am.* 2006;29:113–128.

Freyd JJ. *Betrayal trauma: The logic of forgetting childhood abuse.* Cambridge: Harvard University Press; 1996.

Hornstein N, Putnam FW. Clinical phenomenology of child and adolescent dissociative disorders. *J Am Acad Child Adolesc Psychiatry.* 1992;31:1077–1085.

Hunter ECM, Phillips ML, Chalder T, et al. Depersonalisation disorder: A cognitive-behavioural conceptualization. *Behav Res Ther.* 2003;41:1451–1467.

van Ijzendoorn MH, Schuengel C. The measurement of dissociation in normal and clinical populations: Meta-analytic validation of the Dissociative Experiences Scale (DES). *Clin Child Fam Psychol Rev.* 1996;16:365–382.

Janet P. *The mental state of hystericals.* New York: G.P. Putnam's Sons; 1901.

Johnson JG, Cohen P, Kasen S, et al. Dissociative disorders among adults in the community, impaired functioning, and axis I and II comorbidity. *J Psychiatr Res.* 2006;40:131–140.

Kluft RP. Dissociative identity disorder. In: Gabbard GO, ed. *Treatment of psychiatric disorders*, 3rd ed, Vol. 2. Washington, DC: American Psychiatric Press; 2001:1653–1693.

Kluft RP. Diagnosing dissociative identity disorder. *Psychiatr Ann.* 2005;35:633–643.

Kluft RP. Applications of innate affect theory to the understanding and treatment of dissociative identity disorder. In: Vermetten E, Dorahy M, Spiegel D, eds. *Traumatic dissociation.* Washington, DC: American Psychiatric Press; 2007:301–316.

Lemche E, Surquladze SA, Giampietro VP, et al. Limbic and prefrontal responses to facial emotion expressions in depersonalization. *Neuroreport.* 2007:473–477.

Lewis DO, Yeager CA, Swica Y, et al. Objective documentation of child abuse and dissociation in 12 murderers with dissociative identity disorder. *Am J Psychiatry.* 1997;154:1703–1710.

Lilienfeld SO, Kirsch I, Sarbin TR, et al. Dissociative identity disorder and the sociocognitive model: Recalling the lessons of the past. *Psychol Bull.* 1999;125:507–523.

Loewenstein RJ. An office mental status examination for chronic complex dissociative symptoms and multiple personality disorder. *Psychiatr Clin North Am.* 1991;14:567–604.

Loewenstein RJ. Dissociative amnesia and dissociative fugue. In: Gabbard GO, ed. *Treatment of psychiatric disorders*, 3rd ed., Vol. 2. Washington, DC: American Psychiatric Press; 2001:1625.

Loewenstein RJ. Psychopharmacologic treatments for dissociative identity disorder. *Psychiatr Ann.* 2005; 35:666–673.

Loewenstein RJ. DID 101: A hands-on clinical guide to the stabilization phase of dissociative identity disorder treatment. *Psychiatr Clin North Am.* 2006;29:305–332.

Loewenstein RJ. Dissociative identity disorder: Issues in the iatrogenesis controversy. In: Vermetten E, Dorahy M, Spiegel D, eds. *Traumatic dissociation.* Washington, DC: American Psychiatric Press; 2007:275–299.

Lyons-Ruth K, Dutra L, Schuder MR, et al. From infant attachment disorganization to adult dissociation: Relational adaptations or traumatic experiences? *Psychiatr Clin North Am.* 2006;29:63–86.

Morgan CA, Hazlett G, Wang S, et al. Symptoms of dissociation in humans experiencing acute, uncontrollable stress: A prospective investigation. *Am J Psychiatry.* 2001;158:1239–1247.

Prince M. *The dissociation of a personality: A biographical study of abnormal psychology*, 2nd ed. New York: Longmans, Green and Co; 1908.

Putnam FW. *Diagnosis and treatment of multiple personality disorder*. New York: Guilford; 1989.

Putnam FW. *Dissociation in children and adolescents: A developmental perspective*. New York: Guilford; 1998.

Reinders AA, Nijenhuis ER, Quak J, et al. Psychobiological characteristics of dissociative identity disorder: A symptom provocation study. *Biol Psychiatry*. 2006;60:730–740.

Ross CA. *Dissociative identity disorder: Diagnosis, clinical features, and treatment of multiple personality*. New York: John Wiley & Sons; 1997:109.

Sargent W, Slater E. Amnesic syndromes in war. *Proc R Soc Med*. 1941;34:757–764.

Spanos NP. *Multiple identities and false memories: A sociocognitive perspective*. Washington, DC: American Psychological Association; 1996.

Simeon D, Guralnik O, Hazlett E, et al. Feeling unreal: A PET study of depersonalization disorder. *Am J Psychiatry*. 2000;157:1782–1788.

Simeon D, Guralnik O, Schmeidler J, et al. The role of childhood interpersonal trauma in depersonalization disorder. *Am J Psychiatry*. 2001;158:1027–1033.

Simeon D, Knutelska M, Nelson D, et al. Feeling unreal: A depersonalization disorder update of 117 cases. *J Clin Psychiatry*. 2003;64:990–997.

Steinberg M. *Handbook for the assessment of dissociation: A clinical guide*. Washington, DC: American Psychiatric Press; 1995.

Vermetten E, Schmahl C, Lindner S, et al. Hippocampal and amygdalar volumes in dissociative identity disorder. *Am J Psychiatry*. 2006;163:630–636.

Vermetten E, Dorahy M, Spiegel D, eds. *Traumatic dissociation*. Washington, DC: American Psychiatric Press; 2007.

Waller NG, Ross CA. The prevalence and biometric structure of pathological dissociation in the general population: Taxometric and behavioral genetic findings. *J Abnorm Psychol*. 1997;106:499–510.

Sexual and Gender Identity Disorders

Identification of sexual and gender identity disorders starts with taking an adequate sexual history, but that has proven to be a challenging task for both patients and clinicians. A patient survey showed that 71% of respondents believed that physicians would dismiss concerns about sexual problems, and 68% were afraid of embarrassing their physicians by discussing sexual dysfunction (Marwick, 1999).

Barriers to communication between patients and clinicians include fear of embarrassing each other, general unease with the topic, and difficulty in wording questions and answers. Other system-related barriers include preservation of confidentiality, concerns about medical record documentation of private details, and legal issues stemming from offending patients or misperceived sexual advances. How to take a sexual history will be further detailed in this chapter.

The *Diagnostic and Statistical Manual*, Fourth Edition, Text Revision (DSM-IV-TR) (American Psychiatric Association, 2000), identifies the following sexual and gender identity disorders: sexual desire disorders (hypoactive sexual desire disorder and sexual aversion disorder), sexual arousal disorders, orgasmic disorders, sexual pain disorders, paraphilias (Kafka, 1994), and gender identity disorders (Zucker, 2004). This chapter will discuss each of these disorders.

EPIDEMIOLOGY

According to a 2000 survey (Rosen, 2000), sexual disorders are more prevalent in women (43%) than in men (31%). In men, premature ejaculation is the most common disorder (one third of men report difficulties), followed by male erectile disorder (one fourth of men report difficulties). In women, hypoactive sexual desire disorder is the most common (one third of women report difficulties), followed by female orgasmic disorder (one fourth of women report difficulties).

ETIOLOGY

Various factors play different roles in the etiology of sexual disorders. This mandates the use of the biopsychosocial model for evaluating sexual disorders, which identifies the factors that predispose, precipitate, and/or perpetuate sexual disorders (see Table 15-1).

Biological factors include genetic predisposition, medical problems (systemic and local), and effects of substances (e.g., alcohol, illicit drugs, medications, and herbal supplements), whereas psychosocial factors include psychiatric disorders, conflict within the sexual partnership, and history of sexual and nonsexual traumas.

BIOPSYCHOSOCIAL EVALUATION

The biopsychosocial evaluation comprises evaluating individuals and couples to identify predisposing, precipitating, and perpetuating factors of sexual dysfunction. The evaluation begins with appropriate history taking, followed by a thorough physical examination and obtaining suitable laboratory tests, and ends with reaching an accurate formulation and diagnosis. While going through this entire procedure, the clinician should have in mind a clear target of evaluating biological factors of sexual dysfunction (medical problems or substance effects) before declaring that the psychosocial factors are the main culprit behind the individual's sexual dysfunction. This is crucial because of the differences in the management and prognosis of those two categories.

TABLE 15-1	**Biopsychosocial Evaluation: Identification of Predisposing, Precipitating, and Perpetuating Factors of Sexual Disorders**

I. Evaluation of the individual
  A. Biological factors
    1. Genetic predisposition
    2. Medical problems
      (a) Systemic: diabetes mellitus, anemia, hypertension, hyperlipidemia, heart disease, atherosclerosis, aneurysm, and smoking
      (b) Hormonal and endocrinal: hypothyroidism or hyperthyroidism, hypothalamic-pituitary axis dysregulation (manifested by high or low hormone levels), hypogonadism, pituitary tumors, surgical or medical castration, natural or surgical menopause, and ovarian failure
      (c) Neurologic: spinal cord injury, disease of the central or peripheral nervous system, including diabetes and peripheral neuropathy
      (d) Genital: congenital abnormalities, blunt trauma, Peyronie disease (scarring on the penile dorsum), pelvic fractures, and pelvic surgery
      (e) Illnesses that limit physical activity, such as arthritis and cardiac problems
    3. Substance effects
      (a) Alcohol and illicit drugs such as marijuana, opiates, cocaine, and sedatives
      (b) Prescription medications such as antihypertensives, diuretics, antihistamines, serotonin reuptake inhibitors, and antipsychotics
      (c) Over-the-counter medications such as sleep aids, antihistamines, and cold medicines
      (d) Dietary supplements and herbal preparations with hormonal or anticholinergic effects
      (e) Toxins such as lead and arsenic
  B. Psychosocial factors
    1. Psychiatric disorders such as depressive and anxiety disorders
    2. Trauma, loss, and conflict, such as sexual trauma and relational problems
    3. Financial, vocational, and residential factors (e.g., partners not living together)
II. Evaluation of the couple
  A. Sexual knowledge, skills, and attitude
  B. Relationship, commitment, and motivation

History Taking

Establishing rapport is the first and most important step in caring for a patient with a sexual dysfunction, who would understandably be embarrassed to discuss sexual issues with the clinician. Empathy, genuine concern, and professional style are the basic components of establishing effective rapport. Sexual history is collected in variable settings, such as evaluation of the individual versus the couple, or adolescents' interviews witnessed by their parents. The Association of Reproductive Health Professionals recommends that a third party be present during sexual history taking if a patient is impaired or litigious or acts or speaks in a sexual manner. In the mental health field, ideally the couple would be evaluated together initially, and then individually, followed by another meeting with the couple (IsHak, 2008a).

Obtaining a detailed sexual history is a big challenge to the clinician, with the opening question being the most difficult part. Floyd et al. (1999) studied interviewing techniques for sexual practices using different questions to introduce exploration of sexual problems in a primary care setting (see Table 15-2). The study revealed that participants expressed more comfort with transition using a ubiquity statement than a lifestyle bridge. It also showed that men were more comfortable with the direct statement method, whereas women felt more comfortable with closed-ended questions. Pomeroy (1982) recommended using "gentle assumption," where, in a gentle voice, questions are framed along the lines of "How frequently do you masturbate, if at all?" rather than "Do you masturbate?"

After a successful opening when obtaining a sexual history on a patient with a sexual disorder, the clinician should try to identify a clear chief sexual complaint occurring in one of the phases of the sexual response cycle (desire, arousal, and orgasm) or related to sexual pain, sexual behaviors,

TABLE 15-2	Transition Statements for Beginning to Take the Sexual History

Lifestyle bridge; for example, "You have told me about your lifestyle, your occupation, exercise, and diet; now I am going to ask you some questions about your sexual activities."

Ubiquity statement; for example, "I routinely ask all my patients about their sexual history; I am now going to ask you some questions about your sexual activities."

Eliciting feelings about exploring this area; for example, "How do you feel about answering some questions about your sexual activity?"

Direct statement; for example, "I am now going to ask you about your sexual activities."

Open-ended question; for example, "How would you describe your sexual activities?"

Closed-ended question; for example, "Are you currently sexually active with a partner?"

or gender identity. The clinician should then proceed to eliciting the history of present illness, which includes the onset, course, and duration (lifetime or acquired) of the chief complaint, as well as associated symptoms and signs, effect on functioning, and precipitating factors (generalized or situational). The clinician should also inquire about the past history of the same or different sexual disorders and response to different interventions. The final piece to complete the detailed sexual history is to obtain an adequate personal sexual history that comprises a chronological account of early sexual activities, puberty, sexual orientation issues, masturbatory practices, sexual relationships, pregnancy, abortion, sexual assaults, aging effects, menopause, current relationship details, frequency of sexual activity, preferred sexual practices, and satisfaction level. It is also of utmost importance to identify high-risk situations, such as the presence of sexually transmitted diseases, and unlawful practices, such as pedophilia. The last step in interviewing the patient is to try to exclude biological factors or psychiatric disorders as a cause of the sexual problem. This is accomplished by obtaining adequate psychiatric, substance use, and medical histories. Because different psychiatric disorders could lead to a variety of sexual disorders, the clinician should always screen for other axis I psychiatric disorders.

Substance use is a major cause of sexual dysfunction, which may often not be identified by the patient as a cause. Substances implicated include, but are not limited to, alcohol, illicit drugs, herbal supplements, and prescription and over-the-counter medications.

Obtaining a detailed medical history is essential to complete the evaluation of a patient with sexual dysfunction. This should include any history of medical problems and a review of the various systems. Special attention should be paid to vascular, genital, neurologic, endocrinological, and surgical issues.

Examination

A detailed physical examination is an important step in evaluating a patient with sexual dysfunction. It includes a review of the various systems with special emphasis on secondary sexual characteristics, abdominal examination (aneurysms), pulse (atherosclerosis), neurologic assessment, and external genitalia/pelvic examination. It may be most appropriate for this examination to be conducted by a subspecialist in sexual disorders, urologist, gynecologist, or primary care physician.

Psychiatric examination involves performing a detailed mental status examination to elaborate different findings in the psychiatric history and assess sexual knowledge, skills, and attitude, as well as the patient's current relationship, commitment, and motivation for sexual activity and satisfaction. Assessment instruments have been utilized for this purpose, including the Arizona Sexual Experiences Scale (McGahuey et al., 1998), the Changes in Sexual Functioning Questionnaire, Clinical Version (Clayton et al., 1997), and the International Index of Erectile Function (IIEF) (Rosen et al., 1999).

Laboratory Investigations

Different laboratory investigations are used to evaluate a patient with sexual dysfunction, with the primary aim to identify any biological factor that might be causing or exacerbating the sexual problem. The standard laboratory tests ordered for all patients include complete metabolic panels; complete blood count; lipid profiles; urine analysis; function tests of the thyroid, kidneys, and liver; and hormonal levels.

Checking hormonal levels is a crucial step. Important hormones include total testosterone (normal = 300 to 1,000 ng/dL in men and 30 to 120 ng/dL in women), free testosterone (normal using the equilibrium ultrafiltration method = 5 to 21 ng/dL in men and 0.3 to 0.85 ng/dL in women), prolactin (normal <15 mIU/mL), luteinizing hormone (LH) (normal = 5 to 15 mIU/mL), and follicle-stimulating hormone (FSH) (normal = 5 to 15 mIU/mL).

Subspecialists in sexual disorders may perform specific investigations for the evaluation of male erectile dysfunction, including nocturnal penile tumescence and rigidity analysis. Another test used is direct injection of prostaglandin E1 (PGE1) into the penis, where the patient is expected to develop an erection within minutes if the penile structure is within normal range of functioning.

Other investigations include vascular testing, such as duplex ultrasonography and dynamic infusion (cavernosometry and cavernosography), and neurologic testing, such as biothesiometry (measuring sensory perception threshold of the penis or female genital points), somatosensory evoked potentials, and pudendal electromyography.

Newer investigations for women include pH probes to measure lubrication, a balloon device to evaluate the ability of the vagina to relax and dilate, vibratory and heat and cold sensation measures of the external and internal genitalia, and high frequency Doppler imaging, or ultrasonography, to measure blood flow to the vagina and clitoris during arousal (Berman et al., 2003). Another recent test for women is the measurement of vaginal and minor labial oxygen tension using a modified Clark oxygen electrode to obtain partial oxygen pressure (pO$_2$) (Sommer et al., 2001).

Formulation and Diagnosis

After the examination, the clinician should have a clearer idea about the target sexual symptoms and signs and be capable of identifying the biopsychosocial factors that predispose, precipitate, or perpetuate the sexual disorder (Table 15-1).

The clinician should be able to rule out whether another axis I psychiatric disorder, the use of a substance, or a general medical condition better accounts for the patient's sexual dysfunction. Once this goal is reached, the clinician is left with the remaining diagnoses of sexual disorders listed in DSM-IV-TR, which will be discussed in detail in the subsequent text.

SEXUAL DESIRE DISORDERS

Hypoactive Sexual Desire Disorder

Hypoactive sexual desire disorder is a persistent or recurrent deficiency or absence of desire for sexual activity that results in marked distress or interpersonal difficulty. It is crucial to rule out the medical- and substance-related conditions that reduce sexual desire. General medical conditions such as low testosterone levels, anemia, hypertension, diabetes, thyroid problems, multiple sclerosis, systemic lupus erythematosus, hyperprolactinemia, and hysterectomy can manifest with decreased desire. Medications that can interfere with sexual desire include selective serotonin reuptake inhibitors (SSRIs), antihypertensive agents, estrogens, and progestins.

Dependence on substances such as heroin or alcohol can contribute significantly to loss of libido. Many of the other axis I psychiatric disorders impair desire and therefore might be confused with hypoactive sexual desire disorder if the responsible axis I disorder is not identified, such as major depressive disorder, dysthymia, panic disorder, obsessive-compulsive disorder, anorexia nervosa, and schizophrenia.

The biopsychosocial approach to treatment includes using medications, including hormones such as topical or transdermal testosterone (Shifren et al., 2000) and estrogen replacement therapy around menopause. Note that bupropion may be added to the antidepressant regimen in cases of SSRI-induced sexual dysfunction before considering switching the antidepressant altogether. Segraves et al. (2001) demonstrated the effectiveness of sustained-release bupropion in approximately 29% of nondepressed women with hypoactive sexual desire disorder at doses of 300 mg per day. Interestingly, phosphodiesterase type 5 (PDE-5) inhibitors, such as sildenafil,

A CASE OF FEMALE HYPOACTIVE SEXUAL DESIRE DISORDER

A 29-year-old newly married teacher reported that she feels very little desire to have sex with her husband or anyone since puberty. She does not enjoy having intercourse with her husband and considers it to be a chore. This issue markedly strains their relationship, because it manifests with her recurrent rejection of her husband's sexual invitations or requests. The patient sought medical help after she reports having arguments almost daily with her husband, who feels rejected and alienated. The examination revealed the absence of any axis I disorder, including depression. A diagnosis of hypoactive sexual desire disorder, lifelong type, is given after ruling out medical- and substance-related disorders.

could be effective especially when hypoactive sexual desire disorder coexists with arousal disorders (Hensley, 2002).

Psychosocial treatments include psychotherapy (individual cognitive behavioral therapy, psychodynamic therapy, and sex therapy with the couple), sex education, and self-exploration. Other somatic therapies that can be utilized include vacuum devices such as the Eros Clitoral Therapy Device (Eros-CTD), approved by the U.S. Food and Drug Administration (FDA), to promote desire (Billups et al., 2001). Hypoactive sexual desire disorder improves with age and in highly motivated patients.

Sexual Aversion Disorder

Sexual aversion disorder is the persistent or recurrent aversion to and avoidance of genital sexual contact with a sexual partner, resulting in marked distress or interpersonal difficulty. It is prevalent in patients with anorexia nervosa (Raboch, 1991) and panic disorder (Figueira, 2001).

Treatment modalities are similar to those used for hypoactive sexual desire disorder, with special emphasis on behavior therapy using desensitization, which has shown some effectiveness in case reports (Finch, 2001). Sexual aversion disorder is at times difficult to treat and has a guarded prognosis.

Disorder of Increased Sexual Activity or Desire

The disorder of increased sexual activity or desire is referred to at times as *hyperactive sexual desire disorder* (Leiblum and Rosen, 1988) and is not listed in DSM-IV-TR. It manifests as persistent or recurrent engagement in sexual encounters, masturbation, and pornography that interferes with social and occupational functioning.

Models from addiction, compulsive, and impulse control disorders are used to understand the disorder of increased sexual activity or desire (Gold and Heffner, 1998). There is a high comorbidity between this disorder and addiction, compulsive, and impulse control disorders, such as pathological gambling. Patients with bipolar disorder, anxiety disorders, Kluver-Bucy syndrome, and traumatic brain injury also experience increased sexual activity.

The biopsychosocial approach is applied for treatment by using medications, including higher doses of SSRIs, clomipramine, or naltrexone, as well as psychotherapies, including group psychotherapy, 12-step programs, individual cognitive behavioral therapy, and psychodynamic therapy. Good prognosis is correlated with high motivation, adequate social support, and absence of psychiatric comorbidities.

Male Erectile Disorder

Male erectile disorder manifests as an inability to attain or maintain an erection for the completion of sexual activity, causing marked distress and interpersonal difficulties. This condition may be lifelong or acquired, generalized or situational.

Medical- and substance-related conditions affecting arousal need to be ruled out first. General medical conditions such as diabetes mellitus, hormonal problems, atherosclerosis, multiple sclerosis, spinal injuries, congenital anomalies, renal failure, and morbid obesity can all affect erection. Substances that can interfere with obtaining a satisfactory erection include antihypertensives (especially β-blockers), antipsychotics, nicotine, cocaine, and opioids.

Again, the biopsychosocial approach is applied for treatment where the use of medications is integrated with psychotherapeutic techniques to obtain the maximum therapeutic effect. Medications include an oral PDE-5 inhibitor such as sildenafil, vardenafil, or tadalafil. Alternatively, alprostadil (intracavernosal injections, intraurethral suppositories, or cream) could be utilized. Psychotherapies include sex therapy with the couple using sensate focus exercises, individual cognitive behavioral therapy, and psychodynamic therapy. Other somatic therapies include vacuum devices and penile prosthesis, which is utilized as a last resort. The absence of medical and psychiatric comorbidities signals a good prognosis.

Female Sexual Arousal Disorder

Female sexual arousal disorder is an inability to attain and/or maintain vaginal lubrication, vaginal elongation, and engorgement of the external genitalia for the completion of sexual activity, causing marked distress and interpersonal difficulty. This condition may be lifelong or acquired, generalized or situational. As in male erectile disorder, medical- and substance-related conditions affecting arousal need to be ruled out first. Any comorbid psychiatric disorders need to be addressed. Substances that can interfere with sexual arousal include antihistamines, β-blockers, antipsychotics, cocaine, and opioids.

Treatment involves integrating the use of medications with psychotherapy. Medications include hormone replacement therapy (HRT), estrogen cream, testosterone, and PDE-5 inhibitors. Psychotherapies include sex therapy with the couple using sensate focus exercises, individual cognitive behavioral therapy, and psychodynamic therapy, especially with history of sexual trauma. Other somatic therapies include a vacuum device such as the Eros-CTD, which is FDA approved for this purpose. Prognosis is generally favorable in the absence of psychiatric and medical comorbidities.

ORGASMIC DISORDERS

Premature Ejaculation

Premature ejaculation is persistent or recurrent ejaculation with minimal sexual stimulation or before, on, or shortly after penetration and before the person wishes it, resulting in marked distress or interpersonal difficulty. Recent sexual behavior surveys revealed that one third of men experienced recurrent premature ejaculation, making it the most common sexual disorder in men (Laumann et al., 1999). This condition may be lifelong or acquired, generalized or situational. Medical conditions such as prostatitis, urethritis, diabetes, benign prostatic hyperplasia, and urinary incontinence, as well as substance-related conditions such as cigarette smoking, opiate withdrawal, and using over-the-counter medications for the common cold, all need to be ruled out first. Comorbid psychiatric disorders such as anxiety disorders and social phobia would need to be addressed (Figueira et al., 2001).

An integration of the use of medications with psychotherapy is applied when treating premature ejaculation, following the biopsychosocial approach. Medications include SSRIs (6 to 12 hours before intercourse or fluoxetine 90 mg weekly); PDE-5 inhibitors (such as sildenafil 50 mg 4 hours before intercourse) as sole agents or in combination with SSRIs (Waldinger, 2004); tricyclic antidepressants (e.g., clomipramine 50 mg 2 to 12 hours before intercourse or daily); or topical anesthetic agents (lidocaine or prilocaine 2.5%). Psychotherapies include sex therapy with the couple using sensate focus exercises, behavior therapy (start–stop method, squeeze method, or biofeedback), and individual psychotherapy. Other somatic therapies include the use of condoms, masturbation 1 to 2 hours before sexual activity, and utilizing the partner-on-top sexual position. Prognosis is generally good.

Male Orgasmic Disorder

Male orgasmic disorder is persistent or recurrent delay in or absence of orgasm following a normal sexual excitement phase during sexual activity, resulting in marked distress or interpersonal difficulty. Approximately 8% of men experience orgasmic difficulties as revealed by sexual behavior surveys (Laumann et al., 1999), making it the least common sexual disorder in men. This condition may be lifelong or acquired, generalized or situational. Retrograde ejaculation needs to be ruled out. Medical conditions, such as low testosterone, diabetes, and pelvic conditions,

A CASE OF PREMATURE EJACULATION

A 26-year-old single male photographer is presenting with a chief complaint of "ejaculating very fast, way before I want to." On examination, the man revealed that he has been experiencing first onset ejaculation before penetration consistently since he and his current female roommate started to engage in sexual relations. He appeared mildly anxious, with no relevant medical- or substance-related problems. A diagnosis of premature ejaculation, acquired type, is given.

and substance-related conditions, such as using marijuana, SSRIs, or antipsychotic medications, need to be ruled out as well. Comorbid psychiatric disorders such as obsessive-compulsive disorder and posttraumatic stress disorder would need to be addressed (Figueira et al., 2001).

Medications that treat male anorgasmia are almost nonexistent. However, trials of PDE-5 inhibitors such as sildenafil worked for SSRI-induced delayed or absent orgasm. More recently, trials using cabergoline (a dopaminergic agent) or oxytocin have been published in case reports (IsHak et al., 2008b). Psychotherapies that can be utilized include sex therapy with the couple using sensate focus exercises and individual psychotherapy. Prognosis is generally guarded.

Female Orgasmic Disorder

Female orgasmic disorder is the persistent or recurrent delay in or absence of orgasm following a normal sexual excitement phase, resulting in marked distress or interpersonal difficulty. Sex surveys revealed that approximately 24% of women experience orgasmic difficulties at some point in their lives (Laumann et al., 1999), making it the second most common sexual disorder in women after hypoactive sexual desire disorder. This condition may be lifelong or acquired, generalized or situational. The adequacy of sexual arousal and the presence of other sexual disorders such as desire or arousal problems need to be evaluated before making the diagnosis. It is also important to rule out medical conditions such as hyperprolactinemia, diabetes, and pelvic conditions, as well as substance-related conditions such as use of marijuana, SSRIs, or antipsychotic medications. As in male orgasmic disorder, comorbid psychiatric disorders such as obsessive-compulsive disorder and posttraumatic stress disorder would need to be addressed (Figueira et al., 2001).

No approved medications exist for female anorgasmia. Trials of PDE-5 inhibitors such as sildenafil worked only for SSRI-induced delayed or absent orgasm. More recently, trials using cabergoline (a dopaminergic agent) or oxytocin have been published in case reports (IsHak et al., 2008b). Psychotherapies that can be utilized include sex therapy with the couple using sensate focus exercises and individual psychotherapy. Other somatic therapies that have been shown to be beneficial include delivering mild electrical pulses to stimulate the sacral nerves feeding the bladder, sphincter, and pelvic floor muscles. This was based on the observation that women who received the InterStim neurostimulator implant due to urinary bladder control problems reported improvement in sexual functioning. Somatic therapies also include Kegel exercises, which enhance control of the pubococcygeus muscle. The exercises focus on getting the muscle to contract 10 to 15 times three times per day. Prognosis is generally favorable.

SEXUAL PAIN DISORDERS

Vaginismus

Vaginismus is recurrent or persistent involuntary spasm of the musculature of the outer third of the vagina that interferes with sexual intercourse, resulting in marked distress or interpersonal difficulty. It is caused by contraction of the pelvic floor muscles, leading to the obstruction of the introitus and interfering with penetration. Data from sexual dysfunction clinics showed that 12% to 17% of female patients presented with this complaint (Spector and Carey, 1990). This condition may be lifelong or acquired, generalized or situational. Common etiological factors include genital pain, history of sexual trauma, or extreme fear of sexual intercourse. Persistent vaginismus in a marital relationship may present to clinicians as an unconsummated marriage.

It is crucial to rule out that the cause of vaginismus is pelvic, vaginal, or vulvar pain conditions. Anxiety and somatization disorders also need to be ruled out.

No approved medications exist for vaginismus. Recently, local botulinum toxin has been used with significant success (Ghazizadeh and Nikzad, 2004). Psychotherapies that have been shown to be effective include couples/sex therapy (Biswas and Ratnam, 1995) and cognitive behavioral therapy (Kabakçi and Batur, 2003). Effective somatic therapies for vaginismus include systematic desensitization using dilators. In addition, Kegel exercises, which enhance control of pelvic floor muscles, have shown some effectiveness in the treatment of vaginismus. Prognosis is generally favorable in the absence of history of serious sexual trauma or treatment-resistant pain.

Dyspareunia

Dyspareunia is recurrent or persistent genital pain associated with sexual intercourse in either a male or a female. By definition, it is not caused by vaginismus or lack of lubrication, and it results in marked distress or interpersonal difficulty. Basson (2005) reported that dyspareunia leads to prevention of intercourse in approximately 10% of patients. This condition may be lifelong or acquired, generalized or situational. Vaginismus is mainly due to psychological reasons (e.g., history of sexual trauma, relationship conflicts, and guilt), whereas dyspareunia is mainly caused by medical issues (e.g., endometriosis, pelvic inflammatory disease, and pelvic injury).

Vaginismus, somatoform disorders, pelvic deformities, infections, and endometriosis need to be ruled out. The influence of substances such as antihistamines and marijuana needs to be evaluated.

No approved medications exist for dyspareunia. However, 0.2% nitroglycerin cream applied to the skin at the genital area 5 to 10 minutes before intercourse has been shown to be effective (Walsh et al., 2002). Psychotherapies that have shown effectiveness include couples/sex therapy using sensate focus exercises. Other somatic therapies that have been shown to be relatively effective in the treatment of dyspareunia include hypnosis (Kandyba and Binik, 2003). Prognosis is generally favorable.

PARAPHILIAS

According to DSM-IV-TR, paraphilias are characterized by sexual fantasies, urges, or behaviors involving nonhuman objects (fetishism, transvestic fetishism), suffering or humiliation (sadism, masochism), children (pedophilia), or other nonconsenting persons (voyeurism, frotteurism, and exhibitionism). To meet diagnostic criteria for each disorder, the person should have been experiencing over a period of at least 6 months recurrent, intense, sexually arousing fantasies, sexual urges, or behaviors involving the type of paraphilias to be diagnosed, and the person has acted on these urges or the sexual urges, or fantasies cause clinically significant distress or impairment in social, occupational, or other important areas of functioning (American Psychiatric Association, 2000; Kafka, 1994).

It is important to distinguish paraphilias from other disorders where sexual acting out is manifest, such as bipolar disorder, traumatic brain injury, substance intoxication, chronic or residual psychotic illnesses, mental retardation, and cluster B personality disorders. Diagnostic tests might be needed to confirm the presence of paraphilias, such as the use of the Abel Assessment in detecting pedophilia (Fischer and Smith, 1999). It is also important to distinguish the different types of paraphilias.

No FDA-approved medications exist for paraphilias. However, the SSRIs have been demonstrated to reduce sexual behaviors in paraphilias. Moreover, antiandrogens such as medroxyprogesterone (Depo-Provera) and gonadotropin-releasing hormones have been used with relative success in pedophilia (Brannon, 2005). Psychotherapies that have been implemented include cognitive behavioral therapy; behavioral therapy, such as pairing paraphilic arousal with unpleasant stimuli; and victim empathy therapy, where the focus is on identifying with the victim. Twelve-step programs are viewed as an important adjunct. Other somatic therapies that have been utilized include surgical removal of testicles, especially for repeated sexual offenders. Prognosis is guarded with a high rate of recidivism.

GENDER IDENTITY DISORDERS

DSM-IV-TR defines gender identity disorders as a heterogeneous group of disorders whose common feature is a strong and persistent identification with the opposite sex. In adolescents and adults, the disturbance is manifested by symptoms such as a stated desire to be the other sex, frequent passing as the other sex, desire to live or be treated as the other sex, or the conviction that he or she has the typical feelings and reactions of the other sex. Other symptoms include persistent discomfort with his or her sex or sense of inappropriateness in the gender role of that sex, preoccupation with getting rid of primary and secondary sex characteristics (e.g., request for hormones, surgery, or other procedures to physically alter sexual characteristics to simulate the other sex), or the belief that he or she was born the wrong sex. The above-mentioned symptoms must cause clinically significant distress or impairment in social, occupational, or other important areas of functioning, and the disturbance must not be concurrent with a physical intersex condition such as true or pseudohermaphroditism. Therefore, physical intersex conditions should be ruled out.

No approved medications exist for gender identity disorder; however, hormones might be indicated following adequate psychological preparation. Psychotherapies that can be utilized include individual cognitive behavioral therapy. Other somatic therapies involve sex reassignment surgery following adequate psychological preparation. Prognosis is unknown.

CONCLUSION

This chapter has discussed the importance of taking a complete sexual history of a patient, including how to approach difficult topics, and the various sexual and gender identity disorders listed in DSM-IV-TR. It is essential to establish an open relationship with patients that allows them to talk openly about their sexual issues in a supportive environment. Treatments, both somatic and psychological, are now available for many conditions and can help patients experience greatly enhanced quality of life.

Clinical Pearls

- Always evaluate the presence of medical problems (systemic, supra-spinal, spinal, pelvic, genital), as well as use of substances (alcohol, street drugs, prescriptions, over-the-counter medications, dietary supplements, and toxins) before making the diagnosis of any sexual disorder.
- Order hormonal levels (prolactin, testosterone, and thyroid) in patients with sexual dysfunction and correct hormonal deficiencies if present.
- Add bupropion to antidepressant regimen in cases of SSRI-induced sexual dysfunction before considering switching the antidepressant altogether.
- Engage the patient and his or her partner in a dialogue that includes sex education, pros and cons of proposed interventions, and potentially combining medications with sex therapy, if indicated.
- Vaginismus is mainly due to psychological reasons (e.g., history of sexual trauma, relationship conflicts, and guilt), whereas dyspareunia is mainly caused by medical issues (e.g., endometriosis, pelvic inflammatory disease, and pelvic injury).

Self-Assessment Questions and Answers

15-1. A 67-year-old white man is presenting with new-onset erection problems and urinary frequency. Over the last 12 months, he has been noticing difficulties in maintaining erections that he had attributed to his inability to focus because he is facing financial problems. The patient has not been using any drugs or alcohol and considers himself "pretty healthy" for his age. "What is the best approach?"

A. Do nothing; a decline in erectile stability is expected with age.
B. A complete medical and urological evaluation is needed.
C. Financial counseling would have a significant impact.
D. Treat viral infections that commonly cause such a presentation.

It is imperative to rule out medical and urological (e.g., benign prostatic hypertrophy) issues in patients older than 50 years who are presenting with urinary frequency and sexual dysfunction. Although the ability to obtain and maintain erection decreases with time, treatment with phosphodiesterase-5 inhibitors would be indicated after ruling out medical and urological causes. Financial counseling would be helpful but not necessarily have significant impact on sexual functioning. Viral infections are rarely implicated in these presentations (IsHak, 2008a). *Answer: B*

15-2. In female arousal disorder, which of the following is true?
A. It is the most common sexual problem in women.
B. Individual psychotherapy and/or sex therapy do not influence the outcome.
C. Sexual pain has a direct impact on arousal.
D. Substance-related conditions do not reduce sexual desire.

Female arousal disorder is the third most common sexual problem in women, following hypoactive sexual desire disorder and female orgasmic disorder. Individual psychotherapy and/or sex therapy enhance the outcome. Sexual pain and desire problems have a direct negative impact. Medications that can interfere with sexual desire include selective serotonin reuptake inhibitors (SSRIs), antihypertensive agents, estrogens, and progestins. *Answer: C*

15-3. During sexual history taking
A. Do not allow a third party to participate, due to patient confidentiality issues.
B. It is more important for the clinician to establish authority on matters of sexual health than to establish rapport with the patient.
C. Male patients prefer direct statements and women patients prefer closed-ended questions.
D. The opening question is easiest; the rest become progressively more difficult.

A third party is recommended to be present during sexual history taking if a patient is impaired or litigious or acts or speaks in a sexual manner. Establishing rapport is the first and most important step in caring for a patient with a sexual dysfunction because of understandable embarrassment in discussing sexual issues. Floyd et al.'s (1999) study showed that men were more comfortable with the direct statement method and women with closed-ended questions. The opening question is the most difficult part of taking the sexual history. *Answer: C*

15-4. The treatment models of addiction, obsessive-compulsive, and impulse control disorders are used to understand disorders of
A. Gender identity
B. Increased sexual activity or desire
C. Orgasm
D. Sexual pain

Disorders of increased sexual activity or desire and addiction, compulsive, and impulse control disorders have high comorbidity. *Answer: B*

References

American Psychiatric Association (APA). *Diagnostic and statistical manual of mental disorders*, 4th ed., text revision. Washington, DC: American Psychiatric Publishing; 2000.

Basson R. The optimal discipline for assessing and managing pain during sex. *Arch Sex Behav.* 2005;34(1):23–24, 57–61; author reply 63–7.

Berman JR, Berman LA, Toler SM, et al. Sildenafil Study Group. Safety and efficacy of sildenafil citrate for the treatment of female sexual arousal disorder: A double-blind, placebo controlled study. *J Urol.* 2003;170:2333–2338.

Billups KL, Berman L, Berman J, et al. Goldstein I: A new non-pharmacological vacuum therapy for female sexual dysfunction. *J Sex Marital Ther.* 2001;27:435–441.

Biswas A, Ratnam SS. Vaginismus and outcome of treatment. *Ann Acad Med Singapore.* 1995;24:755–758.

Brannon GE. *Paraphilias. e-Medicine.* http://www.emedicine.com/med/topic3127.htm, WebMD, 2005.

Clayton AH, McGarvey EL, Clavet GJ. The Changes in Sexual Functioning Questionnaire (CSFQ): Development, reliability, and validity. *Psychopharmacol Bull.* 1997;33:731–745.

Figueira I, Possidente E, Marques C, et al. Sexual dysfunction: A neglected complication of panic disorder and social phobia. *Arch Sex Behav*. 2001;30:369–377.

Finch S. Sexual aversion disorder treated with behavioural desensitization. *Can J Psychiatry*. 2001;46: 563–564.

Fischer L, Smith G. Statistical adequacy of the Abel assessment for interest in paraphilias. *Sex Abuse*. 1999; 11(3):195–205.

Floyd M, Lang F, Beine KL, et al. Evaluating interviewing techniques for the sexual practices history. Use of video trigger tapes to assess patient comfort. *Arch Fam Med*. 1999;8(3):218–223.

Ghazizadeh S, Nikzad M. Botulinum toxin in the treatment of refractory vaginismus. *Obstet Gynecol*. 2004;104:922–925.

Gold SN, Heffner CL. Sexual addiction: Many conceptions, minimal data. *Clin Psychol Rev*. 1998;18(3): 367–381.

Hensley PL. Nurnberg HG: SSRI sexual dysfunction: A female perspective. *J Sex Marital Ther*. 2002; 28(Suppl 1):143–153.

IsHak WW. The biopsychosocial evaluation and treatment of sexual disorders. In: IsHak WW, ed. *The guidebook of sexual medicine*. Beverly Hills: A&W Publishing; 2008a.

IsHak WW, Berman D, Peters A. Male anorgasmia treated with oxytocin. *Br J Sex Med*. 2008b;5(4): 1022–1024.

Kabakçi E, Batur S. Who benefits from cognitive behavioral therapy for vaginismus? *J Sex Marital Ther*. 2003;29(4):277–288.

Kafka MP. Paraphilia-related disorders: Common, neglected, and misunderstood. *Harv Rev Psychiatry*. 1994;2(1):39–40, discussion 41-42.

Kandyba K, Binik YM. Hypnotherapy as a treatment for vulvar vestibulitis syndrome: A case report. *J Sex Marital Ther*. 2003;29(3):237–242.

Laumann EO, Paik AM, Rosen RC. Sexual dysfunction in the United States: Prevalence and predictors. *JAMA*. 1999;281:537–544.

Leiblum SR, Rosen RC. *Sexual desire disorders*. New York: Guilford; 1988.

Marwick C. Survey says patients expect little physician help on sex. *JAMA*. 1999;281:2173–2174.

McGahuey CA, Gelenberg AJ, Laukes CA, et al. The Arizona Sexual Experiences Scale (ASEX): Reliability and validity. *J Sex Marital Ther*. 1998;26:25–40.

Pomeroy WB. *Taking a sex history: Interviewing and recording*. New York: Free Press; 1982.

Raboch JS, Faltus F. Sexuality of women with anorexia nervosa. *Acta Psychiatr Scand*. 1991;84:9–11.

Rosen RC. Prevalence and risk factors of sexual dysfunction in men and women. *Curr Psychiatry Rep*. 2000;2:189–195.

Segraves RT, Croft H, Kavoussi R, et al. Bupropion sustained release (SR) for the treatment of hypoactive sexual desire disorder (HSDD) in nondepressed women. *J Sex Marital Ther*. 2001;27:303–316.

Shifren JL, Braunstein GD, Simon JA, et al. Transdermal testosterone treatment in women with impaired sexual function after oophorectomy. *N Engl J Med*. 2000;343:682–688.

Sommer F, Caspers HP, Esders K, et al. Measurement of vaginal and minor labial oxygen tension for the evaluation of female sexual function. *J Urol*. 2001;165(4):1181–1184.

Spector IP, Carey MP. Incidence and prevalence of the sexual dysfunctions: A critical review of the empirical literature. *Arch Sex Behav*. 1990;19:389–408.

Waldinger MD. Lifelong premature ejaculation: From authority-based to evidence-based medicine. *BJU Int*. 2004;93:201–207.

Walsh KE, Berman JR, Berman LA, et al. Safety and efficacy of topical nitroglycerin for treatment of vulvar pain in women with vulvodynia: A pilot study. *J Gend Specif Med*. 2002;5(4):21–27.

Zucker KJ. Gender identity development and issues. *Child Adolesc Psychiatr Clin N Am*. 2004;13:551–568, vii.

Eating Disorders

Cases of women who starved themselves have been reported for hundreds of years, including *anorexia mirabilis* in sainted women of the Middle Ages and the notorious "fasting girls" of the 16th through 19th centuries. Anorexia nervosa as it is currently recognized was first described in the late 1870s. The 1983 death of singer Karen Carpenter from anorexia nervosa resulted in a flood of television programs and magazine articles that brought considerable attention to eating disorders. After popular magazines featured articles suggesting that Jane Fonda, Olympic gymnast Cathy Rigby, and Princess Diana of England may have suffered from anorexia nervosa and/or bulimia nervosa, virtually every woman in the United States became aware of these disorders and their dangers.

Although cultural standards of beauty have shaped ideal body image throughout history, media may play a more powerful role in today's society. The average fashion model is 23% thinner than most women. Media pressure to be thin and a multibillion-dollar dieting industry raise concerns about the increasing rates of eating disorders (Derenne and Beresin, 2006). Entertainment and fashion magazines, television, and the Internet regularly feature stories about prominent actors and models who struggle with eating disorders. Such attention may contribute to increased awareness and recognition of these disorders by clinicians, but case finding is still poor, particularly in identifying bulimia nervosa. Misimpressions may contribute to the continued difficulty many families have in obtaining insurance coverage to evaluate and treat anorexia nervosa and bulimia nervosa (O'Hara and Smith, 2007).

Binge eating disorder, similar in many respects to "compulsive overeating," has been added to the formal diagnoses of anorexia nervosa and bulimia nervosa in the *Diagnostic and Statistical Manual of Mental Disorders*, Fourth Edition, Text Revision (DSM-IV-TR; American Psychiatric Association, 2000), as a diagnosis worthy of additional study. Data from the American Obesity Association (2006) indicate that 15% of children and 30% of adults meet the criteria for obesity. Overly restrictive diets and sedentary lifestyles are likely related to increasing rates of obesity and disordered eating, including binge eating and purging (Derenne and Beresin, 2006). Dieting, media use, body image, and weight-related teasing may also be risk factors for the entire spectrum of eating disorders, including obesity (Haines and Neumark-Sztainer, 2006). Many patients who may not meet the strict diagnostic criteria for any one of these disorders but present with variations of the psychological and behavioral signs and symptoms described in this chapter are considered to have eating disorders not otherwise specified.

EPIDEMIOLOGY

The National Comorbidity Replication Study, a face-to-face, household-based epidemiologic survey, provided recent information on the prevalence of these disorders. Lifetime prevalence estimates of anorexia nervosa, bulimia nervosa, and binge eating disorder are 0.9%, 1.5%, and 3.5% in women, and 0.3%, 0.5%, and 2.0% in men, respectively (Hudson et al., 2007). Individual symptoms of eating disorders are relatively common in general and include body image distortion; extreme fear of being fat out of line with health concerns; the desire to reduce body fat to levels below those ordinarily considered healthy; restrictive and fad dieting; amphetamine and cocaine use for anorectic effects; purging by means of vomiting, laxative abuse, and/or diuretic abuse; and excessive or compulsive exercise among normal-weight and even underweight individuals (Drewnowski et al., 1988; Mond et al., 2006). Those who manifest abnormal eating behaviors do not necessarily develop eating disorders (Steinhausen et al., 2005). Some symptoms may even be seen in most of certain subgroups of women, as in select college sororities or among dance majors.

Men with anorexia nervosa and bulimia nervosa form the minority of cases. In clinical settings 90% to 95% of cases are females. The age of onset for anorexia nervosa peaks in early and late adolescence. Bulimia nervosa occurs in the teenage and early adult years, but cases of anorexia nervosa and bulimia nervosa with prepubertal onset and onset age 40 and older have been reported. Recent evidence suggests these disorders are more prevalent across socioeconomic status and ethnicity and in white, Hispanic, and Asian Americans more so than African Americans.

Binge eating disorder has been reported in 1% to 4% of nonpatient community samples. Similar to other eating disorders, it is more common among women, although rates among men represent a much higher percentage than in other eating disorders, with a female-to-male ratio of 3:2 (Spitzer et al., 1992, 1993). Binge eating disorder is quite common among overweight individuals seeking treatment for weight loss. It has been estimated that approximately 70% of participants in Overeaters Anonymous and 30% in weight loss programs have binge eating disorder (de Zwaan et al., 1992; Devlin, 1996). It appears to affect a more diverse population than anorexia nervosa or bulimia nervosa and does not show differences in prevalence based on ethnicity.

ETIOLOGY AND PATHOGENESIS

Theories regarding the etiology and pathogenesis of eating disorders have implicated virtually every biopsychosocial level.

Biological Theories

One popular biological theory posits the presence of a hypothalamic or suprahypothalamic abnormality to account for the profound disturbances seen in patients with eating disorders in the secretion of luteinizing hormone (LH), follicle stimulating hormone (FSH), growth hormone (GH), response to thyrotropin-releasing hormone (TRH), cortisol, response to corticotropin-releasing hormone (CRH), abnormal dexamethasone suppression test and arginine vasopressin, among other hormones and peptides (Krassas, 2003). In patients with anorexia nervosa, leptin levels are decreased, whereas ghrelin levels are elevated. Many of these levels return to normal after nutrition is resumed. Neuropeptides in the hypothalamic and gut-related systems play a significant role in regulating eating control and homeostasis. Neuropeptide Y and the opioid peptides have shown state-related abnormalities in patients with eating disorders. Those with bulimia nervosa show blunting of postmeal release of cholecystokinin (Jimerson and Wolfe, 2004). Finally, there are significant abnormalities in catecholamine metabolism, most notably serotonin, which may be related to stereotypic core symptoms in anorexia nervosa, including feeding, temperament, and personality; body image distortion; cognition; physical exercise; and onset and gender (Kaye et al., 2005). Biological data obtained from patients who have recovered and been clinically stable for long-enough periods of time virtually always show a return to normal values.

Another theory suggests that some eating disorders, particularly bulimic syndromes, may be variants of mood disorders. Supporting arguments include the frequent comorbidity of affective disturbance with eating disorders, an increased prevalence of mood disturbance in first-degree relatives of patients with bulimia nervosa, and responses of patients with bulimia nervosa to antidepressant medications.

Genetically transmitted vulnerability for eating disorders is probable, with good evidence of heritability from twin studies, but the search for definitive candidate genes has been more inconclusive (Becker et al., 2004). The past decade has seen an explosion of association and linkage studies of eating disorders. Association studies compare people displaying a trait of interest to controls and then determine the genotypes for hypothesized candidate genes related to the phenotype. Linkage studies examine genotypes of large samples of complex pedigrees (Bulik, 2005). Eating disorders have a familial pattern of transmission, but such patterns do not necessarily suggest exclusively genetic influences (Yager, 1982). In fact, the etiology of eating disorders is probably much like that of mood disorders, in which adverse environments interact with genetic vulnerabilities to bring about clinical conditions. Anorexia nervosa and bulimia nervosa may even share transmission with anxiety disorders and major depression. These gene–environment interactions may also affect treatment response. Genes of interest identified from association studies for eating disorders include those in the serotonergic system (both those for receptors 2A and 2C and of the serotonin transporter gene) and norepinephrine transporter, monoamine oxidase A, and estrogen genes. Newer research has also focused on possible associations with polymorphisms of the CLOCK (endogenous oscillator) system, brain-derived neurotropic factor (BDNF), preproghrelin, and the dopamine receptor.

Linkage studies for anorexia nervosa have shown susceptibility on chromosome 1, regions of interest on chromosomes 2 and 13, and possible associations with serotonin 1D and δ-opioid receptor genes (Bulik, 2005). The largest series of twins for both anorexia nervosa and bulimia nervosa show much higher concordance for monozygotic (~50%) than dizygotic (~14%) twins (Crisp et al., 1985; Kendler et al., 1991), suggesting some genetic influences are important. Genetic vulnerability to obesity may play a role in predisposing individuals to bulimia nervosa and binge eating disorders. The only study of linkage for bulimia nervosa involving a large sample of families showed significant linkage on chromosome arm 10p (Bulik, 2005).

Still another theory suggests that the processes of combined dieting and exercise produce an "autointoxication" with endogenous opioids, essentially an altered state of consciousness as a consequence of the starvation state, and that, at a certain point, this autointoxication creates an autoaddiction to internally generated opioids (Marrazzi and Luby, 1986).

Apart from these speculative theories, the primary biological influences in the pathogenesis of eating disorder symptoms are related to starvation and malnutrition. Studies with starving normal volunteers have demonstrated that many of the psychopathological as well as physical signs and symptoms of eating disorders are attributable to starvation. Starvation produces significant organ wasting and laboratory abnormalities (Garfinkel and Garner, 1982). More interesting from the point of view of the pathogenesis of psychopathology are the observations that starved normal volunteers become food preoccupied, depressed, and irritable; hoard food; develop abnormal taste preferences; and binge eat when food is readily available. Furthermore, in one study in which previously normal volunteers who were starved over several months to 25% below their usual healthy weights, full psychological recovery did not occur until 6 months to a year *after* the volunteers had regained all their lost weight. In other words, many of the strange and bizarre psychological symptoms, including compulsive rituals and markedly disturbed personality traits, may *result* from, rather than cause, severe starvation.

Psychological Theories

Hypotheses regarding possible psychological factors in etiology and pathogenesis have been derived from classical, operant, cognitive, and social learning theories; psychodynamic schools, including classical psychoanalysis, ego psychology, object relations, and self-psychology theories; existential psychology; and several schools of family theory (Garner and Garfinkel, 1997).

Maladaptive Learned Responses

On the basis of classical or operant conditioning principles, maladaptive learned responses may be used to reduce anxiety. In the patient with anorexia nervosa, these may take the form of food and/or weight phobias. In the patient with bulimia nervosa, inner tension states may be relieved by excessive eating. Anxiety generated by the shame, guilt, and loss of self-control brought about by the eating binge is in turn relieved by purging.

Cognitive Distortions

Cognitive distortions (misguided and erroneous self-statements) that developed to reduce and manage anxiety in socially awkward and sensitive adolescents (as well as in others) tend to confound self-worth with physical appearance. The self-statements are constantly repeated as preconscious inner thoughts, cycled over and over again in a ruminative manner, and have a self-reinforcing quality, so that they become overlearned shibboleths. The thinking distortions include tendencies to overgeneralize, magnify horrible things, think in all-or-none and black-and-white terms, take everything personally, and think superstitiously.

Distortions of Perceptions and Interceptions

Experiments with photographs, distorting mirrors, and videotape recordings, although not all in agreement, generally tend to support the idea that patients with eating disorders have a greater tendency to distort and misperceive their body widths, seeing themselves as much wider than they are. They also have greater difficulty in clearly identifying inner states such as hunger and satiety (intercepts) and some of their own emotional states.

Perfectionist, Rigid, and Compulsive Coping Styles

Developmentally, children with anorexia nervosa and bulimia nervosa are more likely to have genetically influenced anxiety disorders, including overanxiety, separation anxiety, and depression during the years before adolescence (Silberg and Bulik, 2005). Perfectionist tendencies during latency, such as excessive neatness, orderliness, and a rigid tendency to follow rules, also increase the odds for developing an eating disorder and may represent markers for a specific subgroup of patients with anorexia nervosa (Anderluh et al., 2003).

Weak Sense of Self and Low Self-Worth

Several authorities have suggested that children who will be predisposed to eating disorders suffer developmentally from a weak sense of self and low self-worth. According to one view, these weaknesses may stem from the parents' failure to treat the child as a legitimate and authentic person in his or her own right. Instead, such parents are thought to take their child for granted and value the child primarily for behaving well (so that the parents do not have to be bothered) and satisfying the parents' own needs to feel valuable and show off. The child satisfies the parents' needs by various achievements and accomplishments (which may have little intrinsic satisfaction for the child); hence, some pre–anorexia nervosa children have been characterized as "the best little girl in the world." This character structure may also result from constitutional factors.

Conflicts over Adolescent Development and Psychosexual Maturity

Because anorexia nervosa resembles both psychological and physiological regression from the healthy adolescent state to prepubertal structures, the idea that patients may develop the disorder as a way of putting off the tasks of adolescence has had considerable appeal. In this view patients may avoid the difficult tasks of establishing a separate identity, value system, and life plan; separating from their families; and contending with heterosexual urges and peer pressures.

Family Factors

To start with, it must be stressed that a family cause for eating disorders has not been proved; a reasonable number of patients seem to come from families that are, for all intents and purposes, "normal," and many normal adults grow up in families that manifest the presumed pathogenetic patterns to be described. When family problems are evident, it is far too easy to erroneously attribute the eating disorders to the family's problems; even in such instances, the disorders may result from entirely different factors (Lock and le Grange, 2005; Yager, 1982). Findings suggest that family treatment can be helpful for adolescents with eating disorders.

Some families are thought to be more likely than others to produce a child with an eating disorder, including those in which a parent is enmeshed with a child (i.e., overinvolved to the point of being unable to distinguish the parent's needs and wishes from the child's), overt conflict between the parents or between parent and child is studiously avoided, and rules about how family members communicate with one another are so rigid that it may be impermissible to address the sources and even the existence of tensions in the family (Minuchin et al., 1978).

Other research has pointed out the complexities in parental transactions with anorexic children, involving combinations of high "expressed emotion," in which children are blamed and criticized, together with high parental affective style, in which parents may be emotionally overinvolved, guilt-inducing, and/or intrusive (Cook et al., 1991). A family pattern characterized by high expressed emotion has been empirically linked to poorer outcome for anorexia nervosa (and other psychiatric disorders such as schizophrenia and mood disorders). Patterns of childhood physical and sexual abuse and other forms of parental "boundary violations" have also been cited as contributing factors. Families in which food is used as a salve for emotional problems, to distract from or relieve tensions related to family dysfunctions and other sources, may contribute to the subsequent appearance of binge eating during times of distress. Families where children and adolescents eat excessive sweets and snacks and consume food specially prepared for them may be more likely to foster the development of eating disorders, while regular breakfast consumption is negatively associated with an eating disorder (Fernandez-Aranda et al., 2007). Finally, insecure forms of interpersonal attachment (starting with the relative security or insecurity of how babies "attach" with their primary caregivers) has been found to be common in eating disorders, which may hold promise in terms of therapy and understanding transgenerational transmission (Ward et al., 2000).

Social and Cultural Factors

The prevalence of these disorders seems to have increased dramatically over the past several decades. The current increase in prevalence is concurrent with changing cultural standards of beauty as documented by steadily decreasing weights for height over the past two decades among fashion models, Playboy magazine centerfolds, and beauty pageant winners. Social and cultural dynamics that derive from postindustrialized, more modern and westernized nations likely contribute to environments in which eating disordered practices and beliefs are supported. Emerging population data may be reflecting the role of the modernization of society. Peer environment and media exposure may also play a role in beliefs about body ideals and the value of thinness and body shape (Becker et al., 2004).

Social feminist theorists have suggested that anorexia nervosa may signify the unconscious hunger strikes of women who have been demeaned by society, and the highly skewed sex distribution, with a roughly 9 to 1 preponderance of women to men, has also been interpreted as due to cultural influences. Conflict about transitioning gender-appropriate roles for women balancing or redesigning career and family may link social transition to risk for eating disorders (Becker et al., 2004). Also, men who develop anorexia nervosa may have more conflicts over sexual identity and even a higher prevalence of homosexual behavior. Homosexual male college students' attitudes toward their bodies and food fall midway between those of other men and women in college (Yager et al., 1988a). In general, men also face increasing social and cultural pressures to be thin and more muscular.

ANOREXIA NERVOSA

Primary symptoms for both anorexia nervosa and bulimia nervosa are a preoccupation with weight and a desire to be thinner. The two disorders are *not* mutually exclusive, and there appears to be a continuum among patients of the two symptom complexes of self-starvation and the binge–purge cycle: approximately 50% of patients with anorexia nervosa will also have bulimia nervosa, and many patients with bulimia nervosa may have previously had at least a subclinical form of anorexia nervosa.

Description, Diagnostic Criteria, and Differential Diagnosis

Although the diagnosis of anorexia nervosa requires a loss of weight of at least 15% below normal, many patients have lost considerably more by the time they come to medical attention. Many do not present to practitioners until weight loss, amenorrhea, or other physical and psychiatric complications are severe. Patients engage in a variety of behaviors designed to lose weight, such as refusal to eat in front of others, avoidance of entire classes of food, and unusual spice and flavoring practices (e.g., putting huge quantities of pepper or lemon juice on all foods). Some individuals exercise compulsively for hours each day, and compulsions not related to eating, such as cleaning and counting rituals, are common. Although patients may initially seem cheerful and energetic, approximately half of them will develop an accompanying major depression, and all will become moody and irritable. A lifetime prevalence of obsessive-compulsive disorder of up to 40% has also been reported in anorexia nervosa (Kaye et al., 2004). Many complain of not having any real sense of themselves apart from the anorexia nervosa.

Weight losses of 30% to 40% below normal are not unusual. Accompanying these losses are signs and symptoms indicative of the physical complications of starvation: depletion of fat, muscle wasting (including cardiac muscle loss in severe cases), bradycardia and other arrhythmias, constipation, abdominal pains, leukopenia, hypercortisolemia, osteoporosis, and in extreme cases

---

Clinical Characteristics of Anorexia Nervosa
- Overvalued ideas about shape and weight
- Food restriction, overactivity, and purging
- Body checking and other rituals
- Obsessive, anxious, and/or depressed behaviors
- Common onset during adolescence
- Environment of families with perfectionist traits, overinvolvement, high expressed emotion
- Amenorrhea or infertility
- Osteopenia

---

the development of cachexia and lanugo (fine baby-like hair over the body). Metabolic alterations that conserve energy are seen in thyroid function (low T3 syndrome) and reproductive function, with a marked drop or halt in LH and FSH secretion. All women patients stop menstruating; up to a third stop menstruating even before losing sufficient body fat to account for the onset of amenorrhea. Osteopenia is often noted after only 6 months of amenorrhea. Because anorexia nervosa often begins in the early to mid teens, during the peak age of bone formation, the risk of osteoporosis is significant. Anorexia nervosa patients in their mid-20s have seven times the rate of pathological stress fractures as age-matched controls (Rigotti et al., 1984, 1991).

Anorexia nervosa appears in two general varieties, the restricting and binge eating/purging subtypes, although these may occasionally alternate in the same patient. Those with the restricting subtype tend to exert maximal self-control regarding food intake and be socially avoidant, withdrawn, and isolated, with an obsessional thinking style and ritualistic behavior in nonfood areas. In contrast, those with the binge eating–purging subtype are unable to restrain from frequent food binges and then purge by vomiting or ingesting extremely large quantities of laxatives and/or diuretics to further weight loss; they are also commonly depressed and self-destructive; often display the emotional, dramatic, and erratic personality cluster; and frequently abuse alcohol and drugs.

Full recovery within a few years is seen in up to 50% of patients. Younger onset patients and those with the restricting rather than binge eating–purging subtype appear to have a better prognosis. Death from starvation, sudden cardiac arrhythmias, and suicide occurs in 5% of patients within 10 years of onset and almost 20% of patients within 20 years (Steinhausen, 2002). Of note, the death rate has been estimated to be 12 times higher for women with anorexia nervosa than age-matched comparison groups of women in the community and twice as high as other age-matched groups of women psychiatric patients (Sullivan, 1995). Suicide rates for patients with histories of both eating disorders and alcoholism are more than 50 times higher than among community controls. Anorexia nervosa has the highest mortality rate of any psychiatric disorder.

Treatment

Treatment planning for eating disorders must be based on a comprehensive assessment that includes attention to physical status; psychological and behavioral aspects of the eating disorders; associated psychological problems such as substance abuse and mood and personality disturbances; and the family (American Psychiatric Association, 2006). Each patient will have unique problems, and treatment components should be targeted to each specific problem.

Treatment usually includes attention to weight normalization (restoration of a healthy weight determined by the return of menses) and physical complications, enhancement of motivation to return to healthy eating patterns and participate in treatment, and education about healthy eating and nutrition. Treatment also consists of symptom reduction through cognitive behavioral therapy (CBT) programs (e.g., changing core dysfunctional cognitions and feelings and treating associated psychiatric conditions); enlisting family support and treatment through individual, group, and family psychotherapies; and relieving mood disturbances and eating disorder symptoms through psychopharmacological interventions. It is important to prevent relapse. As is true for many types of disorders, some self-help programs may be useful. The following discussion is organized around the management of specific problems related to eating disorders.

Low Weight

Most controlled studies have dealt with short-term weight restoration rather than long-term treatment, and in current practice, initial attention to weight restoration is followed closely by individual and family psychotherapies (American Psychiatric Association, 2006).

There is general, but not universal, agreement that weight restoration should be a central and early goal of treatment for the emaciated patient. Weight restoration may bring about many psychological benefits, including a reduction in obsessional thinking and disturbances in mood and personality. Although some underweight patients may be successfully treated outside the hospital—up to 50% in some series—such a program usually requires a highly motivated patient, a cooperative family, and good prognostic features such as younger age and brief duration of symptoms. The large majority of severely emaciated patients (those at 25% to 50% below recommended weight) require inpatient treatment in a psychiatric unit, a competently staffed general hospital unit, or a specialized eating disorder unit. The problem is how to encourage, persuade, or, in the case of the preterminal recalcitrant patient, benevolently coerce the patient into gaining weight. Patients find an understanding, psychoeducational, empathic approach useful rather than a complete focus on interventions aimed at weight gain. Adolescents treated with hospitalization may have a good outcome and recovery, but in adults with eating disorders requiring hospitalization is usually predicted a poor prognosis.

Although many clinicians employ supplemental estrogens and progestins, calcium, and vitamin D to combat osteopenia and early osteoporosis, such interventions have not been shown to be effective in reversing these conditions in anorexia nervosa (Golden et al., 2002; Mehler, 2003). Low bone mineral density is a consequence of increased bone resorption and decreased bone formation with possible causes related to hypoestrogenism, hypoandrogenism, poor nutrition, hypercortisolemia, decreased insulin growth factor (IGF-I) with possible GH resistance, and elevated ghrelin and peptide YY levels, all particularly adverse during adolescence when peak bone formation usually occurs. Currently, recommended treatments continue to include sustained weight recovery, adequate calcium and vitamin D intake, and careful education about possible risks of excessive and high impact exercise. Oral estrogen does not improve bone mineral density, but other experimental treatments, such as rhIGF-I with estrogen and low-dose testosterone, may be future therapeutic options (Madhusmita and Klibanski, 2006). Current guidelines suggest that estrogen administration may fuse the epiphyses and should not be administered to girls before their growth is complete (American Psychiatric Association, 2006). Patients should be encouraged to achieve weight gain to restoration of menses prior to being offered hormonal interventions. At this time bisphosphonates are not recommended.

Programs that have the best therapeutic effects on eating and weight gain combine informational feedback regarding weight gain and caloric intake, large meals, and a behavioral program that includes both positive reinforcers (e.g., praise and desired visits) and judiciously applied negative reinforcers that are aimed at reducing caloric expenditures (e.g., bed rest, room and activity restrictions, and prolonged hospital stays that become necessary if severely underweight patients do not make sufficient progress toward nutritional rehabilitation).

Lengths of hospital stays are generally shorter for those treated with behavior therapy. However, strict hospital-based behavior therapy programs have not yet been shown to be any more effective in the long run than less rigidly controlled programs. Nasogastric tube feeding and total parenteral nutrition programs are rarely necessary but may sometimes be lifesaving. Supplemental nasogastric refeeding programs remain controversial as to long-term outcomes. In the short term, supplemental nasogastric feedings may promote more rapid weight restoration without interfering with concurrent behavioral programs, and contrary to previous fears, they do not appear to promote rapid relapse once they are discontinued (Rigaud et al., 2007).

Psychotherapies

The role of individual and family psychotherapy in bringing about weight gain is difficult to evaluate. To the extent that a patient's motivation to change may be increased through such therapies, they may be valuable. Families can benefit from family therapy and counseling as soon as the problems are identified, particularly in the treatment of children and adolescents (Lock and le Grange, 2005; Lock et al., 2002).

Psychopharmacological approaches

Many clinical authorities recommend avoiding medications in severely malnourished patients with anorexia nervosa because such patients may be especially prone to serious side effects and no one has yet demonstrated that medication approaches to gaining and sustaining weight have any convincing long-term advantages over nonmedication programs. In particular, malnourished anorexic patients are sensitive to hypotension and arrhythmias associated with tricyclic antidepressants, seizures with bupropion, and extrapyramidal symptoms from metoclopramide. Low doses of atypical antipsychotic medications or anti-anxiety drugs are sometimes prescribed, but existing studies do not support their general use (Brambilla et al., 2007). Thus far, apart from small case series (Gwirtsman et al., 1990; Kaye et al., 1991), the value of selective serotonin reuptake inhibitors (SSRIs) or other antidepressant medications for weight gain is unproved (Claudino et al., 2006). And a multicenter controlled trial focusing on potential relapse prevention strategies for anorexia nervosa patients after they had regained weight found that adding fluoxetine to well-conducted CBT did not offer additional benefits to CBT alone (Walsh et al., 2006). Medical regimens are sometimes required for patients with refeeding syndrome, laxative abuse, severe constipation and other abdominal symptoms, and for associated medical complications.

Psychological Problems
Psychotherapeutic approaches

For anorexia nervosa, most authorities suggest that individual psychotherapy using a highly empathic and nurturing reality-based perspective is most useful. Combinations of supportive advice, education, and praise for progress may be helpful (McIntosh et al., 2006), as are psychotherapies focusing on cognitive, behavioral, and interpersonal issues. The value of family therapy following hospital discharge has also been demonstrated in controlled studies for younger patients with anorexia nervosa (Russell et al., 1987; Lock and le Grange, 2005).

Psychopharmacological approaches

Antidepressant medication is often used for persistent depression following weight gain and sometimes for depression in still-underweight patients. Although little justification exists by way of controlled trials, many clinicians have started to use SSRIs to treat both depressive and obsessive-compulsive symptoms in low-weight patients with anorexia nervosa who are not responding to psychotherapeutic or behavioral interventions alone. Low-dose atypical antipsychotic medications or antianxiety drugs are sometimes used in patients with anorexia nervosa for specific symptoms such as psychotic thinking and severe anxiety, but their use is based solely on clinical impressions of their occasional value (Attia and Schroeder, 2005).

BULIMIA NERVOSA
Description, Diagnostic Criteria, and Differential Diagnosis

Bulimia nervosa occurs predominantly (90% to 95%) in weight-preoccupied females who engage in marked eating binges and purging episodes at least twice a week for 3 consecutive months. Two subtypes can be distinguished: the purging subtype uses self-induced vomiting or misuses laxatives or diuretics; and the nonpurging subtype uses other inappropriate compensatory behaviors such as excessive exercise or fasting, but does not ordinarily self-induce vomiting or misuse laxatives or diuretics. Patients frequently consume between 5000 and 10,000 calories per binge, and binge–purge cycles may occur as frequently as several times per day. Patients feel as if their eating is out of control, are so ashamed that they are often secretive about their problem, and up to 75% have a concurrent major depression or anxiety disorder. For patients with bulimia nervosa, the odds of having a mood, anxiety, or substance use disorder are increased by 7.8, 10.2, and 4.6 times, respectively, over rates in the population at large (Hudson et al., 2007). Substantially increased rates of personality disorders have also been reported among bulimia nervosa patients.

A CASE OF ANOREXIA NERVOSA

A 24-year-old graduate student at a weight of 76 lb was brought for consultation by her husband because she was fainting repeatedly and would not permit herself to eat in spite of his pleas and concerns for her safety. With a height of 5 ft 4 in., she had never weighed >90 lb over the last 4 years and not had a menstrual period since age 16. She permitted herself to eat only tiny bits of white-colored food and only from someone else's plate. Her exercise pattern included 200 push-ups and sit-ups each morning; if she lost count, she was obliged to start over. In addition, she swam 32 laps each day in the university's pool. On days when she permitted herself an extra morsel and thereby considered herself to have been "bad" with respect to eating, she would force herself to swim an additional even number of laps in multiples of four or she would take handfuls of laxatives to induce severe cramps and diarrhea, both as a punishment and to ensure that she lost the additional weight. In spite of these limitations, she was able to carry out complex and demanding intellectual assignments in her courses. Under duress, she finally agreed to gain weight but could do so only by means of an extremely ritualistic diet of carefully measured amounts of cheese and ice cream.

Patients with both personality disorders and bulimia nervosa do not show differences in the overall natural course of bulimia nervosa (Grilo et al., 2007).

All patients with a known or suspected eating disorder need a thorough medical evaluation as well as consideration of other medical disorders that may cause gastrointestinal symptoms (see Table 16-1).

Physical complications of binge–purge cycles include fluid and electrolyte abnormalities with hypochloremic hypokalemic alkalosis, esophageal and gastric irritation and bleeding, large bowel abnormalities due to laxative abuse, marked erosion of dental enamel with accompanying decay, and parotid and salivary gland hypertrophy (squirrel face) with hyperamylasemia of approximately 25% to 40% over normal values (Mitchell et al., 1987).

The disorder is often chronic when untreated, lasting years to decades, but may tend toward slight spontaneous improvement in symptoms over time (Yager et al., 1988b). Over a period of 5 years approximately three quarters of patients with bulimia nervosa who receive treatments of various types will have a remission of symptoms, but almost half will subsequently relapse (Grilo

TABLE 16-1 Differential Diagnosis of Binge Eating and Vomiting

Binge eating
- Bulimia nervosa
- Binge eating disorder (in obese or nonobese)
- CNS lesions (e.g., Kleine-Levin syndrome, seizures, and rarely tumors)
- Appetite increases because of metabolic conditions or drugs
- Other psychiatric disorders such as atypical depression

Vomiting
- Self-induced purging in bulimia nervosa
- CNS causes (e.g., increased intracranial pressure, tumor, seizure disorder)
- Gastrointestinal causes (e.g., mechanical obstruction, malabsorption, ulcers, infections, toxins, metabolic, allergic, "functional")
- Migraine
- Instrumental (goal-directed) vomiting (e.g., wrestlers before a match to reduce weight)
- Endocrine causes (e.g., early pregnancy with "morning sickness," hyperemesis gravidarum, adrenal disease, diabetes mellitus, pituitary dysfunction, hyperparathyroidism)
- Psychogenic causes (e.g., anxiety, conversion disorders, borderline personality disorder)

CNS, central nervous system.

et al., 2007). After 5 years, between half and two-thirds still have significant symptoms (Fairburn et al., 2000).

Treatment

Binge Eating and Purging

In practice, various treatment approaches are frequently combined, depending on the individual's needs.

Psychotherapeutic approaches

Many controlled studies have shown the value of individual and group CBT in particular, although other psychotherapies may be of value as well.

A cognitive behavioral approach includes several stages, each consisting of several weeks or more of weekly or biweekly individual and/or group sessions. The first stage emphasizes the establishment of control over eating using behavioral techniques such as self-monitoring (e.g., keeping a detailed, symptom-relevant diary) and response prevention (e.g., eating until satiated without being allowed to vomit), the prescription of a pattern of regular eating, and stimulus-control measures (e.g., avoidance of situations most likely to stimulate an eating binge). Patients are actively educated about weight regulation, dieting, and the adverse consequences of bulimia nervosa. The second stage focuses on attempts to restructure the patient's unrealistic cognitions (e.g., assumptions and expectations) and instill more effective modes of problem solving. The third stage emphasizes maintaining the gains and preventing relapse, and often provides 6 months to a year of weekly sessions to provide close follow-up during the time that patients are most likely to relapse (Fairburn, 1981, 1995; Fairburn and Wilson, 1993; Yager and Powers, 2007).

Intensive outpatient programs for patients with bulimia nervosa have also been employed in which patients start by attending various group programs several hours each day for several weeks. For those completing the programs, approximately 50% to 90% experience a substantial reduction in binging and purging rates, averaging approximately 70%, and in approximately one-third of patients these symptoms remit entirely (however, the dropout rate is considerable in many groups). Available follow-up reports, generally for <3 years, indicate that many of the gains are maintained, although some recidivism is seen, particularly at times of severe stress. Recent studies show that many patients can benefit from self-guided CBT provided through structured manuals (Schmidt et al., 2007).

Psychodynamic psychotherapy

In a controlled comparison with a 3-year follow-up, interpersonal psychotherapy proved in many respects as or more effective than CBT for treating bulimia nervosa (Fairburn et al., 1995). This approach focuses on issues of losses and grief and interpersonal conflicts and deficits (i.e., personality problems). Although long-term psychodynamic psychotherapy has often been employed to treat bulimia nervosa, no controlled studies of its effectiveness in comparison to other modalities are available. Most CBT programs utilize important interpersonal and psychodynamically derived therapy principles.

Psychopharmacological approaches

Controlled studies indicate that tricyclic antidepressants (particularly imipramine and desipramine), the SSRIs fluoxetine and sertraline, monoamine oxidase inhibitors (MAOIs) and particularly phenelzine, as well as other antidepressants are useful in reducing binge eating and purging in bulimia nervosa (Mitchell et al., 2007), although they are not by themselves an adequate treatment program and often more than one type will have to be tried before the best one for the patient is found. Currently, fluoxetine is the only medication approved by the U.S. Food and Drug Administration to treat bulimia nervosa. Fluoxetine has been shown with convincing evidence to reduce the core symptoms of bulimia nervosa, particularly binge eating and purging, as well as psychological features, in the short term and may decrease relapse at 1 year (Shapiro et al., 2007). SSRIs are commonly chosen as first-line treatments because they are effective and have relatively few adverse effects.

Common problems include medication compliance and maintaining good blood levels amid persistent vomiting. Fluoxetine and the tricyclic antidepressants imipramine and desipramine

A CASE OF BULIMIA NERVOSA

An 18-year-old athletically built college freshman had been bulimic since the age of 15, gorging an estimated 5,000 to 20,000 calories of junk food each evening after her family went to bed and vomiting repeatedly when she felt painfully full. The disorder began when her mother became seriously depressed about the deteriorating health of her own alcoholic mother. In addition to feeling out of control and despondent about her eating, the patient had been sexually promiscuous since age 16 and had been drinking heavily and using cocaine whenever it was available since starting college. Treatment ultimately required programs that addressed her substance abuse problems as well as the eating and mood disorders.

have been best studied in double-blind placebo-controlled trials and are effective in patients with or without concurrent major depression. Higher doses of fluoxetine than those used for depression are necessary for optimal response (e.g., 60 mg per day rather than the usual antidepressant dose of 20 mg per day) (Goldbloom et al., 1995). Other medications with preliminary evidence for efficacy include trazodone, topiramate, duloxetine and odansetron. A 10-week trial showed significantly greater decreases in binging–purging days, body dissatisfaction, drive for thinness, and EAT scores in patients treated with topiramate (average dose 100 mg/day) than in those given placebo (Shapiro et al., 2007).

Results of medication treatment are similar to those with CBT, and many patients who do not respond to psychological treatment alone benefit from medication; initially symptoms are reduced in 70% to 90% of patients, and approximately only one third entirely stop binge eating and purging (Mitchell et al., 2007). Some evidence suggests that combining medication and CBT is better than either treatment alone (Walsh et al., 1997). In practice, many clinicians utilize a combined approach, particularly for patients who do not respond to available psychotherapeutic and educational interventions within a brief period of time.

Hospitalization

Hospitalization is rarely indicated for uncomplicated bulimia nervosa. Indications include failure to respond to adequate outpatient treatment trials, worrisome medical complications not manageable in the outpatient setting, and a severe mood disorder with suicidality.

BINGE EATING DISORDER

Description, Diagnostic Criteria, and Differential Diagnosis

Patients with binge eating disorder typically manifest the psychological and behavioral aspects of patients with bulimia nervosa, but usually without employing the compensatory behaviors such as vomiting or use of laxatives. Consequently, they tend to be obese, because they do not subject themselves to the self-damaging methods of purging. As the condition is currently construed, binge eating must occur at least twice a week for at least 6 months. Eating binges are triggered by dysphoric feelings of tension or distress, boredom, habit, or attempts to diet excessively. Some individuals describe eating to numb themselves emotionally. In comparison to others of similar weight who do not display these patterns, those with binge eating disorders ordinarily have more self-loathing, depression, anxiety, and sensitivity to interpersonal rejection. Onset usually occurs in the teens or 20s, often after strict attempts to diet. Patients with binge eating disorder are more likely to have comorbid depressive, substance abuse, and personality disorders than comparison groups of obese persons without binge eating disorder, but they may be less likely to have these comorbid problems than patients with bulimia nervosa (Hudson et al., 2007).

Treatment

A recent systematic review identified 26 studies examining the efficacy of various treatment modalities for binge eating disorder. The strength of evidence for medications and behavioral interventions was moderate. Medications may provide some benefits for treatment, whereas CBT

Clinical Characteristics of Binge Eating Disorder

- Binge eating episodes cause distress and occur at least twice a week for 6 months
- Binge eating consists of feeling out of control while eating larger amounts of food than most people would eat in 2 hours
- Binge eating occurs with at least three qualifiers:
  - Eating too rapidly
  - Eating until one feels too full or sick
  - Eating large portions when one is not hungry
  - Eating alone because one feels shame about portions
  - Feeling disgusted or guilty after binge eating

individually or in groups reduces binging and improves abstinence (Brownley et al., 2007). Many clinicians use information and experience gleaned from the treatment of bulimia nervosa to guide their clinical decision making. In addition to binge eating episodes, target symptoms often include obesity.

Binge Eating

Substantial reductions in the frequency of binge eating have been obtained with CBT in individual and group settings and in highly structured programs using intensive self-monitoring, nutritional and behavioral counseling, cognitive restructuring, and relapse prevention. This reduction in binge eating and improvement of psychological features such as feelings of restraint, hunger, and disinhibition may last for 4 months but does not lead to weight loss from treatment with CBT or dialectical behavior therapy (Brownley et al., 2007; Munsch et al., 2007). Self-guided manuals employing these techniques may also be helpful (Perkins et al., 2006). Self-help in various techniques with and without facilitation may decrease binge eating and psychological features associated with binge eating disorder and promote abstinence (Brownley et al., 2007).

Medication trials for binge eating disorder have yielded promising yet preliminary results acutely, but improvements seem to fall short over the long term. Almost all gains made on medication disappear when the medication is stopped (Devlin, 1996). SSRIs are associated with a short-term decrease in binge eating. In one study fluoxetine led to a decrease in binge eating, depression, and weight gain as compared to placebo. Citalopram, sertraline, fluoxetine, and imipramine all produced reductions in binge eating but variable responses to depressive and obsessive symptoms and did not produce significant rates of remission. The placebo effect is very large in studies of binge eating disorder, as are dropout rates (Brownley et al., 2007). The appetite suppressant sibutramine is associated with decreases in binge eating and weight loss (Appolinario et al., 2003), as is the fat absorption blocking medication orlistat (Grilo et al., 2005), but both are associated with bothersome adverse effects. In controlled trials topiramate decreased binge episodes, days, and obsessive-compulsive psychological features (McElroy et al., 2003).

Weight Loss

Results have been mixed regarding weight loss among obese binge eaters. CBT programs designed specifically to help obese binge eaters lose weight are more effective at producing weight loss than those aimed solely at reducing binge eating episodes. Substantial numbers will regain much of their lost weight within 2 to 5 years following such treatments.

Pharmacologic treatments for weight loss among binge eating and non–binge eating obese persons are a matter of considerable interest and some controversy (National Task Force on the Prevention and Treatment of Obesity, 1996). In short-term studies, fluoxetine, citalopram, sertraline, bupropion, and imipramine have been superior to placebo in facilitating weight loss, but only while medication is taken. As noted earlier, the appetite suppressant sibutramine and the fat absorption blocker orlistat are associated with decreases in binge eating and also result

A CASE OF BINGE EATING DISORDER

A 44-year-old married woman, 5 ft 5 in. and 150 lb, complained of being a compulsive overeater for >20 years, since shortly after the birth of her first child. Although she weighed only 125 lb when she got married, she gained 60 lb during her first pregnancy and was never able to return to her earlier weight in spite of multiple diets using everything from Weight Watchers to very low calorie diets to diet pills. She found herself compulsively eating large quantities of chocolate and pastries, her "downfall," several times per week, whenever she was alone in the house, particularly when she felt stressed or irritable. She felt defeated and demoralized and had considerable self-hate in relation to her appearance. Although her husband had been generally supportive, she felt that he was starting to make snide remarks about her figure and her "inability to control" herself, and she feared for her marriage.

in weight loss. Topiramate may be an effective medication for weight loss as well. One study comparing weight loss therapy with CBT and desipramine showed the greatest weight loss in the group that received all three interventions. None of these treatments yield persistent weight loss after medication is discontinued (Brownley et al., 2007).

ROLE OF THE NONPSYCHIATRIC PHYSICIAN IN PATIENT MANAGEMENT

The nonpsychiatric physician should play a major role in the prevention, detection, and management of patients with eating disorders. Pediatricians and family physicians should be alert to excessive concerns about dieting and appearance in preteens and their families and educate them about healthy nutrition and the dangers of eating disorders. Because the prevalence of subclinical and full-blown forms of these disorders is so high, physicians should routinely question young female patients about what they desire to weigh; their dietary, dieting, and exercise practices; and their use of laxatives. Psychological problems in young women should stimulate attention to symptoms of eating disorder as well as problems with mood, anxiety, substance abuse, sexual behavior, and more. Gynecologists, internists, gastroenterologists, dermatologists, and dentists are also likely to encounter in their practices large numbers of patients with eating disorders. Dermatologists may be able to identify those with a hidden eating disorder early in the course of illness, because 40 cutaneous signs have been identified, classified, and associated with variations in an individual's body mass index (BMI) (Strumia, 2005).

Once an eating disorder is detected, patients merit a full physical examination; laboratory tests including electrolytes, complete blood count, thyroid, calcium, magnesium, and (for suspected purging) amylase studies; and, for the very thin patient, blood urea nitrogen (BUN), creatinine, and an electrocardiogram or rhythm strip. Patients who have been amenorrheic for 6 months or more should have a bone densitometry assessment (dual energy x-ray absorptiometry [DEXA] scan). The physician should work with a registered dietician and mental health professional knowledgeable about eating disorders to see if the problems can be ameliorated in outpatient care. This multidisciplinary team approach can be highly successful with motivated patients. The physician's role is to educate, encourage, refer, and monitor the patient's weight and laboratory tests. For the patient with anorexia nervosa, monitoring should include weekly or twice weekly visits to the office for postvoiding weights in a hospital gown (with care taken that the patient has not imbibed large quantities of fluid just before being weighed and is not concealing hidden weights) and for ongoing monitoring of any physiological abnormalities of concern.

The physician should also prescribe and monitor a course of antidepressant medication for young adults with bulimia nervosa and mood or anxiety disorders associated with an eating disorder.

Patients with binge eating disorder should be referred for CBT and dietary counseling. If symptoms of depression or anxiety are severe, treatment with an SSRI should be considered. If the patient's obesity is moderate, carries high risk for medically serious complications, and fails to respond to CBT interventions, treatments using sibutramine or topiramate are the options. For morbidly obese patients, those who are at least 100 lb overweight, and for whom more conventional treatments fail, surgical approaches such as gastroplasties with banding should be considered and may be lifesaving.

INDICATIONS FOR PSYCHIATRIC CONSULTATION AND REFERRAL

Every patient with a serious eating disorder warrants consultation with a psychiatrist knowledgeable about eating disorders for guidance to the patient, family, and referring physician about the nature, severity, and prognosis of the disorder and what treatment options are available. A primary care physician should also enlist the support of a registered dietician in the patient's treatment. The patient and family are educated regarding the nature and severity of the illness; health risks; benefits of treatment, including reducing pathologic behaviors and attitudes; and the need for follow-up (Yager and Andersen, 2005).

Specific indications for mandatory consultation include failure of the patient to respond to attempts at management in the physician's setting with deteriorating status, severe depression with suicidality, or marked family problems. The feasibility of outpatient weight restoration and availability of local resources should also be considered.

Clinical Pearls

- Alerting signs include menstrual irregularities, infertility, desire to weigh 10 to 15 lb less than reasonable, overconcern with weight or physical appearance, vague gastrointestinal complaints, overuse of laxatives or diuretics, and mood or anxiety disturbance.
- Signs of self-induced vomiting include puffy cheeks, scars on the knuckles (Russell sign), and decay of the front teeth.
- Alerting laboratory signs include disturbances in serum electrolytes, magnesium, and amylase.
- Patients with anorexia nervosa are often devious in providing information and getting weighed (e.g., drinking large quantities of fluids or putting weights in their clothing). Alternative informants such as family members are always required.
- Suspect osteopenia in patients amenorrheic for as little as 6 months. Bone densitometry may be indicated to educate patients about the objective seriousness of their condition.

Self-Assessment Questions and Answers

16-1. Patients with bulimia nervosa who engage in binge/purge behaviors are at risk for which of the following medical findings?

A. Hyperkalemia
B. Increased serum amylase
C. Hyperchloremia
D. Hypothyroidism
E. Hypermagnesemia

Serum amylase is often increased 25% to 40% over normal values in individuals who are purging. The primary source is increased secretion from salivary glands that are overstimulated by self-induced vomiting, although pancreatic amylase secretion may also be stimulated by these processes. Patients who vomit gastric secretions and gastric fluids often have hypokalemic, hypochloremic alkalosis as a consequence of losing potassium, chloride, and acid from the stomach, and therefore are very unlikely to have hyperkalemia or hyperchloremia.

Hypothyroidism is not associated with binge eating or purging. Magnesium loss may occur in patients who purge by laxative abuse, but the diarrhea that ensues is likely to produce hypomagnesemia, not hypermagnesemia. *Answer: B*

16-2. A 17-year-old girl is taken to her family physician by her worried parents. In the last 6 months she has become determined to lose weight despite never being overweight at 130 lb and 5 ft 6 in (body mass index [BMI] of 21). She loses weight through dieting and exercise and currently weighs 100 lb (BMI of 16) and stopped menstruating 4 months ago. She has developed some strange rituals, including checking her body in the mirror many times throughout the day and adding large amounts of lemon juice to her food. What first step of treatment should be offered?

A. Initiate bisphosphonates to treat osteopenia secondary to dysmenorrhea from anorexia nervosa and prevent further bone loss.

B. Tell the patient to eat more and gain weight so that she resumes her menses.

C. Educate the patient and her family about anorexia nervosa, the health risks, the benefits of treatment beginning with weight restoration with the help of a registered dietician, and the need for close follow-up.

D. Tell the patient she needs to start an SSRI such as fluoxetine in order to treat her anorexia nervosa and gain weight.

E. As this is a normal presentation in a teenage girl interested in sports and her appearance, no further intervention is necessary at this time.

Anorexia nervosa guidelines suggest that the first important treatment includes education for the individual and family, description of health risks, involvement of a registered dietician, and weight restoration with a close follow-up. Bisphosphonates are not indicated to treat osteopenia in anorexia nervosa. Selective serotonin reuptake inhibitors (SSRIs) are not first-line treatment for anorexia nervosa but are sometimes used after weight restoration and when the individual has significant associated psychological concerns. The young woman meets criteria for anorexia nervosa so this is not a normal presentation and she will not improve if the clinician simply instructs her to gain weight (Yager and Andersen, 2005). *Answer: C*

16-3. A 43-year-old man accompanies his wife to an Overeaters Anonymous meeting at her insistence. He has been unable to stop his binge eating, and she has become more concerned about his obesity, as he has been diagnosed with hypertension. He has started a weight loss program recommended by his doctor but finds himself unable to adhere to it successfully. During periods of discouragement, he has begun to eat large quantities in a binge pattern. Which one of the following is the best choice for treating binge eating disorder?

A. Individual psychodynamic psychotherapy

B. D-thyroxine

C. Cognitive behavioral therapy

D. Dexfenfluramine

E. Dextroamphetamine

There is a strong evidence base showing cognitive behavioral therapy's effectiveness for binge eating disorder. Although psychodynamic psychotherapy may work for some patients, at this point no strong, well-controlled studies of its use for binge eating disorder have been conducted. Dexfenfluramine has been removed from the market after it was found to reduce binge eating but cause increased risk for pulmonary hypertension and heart valve problems. D-thyroxine and dextroamphetamine are not indicated in this hypertensive patient. *Answer: C*

16-4. An 18-year-old woman being evaluated for depression reveals that she worries excessively about her weight. She states that she is unable to diet and consumes large quantities of food about once a month. She appears to have normal weight for her height. What is the most likely diagnosis?

A. Anorexia nervosa

B. Body dysmorphic disorder

C. Bulimia nervosa

D. Eating disorder not otherwise specified

E. Factitious disorder

Although this patient has significant concerns and issues related to eating disorders, she does not have anorexia nervosa, because she has not lost weight to make the criterion of weighing <15% of her healthy weight. She is concerned overall about her weight but, from the available information, is not preoccupied with the shape or appearance of specific body parts, so that she does not appear to have body dysmorphic disorder. Although she appears to have episodes of overeating or binge eating, there is no indication that she is purging, so bulimia nervosa seems less likely. Factitious disorder is not likely because there are no physical signs or symptoms that she might be creating or intentionally provoking. *Answer: D*

16-5. Which of the following psychiatric disorders will up to half of patients with anorexia nervosa experience?

A. Posttraumatic stress disorder

B. Generalized anxiety disorder

C. Major depressive disorder

D. Obsessive-compulsive disorder

E. Social phobia

Although many disorders are in fact comorbid with anorexia nervosa, particularly obsessive-compulsive disorder (40%), major depression is the most common, with a prevalence and lifetime comorbidity of approximately 50%. *Answer: C*

References

American Obesity Association. *Obesity in the U.S.: overall prevalence*. Accessed on June 17, 2006. Available at www.obesity1.tempdomainname.com.

American Psychiatric Association. *Diagnostic and statistical manual*, 4th ed., text revised. Washington, DC: American Psychiatric Association; 2000.

American Psychiatric Association. Practice guidelines for eating disorders. *Am J Psychiatry*. 2006; 163(Suppl):7.

Anderluh MB, Tchanturia K, Rabe-Hesketh S, et al. Childhood obsessive-compulsive personality traits in adult women with eating disorders: Defining a broader eating disorder phenotype. *Am J Psychiatry*. 2003;160:2.

Appolinario JC, Bacaltchuk J, Sichieri R, et al. A randomized, double-blind placebo-controlled study of sibutramine in the treatment of binge-eating disorder. *Arch Gen Psychiatry*. 2003;60:1109–1116.

Attia E, Schroeder L. Pharmacologic treatment of anorexia nervosa: Where do we go from here? *Int J Eat Disord*. 2005;37:S60–S63.

Becker AE, Keel P, Anderson-Fye EP, et al. Genes and/or jeans?: Genetic and socio-cultural contributions to risk for eating disorders. *J Addict Dis*. 2004;23(3):81–103.

Brambilla F, Garcia CS, Fassino S, et al. Olanzapine therapy in anorexia nervosa: Psychological effects. *Int Clin Psychopharmacol*. 2007;22(4):197–204.

Brownley KA, Berkman ND, Sedway JA, et al. Binge eating disorder treatment: A systematic review of randomized controlled trials. *Int J Eat Disord*. 2007;40:337–348.

Bulik C. Exploring the gene-environment nexus in eating disorders. *J Psychiatry Neurosci*. 2005;30(5): 335–339.

Claudino AM, Silva de Lima M, Hay PPJ, et al. Antidepressants for anorexia nervosa. *Cochrane Database Syst Rev*. 2006;(1):CD004365.

Cook WL, Kenny DA, Goldstein MJ. Parental affective style risk and the family system: A social relations model analysis. *J Abnorm Psychol*. 1991;100(4):492–501.

Crisp AH, Hall A, Holland AJ. Nature and nurture in anorexia nervosa: A study of 34 pairs of twins, one pair of triplets and an adoptive family. *Int J Eat Disord*. 1985;4:5–29.

Derenne JL, Beresin EB. Body image, media, and eating disorders. *Acad Psychiatry*. 2006;30:257–261.

Devlin M. Assessment and treatment of binge eating disorder. *Psychiatr Clin North Am*. 1996;19:761–772.

de Zwaan M, Nutziger DO, Schoenbeck G. Binge eating in overweight women. *Compr Psychiatry*. 1992;33:256–261.

Drewnowski A, Hopkins SA, Kessler RC. The prevalence of bulimia nervosa in the US college student population. *Am J Public Health*. 1988;78:1322–1325.

Fairburn CG. A cognitive behavioral approach to the treatment of bulimia. *Psychol Med*. 1981;11: 707–711.

Fairburn CG. *Overcoming binge eating*. New York: Guilford Press; 1995.

Fairburn CG, Wilson GT, eds. *Binge eating: Nature, assessment, and treatment*. New York: Guilford Press; 1993.

Fairburn CG, Norman PA, Welch SL, et al. A prospective study of outcome in bulimia nervosa and the long-term effects of three psychological treatments. *Arch Gen Psychiatry*. 1995;52:304–312.

Fairburn CG, Cooper Z, Doll HA, et al. The natural course of bulimia nervosa and binge eating disorder in young women. *Arch Gen Psychiatry*. 2000;57:659–665.

Fernandez-Aranda F, Krug I, Granero R, et al. Individual and family eating patterns during childhood and early adolescence: An analysis of associated eating disorder factors. *Appetite*. 2007;49(2):476–485.

Garfinkel PE, Garner DM. *Anorexia nervosa: A multidimensional perspective*. New York: Brunner/Mazel; 1982.

Garner DM, Garfinkel PE, eds. *Handbook of psychotherapy for anorexia nervosa and bulimia*, 2nd ed. New York: Guilford Press; 1997.

Goldbloom DJ, Wilson MG, Thompson VL, et al. Fluoxetine Bulimia Nervosa Research Group. Long-term fluoxetine treatment of bulimia nervosa. *Br J Psychiatry*. 1995;166:660–666.

Golden NH, Lanzkowsky L, Schebendach J, et al. The effect of estrogen-progestin treatment on bone mineral density in anorexia nervosa. *J Pediatr Adolesc Gynecol*. 2002;15:135–143.

Grilo CM, Masheb RM, Salant SL. Cognitive behavioral therapy guided self-help and orlistat for the treatment of binge eating disorder: A randomized, double-blind, placebo-controlled trial. *Biol Psychiatry*. 2005;57(10):1193–1201.

Grilo CM, Pagano ME, Skodol AE, et al. Natural course of bulimia nervosa and of eating disorder not otherwise specified: 5-year prospective study of remissions, relapses, and the effects of personality disorder psychopathology. *J Clin Psychiatry*. 2007;68(5):738–746.

Gwirtsman HE, Guze BH, Yager J, et al. Treatment of anorexia nervosa with fluoxetine: An open clinical trial. *J Clin Psychiatry*. 1990;51:378–382.

Haines J, Neumark-Sztainer D. Prevention of obesity and eating disorders: A consideration of shared risk factors. *Health Educ Res*. 2006;21(6):770–782.

Hudson JI, Hiripi E, Pope HG Jr, et al. The prevalence and correlates of eating disorders in the National Comorbidity Survey Replication. *Biol Psychiatry*. 2007;61(3):348–358.

Jimerson DC, Wolfe BE. Neuropeptides in eating disorders. *CNS Spectr*. 2004;9(7):516–522.

Kaye WH, Weltzin TW, Hsu LKG, et al. An open trial of fluoxetine in patients with anorexia nervosa. *J Clin Psychiatry*. 1991;52:464–471.

Kaye WH, Bulik CM, Thornton L, et al. Price Foundation Collaborative Group. Comorbidity of anxiety disorders with anorexia and bulimia nervosa. *Am J Psychiatry*. 2004;161:2215–2221.

Kaye WH, Frank GK, Bailer UF, et al. Neurobiology of anorexia nervosa: Clinical implications of alterations of the function of serotonin and other neuronal systems. *Int J Eat Disord*. 2005;37:S15–S19.

Kendler KS, MacLean C, Neale M, et al. The genetic epidemiology of bulimia nervosa. *Am J Psychiatry*. 1991;148:1627–1637.

Krassas GE. Endocrine abnormalities in anorexia nervosa. *Pediatr Endocrinol Rev*. 2003;1(1):46–54.

Lock J, Grange D, Agras WS, et al., eds. *Treatment manual for anorexia nervosa: A family-based approach*. New York: Guilford Press; 2002.

Lock J, le Grange D. Family-based treatment of eating disorders. *Int J Eat Disord*. 2005;37:S64–S67.

Madhusmita M, Klibanski A. Anorexia nervosa and osteoporosis. *Rev Endocr Metab Disord*. 2006;7: 91–99.

Marrazzi MA, Luby ED. An auto-addiction opioid model of chronic anorexia nervosa. *Int J Eat Disord*. 1986;5:191–208.

McElroy SL, Arnold LM, Shapira NA, et al. Topiramate in the treatment of binge eating disorder associated with obesity: A randomized, placebo-controlled trial. *Am J Psychiatry*. 2003;160:2.

McIntosh VVW, Jordan J, Luty SE, et al. Specialist supportive clinical management for anorexia nervosa. *Int J Eat Disord*. 2006;39:625–632.

Mehler PS. Osteoporosis in anorexia nervosa: Prevention and treatment. *Int J Eat Disord*. 2003;33: 113–126.

Minuchin S, Rosman BL, Baker L. *Psychosomatic families: Anorexia nervosa in context*. Cambridge: Harvard University Press; 1978.

Mitchell JE, Seim HC, Colon E, et al. Medical complications and medical management of bulimia. *Ann Droit Int Med*. 1987;107:71–77.

Mitchell JE, Agras S, Wonderlich S. Treatment of bulimia nervosa: Where are we and where are we going? *Int J Eat Disord*. 2007;40:95–101.

Mond J, Hay P, Rodgers B, et al. Use of extreme weight control behaviors with and without binge eating in a community sample: Implications for the classification of bulimic-type eating disorders. *Int J Eat Disord*. 2006;39:294–302.

Munsch S, Biedert E, Meyer A, et al. A randomized comparison of cognitive behavioral therapy and behavioral weight loss treatment for overweight individuals with binge eating disorder. *Int J Eat Disord*. 2007;40:102–113.

National Task Force on the Prevention and Treatment of Obesity. Long-term pharmacotherapy in the management of obesity. *JAMA*. 1996;276:1907–1915.

O'Hara SK, Smith KC. Presentation of eating disorders in the news media: What are the implications for patient diagnosis and treatment? *Patient Educ Couns*. 2007;68(1):43–51.

Perkins SJ, Murphy R, Schmidt U, et al. Self-help and guided self-help for eating disorders. *Cochrane Database Syst Rev*. 2006;(3):CD004191.

Rigaud D, Brondel L, Poupard AT, et al. A randomized trial on the efficacy of a 2-month tube feeding regimen in anorexia nervosa: A 1-year follow-up study. *Clin Nutr*. 2007;26:421–429.

Rigotti NA, Nussbaum SR, Herzog DB, et al. Osteoporosis in women with anorexia nervosa. *N Engl J Med*. 1984;311:1601–1606.

Rigotti NA, Neer RM, Skates SJ, et al. The clinical course of osteoporosis in anorexia nervosa: A longitudinal study of cortical bone mass. *JAMA*. 1991;265:1133–1138.

Russell GFM, Szmukler GI, Dare C, et al. An evaluation of family therapy in anorexia nervosa and bulimia nervosa. *Arch Gen Psychiatry*. 1987;44:1047–1056.

Schmidt U, Lee S, Beecham J, et al. A randomized controlled trial of family therapy and cognitive behavior therapy guided self-care for adolescents with bulimia nervosa and related disorders. *Am J Psychiatry*. 2007;164:591–598.

Shapiro JR, Berkman ND, Brownley KA, et al. Bulimia nervosa treatment: A systematic review of randomized controlled trials. *Int J Eat Disord*. 2007;40:321–336.

Silberg JL, Bulik CM. The developmental association between eating disorders symptoms and symptoms of depression and anxiety in juvenile twin girls. *J Child Psychol Psychiatry*. 2005;46(12):1317–1326.

Spitzer RL, Devlin MC, Walsh BT, et al. Binge eating disorder: A multi-site field trial of the diagnostic criteria. *Int J Eat Disord*. 1992;11:191–203.

Spitzer RL, Yanovski S, Wadden T, et al. Binge eating disorder: Its further validation in a multisite study. *Int J Eat Disord*. 1993;13:137–153.

Steinhausen H.-Ch. The outcome of anorexia in the 20th century. *Am J Psychiatry*. 2002;159:1284–1293.

Steinhausen HC, Gavez S, Winkler Metzke C. Psychosocial correlates, outcome, and stability of abnormal adolescent eating behavior in community samples of young people. *Int J Eat Disord*. 2005;37:119–126.

Strumia R. Dermatologic signs in patients with eating disorders. *Am J Clin Dermatol*. 2005;6(3):165–173.

Sullivan PF. Mortality in anorexia nervosa. *Am J Psychiatry*. 1995;152:1073–1074.

Walsh BT, Wilson GT, Loeb KL, et al. Medication and psychotherapy in the treatment of bulimia nervosa. *Am J Psychiatry*. 1997;154:523–531.

Walsh BT, Kaplan AS, Attia E, et al. Fluoxetine after weight restoration in anorexia nervosa: A randomized controlled trial. *JAMA*. 2006;295(22):2605–2612.

Ward A, Ramsay R, Treasure J. Attachment research in eating disorders. *Br J Med Psychol*. 2000;73(Pt1): 35–51.

Yager J. Family issues in the pathogenesis of anorexia nervosa. *Psychosom Med*. 1982;44:43–60.

Yager J, Andersen AE. Anorexia nervosa. *N Engl J Med*. 2005;353(1):1481–1488.

Yager J, Powers P, eds. *Clinical manual of eating disorders*. Arlington: American Psychiatric Press; 2007.

Yager J, Kurtsman F, Landsverk J, et al. Behaviors and attitudes related to eating disorders in homosexual male college students. *Am J Psychiatry*. 1988a;145:495–497.

Yager J, Landsverk J, Edelstein CK. A 20-month follow-up study of 628 women with eating disorders, Part I: Course and severity. *Am J Psychiatry*. 1988b;144:1172–1177.

Sleep Disorders

THE SCOPE AND CONSEQUENCE OF SLEEP SYMPTOMS AND SLEEP DISORDERS

Sleep-related symptoms such as insomnia, poor sleep quality, daytime somnolence, fatigue, and lack of energy rank among the most common complaints in all branches of medicine. A survey of the general population by the National Sleep Foundation revealed that 21% of the population polled felt that they had a sleep problem (National Sleep Foundation, 2005). In a home-interview study of 3,030 community dwellers, 15.9% to 22.3% reported some form of insomnia, and in a telephone survey of 982 community dwellers, 37.9% reported insomnia of any kind, with 11.7% meeting criteria for insomnia (Ohayon and Partinen, 2002). Sleep-related symptoms are also widely reported in people with psychiatric and medical conditions.

Sleep disorders are consequential. They lead to significant impairments in quality of life, the magnitude of which equals, and in some areas surpasses, the impairments associated with other chronic medical and psychiatric conditions, such as major depression and congestive heart failure (Katz and McHorney, 2002). They are associated with poor mental functioning, decreased occupational efficiency, reduced industrial productivity, and an increased risk of traffic accidents (Mitler et al., 1988). Some sleep disorders (e.g., sleep apnea syndrome) are associated with an increased risk of cardiovascular disease and death (Gozal and Kheirandish-Gozal, 2008). Persistent insomnia is associated with an increased risk to develop new emotional disorders in the future, in particular depressive, anxiety, and substance-use disorders (Ford and Kamerow, 1989; Tan et al., 1984). The recognition of the potentially deleterious effect of sleep deprivation and shift work sleep disorder on the productivity, safety, and welfare of physicians-in-training, and on their patients' medical care, prompted the Accreditation Council for Graduate Medical Education (ACGME) to approve an 80-hour weekly work limit for resident physicians (Volpp et al., 2007).

Given the fact that many effective interventions are now available for primary and secondary sleep disorders, it behooves physicians of all specialties to become familiar with the evaluation and management of sleep disorders.

NORMAL HUMAN SLEEP

Sleep Stages and Architecture

The milestone discovery of rapid eye movement (REM) sleep by Aerinksy and Kleitman in 1953 made it clear that sleep is not merely the absence of wakefulness, but a complex behavioral, physiological, and psychological state that is the product of active and coordinated brain processes which have correlates throughout the rest of the body. Within the brain, these processes produce an orderly progression through various stages of sleep that repeat in a cyclical manner throughout the night, resulting in the pattern known as *sleep architecture*.

Proper characterization of sleep stages requires simultaneous monitoring of various physiological parameters, a process known as *polysomnography*. Minimally required are the electroencephalogram (EEG), electrooculogram (EOG), and the electromyogram (EMG) of skeletal muscle, typically the submentalis (Rechtshaffen and Kales, 1968). The EEGs of awake and attentive individuals exhibit a pattern of low voltage and mixed ("random") frequencies. However, during relaxed wakefulness or drowsiness, the EEG reveals a preponderance of rhythmic alpha activity (8 to 12 cps). The transition from wakefulness to stage 1 sleep is marked by the disappearance of rhythmic α and the establishment of relatively low voltage and mixed frequency pattern with the prevalence of theta (3 to 7 cps) activity.

During stage 2, two characteristic waveforms are noted: sleep spindles (12 to 14 cps activity lasting 0.5 to 1.5 seconds) and K complexes (negative sharp waves followed by a slower positive component lasting 0.5 second or greater). Low-voltage mixed-frequency activities persist in the background. Sleep spindles are synchronized waveforms, that is, they have a uniform oscillatory pattern resulting from the simultaneous activation of large numbers of neurons by one or more synchronizing pacemakers located in the thalamus. Spindles are found in all mammals and identical in all species. They develop before age 3 months in humans and may be slower to develop in mental retardation. Spindles are generated by the thalamus and thought to promote the closure of the thalamic gate during non–rapid eye movement (NREM) sleep, resulting in the obliteration of synaptic transmission to the cortex. The significance of K complexes is unknown; they may occur spontaneously or in response to environmental noise.

During stages 3 and 4, high amplitude, slow delta activity (<3 cps) dominates the record. During stage 3 sleep, 20% to 50% of the tracing comprises delta waves, whereas during stage 4 sleep, >50% of the record comprises delta waves. Stages 3 and 4 sleep are collectively referred to as *delta sleep, deep sleep,* and *slow wave sleep.* Well-formed delta waves are not seen until 2 to 6 months after birth. The emergence of delta sleep is a reflection of maturation in brain structure and function.

Although the eyes are still (other than occasional eye blinks) during relaxed wakefulness, involuntary ocular activity occurs just before the onset of stage 1 sleep (see Fig. 17-1). On the EOG, this is noted as slow ("rolling") eye movements. These usually persist during the initial portions of stage 1. Eye movements are absent during stages 2, 3, and 4 (see Fig. 17-2). During wakefulness, the EMG reveals phasic (episodic) bursts of activity. However, as individuals wind down before sleep, EMG tone (amplitude) gradually diminishes and continues to do so as sleep progresses through the various stages. Stages 1 through 4 are collectively referred to as *non-REM* (*NREM*) sleep and constitute approximately 75% of total sleep time in adults.

During REM sleep, the EEG again displays low-voltage mixed frequencies. However, characteristic REMs are noted on the EOG, and the EMG displays the lowest amplitude of the night, a reflection of skeletal muscle atonia mediated through active central nervous system (CNS) inhibition (see Fig. 17-3).

Sleep is typically entered through stage 1, and an orderly progression from stages 1 through 4 occurs within 45 minutes of falling asleep. Within 90 minutes, the first REM period occurs. This NREM-REM pattern, referred to as a *sleep cycle*, lasts approximately 90 minutes and recurs

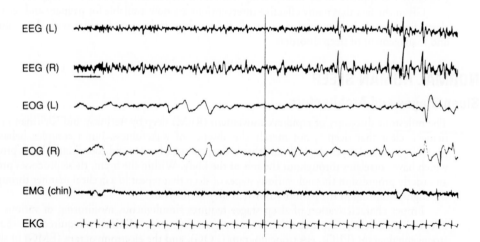

FIGURE 17-1. Stage 1 sleep. EEG, electroencephalogram; EOG, electrooculogram; EMG, electromyogram; EKG, electrocardiogram. L, left; R, right. (Reprinted with permission from Stoudemire, *Clinical Psychiatry for Medical Students*, Third Edition.)

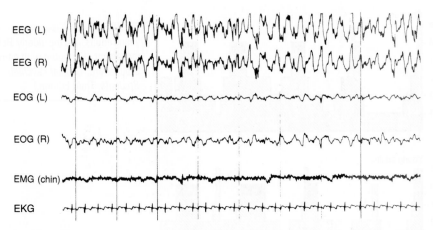

FIGURE 17-2. Stages 2, 3, and 4. (Reprinted with permission from Stoudemire, *Clinical Psychiatry for Medical Students*, Third Edition.)

continuously throughout the night (see Fig. 17-4). Although this cycle is present at birth, each cycle lasts 50 to 60 minutes in neonates and is usually devoid of slow wave sleep.

Delta sleep is most prominent in the first third of the night and virtually disappears during the last third of the night. Greater periods of prior sleep deprivation result in longer periods of delta sleep in the beginning of the night on subsequent nights. In contrast, REM sleep periods, although initially brief in duration, lengthen with each subsequent sleep cycle such that REM sleep is most prominent in the last third of the night. This pattern is relatively independent of prior sleep deprivation and thought to be controlled by a circadian oscillator in the brain, one that also controls body temperature, the concentration of plasma cortisol, and other biological cycles (Tobler, 2005).

The percentage distribution of sleep stages in a young adult is outlined in Table 17-1 (Iglowstein et al., 2003). Many factors alter these percentages. For example, conditions that produce sleep disruption, such as disease states and environmental noise, cause an increase in the proportion of stage 1 sleep and a decrease in delta sleep. Age also has profound effects on sleep. Delta sleep is maximal in children and diminishes markedly with age, especially during adolescence. Seniors may have little or no delta sleep. The loss of delta sleep with age may be a

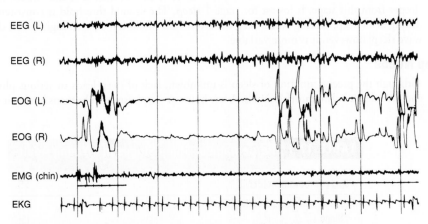

FIGURE 17-3. Rapid eye movement (REM) sleep. (Reprinted with permission from Stoudemire, *Clinical Psychiatry for Medical Students*, Third Edition.)

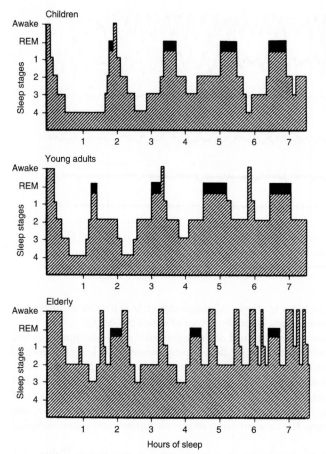

FIGURE 17-4. Sleep cycles in children, young adults, and the elderly. REM, rapid eye movement. (Reprinted with permission from Stoudemire, *Clinical Psychiatry for Medical Students*, Third Edition.)

consequence of the diminution in cortical synaptic activity. In contrast, stage 1 sleep increases with age. With aging, there is a general tendency toward sleep fragmentation, characterized by an increase in the frequency of awakenings and brief arousals.

Sleep Depth

The arousal threshold, as measured by the volume of environmental sound needed to awaken a sleeper from this stage, is lowest for stage 1 sleep. The arousal threshold is consistently highest during delta sleep. During REM sleep the arousal threshold can be even higher than during delta wave sleep; however, it is more variable.

Sleep Needs

Although the precise function of sleep is unknown, lack of sleep leads to serious physical harm and even death in laboratory animals. A few hours of sleeplessness in humans have minimal effects

TABLE 17-1	**Percentage of Sleep Stages in a Young Adult**
Rapid eye movement (REM)	25
Nonrapid eye movement (NREM)	75
Stage 1	(5)
Stage 2	(45)
Stages 3 and 4	(25)

on cognitive function and alertness levels the following day. However, with greater deprivation of sleep, performance on tasks becomes impaired. Although the average nightly sleep duration is approximately 8 hours in adults, children obtain approximately 10 hours and the elderly <7 hours. The situation is complicated by the fact that the need for sleep is highly variable from person to person even within similar age-groups, with some individuals requiring as little as 5 hours of nightly sleep. The most prudent answer to the question "How much sleep do I need?" is the amount of sleep that consistently results in optimal daytime alertness and a sense of mental efficiency and well-being.

When discussing sleep needs, consideration should also be given to the need for optimal sleep quality because this also contributes to daytime alertness. Sleep quality refers to the integrity of the sleep architectural pattern. Impairments in sleep quality appear polysomnographically as an increase in the number of arousals (brief increases in EEG frequency and stage changes), awakenings, and body movements; an increase in the shallow stages of sleep (1 and 2); a decrease in deep (delta) sleep; and a decrease in the number of well-formed sleep cycles. Conditions that lead to impairment in sleep quality and quantity, and treatments that improve these, will be discussed later in this chapter.

Sleep Deprivation and Rebound

On the night following total sleep deprivation, a rebound of delta sleep is noted first; that is, delta sleep is recovered at the expense of other sleep stages. REM rebound occurs later during the night or on subsequent nights. The conservation of slow wave sleep is one of many findings that support the notion that delta sleep is related to the maintenance of important biological and psychological functions. Additionally, selective deprivation of either delta or REM sleep for long periods of time also results in a subsequent rebound in the proportion of that particular sleep stage. For example, REM rebound is often seen following the abrupt discontinuation of drugs that suppress REM activity, such as certain antidepressant agents, and is often experienced as vivid dreaming and nightmares.

COGNITIVE AND BEHAVIORAL ASPECTS OF SLEEP

Cognitive mental processes seem to be at a low level during stage 1 sleep, because sleepers who are awakened from it usually report experiencing thought fragments or vague images. Most individuals awakened from delta sleep report no mental activity at all. In contrast, most sleepers report dreams when awakened from REM sleep. Dreaming is only one facet of a host of complex biological processes that are activated during REM sleep and affect almost every bodily function. These produce, among other things, REMs, bursts of tachycardia, penile tumescence, and peripheral skeletal muscle atonia. The observation of a highly active mind superimposed on a picture of a motionless paralyzed body is one finding among many that led earlier researchers to refer to REM sleep as *paradoxical* sleep.

The onset of sleep is characterized by a reduced responsiveness to environmental stimuli. Individuals asked to respond to sound or light have an increased reaction time as they approach sleep and no longer react following established sleep. Consequently, sleep-deprived automobile drivers tend to react sluggishly to traffic hazards and are more vulnerable to traffic accidents. Nevertheless, responsiveness to certain important stimuli can be maintained during normal sleep, as in the case of a sleeping mother's selective sensitivity to her baby's crying. Sleep also produces retrograde amnesia; memory for events just before the onset of sleep is lost if the ensuing sleep lasts for more than a few minutes. This phenomenon is the basis for not recollecting the moment of sleep onset or the events that occur during brief awakenings during the course of the night.

TESTS COMMONLY UTILIZED TO ASSESS SLEEP AND WAKEFULNESS

Polysomnography

Polysomnography is typically performed in sleep laboratories. Under strictly controlled situations, it can also be performed in the home. Sleep laboratories that employ polysomnography are typically part of larger clinical programs dedicated to the evaluation and treatment of a multitude of sleep disorders and usually referred to as *sleep disorders centers*. These are typically staffed by physicians specializing in sleep medicine. Under current ACGME and American Board of Medical Specialties guidelines, physicians with host specialties in psychiatry, neurology, pediatrics, internal medicine, and otolaryngology are eligible to acquire specialized training in sleep medicine and take certification boards for this specialty.

In preparation for polysomnography, patients are introduced to their sleeping quarters during their initial office-based evaluation, and provisions are made for special needs. Typically, studies are conducted in noise-free and private rooms that are aesthetically appealing to maximize comfort. On the night of the test, patients arrive at the laboratory well in advance of the study time to acclimate to the new environment. Contrary to their commonly expressed concerns, most patients experience their sleep in the laboratory to be the same as, and at times even better than, their sleep at home.

As noted earlier, characterization of sleep stages requires, at the minimum, the EEG, EOG, and EMG of the submentalis. However, a typical clinical polysomnogram also includes monitors for airflow at the nose and mouth, respiratory effort strain gauges placed around the chest and abdomen for the detection of sleep-related breathing disturbances, EMG of the anterior tibialis muscles for the detection of periodic limb movements, electrocardiogram, and pulse oximetry. Finally, patients' gross body movements are continuously monitored by audiovisual means.

Multiple Sleep Latency Test and Maintenance of Wakefulness Test

The Multiple Sleep Latency Test (MSLT) and the Maintenance of Wakefulness Test (MWT) assess objective measures of daytime sleepiness (Doghramji et al., 1997; Mitler et al., 1982). Objective measures of sleepiness are important because sleepy patients often cannot accurately estimate the severity of their own sleepiness. For example, patients who are so sleepy that they regularly succumb to involuntary sleep attacks—sleep episodes that strike without warning—can deny feeling sleepy just before these episodes. Although no tests can directly assess the biological basis of sleepiness, the MSLT does so indirectly by measuring the propensity to fall asleep during the day in a setting that minimizes alerting factors. The sleep latency, or length of time taken to fall asleep, is regarded to be inversely proportional to the magnitude of daytime sleepiness. According to the American Academy of Sleep Medicine, "The MSLT is considered the de facto standard for the measurement of sleepiness since there is no other known biological measurement that directly reflects this clinical phenomenon" (Arand et al., 2005). During this test, the patient is monitored polysomnographically in a darkened room while lying down on a sleep laboratory bed during five nap opportunities, spaced 2 hours apart, and beginning at 10:00 AM. The patient is instructed to not resist the tendency to fall asleep. Sleep latency on the MSLT is defined as the time from turning off the lights to the onset of sleep. Although the MSLT has been utilized to identify the extent of daytime somnolence in diverse populations and diagnoses, it is most useful in the diagnostic assessment of narcolepsy; a sleep latency of <8 minutes and the presence of REM sleep in at least two of the nap subtests, in the context of normal amounts of prior sleep, are regarded as diagnostic of narcolepsy (American Academy of Sleep Medicine, 2005).

The MWT is similar in methodology to the MSLT, yet patients are studied in a dimly lit, quiet room while sitting comfortably. They are instructed to resist the urge to fall asleep (i.e., to stay awake) during the nap opportunities. It was developed to assess the ability to remain awake in soporific conditions, which may be more in parallel with the challenge that sleepy individuals face during their daily lives while engaged in potentially critical tasks such as driving and operating heavy machinery. It is more sensitive than the MSLT in assessing changes in levels of sleepiness in extremely sleepy patients. Through the study of normal individuals undergoing the MWT (Doghramji et al., 1997), the determination has been made that the inability to remain awake for longer than an average of 8 minutes across all nap opportunities is considered abnormal.

Epworth Sleepiness Scale

In office-based clinical settings, sleepiness can be more easily assessed by using subjective scales such as the Stanford Sleepiness Scale (SSS) and the Epworth Sleepiness Scale (ESS) (see Table 17-2) (Hoddes, 1973; Johns, 1991).

The latter measures the self-reported tendency to fall asleep under situations of daily living on a scale of 0 to 3, with 0 representing no chance and 3 representing a high chance of

TABLE 17-2 **The Epworth Sleepiness Scale**

Epworth Sleepiness Scale

Name: _____ Today's date: _____

Your age (Yrs): _____ Your sex (Male = M, Female = F): _____

How likely are you to doze off or fall asleep in the following situations, in contrast to feeling just tired?

This refers to your usual way of life in recent times.

Even if you haven't done some of these things recently try to work out how they would have affected you.

Use the following scale to choose the **most appropriate number** for each situation:

0 = would **never** doze

1 = **slight chance** of dozing

2 = **moderate chance** of dozing

3 = **high chance** of dozing

It is important that you answer each question as best you can.

Situation   **Chance of Dozing (0-3)**

Sitting and reading _____ ___

Watching TV _____ ___

Sitting, inactive in a public place (e.g. a theatre or a meeting) _____ ___

As a passenger in a car for an hour without a break _____ ___

Lying down to rest in the afternoon when circumstances permit _____ ___

Sitting and talking to someone _____ ___

Sitting quietly after a lunch without alcohol _____ ___

In a car, while stopped for a few minutes in the traffic _____ ___

THANK YOU FOR YOUR COOPERATION

© M.W. Johns 1990-97, reproduced with permission

dozing off. A cumulative score of 10 and above indicates an abnormally high level of daytime sleepiness.

Actigraphy

Actigraphy, though not a substitute for polysomnography, measures body movement patterns during sleep and wakefulness with a portable device, such as a wrist monitor. Because actigraphy does not measure sleep itself, nor any of the other physiological measures of a full polysomnogram, it cannot be utilized for most diagnostic purposes. It is, however, useful for the assessment of sleep–wake patterns in patients who cannot report them accurately themselves. It is particularly useful in the diagnostic evaluation of circadian rhythm disorders such as delayed sleep phase syndrome, advanced sleep phase syndrome, and shift work sleep disorder.

EPIDEMIOLOGY OF SPECIFIC SLEEP DISORDERS

Obstructive Sleep Apnea Syndrome

The prevalence of obstructive sleep apnea syndrome (OSAS) is 2% in women and 4% in men. In the United States, 26% of adults are considered to be at high risk of developing OSAS (Hiestand, 2006). The risk is also higher in men (27% to 35% in men vs. 12% in women) (Young et al., 2004). The prevalence of the condition increases with age. Patients typically present for evaluation between ages 40 and 60, yet seniors aged 65 years or older have a 2 to 3 times higher prevalence of OSAS compared to their younger counterparts (Young et al., 2004). Women are more likely to develop OSAS after reaching menopause.

African Americans older than 35 years are more likely to have OSAS than whites irrespective of body weight (Palmer and Redline, 2003). The prevalence of OSAS among Asian cultures is similar to that of whites, despite Asian populations having comparably lower mean body weight (Palmer and Redline, 2003).

Narcolepsy

Narcolepsy is a rare disorder that affects 0.02% to 0.16% of the population worldwide. Its prevalence in Western Europe and North America is 25 to 50 per 100,000 people (Longstreth et al., 2007) and incidence is 0.74 per 100,000 person-years (Longstreth et al., 2007). Onset is typically in the teens and 20s but has been reported as early as age 5 and as late as age 40 (Okun et al., 2002). It is equally common in men and women (Coleman et al., 1982; Ohayon et al., 2002; Silber et al., 2002).

Idiopathic Hypersomnia

The prevalence of idiopathic hypersomnia (IH) is unknown. It is usually diagnosed before age 30 (Billiard and Besset, 2003; Billiard and Dauvilliers, 2001).

Periodic Limb Movement Disorder

The incidence and prevalence of periodic limb movement disorder (PLMD) in the general population are not known but estimated at 1% to 15% in people with insomnia (American Academy of Sleep Medicine, 2005). Found equally in both genders, PLMD is rare in children, is most prevalent in middle age, and increases in prevalence with age. It has been observed in up to 34% of people older than 60 years.

Restless Legs Syndrome

Five percent to 15% of the population has mild symptoms of restless legs syndrome (RLS) (Allen et al., 2005; Hogl and Poewe, 2005; Lavigne and Montplaisir, 1994; Nichols et al., 2003). Its

---

A CASE OF NARCOLEPSY

A 21-year-old single college student was brought to medical attention at the request of her teachers for repeatedly falling asleep in class. The patient noted that she always felt tired but had thought that this was normal. Her grades had deteriorated over the prior 4 to 5 years, and she noted that she was spending increasingly longer periods of time sleeping or just lying around after classes were over. She denied drug use or abuse but reported "jelly-like" legs following laughter or anger and vivid dreams during sleep, followed by awakenings during which she could not move despite attempts to do so. Her roommates had reported to her, repeatedly, that she was a disturbed sleeper and had often heard vocalizations as she slept. During the interview, it was noted that she felt washed out, talked slowly, and had minimal affective modulation.

prevalence has been estimated to be 3.4% of the population and increases with age. It is twice as prevalent in women as men. One study showed 72% of children with RLS had a parent with the illness, usually the mother (Kotagal and Silber, 2004). There may be a genetic basis for RLS when coexisting with PLMD (Hogl and Poewe, 2005; Stefansson et al., 2007).

SPECIFIC SLEEP DISORDERS

The two cardinal symptoms of sleep disorders are insomnia and excessive daytime sleepiness (excessive daytime somnolence; EDS). Sleepiness refers to the increased likelihood of falling asleep. This is considered a normal biological need or drive; an apt analogy is sleep is to sleepiness as food is to hunger. Sleepiness is considered excessive when there is an increased likelihood of falling asleep at inappropriate times, such as when driving or in the middle of a conversation. Insomnia is the inability to fall asleep or stay asleep despite adequate opportunity to do so. Unusual activity during sleep is another cardinal symptom of sleep disorders, more extensively described in the section on parasomnias. Table 17-3 lists sleep disorders that present with insomnia and EDS.

Inadequate Sleep Hygiene

"Sleep hygiene" measures are behaviors and external factors that influence sleep quality and quantity (see Table 17-4). Inadequate sleep hygiene violates one or more of these measures, which, in turn, leads to the complaint of either insomnia or EDS or both. These measures can help at home when given to patients complaining of insomnia or EDS (Hauri, 1991).

Insufficient Sleep Syndrome

Persons affected with insufficient sleep syndrome curtail their time in bed, usually in response to social and occupational demands. It is one of the most common causes of EDS in general and may affect one third of the population (Bonnet and Arand, 1995). Sleep deprivation may be acute, lasting a few hours or days, or chronic, lasting many days, months, or years. It may also be total, encompassing the entire night, or partial, involving a few hours per night. The most common type is chronic and partial. Sleep deprivation by as little as 1 hour per night, over long periods of time, can lead to debilitating EDS, which may necessitate long periods of recovery sleep. Sleep

TABLE 17-3	Commonly Encountered Sleep Disorders and Most Commonly Reported Corresponding Symptom(s)	
Disorder	**Insomnia**	**Excessive Daytime Somnolence**
Inadequate sleep hygiene	*	*
Insufficient sleep syndrome		*
Adjustment sleep disorder	*	
Psychophysiological insomnia	*	
Obstructive sleep apnea syndrome		*
Central sleep apnea syndrome	*	
Narcolepsy		*
Periodic limb movement disorder	*	*
Restless legs syndrome	*	
Drug-dependent and drug-induced sleep disorders	*	*
Circadian rhythm sleep disorders	*	*
Medical/psychiatric sleep disorders	*	*

*, commonly reported symptom.

TABLE 17-4	Sleep Hygiene Measures

The Dos of sleep hygiene
- Increase exposure to bright light during the day
- Establish a daily activity routine
- Exercise regularly in the morning and/or afternoon
- Set aside a worry time
- Establish a comfortable sleep environment
- Do something relaxing before bedtime
- Try a warm bath

The Don'ts of sleep hygiene
- Alcohol
- Caffeine, nicotine, and other stimulants
- Exposure to bright light during the night
- Exercise within 3 h of bedtime
- Heavy meals or drinking within 3 h of bedtime
- Using your bed for things *other than* sleep (or sexual activity)
- Napping, unless a shiftworker
- Watching the clock
- Trying to sleep
- Noise
- Excessive heat/cold in room

logs usually reveal curtailed bedtimes, occasionally with extended bedtime hours on weekends and holidays. Treatment with stimulant agents is rarely warranted because no degree of chronic curtailment in sleep needs can be soundly overcome by the habitual use of stimulant agents. Instead, sufferers, usually younger adults, should be urged to extend bedtimes on a daily basis.

Insomnia

Adjustment Insomnia

The common disorder of adjustment insomnia is caused by acute emotional stressors, such as a job loss or a hospitalization, that result in insomnia. Symptoms usually remit shortly following the abatement of the stressors. Treatment is warranted if daytime sleepiness and fatigue interfere with functioning or if the disorder lasts for more than a few weeks. Treatment modalities are similar to those outlined for psychophysiological insomnia (see the following text).

Psychophysiological Insomnia

Although insomnia may be *initiated* by a wide variety of stressors and conditions, it may persist well beyond the resolution of these factors due to the emergence of *perpetuating* factors, such as learned mental associations ("I'll never be able to fall asleep") or somatized tension, which, in turn, cause arousal and prevent sleep. Patients then develop an excessive concern about the inability to fall asleep, mostly felt as bedtime approaches, leading to *anticipatory* anxiety over the prospect of another night of sleeplessness followed by another day of fatigue. A vicious cycle is set up, therefore, where excessive focus on sleep and the "trying" to sleep cause greater tension and diminished sleep.

The diagnosis of psychophysiological insomnia is supported by a history of difficulty in falling asleep that is situational, occurring only in the context of the patient's own bedroom. Sleep may be normal in other situations such as hotel rooms. Patients also report that they can fall asleep when they are not trying to, like when they are watching TV or reading. Patients also report approaching bedtimes at home with intense anxiety and dread. Although they may have "hard driving" personalities, psychiatric evaluation usually does not uncover diagnosable psychopathology.

During the clinical examination, patients may appear tense. Although polysomnography is not usually necessary to confirm the diagnosis, it can be useful in ruling out other, concurrent, sleep disorders.

Cognitive behavioral and pharmacologic treatments are well suited for this disorder. The former usually take a longer time to implement, yet have the advantage of longer-lasting benefit. Pharmacologic treatments, in contrast, provide rapid relief from symptoms, yet may not provide definitive resolution following discontinuation of treatment unless combined with behavioral and psychotherapeutic measures.

Cognitive behavioral therapies for psychophysiological insomnia are also employed for other forms of insomnia. They include sleep hygiene education, described earlier, and stimulus control therapy. Patients are instructed to get out of bed following 15 to 20 minutes of sleeplessness while in bed, go to another room, engage in relaxing activities, but remain awake. They then return to bed only when sleepy. This therapy strives to reassociate the bedroom and bed with sleep and break the mental association between the bedroom and wakefulness. In addition, relaxation training strives to diminish tension and anxiety with various strategies including progressive muscle relaxation, biofeedback, guided imagery, autogenic training, abdominal breathing exercises, and meditation. Sleep restriction strives to curtail sleep, thereby producing a state of sleep debt, which aids in consolidating subsequent sleep. Patients are instructed initially to limit the time spent in bed to the amount of actual time they habitually sleep, as determined using sleep logs. The sleep efficiency, which is the ratio of actual sleep time to time spent in bed, is calculated over 5 days. When sleep efficiency increases >90%, patients are allowed 15 to 20 minutes of additional time in bed by going to bed earlier. If sleep efficiency decreases below 85%, then their time in bed is further curtailed by a similar amount. Morning rising time is kept constant, and napping is disallowed. Over time, sleep becomes more consolidated and productive.

Cognitive therapy strives to identify and dispel thoughts that are tension producing and have a negative effect upon sleep. Many involve misperceptions about sleep, such as unrealistic expectations ("I must get 8 hours of sleep every night"), etiologic misconceptions ("a chemical imbalance prevents me from sleeping"), amplifications of consequences ("insomnia is incurable"), and sleep performance anxiety ("if I do not sleep well, my performance tomorrow will be seriously jeopardized"). Once identified, misperceptions are consciously challenged, and positive perceptions about sleep are substituted. Paradoxical intention attempts to dissolve performance anxiety that prevents sleep by asking patients to stop trying to sleep and deliberately attempt to remain awake.

Hypnotic agents are also utilized for psychophysiological insomnia and discussed in the following text.

Sleep Apnea Syndrome

There are two types of sleep apnea syndrome, obstructive (OSA) and central (CSA). The defining pathologic events in OSA are apneas, or pauses in ventilation (apnea), during sleep that are due to a closure of the upper airway. In CSA apneas are due to impaired inspiratory effort despite a patent upper airway. Isolated cases of pure CSA are rare; instead, CSA usually coexists with OSA, in which case the latter is considered the primary pathologic entity.

Upper airway closure in OSA is thought to occur because of failure of the genioglossus and other upper airway dilator muscles. Apneas are accompanied by cyclic asphyxia (hypoxemia, hypercarbia, and acidosis), which in turn, can cause cardiac arrhythmias, pulmonary and systemic

A CASE OF PSYCHOPHYSIOLOGICAL INSOMNIA

A 46-year-old salesman presented to his primary care physician with the complaint of poor sleep over the past year. He dated the onset of symptoms to a few international trips, during which he was unable to sleep well due to prolonged travel. However, his sleep remained poor following his return and until the present time. He would approach bedtime with dread and worry. Despite a regular bedtime of 11:00 PM, he reported spending 2 to 3 hours in bed, tossing and turning, with his mind racing. After falling asleep, he also reported awakening at least five times, with each awakening lasting an average of 30 minutes, during which he would lie in bed anxiously awaiting the oncoming day, checking the clock repeatedly. On examination, he appeared well dressed yet fatigued and tense.

Clinical Characteristics of Obstructive Sleep Apnea Syndrome
- Loud snoring
- Reports of pauses in respiration during sleep
- Excessive daytime somnolence (EDS)
- Disturbed, nonrefreshing sleep
- Weight gain
- Morning headaches
- Morning dry mouth

---

hypertension, and a fall in cardiac output, which rises to normal levels following the termination of apneas.

Apneas are terminated by arousals, episodes of sudden brain activation that are reflected by an increase in EEG frequency to the alpha range during sleep; in turn, they cause sleep fragmentation and poor sleep quality, which are thought to be responsible for the EDS and emotional consequences of the disorder, discussed further in the following text.

Patients commonly present for clinical attention at the behest of the bed partner who may be concerned about sleep-related gaps in breathing or loud snoring, or because sleepiness interferes with daytime function. Because patients are unaware of their own snoring, bed partners and family members must be questioned in this regard during a new patient evaluation. Snoring can be exacerbated by weight gain, alcohol ingestion near bedtime, and lying on one's back. It is often a source of embarrassment and may place significant strain on interpersonal relationships as spouses resort to sleeping in separate beds or bedrooms. Bed partners also often observe whole body movements, occasionally violent, during apneic episodes. Many patients talk and yell during sleep and assume unusual body positions as they attempt to inspire, yet sleepwalking is uncommon. Despite obvious discontinuous sleep, it is striking that most patients report sleep to be continuous, with the notable exception of the elderly, who may report insomnia. The consequences of, and symptoms associated with, OSA are a consequence of fragmented nocturnal sleep and asphyxia. Factors that predispose individuals to OSA are summarized in Table 17-5 (Nuckton et al., 2006; Young et al., 2004). Historical risk factors include a history of snoring, breathing pauses during sleep, and EDS.

Approximately 25% of the prevalence of OSA is due to genetic inheritance (Palmer and Redline, 2003). OSA is three times more likely in active smokers than people who have never smoked (Zhang et al., 2006). Also, people with chronic nocturnal nasal congestion due to any cause have a two-fold higher prevalence of OSA (Young et al., 1997, 2002, 2004). A variety of medical conditions, such as diabetes mellitus, increase the risk (West et al., 2006).

TABLE 17-5 **Predisposing Factors for Obstructive Sleep Apnea Syndrome**

Obesity (body mass index >30)
Neck circumference >17″ in men and >16″ in women
Upper airway occlusion as judged by the Mallampati score
Adenotonsillar hypertrophy
Large uvula
Low-lying soft palate
Tonsillar hypertrophy
Narrow or obstructed nasal passages
Retrognathia, micrognathia, and other craniofacial abnormalities

The most apparent consequence of sleep fragmentation is EDS, which is reported regardless of the extent of nocturnal sleep. This is most evident in relaxing situations (like reading) and can interfere with activities of daily life as sufferers fall asleep in meetings or at movies. It can result in breaches in marital and family relationships and diminished job productivity and school performance. In extreme sleepiness, patients can fall asleep while speaking, walking, or driving. Patients with OSA are at increased risk of traffic accidents. In contrast to patients with narcolepsy, OSA sufferers do not obtain relief from EDS by napping; in fact, naps in patients with OSA are typically followed by greater sleepiness and headaches.

Depression is common, and its severity is related to the severity of the OSA; therefore, OSA should be considered in the differential diagnosis of major depression. Sudden awakenings associated with intense anxiety have also been reported. Lapses in memory and judgment, personality changes and irritability, and aggressiveness leading to violent outbursts (Ohayon et al., 2000) have all been reported in association with OSA. Many patients misuse alcohol to control anxiety and stimulants to stay awake. Cognitive changes include deficiencies in attention, concentration, complex problem solving, and short-term recall (Beebe et al., 2003; Findley et al., 1986). Occupational and academic productivity is impaired (Engleman and Joffe, 1999). Inhibited sexual desire, impotence, and ejaculatory impairment are reported by approximately a third of patients.

Bradycardia occurs during the apneic phase, alternating with tachycardia after resumption of ventilation. Other cardiac dysrhythmias, including atrioventricular block, premature ventricular contractions, and sinus arrest, have been described during apneas. OSA increases the risk of future systemic hypertension, congestive heart failure, and stroke. If left untreated, OSA may be associated with increased mortality (He et al., 1988).

Dull, frontal headaches are thought to be a result of episodic asphyxia and consequent cerebral vasodilatation. These headaches that begin upon awakening can last for 1 to 2 hours. Gastroesophageal reflux is a consequence of decreased intrathoracic pressure during apneas. Sleep-related enuresis is occasionally reported. Sedating pharmacologic agents, including alcohol and benzodiazepine, and anxiolytic agents such as diazepam and alprazolam tend to increase the duration and frequency of apneas. Therefore, benzodiazepines are contraindicated for untreated patients.

In children, snoring may not be present at all, while some children will exhibit rib flaring and pectus excavatum. Other symptoms in children include agitated awakenings, unusual sleeping postures, and nocturnal enuresis. Daytime somnolence does not occur as often in children with OSA. Rather, behavioral problems, developmental delay, and worsening school performance are seen. Enlarged tonsils and adenoids may result in a characteristic "adenoidal face" appearance, as well as periorbital edema, mouth breathing, and dull expression. Poor speech articulation, problems swallowing, and daytime mouth breathing are all common.

Differential Diagnosis

The differential diagnosis for OSA includes other causes of EDS, primary snoring, affective disorders, Cheyne-Stokes respiration, and central sleep apnea syndrome. All of these can be differentiated from OSA by polysomnography.

The diagnosis is established by polysomnography. OSA is defined as greater than five apneas (cessation of ventilation lasting 10 seconds or longer) or hypopneas (shallow ventilation lasting 10 seconds or longer associated with a decrement of oxyhemoglobin saturation by 4% or more) per hour of sleep (Netzer et al., 2003; Young et al., 2004).

Treatments

The first-line treatment for OSA is continuous positive airway pressure (CPAP) due to greatest efficacy and least potential for adverse effects. CPAP is an ambulatory device that introduces room air at a high flow rate into the upper airway by a nasal mask and dissipates apneas in a "pneumatic splint" mechanism. The optimum pressure required to eliminate apneas is determined through polysomnography with a variable pressure device, following which patients utilize CPAP at a constant pressure at home while asleep. The primary complication in the use of CPAP is nonadherence; half of patients prescribed it actually use it regularly (Kribbs et al., 1993). Reasons include upper airway irritation, discomfort at the mask site, and feelings of suffocation, among others. Various methods can enhance adherence, including in-line air humidification, mask shapes and sizes that are tailored to patients' preferences, bilevel positive airway pressure devices that deliver lower pressures during expiration than inspiration, and demand-pressure devices that tailor the pressure delivered to the severity of apneas on an ongoing basis.

Oral appliances that prevent mandibular collapse or tongue protrusion during sleep have also seen a recent increase in popularity, although efficacy rates are lower than with CPAP. Their side effects include excessive salivation and jaw pain.

If apneas are found to be more frequent in the supine position, positioning devices that promote sleep in the nonsupine position can be helpful in mild OSA cases.

Laser-assisted uvuloplasty (LAUP) is an office-based surgical procedure performed with local anesthesia that has largely replaced uvulopalatopharyngoplasty (UPPP) surgery, an intraoperative procedure performed under general anesthesia. In both, portions of the uvula are removed, and in the latter, part of the soft palate is removed as well. Although both are highly effective for the elimination of snoring, both also suffer from lower efficacy than that of CPAP for pathogenic apneas. Nevertheless, combining these with more invasive procedures, such as genioglossus advancement–hyoid myotomy and suspension, bimaxillary advancement, or maxillary and mandibular osteotomy, yields higher success rates. Although tracheostomy can provide definitive resolution of pathogenic apneas, it is reserved for cases of severe apnea that cannot be managed by CPAP or LAUP. Nasal surgery can be helpful in patients with mild-to-moderate OSA who also have some degree of nasal airway compromise.

Weight reduction should be encouraged, although its results are often unpredictable. Therefore, it should not be relied upon as the sole treatment modality for more severe cases. Similarly, bariatric surgery may be considered; however, it is associated with complications and recurrence of OSA even if weight has not been regained.

Pharmacologic agents have not met with predictable success. Modafinil, a stimulant, may be utilized in treating residual EDS when the OSA is effectively treated by other methods.

Concurrent depression, anxiety, and psychosocial and marital difficulties can be addressed by psychotherapy and antidepressants that are alerting, such as fluoxetine and bupropion. Benzodiazepines should be avoided in patients whose OSA is not effectively managed; instead, the nonbenzodiazepine anxiolytic buspirone, selective serotonin reuptake inhibitors (SSRIs), and the hypnotic ramelteon can be more safely utilized.

If CSA is diagnosed, its underlying conditions should be investigated, such as congestive heart failure, nasal obstruction, CNS lesions, and high altitude travel, and treatment directed at the specific abnormality. Treatment of the idiopathic variety is often inadequate. Acetazolamide, protriptyline, clomipramine, medroxyprogesterone, theophylline, CPAP, and oxygen have met with variable results. Diaphragmatic pacing or mechanical ventilation must be considered in refractory cases. Regardless of the approach chosen, monitoring the course of treatment with polysomnography is essential because some treatments, such as oxygen therapy, may actually exacerbate the condition. CNS depressants such as hypnotic agents and alcohol may have a similar effect and must be avoided.

NARCOLEPSY

The five major symptoms of narcolepsy are persistent daytime sleepiness, cataplexy, hypnagogic (or hypnopompic) hallucinations, sleep paralysis, and disturbed and restless sleep. Persistent daytime sleepiness is present in all patients with narcolepsy and usually accompanied by daytime naps that, unlike in OSA, are brief (typically 15 minutes) and refreshing. Naps are often accompanied by vivid dreams.

Cataplexy, an abrupt paralysis or paresis of skeletal muscles, usually follows emotional experiences such as anger, surprise, laughter, or physical exercise. It can be generalized, in which case the patient typically collapses, or isolated to an individual muscle group, resulting in transient loss of function. The episode typically lasts a few minutes, during which the patient is awake. Following its termination, the patient typically regains function without any residual impairment. Although cataplexy is the pathognomic symptom of narcolepsy, it can only be elicited in up to

70% of interviews. Cataplexy should not be confused with its near-homonym catalepsy, or waxy flexibility, an unrelated phenomenon noted in schizophrenia of the catatonic type.

Hypnagogic (or hypnopompic) hallucinations are vivid and often frightening dreams that occur shortly after falling asleep (or upon awakening), and sleep paralysis, a transient global paralysis of voluntary muscles, usually occurs shortly after falling asleep and lasts a few seconds or minutes.

Cataplexy, hypnagogic hallucinations, and sleep paralysis are thought to be manifestations of an underlying aberration in the control of the timing of REM sleep, which, in turn, results in "attacks" of REM sleep during wakefulness. These then result in the occurrence of the physical (paralysis) and cognitive (vivid hallucinations) manifestations of REM sleep while individuals are awake.

The disturbed and restless sleep of narcolepsy is characterized by numerous awakenings and arousals.

Narcolepsy is a lifelong condition. Its peak age of onset is the second decade, yet diagnosis is established an average of 10 years later. People with narcolepsy develop significant psychosocial impairments as a result of EDS, such as job loss and interpersonal difficulties. They are also susceptible to auto accidents and sustaining injuries as a result of falling asleep in inappropriate situations. Many develop depression, anxiety, and substance use difficulties.

Narcolepsy is idiopathic. A genetic factor is thought to be involved because 1% to 2% of first-degree relatives have narcolepsy, which is 20 to 40 times higher than the population risk. However, most cases are sporadic, and only 17% to 36% of monozygotic twins are concordant for narcolepsy (Mignot, 1998). Therefore, it cannot be explained solely on the basis of genetics; environmental triggers are thought to be involved, such as head trauma, viral illness, exposure to toxins, sleep deprivation, change in the sleep–wake cycle, and developmental factors such as puberty and aging.

There is a strong association of narcolepsy with human leukocyte antigens (HLA). The first marker identified was HLA-DR2, occurring in 85% to 98% of all white patients with narcolepsy-cataplexy. The association is weaker in the African American population. The strongest association across all ethnic groups has been found with HLA DQB1*0602, occurring in 85% to 100% (Hayduk et al., 1997; Mignot et al., 2002; Taheri and Mignot, 2002). Other HLA-associated disorders, such as multiple sclerosis, myasthenia gravis, and systemic lupus erythematosus, are autoimmune in nature, raising the suspicion of a similar etiology in narcolepsy (Mignot et al., 1994). Recently, abnormalities in hypocretin (orexin)–containing neurons were found in narcoleptic animals and humans, and cerebrospinal fluid (CSF) hypocretin-1 levels were noted to be lower in narcoleptics than in normal controls and patients with other neurologic conditions (Ripley et al., 2001). Hypocretin neuron perikarya in the human brain are localized to the perifornical region of the posterior hypothalamus, extending into the lateral hypothalamus. These neurons densely innervate the hypothalamus, histaminergic tuberomammillary nucleus, noradrenergic locus coeruleus, serotonergic raphe nuclei, dopaminergic ventral tegmental area, midline thalamus, and nucleus of the diagonal band–nucleus basalis complex of the forebrain and are thought to be important in maintaining wakefulness. Collectively, these findings suggest that narcolepsy is caused by an autoimmune destruction of wakefulness-controlling hypocretin cells.

Other than the obvious behavioral manifestations of EDS (yawning, drooping eyelids, psychomotor retardation), physical examination is typically unrevealing. The diagnosis must be confirmed by nocturnal polysomnography (NPSG), followed by MSLT. The former is performed to ensure adequate nocturnal sleep and the lack of other intrinsic sleep disorders. The NPSG often reveals a short REM latency and sleep fragmentation caused by numerous awakenings and arousals. To establish the diagnosis, the average MSLT sleep latency should be 8 minutes or less (Arand et al., 2005) and reveal REM episodes during at least two nap opportunities.

Treatment of narcolepsy is directed at daytime somnolence, REM-related aberrations, and psychosocial consequences. In milder cases, excessive sleepiness can be managed with conservative measures such as spending an adequate time in bed, taking two or three short naps, and avoiding alcohol and other sedating agents. Even in more severe cases, judiciously timed naps can minimize the dosage of medication required to control symptoms. Commonly utilized medications for excessive sleepiness and cataplexy are listed in Table 17-6. Pemoline had previously been used for

TABLE 17-6	Medications Used to Treat Narcolepsy	
For EDS	**For Cataplexy**	**For Both EDS and Cataplexy**
Methylphenidate	Protriptyline	Sodium oxybate (γ-hydroxybutyrate)
Methamphetamine	Fluoxetine	
Amphetamine	Venlafaxine	
Modafinil	Clomipramine	

EDS, excessive daytime somnolence.
(Mignot, 2005.)

EDS, but because it has been associated with life-threatening hepatic failure, its use has fallen out of favor. Tolerance may be minimized by prescribing the lowest effective dose and asking patients to take regular drug holidays on days when their need for alertness is lowest.

Many patients with narcolepsy also require emotional support. Education plays a key role in management because peers, parents, teachers, and patients themselves may confuse the effects of drowsiness with laziness or lack of motivation.

Idiopathic Hypersomnia

IH is a lifelong and incurable disorder that has a variable age of onset. The most prominent symptom is unrelenting daytime somnolence. Unlike patients with narcolepsy, patients with IH do not report the REM-related symptoms of cataplexy, hypnagogic/hypnopompic hallucinations, or sleep paralysis and have unrefreshing naps that are rarely accompanied by dreams.

Polysomnography reveals either prolonged or normal nocturnal sleep without evidence of other sleep pathology. The MSLT reveals a mean sleep latency of 8 minutes or less without sleep-onset REM periods. Treatment principles are similar to those outlined for narcolepsy, yet anticataplectic agents are not utilized.

Periodic Limb Movement Disorder and Restless Legs Syndrome

Periodic limb movement disorder (PLMD) is characterized by the repetitive (usually every 20 to 40 seconds) twitches of the legs and, less commonly, arms during sleep. Patients usually present with the complaint of unrelenting insomnia, most often characterized by repeated awakenings following sleep onset. A minority complain of EDS. In either case, they are usually unaware of the movements and the brief arousals that follow and have no lasting sensation in their extremities.

Also known as *Ekbom disease* (Ekbom, 1960), RLS is an irresistible urge to move the extremities, typically the legs, but occasionally also the arms. This is often accompanied by uncomfortable and unpleasant sensations in the extremities, which are described as creepy-crawly, painful, tugging, and tingling, among others. These symptoms begin, or are worsened, during periods of rest or inactivity, such as while attending the theater or reading quietly, and peak in the evening. As a result, patients commonly complain of difficulty in falling and staying asleep. They are also partially or totally relieved by movement, such as walking or stretching, although relief is usually temporary. Many patients are depressed, irritable, and angry. Psychosocial impairments such as job loss and relationship difficulties are quite common.

The two disorders are believed to be related. Approximately 80% of patients with RLS also have PLMD, yet only 30% of individuals who have PLMD have RLS symptoms.

Both periodic leg movements during sleep (PLMS) and RLS are more common in middle and older age. The disorders can be primary (idiopathic), in which case the etiology is thought to be due to an abnormality of brain dopamine receptors. They can also be secondary, in which case they coexist with a wide variety of conditions (e.g., pregnancy), the intake of certain drugs (e.g., caffeine and various antidepressants), drug withdrawal states, iron deficiency, uremia, leukemia, neuropathy, and rheumatoid arthritis and following gastric surgery. They are exacerbated by stress.

TABLE 17-7	Treatments for Restless Legs Syndrome (RLS) and Periodic Limb Movement Disorder (PLMD)
Dopamine agonists and precursors	Ropinirole, pramipexole, levodopa with carbidopa or benserazine
Benzodiazepines	Clonazepam, temazepam
Opiates	Oxycodone, codeine
Other medications	Carbamazepine, gabapentin

(Montplaisir et al., 2005.)

A genetic basis for the primary form was recently established by the discovery of an RLS susceptibility gene. The prevalence in first-degree relatives is three to five times greater than in those without RLS.

Polysomnography is not necessary to establish the diagnosis in RLS; its diagnosis is based on symptoms alone. However, polysomnography is necessary to confirm the diagnosis of PLMD and reveals periodic leg muscle bursts during quiet wakefulness and sleep, the latter associated with arousals and awakenings. RLS should be distinguished from nocturnal leg cramps, which involve pain in the deep muscles of the lower extremities and are independent of sleep and usually worsen with movement, and from akathesia, a motor restlessness that occurs in the context of treatment with neuroleptics and antidepressants.

Once the diagnosis is established, the first goal is to identify underlying causes. Therefore, a thorough physical examination, chemistry panel, complete blood count, and serum ferritin should be performed and underlying abnormalities treated. If the serum ferritin is <50 μg per L, supplementation with ferrous sulfate should be instituted. Sleep hygiene principles should be followed. For the primary disorder, treatment choices are outlined in Table 17-7.

Drug-Related Sleep Disorders

Recreational, over-the-counter, and prescription drugs can cause disturbed sleep and EDS, as summarized in Tables 17-8 and 17-9. It should be noted that although the agents listed in Table 17-8 are associated with insomnia following short-term use, their cessation following long-term administration at high dosages often results in withdrawal symptoms, including sleepiness, lassitude, and irritability. Similarly, the cessation of agents associated with daytime sleepiness

TABLE 17-8	Pharmacologic Agents That Can Cause Insomnia
Monoamine oxidase inhibitors
Selective serotonin and norepinephrine reuptake inhibitor antidepressants
Bupropion
Anticancer agents
Steroids
Decongestants
Bronchodilators
Weight loss agents
Thyroid preparations
Xanthine derivatives (caffeine, theophyilline, etc.)
Nicotine
Stimulants (cocaine, ephedrine, methylphenidate, amphetamines, etc.)

TABLE 17-9	Pharmacologic Agents That Can Cause Excessive Daytime Sleepiness
Alcohol	
Antihypertensive agents	
Anxiolytic agents	
Antipsychotic agents	
Trazodone, some tricyclic antidepressants	
Opioids and other analgesic agents	
Cannabis	

(Table 17-9) can, after prolonged use, result in insomnia. It should also be noted that although caffeine has a half-life in plasma of 3 to 7 hours, its absorption from the gastrointestinal tract can be erratic, and there are wide variations in individual sensitivity to it. Therefore, caffeinated beverages consumed even early in the day can still negatively affect sleep quality at night.

Circadian Rhythm Sleep Disorders

The circadian rhythm sleep disorders feature a disturbance in the coordination between the timing of internal circadian sleep–wake cycle and the environmental light–dark cycle. In all the disorders discussed in the following text, core symptoms include insomnia, EDS, or both.

Jet Lag Syndrome

Jet lag syndrome is caused by rapid travel across two or more time zones, resulting in a mismatch between the sleep schedule of the body and that of the new environment. Symptoms include malaise, gastrointestinal disturbances, and fatigue. The severity is related to the direction of travel (eastward) and number of time zones crossed (more than two). Symptoms are related to the resulting desynchronization between internal body rhythms with respect to one another, such as those of sleep–wakefulness, temperature, sleep, and hormone secretion, and travel-related factors such as discomfort on board an aircraft, poor diet, and use of caffeinated and alcoholic beverages, all of which result in curtailed sleep length and poor sleep quality.

Jet lag countermeasures include adherence to proper sleep hygiene measures. Maximizing exposure to daylight at the new locale can hasten the synchronization of circadian rhythms to the environmental light–dark cycle and to one another. Individuals should also be urged to shift their sleep–wake schedules gradually in the direction of the destination time zone before travel. If these methods are not effective or only minimally effective, treatment can be augmented with short-acting hypnotics and stimulants for a brief period following arrival in the new locale.

Shift Work Sleep Disorder

Shift work sleep disorder results from shifts in bedtimes in response to changes in work shift. This leads to poor sleep quality immediately following the transition to the new shift, which is followed by a period of adaptation. Most problematic is variable shift work, in which shifts are rotated or changed frequently; sleep times typically must be changed accordingly. The severity of symptoms is proportional to the frequency with which shifts are changed, the magnitude of each change, and the frequency of counterclockwise (phase-advancing) changes. However, even fixed-shift workers who must sleep during the day experience difficulties because daytime noise and light can interfere with the quality of their sleep and they often change their sleep times for social or family events.

The elderly are more profoundly affected by rapidly changing shifts. Shift work is associated with impaired job productivity and performance (Metlaine et al., 2005), which are most impaired during the bimodal circadian nadirs of alertness, that is, early morning (approximately 2:00 AM to 7:00 AM) and midafternoon (approximately 2:00 PM to 5:00 PM) in externally synchronized individuals.

Shift workers should be advised to maximize their exposure to sunlight at times when they should be awake and ensure that the bedroom is as dark and quiet as possible when they are asleep, which is often during the day. Bright artificial light emanating from specially constructed boxes, when administered at critical times, can enhance adaptation of internal rhythms to the new shift (Czeisler et al., 1990). If symptoms are not responsive to conventional countermeasures, it may be necessary to devise more rational shift schedules.

Delayed Sleep Phase Syndrome

Individuals with delayed sleep phase syndrome fall asleep later than normal evening bedtime hours, regardless of how early they go to bed, and awaken later than desired, often extending their bedtimes well into the afternoon. Sufferers are usually young adults who present for treatment because of diminished school performance resulting from daytime sleepiness or missed morning classes. Prior history reveals a tendency for individuals to be "night owls." They can be distinguished from people who stay up late by choice because of social or occupational needs in that they cannot fall asleep earlier even if they try.

Attempts to advance the sleep–wake cycle by retiring earlier are uniformly unsuccessful. Instead, it is more productive to delay bedtimes even further by increments of 3 hours a day, until the desired sleep–wake schedule is reached, a process referred to as *chronotherapy* (Weitzman et al., 1981). An alternative method (Rosenthal et al., 1990) is to administer bright light therapy for a duration of 2 hours early in the morning with melatonin at bedtime, which results in a phase advance of biological rhythms on subsequent nights and progressively earlier sleep times.

Advanced Sleep Phase Syndrome

Sleep–wake times are advanced in relationship to socially desired schedules in advanced sleep phase syndrome. The disorder is more common in the elderly and responsive to treatment with bright lights administered in the evening.

Parasomnias

Parasomnias are disturbing events that occur during sleep or are aggravated by sleep. Clinical aspects of the most common parasomnias are summarized in Table 17-10.

Medical/Psychiatric Sleep Disorders

Depression

There is a close association between disturbed sleep and psychiatric disorders, most notably depression. For example, 90% of patients affected by major depression demonstrate clinical evidence of sleep disturbances (Reynolds and Kupfer, 1987). Conversely, most chronic insomnias (between 60% and 69%) are affected by at least one major psychiatric disorder, most commonly mood disorders, which include depression (Jacobs et al., 1988; Tan et al., 1984). Therefore, it is imperative that physicians keep a high index of suspicion for underlying psychopathology with an emphasis on mood disturbances whenever confronted with the complaint of insomnia. This is also true for patients assessed as having a "routine" or "primary" insomnia, who often suffer from undetected depression. For example, symptomatic management of insomnia in such patients with hypnotic agents alone can lead to treatment failure because the underlying disorder, in this case depression, remains unaddressed.

Although it was once thought that early morning awakenings were the hallmark sleep-related symptom of depression, more recent data from large groups of patients with depression have shown that difficulties in falling asleep in the beginning of the night, repeated nocturnal awakenings, and early morning awakenings are equally prevalent (Perlis et al., 1997). The absence of early morning awakenings should not, therefore, rule out a diagnosis of depression, and the presence of initial insomnia as the only sleep-related symptom is consistent with a diagnosis of depression. In contrast, in certain depressive conditions such as bipolar mood disorder and seasonal affective disorder, sleep is uninterrupted, yet patients complain of unrelenting

TABLE 17-10	Clinical Aspects of Selected Parasomnias		
Parasomnia	**Clinical Features**	**Polysomnographic Findings**	**Treatment**
Sleep walking	Ambulation in sleep Age affected: prepubertal children Difficulty in arousal during episode Amnesia for the episode Episodes occur in the first third of night	Sleep walking out of slow wave sleep	Prevention: removal of sharp objects, floor mattress; reassurance of parents, psychiatric evaluation for adults; benzodiazepines in refractory cases
Sleep terror	Sudden, intense scream during sleep with evidence of intense fear	Sleep terror beginning during slow wave sleep	Reassurance Psychiatric evaluation for adults
Nightmares	Sudden awakening with intense fear Recall of frightening dream content Full alertness on awakening Usually occur in latter half of night Frequent nightmares can be indicative of psychiatric conditions	Abrupt awakening from REM Tachycardia and tachypnea during episode	Psychotherapy Hypnosis
REM sleep behavior disorder	Violent or injurious behavior during sleep Body movement associated with dreams Dreams are enacted while they occur Neurologic evaluations with MRI of the brain and evoked potentials rarely reveal structural lesions; most cases idiopathic	Excessive EMG tone or phasic twitching in REM	Clonazepam Protective measures Psychotherapy
Sleep bruxism	Tooth grinding or clenching during sleep Tooth wear and jaw discomfort	Bursts of jaw EMG activity	Dental examination Mouth guards Relaxation training Psychotherapy

REM, rapid eye movement; EMG, electromyogram; MRI, magnetic resonance imaging.

TABLE 17-11	Polysomnographic Findings in Major Depression

Increased sleep latency and frequent awakenings during sleep
Diminished proportion, and absolute amount, of delta sleep
Shift of delta sleep activity from the first to the second sleep cycle
Shortened REM latency
Reversal of the temporal distribution of REM sleep (longer first REM period)

REM, rapid eye movement.

daytime sleepiness. Hypersomnia is also characteristic of the sleep of younger patients with depression.

Depression has profound and predictable effects upon objectively monitored sleep, as well. Polysomnographic patterns of patients with major depression in the acute phase of the illness are summarized in Table 17-11. Many of these patterns are so characteristic that they can be utilized diagnostically with a high degree of accuracy. In addition to being indicative of current depression, some are thought to be trait markers, that is, indicative of the potential for future depression in otherwise healthy individuals. The persistence of polysomnographic abnormalities following the resolution of depressive episodes has also been noted to correlate with a greater probability of relapse.

Although sleeplessness is often thought of as a consequence of depression, emerging evidence suggests it can also herald the emergence of a new depressive episode. Results of the hallmark study of the prevalence of emotional disorders (Ford and Kamerow, 1989) indicated that patients with insomnia who had no evidence of baseline depressive disorders yet whose insomnia persisted over the course of a year were much more likely to develop depression at the end of that year compared to patients with depression in whom the insomnia resolved. Such evidence suggests insomnias caused by disorders other than depression may, if left unaddressed, eventually lead to new depression. Although studies have not conclusively demonstrated that treatment of insomnia itself can avert the onset of future depressive episodes, such studies suggest clinicians should be attentive to insomnia in patients with depression.

If depression is accompanied by sleeplessness, one pharmacologic approach is to select an antidepressant agent that promises to ameliorate sleep-related symptoms. The effects of antidepressants on polysomnographic sleep vary (Gursky and Krahn, 2000; Thase, 1998). In general, the sedating tricyclic antidepressants (e.g., nortriptyline, doxepin) enhance sleep continuity and depth but, because of long half-lives, tend to cause daytime drowsiness. The monoamine oxidase inhibitors, in contrast, can enhance nocturnal awakenings and diminished sleep continuity, but their activating properties make them better suited for the depressive with hypersomnia. The selective serotonin reuptake inhibitors (fluoxetine, paroxetine, sertraline, citalopram, escitalopram) tend to worsen sleep discontinuity and, in the case of fluoxetine, produce an excessive amount of slow-rolling eye movements and arousals (Armitage et al., 1995; van Bemmel et al., 1993; Waugh and Goa, 2003). Bupropion and venlafaxine also tend to have sleep-disruptive effects. In contrast, trazodone, nefazodone, and mirtazapine enhance sleep continuity and diminish the proportion of shallow sleep stages like stage 1. Cases of life-threatening hepatic failure have led to a reduction in the use of nefazodone in the United States. These effects of antidepressants have been evaluated, in general, only in the acute (8 weeks) stages of treatment, and little is known about their effects on sleep over longer periods of time.

On one hand, the use of a single antidepressant to resolve both depression and insomnia has advantages over multiple medications to achieve the same purpose, namely, a diminished potential for pharmacologic interactions and additive side effects, such as daytime somnolence and paradoxical activation with autonomic changes, referred to as *serotonin syndrome*, and diminished cost. On the other hand, it also has the disadvantage of inflexibility, because the same dosage of one drug may achieve efficacy in one arena but leave the other poorly addressed. The addition of a hypnotic agent is also a valid clinical practice; hypnotics are discussed in the following text. When patients require this degree of complex medication management, a psychiatrist should be involved.

Mania

Mania, in the acute phase, is associated with a decrease in total sleep time. Decreased sleep in a depressed bipolar patient can herald an impending switch into mania and signals the need for close observation. Some researchers have presented evidence indicating that decreased sleep may itself be a precipitant and not just a consequence of mania; therefore, situational stressors such as a relationship failure that results in an adjustment sleep disorder can precipitate a manic episode in a depressed bipolar patient (Wehr et al., 1987).

Other Disorders

Sleep in other psychiatric disorders has been extensively studied but is of greater interest to researchers than clinicians. Almost any disorder, however, that is associated with psychic activation or anxiety can produce sleep loss and fragmentation. In addition, many medical and neurologic conditions cause sleep disturbances. For a review of these disorders, readers are referred to Ancoli-Israel (2006).

The Clinical Approach to Sleep-Related Complaints

Most sleep-disordered patients present for clinical attention with the complaints of insomnia and EDS. Although both can be primary disorders, the first task is to identify the underlying disorder(s) before symptomatic treatment. Following their identification, specific treatments can be instituted with confidence.

The diagnostic process, summarized in Table 17-12, begins with a thorough history, with particular attention directed toward the hallmark symptoms of the major sleep disorders outlined earlier. In most cases, it is beneficial also to interview the bed partner, who is more likely than the patient to be aware of unusual events during sleep. If the presenting symptom is daytime sleepiness, its severity should be carefully evaluated. Patients almost invariably misjudge the extent of sleepiness; therefore, direct questioning regarding how sleepy an individual feels often is not helpful. The propensity for falling asleep is a more accurate measure; in severe cases, individuals fall asleep while actively engaged in complex tasks such as speaking, writing, or even eating. They may also experience sleep attacks, which mandates rapid clinical intervention. Milder levels of daytime sleepiness result in falling asleep in passive situations, such as while reading or watching television. The ESS (Johns, 1991) is a useful office-based test for daytime sleepiness (see the preceding text).

If the history is positive for naps, the possibility that they are related to narcolepsy should be examined by determining whether they are refreshing, brief in duration, or accompanied by

TABLE 17-12	The Clinical Evaluation of Sleep Disorders
Patient interview
Chief complaint: insomnia, EDS, or parasomnia?
History of present illness
Sleep–wake habit history
Sleep hygiene history: meal and exercise times, ambient noise, light and temperature, etc.
Pattern of consumption of recreational substances (especially caffeine and alcohol) and medications
Medications
General medical, psychiatric, and surgical history
Sleep diary
Inventories for daytime sleepiness/alertness
Psychological inventories
Bed partner interview
Physical and mental status examination
Serum laboratory tests
Polysomnography

EDS, excessive daytime somnolence.

dreams. The timing of naps also should be determined because this may alert the physician to the possibility of circadian rhythm disorders.

If the presenting symptom is insomnia, its duration should be determined. Disorders causing acute insomnia are usually transient in nature and more likely to resolve with conservative intervention and treatment with hypnotic agents. Chronic and unrelenting insomnia, which lasts more than a few months, usually requires a more careful investigation and complex treatment. A determination also should be made as to whether the patient's difficulty is in falling asleep or maintaining sleep. The former may be related to circadian rhythm disorders, and the latter is more consistent with gastroesophageal reflux disease, central sleep apnea syndrome, and PLMD, among others.

Sleep habits should be carefully reviewed, including the patient's usual bedtime, times spent awake in bed before and following the onset of sleep, and final morning awakening and arising times. Sleep logs completed daily over 2 weeks before the evaluation often are more revealing and accurate in this regard. The history also should include the pattern of drug, medication, and recreational substance use, as well as potential sleep hygiene difficulties.

Most intrinsic disorders of sleep do not exhibit diagnostic signs on physical examination. However, a physical examination should be performed to assess the potential for contributory medical and neurologic illnesses. A thorough psychiatric history and mental status examination are also important. Finally, serum laboratory tests, including thyroid function studies, should be considered if they have not been performed within 6 months before the evaluation.

If the above office-based process raises the possibility of intrinsic sleep disorders, polysomnography should be considered. Circumstances when polysomnography can be useful are outlined in Table 17-13.

Hypnotic Agents

A wide array of compounds have been utilized for their sleep-promoting qualities over the years. Alcohol may be one of the most widely utilized agents by patients with insomnia because it enhances sleepiness and decreases sleep latency. However, it is a poor choice because it is associated with increased nocturnal awakenings and greater daytime somnolence (Roehrs and Roth, 2001). As noted earlier, alcohol can also result in further impairment in sleep-related respiration in patients with OSA. Antihistamines and over-the-counter products cannot be wholeheartedly recommended either because they have unpredictable effects on sleep and can cause adverse systemic effects due to their anticholinergic, sympathomimetic, and other properties. Although barbiturates and barbiturate-like drugs (choral hydrate, glutethimide, among others) were utilized as hypnotics in the past, they too can no longer be recommended because they have a far greater potential for significant sedation and even death in overdoses when compared to benzodiazepines.

TABLE 17-13   Circumstances When Appropriate to Refer to a Sleep Disorders Center

1. Need for nocturnal or daytime polysomnography in the following situations:
   a. Suspicion of a sleep-related breathing disorder
   b. Assessment of efficacy of treatment for a sleep-related breathing disorder
   c. Suspicion of periodic limb movement disorder or another sleep-related neuromuscular disorder which cannot be fully diagnosed by clinical interview
   d. Paroxysmal arousals or other sleep-related behaviors thought related to a seizure disorder and an EEG and clinical evaluation are inconclusive
   e. Suspicion of narcolepsy
   f. When the diagnosis of insomnia is uncertain, if previous treatments have failed, or if that patient experiences abrupt arousals associated with violent behavior (Littner, 2001)
2. Need for a consultation by a physician specializing in sleep medicine

EEG, electroencephalogram.

TABLE 17-14	Most Commonly Prescribed Medications Indicated for Insomnia

1. Benzodiazepine-GABA receptor agonists
   a. Benzodiazepines
      i. Long half-life: flurazepam (Dalmane) and quazepam (Doral)
      ii. Intermediate half-life: estazolam (ProSom) and temazepam (Restoril)
      iii. Short half-life: triazolam (Halcion)
   b. Non-benzodiazepines that act at the benzodiazepine receptor
      i. Zolpidim (Ambien)
      ii. Zolpidem extended release (Ambien CR)
      iii. Zaleplon (Sonata)
      iv. Eszopiclone (Lunesta)
2. Melatonin receptor agonists
   a. Ramelteon (Rozerem)

GABA, γ-aminobutyric acid.

Melatonin, a hormone released by the pineal gland whose secretion peaks during sleep, has long been suspected as helpful for sleep and witnessed extraordinary popularity in recent years among patients with insomnia as an over-the-counter sleep aid. Unfortunately, the evidence for its efficacy as a general sleep aid is scant (Stone et al., 2000). Melatonin may, however, be useful in affecting positive changes in circadian rhythm disorders, although more definitive studies are necessary. In addition, concerns exist regarding its safety, and questions have been raised regarding the purity of certain melatonin preparations. Because of the lack of methodologically rigorous dose-response studies, the proper dosage is unknown as well.

Hypnotic agents have proved to be far safer and more efficacious than previously available agents. Table 17-14 summarizes the most commonly prescribed medications that are indicated for insomnia.

Desirable clinical properties for hypnotics include the ability to diminish sleep latency (the time required to fall asleep), reduce nocturnal awakenings, diminish the time spent awake, and increase the time spent asleep. On one hand, agents with short half-lives (e.g., ramelteon, zaleplon) are suitable for reduction of sleep latency but less efficacious for reduction of all-night awakenings. On the other hand, they are also less likely to produce potentially dangerous next-day carry-over effects.

Hypnotics should be administered at the lowest effective dose and for brief periods of time to avoid tolerance and rebound insomnia, the latter referring to a transient increase in sleep disturbance (relative to baseline sleep) that occurs with abrupt discontinuation of the medication. Rebound can be mitigated by gradually tapering when discontinuing the drug. More recently introduced medications such as eszopiclone and zolpidem ER have demonstrated no appreciable tolerance or rebound effects after 6 months of administration. All hypnotics carry the risk of abuse, with the exception of ramelteon. Caution should be exercised in individuals with respiratory disturbances, and lower dosages should be utilized in the elderly. Details on the comparative use of these medications are found elsewhere in this book.

CONCLUSIONS

Sleep-related complaints such as insomnia and EDS are often symptoms of a variety of neurologic, psychiatric, and medical disorders and can represent primary disorders as well. Therefore, the evaluation of insomnia and EDS should include systematic assessment of the specific sleep-related complaint, guided by knowledge of the many possible pathologic entities. Once the diagnosis is established, treatment can be conducted with confidence. This approach is the most gratifying not only for physicians but for patients as well.

Clinical Pearls

- Sleepy patients are often unaware of their own sleepiness levels; the best way to assess sleepiness is to ask about the propensity to fall asleep at undesirable times.
- Interview the bed partner about the patient's sleep habits, snoring, and unusual body movements during sleep.
- Sleep logs completed over a 2-week period are more accurate than the patient's remembered account of sleep–wake times and habits.
- Sleep is not the same as rest; it is a complex, actively generated state that involves the participation of many brain and body processes.
- Sleep apnea syndrome can be diagnosed only by polysomnography; if a patient's symptoms suggest the disorder, refer for testing before instituting treatment.
- The best treatment for psychophysiological insomnia is the combination of pharmacologic agents and cognitive behavioral techniques.
- Daytime sleepiness is not a salient feature of children with sleep apnea syndrome; rather, they experience behavioral deterioration, developmental delay, and worsening school performance.
- Avoid sedatives and hypnotics in a patient with untreated sleep apnea.
- Do not treat sleep deprivation with medication; the best treatment for sleep deprivation is sleep!
- Think outside the box! The causes of sleep complaints transcend the bounds of traditional medical specialties.

Self-Assessment Questions and Answers

17-1. The transition from wakefulness to stage 1 sleep is marked by
- A. Appearance of rhythmic alpha activity
- B. Establishment of relatively high voltage
- C. Mixed frequency pattern
- D. Absence of theta (3 to 7 cps) activity

The transition from wakefulness to stage 1 sleep is marked by the disappearance of rhythmic alpha and the establishment of relatively low voltage and mixed frequency pattern with the prevalence of theta (3 to 7 cps) activity. *Answer: C*

17-2. Spindles
- A. Are not found in all mammals
- B. Are identical in all species of mammals
- C. Develop before birth in humans
- D. May be faster to develop in mental retardation

Spindles are found in all mammals and identical in all species. They develop before the age of 3 months in humans and may be slower to develop in mental retardation. *Answer: B*

17-3. The multiple sleep latency test (MSLT)
- A. Directly assesses the biological basis of sleepiness
- B. Is most useful in the diagnostic assessment of narcolepsy
- C. Measures the propensity to fall asleep during the day in a setting that maximizes alerting factors
- D. Monitors a patient polysomnographically in a darkened room during 2 nap opportunities, spaced 5 hours apart, and beginning at 10:00 AM

Although no tests can directly assess the biological basis of sleepiness, the MSLT does so indirectly by measuring the propensity to fall asleep during the day in a setting that minimizes alerting factors. During this test, the patient is monitored polysomnographically in a darkened room while lying down on a sleep laboratory bed during five nap opportunities, spaced 2 hours apart, and beginning at 10:00 AM. Although the MSLT has been utilized to identify the extent of daytime somnolence in diverse populations and diagnoses, it is most useful in the diagnostic assessment of narcolepsy. *Answer: B*

17-4. The prevalence of obstructive sleep apnea syndrome
- A. Is higher in women than in men
- B. Decreases with age
- C. Is higher in African Americans than whites
- D. Is higher in Asians than in African Americans

The prevalence of obstructive sleep apnea syndrome (OSAS) is 2% in women and 4% in men. The prevalence of the condition increases with age. African Americans older than 35 years are more likely to have OSAS than whites irrespective of body weight. The prevalence of OSAS among Asian cultures is similar to that of whites, despite Asian populations having comparably lower mean body weight. *Answer: C*

References

Allen RP, Walters AS, Montplaisir J, et al. Restless legs syndrome prevalence and impact: REST General Population Study. *Arch Intern Med*. 2005;165(11):1286–1292.

American Academy of Sleep Medicine. *ICSD—international classification of sleep disorders*, 2nd ed. American Academy of Sleep Medicine; 2005.

Ancoli-Israel S. The impact and prevalence of chronic insomnia and other sleep disturbances associated with chronic illness. *Am J Manag Care*. 2006;12(Suppl 8):S221–S229.

Arand D, Bonnet M, Hurwitz T, et al. The clinical use of the MSLT and MWT. *Sleep*. 2005;28(1):123–144.

Armitage R, Yonkers K, Rush AJ, et al. Nefazodone improves sleep efficiency and has little effect on REM sleep in depressed patients. *Sleep Res*. 1995;24A:392.

Beebe DW, Groesz L, Wells C, et al. The neuropsychological effects of obstructive sleep apnea: A meta-analysis of norm-referenced and case-controlled data. *Sleep*. 2003;26:198–307.

Billiard M, Besset A. Idiopathic hypersomnia. In: Billiard M, ed. *Physiology, investigations and medicine*. New York: Kluwer Academic Publishers, Plenum Publishing; 2003:429–435.

Billiard M, Dauvilliers Y. Idiopathic hypersomnia. *Sleep Med Rev*. 2001;5:349–358.

Bonnet MH, Arand DL. We are chronically sleep deprived. *Sleep*. 1995;18(10):908–911.

Coleman RM, Roffwarg HP, Kennedy SJ, et al. Sleep-wake disorders based on a polysomnographic diagnosis. A National Cooperative Study. *JAMA*. 1982;247(7):997–1003.

Czeisler CA, Johnson MP, Duffy JR, et al. Exposure to bright light and darkness to treat physiologic maladaptation to night work. *N Engl J Med*. 1990;322:1253–1259.

Doghramji K, Mitler MM, Sangal RB, et al. A normative study of the maintenance of wakefulness test (MWT). *Electroencephalogr Clin Neurophysiol*. 1997;103(5):554–562.

Ekbom KA. Restless legs syndrome. *Neurology*. 1960;10:868.

Engleman H, Joffe D. Neuropsychological function in obstructive sleep apnoea. *Sleep Med Rev*. 1999;21:701–706.

Findley L, Barth J, Powers D. Cognitive impairment in patients with obstructive sleep apnea and associated hypoxemia. *Chest*. 1986;90(5):686–690.

Ford DE, Kamerow DB. Epidemiologic study of sleep disturbances and psychiatric disorders. *JAMA*. 1989;262:1479–1484.

Gozal D, Kheirandish-Gozal L. Cardiovascular morbidity in obstructive sleep apnea. Oxidative stress, inflammation, and much more. *Am J Respir Crit Care Med*. 2008;177:369–375.

Gursky J, Krahn L. The effects of antidepressants on sleep: A review. *Harv Rev Psychiatry*. 2000;8(6):298–306.

Hauri PJ. In: Hauri PJ, ed. *Case studies in insomnia*. New York: Plenum Publishing; 1991:65.

Hayduk R, Flodman P, Spence MA, et al. HLA haplotypes, polysomnography, and pedigrees in a case series of patients with narcolepsy. *Sleep*. 1997;20(10):850–857.

He J, Kryger M, Zorick FJ, et al. Mortality and apnea index in obstructive sleep apnea. Experience in 385 male patients. *Chest*. 1988;94(1):9–14.

Hiestand DM, Britz P, Goldman M, et al. Prevalence of symptoms and risk of sleep apnea in the US population: Results from the national sleep foundation sleep in America 2005 poll. *Chest*. 2006;130(3):780–786.

Hoddes E, Zarcone V, Smythe H, et al. Quantification of sleepiness: A new approach. *Psychophysiology*. 1973;10:431–436.

Hogl B, Poewe W. Restless legs syndrome. *Curr Opin Neurol*. 2005;18(4):405–410.

Iglowstein I, Jenni OG, Molinari L, et al. Sleep duration from infancy to adolescence: Reference values and generational trends. *Pediatrics*. 2003;111(2):302–307.

Jacobs EA, Reynolds CF, Kupfer DJ, et al. The role of polysomnography in the differential diagnosis of chronic insomnia. *Am J Med Genet B Neuropsychiatr Genet*. 1988;145:346–349.

Johns MW. A new method for measuring daytime sleepiness: The Epworth Sleepiness Scale. *Sleep*. 1991;14: 540–545.

Katz DA, McHorney CA. The relationship between insomnia and health-related quality of life in patients with chronic illness. *J Fam Pract*. 2002;51:229–235.

Kotagal S, Silber MH. Childhood-onset restless legs syndrome. *Ann Neurol*. 2004;56(6):803–807.

Kribbs N, Pack A, Kline L, et al. Objective measurement of patterns of nasal CPAP use by patients with obstructive sleep apnea. *Am Rev Respir Dis*. 1993;147(4):887–895.

Lavigne GJ, Montplaisir JY. Restless legs syndrome and sleep bruxism: Prevalence and association among Canadians. *Sleep*. 1994;17(8):739–743.

Littner M, Johnson SF, McCall WV, et al. Standards of Practice Committee. Practice parameters for the treatment of narcolepsy: An update for 2000. *Sleep*. 2001;1524(4):451–466.

Longstreth WT Jr, Koepsell TD, Ton TG, et al. The epidemiology of narcolepsy. *Sleep*. 2007;30(1): 13–26.

Metlaine A, Leger D, Choudat D. Socioeconomic impact of insomnia in working populations. *Ind Health*. 2005;43(1):11–19.

Mignot E. Narcolepsy: Pharmacology, pathophysiology, and genetics. In: Kryger M, Thomas R, Dement W, eds. *Principles and practice of sleep medicine*. Philadelphia: Elsevier Science, WB Saunders; 2005:761–779.

Mignot E, Lammers GJ, Ripley B, et al. The role of cerebrospinal fluid hypocretin measurement in the diagnosis of narcolepsy and other hypersomnias. *Arch Neurol*. 2002;59(10):1553–1562.

Mignot E, Lin X, Arrigoni J. DQB1*0602 and DQA1*0102 (DQ1) are better markers than DR2 for narcolepsy in Caucasian and black Americans. *Sleep*. 1994;17(8 suppl):S60–S76.

Mignot E. Genetic and familial aspects of narcolepsy. *Neurology*. 1998;50(2 Suppl 1):S16–S22.

Mitler MM, Gujavarty KS, Sampson MG, et al. Multiple daytime nap approaches to evaluating the sleepy patient. *Sleep*. 1982;5:S119–S127.

Mitler MM, Carskadon MA, Czeisler CA, et al. Catastrophes, sleep, and public policy: Consensus report. *Sleep*. 1988;11(1):100–109.

Montplaisir J, Allen R, Walter A, et al. Restless legs syndrome and periodic limb movements during sleep. In: Kryger M, Thomas R, Dement W, eds. *Principles and practice of sleep medicine*. Philadelphia: Elsevier Science, WB Saunders; 2005:839–852.

National Sleep Foundation. *Sleep in America poll*, 2005:19. Available at http://www.sleepfoundation.org/site/c.huIXKjM0IxF/b.2419039/k.14E4/2005_Sleep_in_America_Poll.htm. http://www.kintera.org/atf/cf/{F6BF2668-A1B4-4FE8-8D1A-A5D39340D9CB}/2005_summary_of_findings.pdf. Accessed July 14, 2008.

Netzer NC, Hoegel JJ, Loube D, et al. Prevalence of symptoms and risk of sleep apnea in primary care. *Chest*. 2003;124(4):1406–1414.

Nichols DA, Allen RP, Grauke JH, et al. Restless legs syndrome symptoms in primary care: A prevalence study. *Arch Intern Med*. 2003;163(19):2323–2329.

Nuckton TJ, Glidden DV, Browner WS, et al. Physical examination: Mallampati score as an independent predictor of obstructive sleep apnea. *Sleep*. 2006;29(7):903–908.

Ohayon MM, Partinen M. Insomnia and global sleep dissatisfaction in Finland. *J Sleep Res*. 2002;11(4): 339–346.

Ohayon MM, Priest RG, Zulley J, et al. Prevalence of narcolepsy symptomatology and diagnosis in the European general population. *Neurology*. 2002;58(12):1826–1833.

Ohayon M, Priest R, Zulley J, et al. The place of confusional arousals in sleep and mental disorders: Findings in a general population sample of 13,057 subjects. *J Nerv Ment Dis*. 2000;188(6):340–348.

Okun ML, Lin L, Pelin Z, et al. Clinical aspects of narcolepsy-cataplexy across ethnic groups. *Sleep*. 2002; 25(1):27–35.

Palmer LJ, Redline S. Genomic approaches to understanding obstructive sleep apnea. *Respir Physiol Neurobiol*. 2003;135(2-3):187–205.

Perlis ML, Giles DE, Buysse DJ, et al. Which depressive symptoms are related to which sleep electroencephalographic variables? *Biol Psychiatry*. 1997;42(10):904–913.

Rechtshaffen A, Kales A. *A manual of standardized terminology, techniques, and scoring systems of sleep stages of human subjects*. Los Angeles: UCLA Brain Information Service/Brain Research Institute; 1968.

Reynolds CF, Kupfer DJ. Sleep research in affective illness: State of the art circa 1987. *Sleep*. 1987;10: 199–215.

Ripley B, Overeem S, Fujiki N, et al. *Neurology*. 2001;57:2253–2258.

Roehrs T, Roth T. Sleep, sleepiness, sleep disorders and alcohol use and abuse. *Sleep Med Rev*. 2001;5(4): 287–297.

Rosenthal NE, Joseph-Vanderpool JR, Levendosky AA, et al. Phase-shifting effects of bright morning light as treatment for delayed sleep phase syndrome. *Sleep*. 1990;13:354–361.

Silber MH, Krahn LE, Olson EJ, et al. The epidemiology of narcolepsy in Olmsted County, Minnesota: A population-based study. *Sleep*. 2002;25(2):197–202.

Stefansson H, Rye DB, Hicks A, et al. A genetic risk factor for periodic limb movements in sleep. *N Engl J Med*. 2007;357:639–647.

Stone BM, Tuerner C, Mills SL, et al. Hypnotic activity of melatonin. *Sleep*. 2000;23:663–669.

Taheri S, Mignot E. The genetics of sleep disorders. *Lancet Neurol*. 2002;1(4):242–250.

Tan TL, Kales JD, Kales A, et al. Biopsychobehavioral correlates of insomnia, IV: Diagnosis based on DSM-III. *Am J Med Genet B Neuropsychiatr Genet*. 1984;141:357–362.

Thase M. Depression, sleep, and antidepressants. *J Clin Psychiatry*. 1998;59(Suppl 4):55–65.

Tobler I. Phylogeny of sleep regulation. In: Kryger M, Thomas R, Dement W, eds. *Principles and practice of sleep medicine*. Philadelphia: Elsevier Science, WB Saunders; 2005:77–90.

van Bemmel A, van den Hoffdakker R, Beersma D, et al. Changes in sleep polygraphic variables and clinical state in depressed patients during treatment with citalopram. *Psychopharmacology*. 1993;113:225–230.

Volpp KG, Rosen AK, Rosenbaum PR, et al. Mortality among hospitalized Medicare beneficiaries in the first 2 years following ACGME resident duty hour reform. *JAMA*. 2007;298:975–983.

Waugh J, Goa KL. Escitalopram: A review of its use in the management of major depressive and anxiety disorders. *CNS Drugs*. 2003;17:343–362.

Wehr TA, Sack DA, Rosethal NE. Sleep reduction as a final common pathway in the genesis of mania. *Am J Psychiatry*. 1987;144:201–204.

Weitzman ED, Czeisler CA, Coleman RM, et al. Delayed sleep phase syndrome. A chronobiological disorder with sleep-onset insomnia. *Arch Gen Psychiatry*. 1981;38:737–746.

West SD, Nicoll DJ, Stradling JR. Prevalence of obstructive sleep apnoea in men with type 2 diabetes. *Thorax*. 2006;61(11):945–950.

Young T, Finn L, Kim H. The University of Wisconsin Sleep and Respiratory Research Group. Nasal obstruction as a risk factor for sleep-disordered breathing. *J Allergy Clin Immunol*. 1997;99(2):S757–S762.

Young T, Peppard PE, Gottlieb DJ. Epidemiology of obstructive sleep apnea: A population health perspective. *Am J Respir Crit Care Med*. 2002;165(9):1217–1239.

Young T, Skatrud J, Peppard PE. Risk factors for obstructive sleep apnea in adults. *JAMA*. 2004;291(16): 2013–2016.

Zhang L, Samet J, Caffo B, et al. Cigarette smoking and nocturnal sleep architecture. *Am J Epidemiol*. 2006;164(6):529–537.

CHAPTER 18

Jon E. Grant and Emil F. Coccaro

Impulse Control Disorders

Impulsivity has been defined as a predisposition toward rapid, unplanned reactions to either internal or external stimuli without regard for negative consequences. Given this definition, multiple psychiatric disorders might be characterized as exhibiting problems with impulse control. In the text revision of the Fourth Edition of the *Diagnostic and Statistical Manual* of the American Psychiatric Association (DSM-IV-TR) (2000), the category of impulse control disorders not elsewhere classified includes intermittent disorder, pathological gambling (PG), kleptomania, trichotillomania, and pyromania.

Although the extent to which the impulse control disorders (ICDs) share clinical, genetic, phenomenological, and biological features is incompletely understood, ICDs share common core qualities: (a) repetitive or compulsive engagement in a behavior despite adverse consequences, (b) diminished control over the problematic behavior, (c) an appetitive urge or craving state before engagement in the problematic behavior, and (d) a hedonic quality during the performance of the problematic behavior (Grant and Potenza, 2005).

Clinical similarities exist between ICDs and substance use disorders, which is why many of these disorders have been referred to as *behavioral addictions*. Both include aspects of tolerance, withdrawal, repeated unsuccessful attempts to cut back or stop, and impairment in major areas of life functioning. Phenomenological data further support a relationship between ICDs and drug addictions; for example, high rates of certain ICDs (e.g., PG) and substance use disorders have been reported during adolescence and young adulthood, and the telescoping phenomenon (reflecting the rapid rate of progression from initial to problematic behavioral engagement in women as compared with men) initially described for alcoholism has been applied to PG (Potenza et al., 2001). Emerging biological data, such as those identifying common genetic contributions to alcohol use and gambling disorders (Slutske et al., 2000) and common brain activity changes underlying gambling urges and cocaine cravings (Potenza et al., 2002), provide further support for a shared relationship between certain ICDs and substance use disorders.

Although many data from diverse sources support a close relationship between ICDs and substance use disorders, other nonmutually exclusive models proposed for ICDs include categorizations as obsessive-compulsive disorders (OCD) and affective spectrum disorders (Potenza and Hollander, 2002; McElroy et al., 1996).

Conceptualization of ICDs within an obsessive-compulsive spectrum is based on common features of repetitive thoughts and behaviors (Potenza and Hollander, 2002). Although clinical aspects, such as ritualistic behaviors, are shared between OCDs and ICDs, other aspects seem different, such as the egosyntonic nature of behaviors in ICDs and the egodystonic nature of compulsions in OCD. Although some evidence supports high rates of co-occurring OCD and ICDs (McElroy et al., 1992), multiple studies do not report an association (Grant and Potenza, 2006). Personality features of individuals with ICDs (impulsive, reward- and sensation-seeking) differ from those with OCD (harm-avoidant) (Grant and Potenza, 2006). Biological differences also exist; for example, whereas increased activity in corticobasal ganglionic-thalamic circuitry has been described during symptom provocation studies of OCD, relatively decreased activity in these brain regions was observed in cue elicitation studies in ICDs (Potenza et al., 2003). Family history and large-scale epidemiologic studies have also not demonstrated associations between ICDs and OCD (Potenza et al., 2002).

The association of ICDs with mood disorders has led to their proposed grouping as an affective spectrum disorder (McElroy et al., 1996). Many people with ICDs report that the pleasurable yet problematic behaviors alleviate negative emotional states. Because the behaviors are risky and self-destructive, the question has been raised whether ICDs reflect some form of hypomania or mania. The elevated rates of co-occurrence between ICDs and depression and bipolar disorder support their inclusion within an affective spectrum, as do early reports of treatment response to serotonin reuptake inhibitors, mood stabilizers, and electroconvulsive therapy (McElroy et al., 1996). However, depression in ICDs may be distinct from primary or uncomplicated depression; it may represent a response to shame and embarrassment. In addition, rates of co-occurrence of ICDs and bipolar disorder may not be as high as initially thought (Grant et al., 2006). Nonetheless, brain imaging studies have found common regional brain activity differences distinguishing bipolar and ICD subjects from controls during a cognitive task involving attention and response inhibition (Potenza et al., 2003). For these reasons, the relationship between ICDs and mood disorders requires clarification, particularly because appropriate classification has implications for treatment development.

EPIDEMIOLOGY

Arguably the best data on the prevalence of ICDs exist for PG. A recent meta-analysis of 120 published studies and a national prevalence study estimate that the lifetime prevalence of serious gambling (meeting DSM-IV-TR criteria) among adults ranges from 0.45% to 1.6% with past-year rates for adults ranging from 0.6% to 1.1% (Petry et al., 2005; Shaffer et al., 1999). Studies have consistently shown that the rate of PG is twice as high among men as compared with women.

Both intermittent explosive disorder (IED) and trichotillomania appear common in community samples. Recent research suggests that upward of 5% to 6% of community samples meet criteria for lifetime IED (Coccaro et al., 2004; Kessler et al., 2006). Clinically significant hair pulling has been reported in 0.6% to 3.4% of college students, and hair pulling that meets DSM-IV-TR criteria for trichotillomania appears relatively common, with an estimated prevalence between 1% and 3% (Christenson et al., 1991). Trichotillomania appears to be more common in females (93.2% of a recent community sample of 1,697 individuals with trichotillomania) (Woods et al., 2006).

Although the precise prevalence rates of kleptomania and pyromania remain unknown, rates of both disorders in treatment-seeking samples suggest that they may be fairly common. One study of 107 patients with depression found that 2.8% ($n = 3$) met current DSM-IV-TR criteria for pyromania (Lejoyeux et al., 2002), and a recent study of 204 psychiatric inpatients revealed that 3.4% ($n = 7$) endorsed current and 5.9% ($n = 12$) had lifetime symptoms meeting DSM-IV-TR criteria for pyromania (Grant et al., 2005). Kleptomania is also experienced by a broad range of psychiatric patient populations, including 3.7% of patients with depression ($n = 107$) (Lejoyeux et al., 2002) and 24% of bulimics (Hudson et al., 1987). A recent study of psychiatric inpatients ($n = 204$) with a range of admitting disorders revealed that 7.8% ($n = 16$) endorsed current kleptomania and 9.3% ($n = 19$) met lifetime criteria (Grant et al., 2005). Although the gender ratio in pyromania is unknown, approximately two-thirds of individuals with kleptomania, in clinical samples, are women.

ETIOLOGY

Multiple theories have been raised over the centuries for what causes a psychiatric disorder. Although there have been no absolute answers, a variety of hypotheses have been proposed. In the last two decades, the advent of neuroimaging and genetics and advances in pharmacotherapies have provided the means by which finding the cause of psychiatric disorders appears possible. Multiple advances have been made to understand the etiology of ICDs. Attempting to understand the etiology of all ICDs may be complicated by differences among these disorders as well as the heterogeneity within an ICD.

A growing body of literature implicates multiple neurotransmitter systems (e.g., serotonergic, dopaminergic, noradrenergic, opioidergic), as well as familial and inherited factors, in the pathophysiology of ICDs (Potenza and Hollander, 2002).

Neurobiology

Serotonin

From a biochemical perspective, serotonin has been a primary focus of inquiry, given its role in behavioral inhibition. A variety of studies suggest a strong role for serotonin (5-HT) in the aggressive behavior seen in patients with IED. For example, numerous neurochemical, 5-HT pharmacologic challenge, and even 5-HT platelet studies demonstrate an inverse correlation between various measures of 5-HT activity and aggressive behavior. This relationship appears to be due primarily to impulsive aggressive behavior, as opposed to aggressive behavior in general. Pharmacologic challenge studies and studies examining the platelet serotonin transporter suggest serotonin (5-HT) dysfunction also plays a role in PG and kleptomania.

Dopamine

Multiple lines of evidence support the mesocorticolimbic (MCL) dopamine system in the mediation of reinforcing behaviors (Kalivas and Volkow, 2005), and it may also mediate some of the rewarding or reinforcing aspects of ICDs. One study found decreased levels of dopamine and increased levels of 3,4-dihydroxyphenylacetic acid (DOPAC) and homovanillic acid (HVA), two dopamine metabolites, in cerebral spinal fluid of men with PG compared to sex-matched controls (Bergh et al., 1997). Another study found that amphetamine, which enhances dopamine synthesis, increases motivation for gambling in pathological gamblers (Zack and Poulos, 2004). These results lend further evidence for the involvement of dopaminergic pathways in the pathophysiology of PG.

Endogenous Opioid System

The endogenous opioid system influences the experiencing of pleasure. Opioids modulate mesolimbic dopamine pathways through disinhibition of γ-aminobutyric acid input in the ventral tegmental area (Kim, 1998). Gambling and related behaviors have been associated with elevated blood levels of the endogenous opioid β-endorphin (Shinohara et al., 1999). Given its mechanism of action and efficacy in the treatment of alcohol and opiate dependence, opioid receptor antagonists have been tested in the treatment of PG and other ICDs and have shown promise in reducing symptoms.

Norepinephrine

Norepinephrine (NE) has been hypothesized to mediate arousal and attention- and sensation-seeking in ICDs. Studies examining NE function in aggression, for example, have found direct relationships between the growth hormone response to the α_2 agonist clonidine and to irritability (i.e., the tendency to explode with negative affect). Although this measure is reflective of postsynaptic NE receptors, plasma levels of NE metabolites such as MHPG (3-methoxy-4-hydroxyphenyl glycol, a metabolite and a presynaptic measure of NE) demonstrate an inverse correlation with aggression. Taken together, there appears to be some initial evidence for a dysregulation in the NE system in regard to aggression. This is in some contrast to studies of pathologic gamblers (Roy et al., 1988), where such individuals were noted to have higher cerebral spinal fluid levels of MHPG and higher urine levels of NE. A different study measured plasma levels of NE in subjects playing Pachinko, a gaming machine that combines elements of pinball and slot machines (Shinohara et al., 1999). Researchers found that plasma levels rose during play, with statistically significant differences in levels in six regular players at the beginning and end of a winning streak.

Stress Pathways

Cortisol changes have been associated with ICDs. A study of male and female aborigines from Kimberley, Australia, whose urine was collected during a 2-day period just after receiving their wages (after which the community members typically gamble) showed significantly higher rates of cortisol and epinephrine excretion than in separate volunteers whose urine was collected several days later (Schmitt et al., 1998). A study of salivary cortisol and heart rate in 19 volunteers recruited from casinos during blackjack versus card play without monetary stakes found statistically significant elevations in both measures during blackjack compared to the control condition (Meyer et al., 2000).

Neuroimaging

There have been a growing number of neuroimaging studies in ICDs. Several studies demonstrate abnormalities in corticolimbic pathways in aggression. In positron emission tomography (PET) studies, glucose utilization has been reported as low in cortical areas and high in subcortical areas in the brains of impulsive violent offenders compared with healthy volunteers. This suggests a possible imbalance between inhibitory cortical areas and excitatory subcortical areas. PET studies examining 5-HT function have reported a reduction in orbitofrontal areas and anterior cingulate cortex in subjects with IED compared to controls. Recent studies using functional magnetic resonance imaging (fMRI) have demonstrated a heightened response of amygdala and a reduced response of orbitofrontal cortex to exposure to angry faces in subjects with IED compared with healthy volunteers (Coccaro et al., 2007). This suggests an imbalance in the function of corticoamygdala circuits in the context of relevant (threat) social stimuli.

In addition to the relevance of orbitofrontal cortex to ICDs, the ventromedial prefrontal cortex (vmPFC) has been implicated as a critical component of decision-making circuitry in risk-reward assessment in addiction (Kalivas and Volkow, 2005). Decreased activation of vmPFC has been observed in participants with PG during presentation of gambling cues (Potenza et al., 2003) and simulated gambling (Reuter et al., 2005). These data support a role for vmPFC dysfunction in ICDs, possibly of a serotonergic nature.

Dopamine and its neurocircuitry have also been implicated in ICDs. In a study of unmedicated participants with PG, investigators measured relative metabolic rate using ^{18}F-deoxyglucose in PET imaging to compare computer blackjack for monetary rewards versus points only (Hollander et al., 2005). They noted significantly higher relative metabolic rates in the primary visual cortex, cingulate gyrus, putamen, and prefrontal cortex in the monetary condition compared to points only, suggesting heightened sensory and limbic activation with increased risk.

The neuroimaging data suggest a complex network of brain regions are activated during ICD behaviors. Consistent with vmPFC's dysfunctional role in other addictive processes and psychiatric conditions (e.g., impulsivity in bipolar disorder), multiple studies using different experimental paradigms provide consistent evidence for its involvement. Similarly, studies suggest a role for the ventral striatum, which is not surprising, given the importance of the nucleus accumbens in addictive processes. PET studies provide evidence for the possible involvement of dopamine and 5-HT, although more extensive research is needed to confirm and extend these preliminary studies.

Genetics

With the rapid rate of discovery of genetic contributions to psychiatric disorders, the importance of genetics in understanding the neurobiology of ICDs is becoming increasingly apparent. However, genetics studies are currently lacking for most ICDs other than PG. Many data from twin studies support the role of genetics in aggression, but twin studies of IED have not yet been performed. However, two family history studies of IED have been published, both supporting familial transmission. Data from the Vietnam Era Twin (VET) Registry have identified common genetic and environmental contributions to PG, alcohol dependence, and antisocial behaviors (Slutske et al., 2000, 2001). Investigations into specific genes relating to NE, serotonin, and dopamine neurotransmitter systems and their contribution to ICDs are being performed.

PSYCHOLOGY OF IMPULSE CONTROL DISORDERS

In addition to neurobiology, behavioral and cognitive attitudes may play a role in the etiology of ICDs. Behavioral and social learning theorists have focused on the role of direct and vicarious reinforcement in developing and maintaining behaviors. Cognitive theorists have focused on information processing biases that inflate subjective estimates of succeeding in various behaviors (e.g., winning in gambling, successfully shoplifting) or that otherwise promote impulse behavior persistence.

Deficits in social information processing represent a critical factor in the development and maintenance of human aggression. Research in children and adolescents has confirmed that impulsive, aggressive children, particularly those with a history of abuse, demonstrate a reduction in the encoding of socially relevant information and the presence of a hostile attribution bias, especially in cases of ambiguous social interaction (Crick and Dodge, 1996). Encoding is the process of absorbing information from the environment, and attribution involves interpreting others' behaviors. A recent study indicated that individuals with IED have difficulty in identifying facial emotions and are more likely to code a neutral face as "negative." When presented with socially ambiguous story vignettes, in which two people have an aggressive encounter, individuals with IED are more likely than healthy controls to attribute hostile intent to the "aggressor."

Positive reinforcement refers to the introduction of a hedonically positive consequence that strengthens a preceding response. The quintessential positive reinforcer of many ICDs is acquiring something rewarding (e.g., winning money, stealing an item). The intermittent reinforcement (e.g., winning money, stealing items) of ICD behaviors describes a schedule of reinforcement that is particularly resistant to extinction.

A range of reinforcers (other than an item of reward) may be available to people with ICDs to initiate and perpetuate the behavior. These include social reinforcers (e.g., interaction with store employees for the kleptomaniac), material reinforcers (e.g., drinks and other goods and services provided for pathological gamblers), ambient reinforcers (e.g., a wide array of visual and auditory stimuli present in stores for the kleptomaniac), cognitive reinforcers (e.g., "near misses" such as being one card away from a large payout for the pathological gambler), and even physiological arousal itself (e.g., the "rush" reported by people who set fires).

A negative reinforcement theory (i.e., involving the removal of a punishing stimulus) hypothesizes that initiating, but not completing, a habitual behavior leads to uncomfortable states of arousal. Applied to kleptomania, this would imply that a frequent shoplifter who has begun but not yet accrued a significant number of items (i.e., "completed" the behavior) may continue shoplifting to experience relief from aversive arousal. The negative reinforcement–based model argues that addictions in general may allow individuals who are chronically either over- or under-aroused to achieve optimal arousal level (Jacobs, 1986).

Another negative reinforcement model is based on the "self-medication" model. A number of studies have found elevated rates of depression and anxiety disorders in individuals with ICDs, who may engage in the behavior to distract themselves from life stressors and unpleasant cognitions. Ironically, problems resulting directly from ICDs (e.g., financial distress, relationship difficulties, and criminal activity) may, in turn, lead to even more ICD behaviors as a misguided attempt of symptom management.

One explanation for why all individuals who engage in various behaviors do not succumb to an ICD may be due to differences in biological constraints surrounding reinforcement sensitivity. For some people, negative or positive reinforcement from an ICD may have a more powerful influence on future behavior. Alternatively, some people may be more or less sensitive or responsive to the punishment associated with the related risks, losses, and/or social opprobrium. Searching for such individual differences may ultimately refine both psychological and biological understanding of the etiology and maintenance of ICDs.

INTERMITTENT EXPLOSIVE DISORDER

Phenomenology

Aggressive outbursts in IED have a rapid onset, often without a recognizable prodromal period. They are short-lived (<30 minutes) and involve verbal assault, destructive and nondestructive property assault, or physical assault. They most commonly occur in response to a minor provocation by a close intimate or associate, and people with IED may have less severe episodes of verbal and nondestructive property assault in between more severe assaultive/destructive episodes. Episodes are associated with substantial distress, impairment in social functioning, occupational difficulty, and legal or financial problems. In a recent community sample study of >9,200 individuals, participants meeting a "narrow" definition of IED (i.e., three high-severity episodes in the current year) had a mean number of approximately 28 aggressive outbursts per year.

IED appears as early as childhood (e.g., prepubertal) and peaks in mid-adolescence, with a mean age of onset ranging from approximately 13 to 18 years. The average duration of symptomatic IED ranges from approximately 12 to 20 years to nearly the whole lifetime. Although IED has been previously reported to occur much more commonly in males (e.g., 3:1) and its age of onset is earlier in males than females by approximately 6 years, recent data suggest

A CASE OF INTERMITTENT EXPLOSIVE DISORDER

James, a 35-year-old single male, reported the occurrence of aggressive outbursts since he was 17. Typically they began suddenly in response to frustration or a threat to his self-esteem. The episodes involved screaming at the "offending" person and escalation, in many cases, to physical assault against this person or some object (e.g., ashtray, phone, wall) in the immediate environment. James would typically have small aggressive outbursts several times weekly and large aggressive outbursts involving property damage or assault against another person several times a year. Although James was good at beginning relationships, they would typically end as these new friends began to witness his volatility. After several years and several breaks in relationships, James began to wonder if his temper was a critical problem. He sought an evaluation and was diagnosed with intermittent explosive disorder. At first, CBT for "anger" was begun. After 12 weeks of therapy and a good, but partial, response, a selective serotonin reuptake inhibitor was begun. Over the next few months, James' aggressive outbursts diminished further to the point where they were limited to very mild aggressive outbursts (e.g., snapping at others when angered) only a few times a week.

the gender difference may be closer to 1:1. Importantly, sociodemographic variables (e.g., sex, age, race, education, marital and occupational status, family income) do not seem to differ as a function of the presence or absence of IED. IED is often comorbid with other lifetime disorders, such as depressive, anxiety, and substance use disorders. However, in most cases, the age of onset precedes that of these other lifetime comorbid disorders, suggesting that IED is not a consequence of them.

Pharmacologic Treatment

Although the U.S. Food and Drug Administration (FDA) has not approved medications to treat IED, several psychopharmacologic agents appear to have effects on aggression. Classes of agents shown to have "antiaggressive" effects in double-blind, placebo-controlled trials of individuals with "primary" aggression (i.e., not secondary to psychosis, severe mood disorder, or organic brain syndromes) include mood stabilizers (e.g., lithium), 5-HT uptake inhibitors (e.g., fluoxetine), and anticonvulsants (e.g., diphenhydantoin, carbamazepine). Although NE β-blockers (e.g., propanolol/nadolol) have also been shown to reduce aggression, these agents have exclusively been tested in patient populations with "secondary" aggression (e.g., mental retardation, organic brain syndromes). Classes of agents that may have "proaggressive" effects include tricyclic antidepressants (e.g., amitriptyline), benzodiazepines, and stimulant and hallucinatory drugs of abuse (e.g., amphetamines, cocaine, phencyclidine). Findings from double-blind, placebo-controlled clinical trials suggest that antiaggressive efficacy is specific to impulsive, rather than nonimpulsive, aggression.

Psychological Treatment

Numerous studies and meta-analytic reviews suggest that relaxation training, skills training, cognitive therapy, and multicomponent treatments all have moderate to large effects in treating anger and that the anger-reducing effects remain at follow-up. Of the different approaches for treating individuals with anger and aggression problems, cognitive restructuring, skills training, multicomponent treatments, and relaxation skills appear to have the strongest influence on aggression (McCloskey, 2008). Notably, however, the anger treatment literature does not discriminate between clinical anger problems *without* aggression and pathological aggression; therefore, these findings may not generalize to more severely aggressive individuals with IED.

PATHOLOGICAL GAMBLING

Phenomenology

Some form of gambling addiction or compulsivity has been recognized since the ancient Romans and discussed in the medical literature since the early 1800s. With recognition of the problem came various attempts to control it (e.g., laws and prison terms, limits on bets), but the problem and the resultant personal and social consequences (e.g., criminal behavior, suicide) have continued for centuries.

PG is characterized by persistent and recurrent maladaptive patterns of gambling behavior and associated with impaired functioning, reduced quality of life, and high rates of bankruptcy, divorce, and incarceration (Argo and Black, 2004). PG usually begins in adolescence or early adulthood, with males tending to start at an earlier age (Argo and Black, 2004). It appears to follow a similar trajectory as substance dependence, with high rates in adolescent and young adult groups, lower rates in older adults, and periods of abstinence and relapse (Grant and Potenza, 2005).

Unique gender differences are seen in individuals with PG. On the one hand, males with PG appear more likely to report problems with strategic or "face-to-face" forms of gambling, such as blackjack or poker. On the other hand, females with PG tend to report problems with non-strategic, less interpersonally interactive forms of gambling, like slot machines or bingo (Potenza et al., 2001). Both female and male gamblers report that advertisements are a common trigger of their gambling urges, although females are more likely to report that feeling bored or lonely may also trigger them (Argo and Black, 2004).

Many pathological gamblers engage in illegal behavior, such as stealing, embezzlement, and writing bad checks, to fund their gambling (Potenza et al., 2000) or attempt to fix past gambling losses (Argo and Black, 2004). Usually due to financial and legal problems, suicide attempts are common and have been reported in 17% of individuals in treatment for PG (Petry and Kiluk, 2002).

Studies consistently find that patients with PG have high rates of lifetime mood (60% to 76%), anxiety (16% to 40%), and personality (87%) disorders, particularly antisocial personality disorder (Argo and Black, 2004). High rates of co-occurrence have been reported for PG and substance use disorders (including nicotine dependence) (Cunningham-Williams et al., 1998).

Pharmacologic Treatment

There are no FDA-approved medications to treat PG. Trials examining the use of antidepressants (clomipramine, sertraline, bupropion, paroxetine, fluvoxamine) have been mixed, with some demonstrating superiority to placebo whereas others did not. Although the results have been mixed, treatment data from these trials suggest that serotonergic antidepressants may be beneficial for some individuals with PG. There is also some indication that individuals with PG and anxiety may preferentially respond to these agents, but which variables predict response to serotonergic agents has not been fully examined. Given the limitations of the existing literature, it is not yet possible to conclude which antidepressants should be recommended and which individuals with PG are more likely to respond to these agents.

Mood stabilizers (e.g., lithium, valproic acid, carbamazepine) have also been examined for the treatment of PG because they have shown promise in treating bipolar disorder as well as general impulsivity. However, only one randomized, placebo-controlled trial of a mood stabilizer has been tested in PG. In that study, sustained release lithium carbonate was shown to be superior to placebo in reducing gambling symptoms (Hollander et al., 2005).

Opiate antagonists are thought to decrease dopamine neurotransmission in the nucleus accumbens and linked motivational neurocircuitry, thereby dampening gambling-related excitement and cravings (Kim, 1998). Two double-blind studies of opiate antagonists (e.g., naltrexone and nalmefene) have demonstrated superiority to placebo in reducing gambling urges and behavior (Grant et al., 2006; Kim et al., 2001).

Psychological Treatments

Most of the psychosocial treatment literature for PG have focused on cognitive behavioral therapy (CBT) techniques. The cognitive aspect includes psychoeducation, increased awareness of irrational cognitions, and cognitive restructuring. The behavioral techniques include identifying gambling triggers and developing nongambling sources to compete with the reinforcers associated with gambling. Studies using either individual cognitive therapy or CBT have demonstrated improvement in PG symptoms compared to a wait-list or referral to Gamblers Anonymous (Ladouceur et al., 2001; Petry et al., 2006). Group cognitive therapy and self-help workbooks

A CASE OF GAMBLING ADDICTION

Michael, a 45-year-old man, started gambling at age 26. He began playing poker with friends for money, and by age 30 he was gambling alone at casinos. Michael reported that his urges to gamble were often triggered by advertisements for the local casino and fantasies of winning large amounts of money. For the last 2 years, he has played blackjack approximately 4 nights a week, usually spending 6 hours a night and losing up to $400 each time. In addition, he began gambling with larger amounts of money. Although a successful self-employed businessman, his work suffered as a result of his gambling. In addition, because of the financial strain, he began embezzling money from work. Because of the lying and time spent away from home, Michael's wife filed for divorce.

have also shown promise in reducing symptoms (Dickerson et al., 1990; Hodgins et al., 2001; Ladouceur et al., 2003). Imaginal desensitization has also been used. Patients are taught relaxation and then instructed to imagine experiencing and resisting triggers to gambling. Imaginal desensitization resulted in significantly greater reduction in gambling symptoms compared to traditional aversion therapy (McConaghy et al., 1983, 1991).

TRICHOTILLOMANIA

Phenomenology

Trichotillomania has been defined as repetitive hair pulling that causes noticeable hair loss and results in clinically significant distress or functional impairment. Accounts of hair pulling are found in the Bible, Homer's the *Iliad*, and the plays of William Shakespeare (Christenson and Mansueto, 1999). The term *trichotillomania* dates back to Hallopeau's 1889 account of a young man who pulled out every hair of his body (Hallopeau, 1889).

The mean age at onset is approximately 13 years (Christenson and Mansueto, 1999). Although prospective studies are lacking, the onset of trichotillomania has been associated with scalp disease and stressful life events (Christenson and Mansueto, 1999). People report pulling hair from any body area, although the scalp is the most common. The feel of the hair's texture is a frequent trigger. Hair pulling is subject to great fluctuations in severity, with worsening of symptoms often related to stress. Individuals often pull for >1 hour each day, may pull hair from spouses or children, and often have rituals surrounding the pulling. For example, they may play with the hair, rub it on their faces, and occasionally eat the root or hair shaft. Significant social and occupational disability is common, with 34.6% of individuals reporting daily interference with job duties and 47% reporting avoidance of social situations such as dating or participating in group activities (Woods et al., 2006).

Pharmacologic Treatment

There are no FDA-approved medications to treat trichotillomania. Several controlled pharmacologic trials using antidepressants (e.g., clomipramine, fluoxetine) have been conducted in trichotillomania, with several studies failing to show superiority to placebo. One study comparing fluoxetine to behavioral therapy or a wait list found that although behavioral therapy demonstrated improvement in hair pulling compared to the wait-list condition, fluoxetine did not (van Minnen et al., 2003).

A placebo-controlled, randomized trial of the opioid antagonist naltrexone demonstrated significant improvement on one measure of trichotillomania symptoms in those assigned to the active agent as compared to placebo (O'Sullivan et al., 1999). Approximately half of those taking naltrexone (compared to none on placebo) reduced hair pulling by >50%.

A recent study examined the efficacy of using an atypical antipsychotic (olanzapine) in the treatment of trichotillomania based on the hypothesis that antipsychotics are beneficial for motor tics. The study found that 85% of those assigned to olanzapine, compared to 17% of those on placebo, improved during the trial (Van Ameringen et al., 2006).

A CASE OF TRICHOTILLOMANIA

Jane, a 37-year-old married woman, presented with hair pulling of 20 years' duration. When she began pulling, the frequency was approximately one time per week and only for a few minutes. She reports that pulling relieves anxiety and brings her pleasure and that, over time, the frequency needed to increase to produce the same feelings. Currently, Jane pulls her hair at least once daily. She may pull several times a day if she experiences a particularly stressful or unfulfilling day. She reports urges to pull her hair during the day but resists them when around other people. When alone at night, she often pulls for as long as 2 hours. After pulling a hair, she caresses her face with it, analyzes each hair to see if she has pulled the root, and then eats the root and throws the hair shaft away. Jane has developed a bald spot on the crown of her head that makes her avoid social situations and friends.

Psychological Treatments

Few controlled psychological treatment studies for trichotillomania have been published to date. Azrin et al. (1980) randomized 34 subjects to either habit reversal therapy or negative practice (where participants were instructed to stand in front of a mirror and act out motions of hair pulling without actually pulling). Habit reversal reduced hair pulling by >90% for 4 months, compared with 52% to 68% reduction for negative practice at 3 months.

A recent study examined 25 participants randomized to either acceptance and commitment therapy/habit reversal or wait-list (Woods et al., 2005). Those assigned to therapy experienced significant reductions in hair pulling severity and impairment compared to those assigned to the wait-list, and improvement was maintained at 3-month follow-up.

One study comparing CBT and clomipramine (Ninan et al., 2000) found that CBT was significantly more effective in reducing symptoms than either clomipramine or placebo. A second study comparing behavioral therapy to fluoxetine found that behavioral therapy resulted in statistically significant reductions in symptoms compared to either fluoxetine or wait-list (van Minnen et al., 2003).

KLEPTOMANIA

Phenomenology

Kleptomania is characterized by repetitive, uncontrollable stealing of items not needed for personal use. Although it typically has its onset in early adulthood or late adolescence (McElroy et al., 1991), the disorder has been reported in children as young as 4 years and adults as old as 77 (Grant, 2006). The literature clearly suggests that most patients with kleptomania are women (McElroy et al., 1991). Items stolen are typically hoarded, given away, returned to the store, or thrown away (McElroy et al., 1991). Many individuals with kleptomania (64% to 87%) have been apprehended at some time due to their stealing behavior, and 15% to 23% report having been incarcerated (Grant, 2006). Most try unsuccessfully to stop. The diminished ability to stop often leads to feelings of shame and guilt. Of those who are married, less than half disclosed their behavior to their spouses due to shame and guilt (Grant, 2006). High rates of other psychiatric disorders (depression, bipolar disorder, anxiety, substance use, and eating disorders) are common in individuals with kleptomania (Grant, 2006; McElroy et al., 1991).

Pharmacologic Treatment

There have been only two pharmacologic trials for kleptomania. One examined escitalopram treatment (Koran et al., 2007). Every participant received the medication and then those who responded were randomized to either continue on escitalopram or be switched to placebo. When the responders were randomized, 43% of those on escitalopram relapsed, compared with 50% on placebo, thereby showing no drug effect in response.

The only formal trial of medication examined naltrexone in a small number of participants, with all aware that they were receiving active medication. Naltrexone resulted in a significant decline in the intensity of urges to steal and stealing thoughts and behavior (Grant, 2006).

A CASE OF SHOPLIFTING

Shirley, a 54-year-old married woman, described a history of uncontrollable shoplifting that began in early adulthood. Over the course of a few months, she reports that she thought about stealing daily and was only rarely able to control her behavior when she entered a store. She currently shoplifts one to two times each week. She describes a "rush" each time she steals, but it is short-lived and when she leaves the store she usually throws away the stolen item or leaves it outside the store. She steals various items, none of which she cares about and all of which she could easily afford. In addition, Shirley lies to her husband, telling him that she buys the items she steals. The behavior and the lying cause significant depression and feelings of worthlessness. She has tried to commit suicide on three occasions, never telling anyone the reason behind her suicide attempts.

Psychological Treatments

No controlled studies of psychological treatments exist for kleptomania. Case reports suggest that CBTs may be effective in treating it. Covert sensitization, where a person is instructed to imagine stealing as well as its negative consequences (e.g., being handcuffed, feeling embarrassed), has been successful in reducing symptoms. Imaginal desensitization, where a person imagines the steps of stealing but also the ability to resist the behavior, has also successfully reduced kleptomania.

PYROMANIA
Phenomenology

DSM-IV-TR (American Psychiatric Association, 2000) describes pyromania as a preoccupation with fire setting and characterizes the behavior with the following diagnostic criteria: (a) deliberate and purposeful fire setting on more than one occasion; (b) tension or affective arousal before the act; (c) fascination with, interest in, curiosity about, or attraction to fire and its situational contexts; and (d) pleasure, gratification, or relief when setting fires or when witnessing or participating in their aftermath.

Although long thought to primarily affect men, recent research suggests that the gender ratio is equal in adults and may be slightly higher among females in adolescence (Grant and Kim, 2007). Mean age of onset is generally late adolescence, and the behavior appears chronic if left untreated (Grant and Kim, 2007). Urges to set fires are common in individuals with this behavior, and the fire setting is almost always pleasurable. Severe distress follows the fire setting, and individuals with pyromania report significant functional impairment (Grant and Kim, 2007).

Treatment

There are no controlled pharmacologic or psychological treatment data regarding pyromania. Clinicians should, therefore, consider the psychosocial and pharmacologic approaches to other ICDs when developing a treatment plan for pyromania.

A CASE OF PYROMANIA

Blake, a 22-year-old single male, reported a 7-year history of setting fires. Initially starting by burning things in his room or backyard, his behaviors gradually progressed to burning small, empty buildings throughout the town. Blake described the fires as exciting. He would spend hours planning, setting, and watching the fires and set a fire approximately once every 2 months. Although he enjoyed the fires, the behavior left him feeling guilty. Owing to the time spent on planning fires, Blake quit spending time with friends, became socially isolated, and felt depressed.

CONCLUSIONS

Clinicians evaluating patients with ICDs should assess the circumstances that led them to seek help. In most psychiatric disorders, patients seek treatment because they are troubled by their symptoms. Patients with ICDs, however, continue to struggle with the desire to engage in the behavior and their need to stop because of mounting social, occupational, financial, or legal problems.

The systematic study of treatment efficacy and tolerability is in its infancy for ICDs. With few studies published, it is not possible to make treatment recommendations with a substantial degree of confidence. No drugs are currently approved by the FDA for treating any of the ICDs. Nonetheless, specific drug and behavioral therapies offer promise for the effective treatment of PG and trichotillomania. Opioid antagonists and lithium currently appear to be the most promising pharmacologic treatments for PG, and both CBT and imaginal desensitization appear beneficial from a psychotherapeutic approach. For trichotillomania, habit reversal therapy may be beneficial.

For other ICDs, fewer data are available to generate empirically supported treatment recommendations. Various forms of CBT generally appear promising. In medication treatment, opioid antagonists also have support for use in these disorders, but the results for serotonergic medications appear mixed.

Clinicians should be aware of the limitations of our treatment knowledge. Most published studies have employed relatively small sample sizes, are of limited duration, and involve possibly nonrepresentative clinical groups (e.g., those without co-occurring psychiatric disorders). Heterogeneity of treatment samples may also complicate identification of effective treatments. At present, issues such as which medication to use and for whom or the duration of pharmacotherapy or CBT cannot be sufficiently addressed with the available data.

Clinical Pearls

- Impulse control disorders are fairly common, disabling behaviors.
- Certain impulse control disorders appear to have clinical, genetic, and neurobiological similarities to substance use disorders.
- Certain impulse control disorders—pathological gambling, intermittent explosive disorder—occur more commonly in men, whereas others—trichotillomania, kleptomania—are more common in women.
- The etiology of impulse control disorders appears to be multifactorial with genetic, neurochemical, psychological, and developmental contributions.
- Intermittent explosive disorder, characterized by short-lived, assaultive outbursts of aggression, generally has its onset in adolescence.
- Serotonergic medications, lithium, and antiepileptic medications have all shown early promise in the treatment of intermittent explosive disorder.
- Pathological gambling, characterized by a maladaptive pattern of gambling behavior, affects approximately 1% of adults and generally has its onset in adolescence or early adulthood.
- Cognitive behavioral therapy, opiate antagonists, and lithium have all shown effectiveness in reducing the symptoms of pathological gambling.
- Trichotillomania, defined as repetitive hair pulling that causes noticeable hair loss, appears to respond to habit reversal therapy but has demonstrated inconsistent responses to medication.
- Kleptomania and pyromania appear to be fairly common among psychiatric patients but both currently lack sufficient treatment data.

Self-Assessment Questions and Answers

18-1. Which of the following medications have shown benefit in treating intermittent explosive disorder?

A. Famciclovir
B. Fluconazole
C. Flumazenil
D. Fluoxetine
E. Fluvastatin

Fluoxetine is a selective serotonin reuptake inhibitor. Given the role of serotonin in behavioral inhibition, agents that increase serotonin have been shown to be helpful in controlling impulsive aggressive behavior. Famciclovir is an antiviral agent for herpes; flumazenil is a benzodiazepine antagonist used to treat benzodiazepine overdose; fluvastatin is an antihyperlipidemic agent used to treat high cholesterol; and fluconazole is an antifungal agent often used for the treatment of candidiasis or cryptococaal meningitis. *Answer: D*

18-2. Which of the following reflects one way in which men and women with pathological gambling differ?

    A. Pathological gambling starts at an earlier age in men.

    B. Pathological gambling starts at an earlier age in women.

    C. Onset of pathological gambling is similar in men and women.

    D. Women with pathological gambling prefer strategic forms of gambling.

    E. Men with pathological gambling are more likely to report feelings of boredom or loneliness as triggers to gambling.

There are important clinical differences in men and women with pathological gambling. Pathological gambling usually begins in adolescence or early adulthood, and males tend to start at an earlier age. Men also report more problems with strategic or "face-to-face" forms of gambling (blackjack or poker) and are less likely to report that feeling bored or lonely triggers their urge to gamble. *Answer: A*

18-3. Which statement concerning kleptomania is true?

    A. Currently only one medication is U.S. Food and Drug Administration (FDA) approved for kleptomania.

    B. Other psychiatric disorders are uncommon among individuals with kleptomania.

    C. Stolen items are typically hoarded, given away, returned to the store, or thrown away.

    D. Most individuals with kleptomania appear to be men.

    E. There have been several controlled psychotherapy studies in kleptomania.

Studies show that the items stolen by individuals with kleptomania are usually hoarded, given away, returned, or thrown out. Most individuals with kleptomania are women, and other psychiatric problems, such as depression, bipolar disorder, anxiety disorders, and substance abuse, are quite common in individuals with kleptomania. There is no FDA-approved medication for kleptomania, and there have been no controlled psychotherapy studies for the treatment of kleptomania. *Answer: C*

18-4. Which statement concerning pyromania is true?

    A. Few individuals with pyromania have urges to set fires.

    B. Individuals with pyromania generally report no functional impairment due to their behavior.

    C. One incident of setting a fire will satisfy diagnostic criteria for pyromania.

    D. The behavior of pyromania appears chronic if left untreated.

    E. The mean age of onset of pyromania is generally after age 50.

Although there are few data on pyromania, research suggests that if left untreated, the behavior appears chronic. The diagnosis requires fire setting on more than one occasion. The mean age of onset is generally late adolescence. Individuals with pyromania report frequent urges to set fires and significant functional impairment due to the behavior. *Answer: D*

18-5. On the basis of current evidence, which reflects the most effective treatment for trichotillomania?

    A. Fluoxetine

    B. Habit reversal therapy

    C. Imaginal desensitization

    D. Lithium

    E. Self-help workbook

Only habit reversal therapy has proven effectiveness in two controlled studies of trichotillomania. Fluoxetine has produced mixed results in placebo-controlled studies, with two studies showing that it was no better than placebo. Lithium has not been studied in placebo-controlled trials. Imaginal desensitization and self-help workbooks have not been examined in controlled studies of trichotillomania. *Answer: B*

References

American Psychiatric Association. *Diagnostic and statistical manual of mental disorders*, 4th ed., text revision. Washington, DC: American Psychiatric Publishing; 2000.

Argo TR, Black DW. Clinical characteristics. In: Grant JE, Potenza MN, eds. *Pathological gambling: A clinical guide to treatment*. Washington, DC: American Psychiatric Publishing; 2004:39–53.

Azrin NH, Nunn RG, Frantz SE. Treatment of hairpulling (trichotillomania): A comparative study of habit reversal and negative practice training. *J Behav Ther Exp Psychiatry*. 1980;11:13–20.

Bergh C, Eklund T, Sodersten P, et al. Altered dopamine function in pathological gambling. *Psychol Med*. 1997;27(2):473–475.

Christenson GA, Mansueto CS. Trichotillomania: Descriptive characteristics and phenomenology. In: Stein DJ, Christenson GA, Hollander E, eds. *Trichotillomania*. Washington, DC: American Psychiatric Publishing; 1999:1–42.

Christenson GA, Pyle RL, Mitchell JE. Estimated lifetime prevalence of trichotillomania in college students. *J Clin Psychiatry*. 1991;52:415–417.

Coccaro EF, McCloskey MS, Fitzgerald DA. et al. Amygdala and orbitofrontal reactivity to social threat in individuals with impulsive aggression. *Biol Psychiatry*. 2007;62:168–178.

Coccaro EF, Schmidt CS, Samuels J, et al. Lifetime and one-month prevalence rates of intermittent explosive disorder in a community sample. *J Clin Psychiatry*. 2004;65:820–824.

Crick NR, Dodge KA. Social information-processing mechanisms in reactive and proactive aggression. *Child Dev*. 1996;67:993–1002.

Cunningham-Williams RM, Cottler LB, Compton WM III, et al. Taking chances: Problem gamblers and mental health disorders—results from the St. Louis Epidemiologic Catchment Area study. *Am J Public Health*. 1998;88:1093–1096.

Dickerson M, Hinchy J, England SL. Minimal treatments and problem gamblers: A preliminary investigation. *J Gambl Stud*. 1990;6:87–102.

Grant JE. Kleptomania. In: Hollander E, Stein DJ, eds. *A clinical manual of impulse control disorders*. Washington, DC: American Psychiatric Publishing; 2006:175–201.

Grant JE, Kim SW. Clinical characteristics and psychiatric comorbidity of pyromania. *J Clin Psychiatry*. 2007;68:1717–1722.

Grant JE, Potenza MN. Pathological gambling and other "behavioral addictions." In: Frances RJ, Miller SI, Mack AH, eds. *Clinical textbook of addictive disorders*, 3rd ed. New York: Guilford Press; 2005: 303–320.

Grant JE, Potenza MN. Compulsive aspects of impulse control disorders. *Psychiatr Clin North Am*. 2006;29:539–551.

Grant JE, Levine L, Kim D, et al. Impulse control disorders in adult psychiatric inpatients. *Am J Psychiatry*. 2005;162:2184–2188.

Grant JE, Potenza MN, Hollander E, et al. A multicenter investigation of the opioid antagonist nalmefene in the treatment of pathological gambling. *Am J Psychiatry*. 2006;163:303–312.

Hallopeau M. Alopecie par grattage: Trichomanie ou Trichotillomanie. *Ann Dermatol Syphiligr (Paris)*. 1889;10:440.

Hodgins DC, Currie S, el-Guebaly N. Motivational enhancement and self-help treatments for problem gambling. *J Counsel Clin Psychol*. 2001;69:50–57.

Hollander E, Pallanti S, Baldini Rossi N, et al. Imaging monetary reward in pathological gamblers. *World J Biol Psychiatry*. 2005;6(2):113–120.

Hudson JI, Pope HG, Yurgelun-Todd D, et al. A controlled study of lifetime prevalence of affective and other psychiatric disorders in bulimic outpatients. *Am J Psychiatry*. 1987;144:1283–1287.

Jacobs DF. A general theory of addictions: A new theoretical model. *J Gambl Behav*. 1986;2:15–31.

Kalivas PW, Volkow ND. The neural basis of addiction: A pathology of motivation and choice. *Am J Psychiatry*. 2005;162:1403–1413.

Kessler RC, Coccaro EF, Fava M, et al. The prevalence and correlates of DSM-IV intermittent explosive disorder in the national comorbidity survey replication. *Arch Gen Psychiatry*. 2006;63:669–678.

Kim SW. Opioid antagonists in the treatment of impulse-control disorders. *J Clin Psychiatry*. 1998;59: 159–164.

Kim SW, Grant JE, Adson DE, et al. Double-blind naltrexone and placebo comparison study in the treatment of pathological gambling. *Biol Psychiatry*. 2001;49:914–921.

Koran LM, Aboujaoude EN, Gamel NN. Escitalopram treatment of kleptomania: An open-label trial followed by double-blind discontinuation. *J Clin Psychiatry*. 2007;68:422–427.

Ladouceur R, Sylvain C, Boutin C, et al. Cognitive treatment of pathological gambling. *J Nerv Ment Dis*. 2001;189(11):774–780.

Ladouceur R, Sylvain C, Boutin C, et al. Group therapy for pathological gamblers: A cognitive approach. *Behav Res Ther*. 2003;41:587–596.

Lejoyeux M, Arbaretaz M, McLoughlin M, et al. Impulse control disorders and depression. *J Nerv Ment Dis*. 2002;190:310–314.

McCloskey MS, Noblett KL, Deffenbacher JL, et al. Cognitive-behavioral therapy for intermittent explosive disorder: A pilot randomized clinical trial. *J Consult Clin Psychol*. 2008 October;76(5):876–886.

McConaghy N, Armstrong MS, Blaszczynski A, et al. Controlled comparison of aversive therapy and imaginal desensitization in compulsive gambling. *Br J Psychiatry*. 1983;142:366–372.

McConaghy N, Blaszczynski A, Frankova A. Comparison of imaginal desensitization with other behavioral treatments of pathological gambling: A two- to nine-year follow-up. *Br J Psychiatry*. 1991;159: 390–393.

McElroy SL, Pope HG, Hudson JI, et al. Kleptomania: A report of 20 cases. *Am J Psychiatry*. 1991;148: 652–657.

McElroy SL, Hudson JI, Pope HG, et al. The DSM-III-R impulse control disorders not elsewhere classified: Clinical characteristics and relationship to other psychiatric disorders. *Am J Psychiatry*. 1992;149:318–327.

McElroy SL, Pope HG Jr, Keck PE, et al. Are impulse-control disorders related to bipolar disorder? *Compr Psychiatry*. 1996;37:229–240.

Meyer G, Hauffa BP, Schedlowski M, et al. Casino gambling increases heart rate and salivary cortisol in regular gamblers. *Biol Psychiatry*. 2000;48(9):948–953.

Ninan PT, Rothbaum BO, Marsteller FA, et al. A placebo-controlled trial of cognitive-behavioral therapy and clomipramine in trichotillomania. *J Clin Psychiatry*. 2000;61:47–50.

O'Sullivan RL, Christenson GA, Stein DJ. Pharmacotherapy of trichotillomania. In: Stein DJ, Christenson GA, Hollander E, eds. *Trichotillomania*. Washington, DC: American Psychiatric Publishing; 1999:93–123.

Petry NM, Kiluk BD. Suicidal ideation and suicide attempts in treatment-seeking pathological gamblers. *J Nerv Ment Dis*. 2002;190:462–469.

Petry NM, Stinson FS, Grant BF. Comorbidity of DSM-IV pathological gambling and other psychiatric disorders: Results from the National Epidemiologic Survey on Alcohol and Related Conditions. *J Clin Psychiatry*. 2005;66:564–574.

Petry NM, Ammerman Y, Bohl J, et al. Cognitive-behavioral therapy for pathological gamblers. *J Consult Clin Psychol*. 2006;74(3):555–567.

Potenza MN, Hollander E. Pathological gambling and impulse control disorders. In: Coyle JT, Nemeroff C, Charney D, et al., eds. *Neuropsychopharmacology: The 5th generation of progress*. Baltimore: Lippincott Williams & Wilkins; 2002:1725–1741.

Potenza MN, Steinberg MA, McLaughlin SD, et al. Illegal behaviors in problem gambling: Analysis of data from a gambling helpline. *J Am Acad Psychiatry Law*. 2000;28:389–403.

Potenza MN, Steinberg MA, McLaughlin SD, et al. Gender-related differences in the characteristics of problem gamblers using a gambling helpline. *Am J Psychiatry*. 2001;158:1500–1505.

Potenza MN, Fiellin DA, Heninger GA, et al. Gambling: An addictive behavior with health and primary care implications. *J Gen Intern Med*. 2002;17:721–732.

Potenza MN, Leung HC, Blumberg HP, et al. An fMRI Stroop study of ventromedial prefrontal cortical function in pathological gamblers. *Am J Psychiatry*. 2003;160(11):1990–1994.

Reuter J, Raedler T, Rose M, et al. Pathological gambling is linked to reduced activation of the mesolimbic reward system. *Nat Neurosci*. 2005;8(2):147–148.

Roy A, Adinoff B, Roehrich L, et al. Pathological gambling. A psychobiological study. *Arch Gen Psychiatry*. 1988;45(4):369–373.

Schmitt LH, Harrison GA, Spargo RM. Variation in epinephrine and cortisol excretion rates associated with behavior in an Australian Aboriginal community. *Am J Phys Anthropol*. 1998;106(2):249–253.

Shaffer HJ, Hall MN, vander Bilt J. Estimating the prevalence of disordered gambling behavior in the United States and Canada: A research synthesis. *Am J Public Health*. 1999;89:1369–1376.

Shinohara K, Yanagisawa A, Kagota Y, et al. Physiological changes in Pachinko players; beta-endorphin, catecholamines, immune system substances and heart rate. *Appl Human Sci*. 1999;18(2):37–42.

Slutske WS, Eisen S, True WR, et al. Common genetic vulnerability for pathological gambling and alcohol dependence in men. *Arch Gen Psychiatry*. 2000;57:666–673.

Slutske WS, Eisen S, Xian H, et al. A twin study of the association between pathological gambling and antisocial personality disorder. *J Abnorm Psychol*. 2001;110(2):297–308.

Van Ameringen M, Mancini C, Patterson B, et al. A randomized placebo controlled trial of olanzapine in trichotillomania. *Eur Neuropsychopharmacol*. 2006;16(Suppl 4):S452, Papers of the 19th ECNP Congress; Paris, France: September 16-20,

van Minnen A, Hoogduin KA, Keijsers GP, et al. The treatment of trichotillomania with behavioral therapy or fluoxetine: A randomized, waiting-list controlled study. *Arch Gen Psychiatry*. 2003;60(5):517–522.

Woods DW, Wetterneck CT, Flessner CA. A controlled evaluation of acceptance and commitment therapy plus habit reversal for trichotillomania. *Behav Res Ther*. 2005;44(5):639–656.

Woods DW, Flessner CA, Franklin ME, et al. The trichotillomania impact project (TIP): Exploring phenomenology, functional impairment, and treatment utilization. *J Clin Psychiatry*. 2006;67(12): 1877–1888.

Zack M, Poulos CX. Amphetamine primes motivation to gamble and gambling-related semantic networks in problem gamblers. *Neuropsychopharmacology*. 2004;29:195–207.

Adjustment Disorders

Adjustment disorders are short-lived maladaptive responses to stress. They occur in response to an identifiable stressor (or stressors) and cause emotional and behavioral symptoms out of proportion to what would be expected or impair a person's ability to function. Common stressors leading to an adjustment disorder in adults may include marital problems, separation, divorce, and financial problems. Stressors potentially leading to an adjustment disorder in adolescents include school problems, parental rejection, alcohol or drug problems, parental separation or divorce, and problems with girlfriends or boyfriends (Andreasen and Wasek, 1980). People with adjustment disorders may suffer a range of symptoms that cause distress or impairment—such as crying spells, insomnia, binge eating and drinking, or inability to focus on important tasks. The adjustment disorder diagnosis is a subthreshold diagnosis in that it is considered less serious in intensity and scope than most axis I and II disorders (e.g., major depressive disorder or posttraumatic stress disorder) but more significant than a problem-level diagnosis (V code diagnoses such as relational problems).

As characterized in the text revision of the Fourth Edition of the *Diagnostic and Statistical Manual of Mental Disorders* (DSM-IV-TR) (American Psychiatric Association, 2000), an adjustment disorder occurs when a stressful event either causes marked distress in excess of what would be expected or significant impairment in the social, occupational, or academic functioning of an individual. For such a diagnosis, symptoms need to begin within 3 months after the onset of a stressor or stressors. After a stressor or its consequences remit, adjustment disorder symptoms must resolve within 6 months. Symptoms can persist beyond 6 months if they occur in response to a chronic stressor (e.g., taking care of a chronically ill child) or in response to a stressor that has enduring consequences (e.g., a traumatic hand injury that leads to long-term maladaptive coping) (American Psychiatric Association, 2000).

A nonpathological response to stress could cause emotional or behavioral symptoms but is not characterized by marked distress in excess of what would be expected or significant impairment in functioning. For example, it is to be expected that a person who has recently suffered the death of a loved one may feel deep sadness, anger, anxiety, and/or detachment, especially in the first weeks and months after the death. A person who develops an adjustment disorder, on the other hand, may feel completely overwhelmed by distressing emotional symptoms—suffering repeated panic attacks, rages, or crying episodes—that make it difficult or impossible to function normally. DSM-IV-TR also stipulates that an adjustment disorder diagnosis should not be made if the disorder qualifies for another axis I disorder (e.g., major depression) or is an exacerbation of a pre-existing axis I or II disorder. An adjustment disorder may be diagnosed in the presence of another axis I or axis II disorder only if the latter does not account for the pattern of symptoms that have occurred as a result of the stressor.

EPIDEMIOLOGY

DSM-IV-TR states that adjustment disorders are common, although prevalence rates vary widely depending on the population studied and the assessment methods used. Women receive this diagnosis twice as often as men, but in children and adolescents, boys and girls receive the diagnosis equally (Andreasen and Wasek, 1980). Adjustment disorders can occur at any age but are diagnosed most frequently in adolescents. An admitting diagnosis of adjustment disorder was given to 7% of adults and 34% of adolescents in one psychiatric emergency service (Greenberg et al., 1995). In another study, approximately 5% of patients admitted for psychiatric reasons over a 4-year period received the diagnosis (Andreasen and Wasek, 1980). In mental health outpatient settings, adjustment disorder was diagnosed in 10% to 30% of the cases studied and in as many as 50% in population sectors experiencing a specific stressor (e.g., following cardiac surgery) (American Psychiatric Association, 2000). In a general medical hospital, the diagnosis was made in 12% of patients and considered a rule-out diagnosis in another 11% (Strain et al., 1998).

ETIOLOGY

Assessment of the stressor (or stressors), the individual, and the interaction between them is important in understanding how an adjustment disorder develops. The stressor may be a single event (e.g., the termination of a romantic relationship) or multiple events (e.g., a business failure occurring while caring for an ill parent). Stressors may be recurrent (e.g., coping with a family member with seasonal affective disorder) or continuous (e.g., living in a war zone). Stressors may also accompany specific developmental stages such as going to school, leaving the parental home, getting married, becoming a parent, failing to attain occupational goals, and retirement (American Psychiatric Association, 2000). Stressors are more likely to be chronic in adolescents than in adults (Andreasen and Wasek, 1980). Individuals from disadvantaged life circumstances experience a high rate of stressors and may be at an increased risk for an adjustment disorder (American Psychiatric Association, 2000).

Because DSM-IV-TR does not provide criteria for what constitutes a stressor, careful attention to the patient's subjective experience is critical for diagnosis and treatment. What may not appear stress inducing to an outside observer may be an overwhelming source of stress for a patient. For example, a 25-year-old graduate student with depressed mood reports numerous psychosocial stressors to a mental health provider, including the deteriorating health of his mother, academic difficulties, being unexpectedly left by his girlfriend for another man, and the recent loss of a stuffed animal he has had since childhood. When asked which of these has been the hardest for him, he states that the loss of his teddy bear is "by far" the most difficult life event he has had to deal with, a response that surprised the clinician. It is important, therefore, to learn from patients what specific stressors they are experiencing and how precisely they are coping with each one.

Insights into the biological, psychological, and sociocultural aspects of an individual and how these factors interact with stress are crucial to understanding the development of an adjustment disorder. Regarding genetics, a British study of twins indicated a significant contribution of heritability to the experience of psychosocial distress (Rijsdijk et al., 2003). A person's temperament has also been found to be a major contributor to the variability of response displayed in reaction to similar stressors. Three temperament clusters have been reported: easy, difficult, and slow to warm up. Children with easy temperaments tend to calm and soothe themselves, whereas children with difficult temperaments appear to be much more sensitive to stimuli (Woolston, 1988).

A person's psychological makeup and unique set of defense mechanisms (e.g., denial, minimization, rationalization, and humor) are also important in determining the response to stress (Vaillant, 1971). A person who uses mature defense mechanisms such as anticipation (planning and preparing for a stressful event) is more likely to successfully cope with a stressor than a person who uses less mature defense mechanisms such as acting out (e.g., eating excessive amounts of junk food and then vomiting). For example, a person who becomes distressed after failing a midterm examination in a class and reacts by assessing why he or she did poorly, speaking with the professor, and increasing study time is more likely to master this stressor and perform better in the class than a person who responds by binge drinking on the following weekends.

In a study of adjustment disorders in a general medical hospital setting, patients with an adjustment disorder, when compared with other axis I and II diagnoses, were more likely to be married and employed full time (Strain et al., 1998). Such social factors can help protect a person from the development of a more serious mental condition (e.g., major depression). Likewise, individuals lacking a strong social support system tend to be more vulnerable to the effects of stress and therefore, more likely to develop an adjustment disorder (or other mental disorders).

Finally, an individual's cultural context is another important variable to consider when making the clinical judgment of whether the response to a stressor is maladaptive and the associated distress in excess of what would be expected (American Psychiatric Association, 2000). For example, there is great variance in how different cultures react and respond to death. A lack of appreciation for a person's cultural context in this regard could lead a clinician to either over- or underestimate the degree to which a person is adaptively coping with a loss.

CHARACTERISTICS OF ADJUSTMENT DISORDER

Signs and Symptoms

By definition, adjustment disorders develop within 3 months of the onset of an identifiable stressor and remit within 6 months after the stressor or its consequences have terminated. The disorder can occur at any age and is associated with suicide attempts, suicide, excessive substance use, and somatic complaints and may complicate the course of illness in individuals who have a general medical condition (American Psychiatric Association, 2000).

DSM-IV-TR identifies six adjustment disorder subtypes, which are diagnosed based on the predominant presenting symptoms:

1. *Adjustment disorder with depressed mood* is diagnosed when the predominant symptoms are depressed mood, tearfulness, or feelings of hopelessness.
2. *Adjustment disorder with anxiety* is diagnosed when the predominant manifestations are nervousness, worry, or jitteriness.
3. *Adjustment disorder with mixed anxiety and depressed mood* is the appropriate diagnosis when the symptoms are predominantly a combination of anxiety and depression.
4. *Adjustment disorder with disturbance of conduct* should be diagnosed when the manifestation results primarily in a violation of the rights of others or of major age-appropriate societal norms and rules (e.g., truancy, vandalism, reckless driving, fighting, and defaulting on legal responsibilities).

Clinical Characteristics of Adjustment Disorders

Behavioral or emotional symptoms
- In response to an identifiable stressor
- Within 3 months of onset of the stressor
- Not for more than an additional 6 months once stressor or consequences terminated
- *Acute* if <6 months
- *Chronic* if 6 months or longer
- Classified by subtype, selected by predominant symptoms
  - Depressed mood
  - Anxiety
  - Mixed anxiety and depressed mood
  - Disturbance of conduct
  - Mixed disturbance of emotions and conduct
  - Unspecified
- Clinically important if
  - In excess of what would be expected from exposure to the stressor
  - Significant impairment in psychosocial functioning
  - Not better accounted for by another axis I disorder or bereavement

5. *Adjustment disorder with mixed disturbance of emotions and conduct* is the diagnosis when the predominant manifestations are both emotional symptoms and conduct disturbance.

6. *Adjustment disorder unspecified* can be used when the maladaptive reaction is not classifiable as one of the aforementioned subtypes.

In general, there is an expectation of good outcome with adjustment disorder with symptom resolution occurring once the stressor remits (Andreasen and Hoenk, 1982). Persistence of an adjustment disorder or its progression to a more severe mental disorder may be more likely in children and adolescents than in adults. However, some or all of this increased risk may be attributable to the presence of comorbid conditions (e.g., oppositional defiant disorder or an incipient personality disorder) or to the possibility that the adjustment disorder actually represented a subclinical manifestation of a more severe mental disorder (American Psychiatric Association, 2000). Adjustment disorders are frequently comorbid with other axis I and II disorders. According to one study, 70% of child and adult inpatients with a diagnosis of adjustment disorder had another axis I or II disorder (Strain et al., 1998). Depressed mood is the most frequently occurring symptom of an adjustment disorder, being present in 76% of cases (Fabrega et al., 1987). Behavioral symptoms such as vandalism, thefts, school suspension or expulsion, temper outbursts, lying, and physical fights occurred in 77% of adolescents but in only 25% of adults in one study (Andreasen and Wasek, 1980).

Suicide attempts and completed suicides are relatively common in patients with adjustment disorders. Twenty-nine percent of patients with an adjustment disorder have suicidal thoughts (Fabrega et al., 1987). A retrospective study found that patients with adjustment disorders were significantly more suicidal at admission than patients without an adjustment disorder diagnosis (Kryzhanovskaya and Canterbury, 2001). Psychological autopsy studies have shown a prevalence of adjustment disorder among suicide victims ranging between 5% and 36% (Cavanagh et al., 1999; Henriksson et al., 1993; Marttunen et al., 1991, Rich et al., 1990; Schaffer et al., 1996). Significantly, psychological autopsies of adolescents diagnosed with adjustment disorder who committed suicide revealed a rapidly evolving suicidal process without any prior indication of emotional or behavioral problems (Portzky et al., 2005). In an outpatient study of adolescents referred for psychiatric treatment, those who were diagnosed with an adjustment disorder and suicidal thoughts were characterized by severe psychosocial impairment, dysphoric moods, psychomotor restlessness, and a previous history of psychiatric difficulties (Pelkonen et al., 2005).

A CASE OF ADJUSTMENT DISORDER IN A YOUNG GIRL

Sarah, a 14-year-old girl, becomes emotionally distraught after her boyfriend of 2 months abruptly ends their relationship to date another girl. She leaves school early and withdraws to her room at home, experiences depressed mood, and ruminates about the end of the relationship throughout the evening and night. The next day Sarah feels as if she wants to fall asleep and never wake up but manages to go to school. A minor argument with a female peer escalates into a physical altercation in which punches are exchanged. Sarah has had no prior history of fighting or aggressive behavior or of depression or anxiety. The school sends her home and suspends her for 2 days. Her parents become frustrated because she wishes to be left alone and refuses to talk to them. Three days after the breakup, she experiences thoughts of wanting to kill herself with her father's amitriptyline prescription. She writes a suicide note, calls her mom, and says that she is planning to kill herself by overdosing. Her mom immediately calls the police, who take Sarah to an emergency room. She is then transferred to a psychiatric crisis center for further evaluation, hospitalized for one night, and discharged the next day. Over the following week, Sarah meets with a psychologist twice and experiences a significant improvement in mood and an absence of suicidal thoughts. She realizes that the breakup is not the end of the world. She meets with the psychologist several more times over the next month.

A CASE OF ADJUSTMENT DISORDER IN AN ADULT MALE

Bruce, a 27-year-old male graduate student with no prior psychiatric history, presents to a psychiatric crisis service requesting medication to help him sleep. He reports poor sleep for 3 days in addition to crying spells and fleeting thoughts of wishing he were dead. He has never experienced suicidal thoughts before and tells the psychiatrist that they are freaking him out. He has not taken action toward ending his life and does not have a plan for suicide. He is a teaching assistant but has been too depressed to work for the last 2 days. Three days before presentation, his girlfriend of 2 years unexpectedly ended their relationship without an explanation. A sleep aid is prescribed, and Bruce agrees to short-term psychotherapy as an outpatient. One week later he reports some sadness about the loss of his girlfriend but states that he is coping better. His sleep has improved, and he denies suicidal ideation or thoughts of death. Although he still feels somewhat sluggish, he has returned to work.

Differential Diagnosis

According to DSM-IV-TR, the adjustment disorder diagnosis is a residual category used to describe presentations that are a response to an identifiable stressor and do not meet criteria for another specific axis I disorder. For example, if an individual has symptoms that meet criteria for a major depressive episode in response to a stressor, the diagnosis of adjustment disorder is not applicable. Psychiatric disorders that need to be differentiated from adjustment disorder include major depressive disorder, dysthymia, oppositional defiant disorder, conduct disorder, substance use disorders, anxiety disorders, and personality disorders.

A study comparing major depression and adjustment disorder with depressed mood in a general medical hospital setting found that adjustment disorder with depressed mood is characterized by better recent functioning, greater severity of stressors, and decreased severity of psychiatric impairment than major depression (Snyder et al., 1990).

Adjustment disorder can be diagnosed in addition to another axis I disorder only if the latter does not account for the particular symptoms that occur in reaction to the stressor. Because personality disorders are frequently exacerbated by stress, the additional diagnosis of adjustment disorder is usually not made. However, if symptoms uncharacteristic of the personality disorder appear in response to a stressor, the additional diagnosis of adjustment disorder may be appropriate (American Psychiatric Association, 2000). For example, an adolescent patient with avoidant personality disorder becomes irritable and aggressive after the death of his father. Although usually very shy and timid, he has been getting into fights at school and committing minor acts of vandalism since the loss of his father, symptoms uncharacteristic of avoidant personality disorder.

Adjustment disorder, posttraumatic stress disorder, and acute stress disorder all require the presence of a stressor. Posttraumatic stress disorder and acute stress disorder are characterized by the presence of an extreme stressor and specific clusters of symptoms (e.g., re-experiencing trauma, hyperarousal, and avoidance; see Chapter 12). Bereavement is generally diagnosed instead of adjustment disorder when the reaction is an expected response to the death of a loved one (see Chapter 28). Adjustment disorders should also be distinguished from other nonpathological reactions to stress that do not lead to marked distress in excess of what is expected and do not cause significant impairment in social or occupational functioning (American Psychiatric Association, 2000).

TREATMENT

Psychotherapy is the mainstay of treatment for adjustment disorders. Providing patients with a rationale for the problems they experience is a powerful form of intervention. A rationale should offer a plausible explanation of the situation a patient has encountered and provide a favorable perspective of the problem (van der Klink and van Dijk, 2003). Individual dynamic psychotherapy can help patients understand the meaning a stressor holds for them as well as what conflicts it creates in them, which can lead to more adaptive coping. In addition to interpersonal support and reassurance, supportive psychotherapy can give patients practical guidance in ways to reduce stressors. Cognitive behavior therapy can reframe stressors, challenge cognitive distortions associated with distress, and motivate adaptive coping behaviors. Interpersonal psychotherapy may be a treatment option for adjustment disorders that arise from stressful interpersonal relationships. Family therapy may be helpful in decreasing family conflict that has contributed either to the development or maintenance of an adjustment disorder and can also galvanize a patient's social support network. Group therapy and support groups may be helpful to patients sharing similar experiences. Crisis intervention, a brief intervention intended to restore individuals to their previous level of functioning and prevent long-term consequences, is a treatment option as well (see also Chapter 23).

No comprehensive guidelines exist for using psychotropic medication to treat adjustment disorders. Depending upon the predominant symptoms a patient is experiencing, brief trials of an antidepressant or antianxiety medication may be used. In a retrospective review of primary care patients, patients with adjustment disorder with depressed mood had a better response to antidepressant medication than patients with major depression (Hameed et al., 2005). Sleep aids can be useful for patients with insomnia. Providing information about prescribed medication can help reduce patient anxiety and improve medication adherence. Patients with more symptoms or greater symptom intensity may benefit from both psychotherapy and pharmacotherapy (see also Chapter 22).

Given the risk of suicidality that can accompany adjustment disorders, a comprehensive evaluation of a patient's risk for suicide is imperative. Inpatient psychiatric hospitalization is warranted if suicide risk is sufficiently high or if no suitable outpatient treatment plan can be developed.

PROGNOSTIC FACTORS

Compared with patients who have a more specific psychiatric disorder (e.g., major depressive disorder), patients with an adjustment disorder require less treatment, are able to return to work sooner, and are less likely to manifest a recurrence of the disorder (Bronisch, 1991; Greenberg et al., 1995; Jones et al., 1999; Looney and Gunderson, 1978).

Patients with a poor outcome tend to have more behavioral symptoms, precipitants, and chronicity. Adolescents have a somewhat poorer outcome compared with adults (Andreasen and Hoenk, 1982). A study comparing readmission rates among patients diagnosed with adjustment disorders, depressive disorders, and anxiety disorders found that those with adjustment disorders were significantly less likely to be readmitted within the first year after an initial psychiatric hospitalization (Jones et al., 2002). In a psychiatric outpatient population, 5 years after an initial diagnosis of an adjustment disorder, 71% of adults, compared with 44% of adolescents, were found to be completely well (Andreasen and Hoenk, 1982). However, another study in children aged 8 to 13 years, which controlled for comorbid conditions, found no compelling evidence for a negative long-term prognosis attributable to a diagnosis of adjustment disorder during a 7- to 8-year follow-up period (Kovacs et al., 1994).

CONCLUSION AND FUTURE DIRECTIONS

Adjustment disorder remains an under-researched diagnostic category compared with other mental disorders. It has not been included in most major epidemiologic studies of mental illness. Despite reportedly being a common psychiatric diagnosis, its prevalence of only 1% in a recent study of depressive syndromes led the researchers to speculate that adjustment disorders may be getting categorized as depressive disorders (Casey et al., 2006). Because the adjustment disorder diagnosis lacks clear operational criteria, the boundaries among adjustment disorders, specific mental disorders (such as major depressive disorder), and normal homeostatic responses to stress are not clear. The reliability of the diagnosis is consequently thought by some to be poor. More specific diagnostic criteria would improve its reliability and validity. More research is also necessary to establish which interventions are most successful in treating adjustment disorders.

Clinical Pearls

- An adjustment disorder diagnosis is not made if the symptom pattern is more consistent with another mental disorder (e.g., major depressive disorder or generalized anxiety disorder).
- Do not assume to know how a patient is experiencing a stressor. Ask patients to describe what impact the stressor is having on them.
- Children and adolescents are more likely to have behavioral manifestations of an adjustment disorder than adults.
- Children and adolescents diagnosed with an adjustment disorder may be at risk for later development of a major psychiatric disorder (e.g., major depressive disorder, schizophrenia, substance use disorder).
- Suicidal ideation, suicide attempts, and suicide can occur in adjustment disorders.
- Adolescents with an adjustment disorder can have a rapidly evolving suicidal process without any apparent indication of emotional or behavioral problems.

Self-Assessment Questions and Answers

19-1. According to DSM-IV-TR, to diagnose an adjustment disorder, emotional or behavioral symptoms need to begin within how many months after the onset of a stressor?

A. 1
B. 3
C. 4
D. 6
E. 12

For an adjustment disorder diagnosis, symptoms need to begin within 3 months after the onset of a stressor or stressors. *Answer: B*

19-2. After an acute stressor or its consequences remit, adjustment disorder symptoms must resolve within how many months?

A. 1
B. 3
C. 4
D. 6
E. 12

Symptoms of an adjustment disorder must resolve within 6 months after a stressor or its consequences remit but can persist beyond 6 months if they occur in response to a chronic stressor or one that has enduring consequences. *Answer: D*

19-3. Which of the following is true regarding the epidemiology of adjustment disorders?

A. Adjustment disorders do not occur in the geriatric population.
B. Adolescent boys receive the diagnosis less commonly than girls.
C. Adolescent girls receive the diagnosis twice as commonly as boys.
D. Men receive the diagnosis three times as commonly as women.

E. Women receive the diagnosis twice as often as men.

Women receive the diagnosis of adjustment disorder twice as often as men, but in children and adolescents, boys and girls receive the diagnosis equally (Andreasen and Wasek, 1980). Adjustment disorders can occur at any age but are most frequently diagnosed in adolescents. *Answer: E*

19-4. Which of the following is true regarding adjustment disorders in adolescents?

A. Adjustment disorders in adolescents can be characterized by a rapidly evolving suicidal process without any prior indication of emotional or behavioral problems.
B. Adjustment disorders are less common in adolescents than in adults.
C. Behavioral symptoms of an adjustment disorder are more common in adults than adolescents.
D. Adjustment disorders in adolescents rarely are comorbid with other axis I and II disorders.
E. Adjustment disorders are more common in adolescent girls than boys.

Adjustment disorders can occur at any age but are most frequently diagnosed in adolescents. In children and adolescents, boys and girls receive the diagnosis equally (Andreasen and Wasek, 1980). Behavioral symptoms such as vandalism, thefts, school suspension or expulsion, temper outbursts, lying, and physical fights occurred in 77% of adolescents but in only 25% of adults in one study (Andreasen and Wasek, 1980). Adjustment disorders are frequently comorbid with other axis I and II disorders. According to one study, 70% of child and adult inpatients with a diagnosis of adjustment disorder had

another axis I or II disorder (Strain et al., 1998).
Answer: A

19-5. A 17-year-old adolescent male experiences depressed mood upon finding out that his parents are filing for divorce. He is unable to sleep and feels "on edge" while at school the next day. In a math class he became irritable with the teacher over a minor matter and left the class while shouting obscenities at the teacher. On his way out of school, he impulsively picked up a large rock and broke one of the classroom windows with it. He has no prior history of such behavior or depression. One week later, he is still unhappy with the divorce, but calmer and more in control of his behavior. This is an example of which adjustment disorder subtype?

A. Adjustment disorder with depressed mood
B. Adjustment disorder with anxiety
C. Adjustment disorder with mixed anxiety and depressed mood
D. Adjustment disorder with disturbance of conduct
E. Adjustment disorder with mixed disturbance of emotions and conduct

Adjustment disorder with mixed disturbance of emotions and conduct is the diagnosis when the predominant manifestations are both emotional symptoms and conduct disturbance. *Answer: E*

References

American Psychiatric Association. *Diagnostic and statistical manual of mental disorders*, 4th ed., text revision. Washington, DC: American Psychiatric Association; 2000.

Andreasen NC, Hoenk PR. The predictive value of adjustment disorders: A follow-up study. *Am J Psychiatry*. 1982;139(5):584–590.

Andreasen NC, Wasek P. Adjustment disorders in adolescents and adults. *Arch Gen Psychiatry*. 1980;37: 1166–1170.

Bronisch T. Adjustment reactions: A long-term prospective and retrospective follow-up of former patients in a crisis intervention ward. *Acta Psychiatr Scand*. 1991;84:86–93.

Casey P, Maracy M, Kelly BD, et al. Can adjustment disorder and depressive episode be distinguished? Results from ODIN. *J Affect Disord*. 2006;92:291–297.

Cavanagh JT, Owens DG, Johnstone EC. Suicide and undetermined death in south east Scotland. A case-control study using the psychological autopsy method. *Psychol Med*. 1999;29:1141–1149.

Fabrega H Jr, Mezzich JE, Mezzich AC. Adjustment disorder as a marginal or transitional illness category in DSM-III. *Arch Gen Psychiatry*. 1987;44:567–572.

Greenberg WM, Rosenfeld DN, Ortega EA. Adjustment disorder as an admission diagnosis. *Am J Psychiatry*. 1995;152:459–461.

Hameed U, Schwartz TL, Malhotra K, et al. Antidepressant treatment in the primary care office: Outcomes for adjustment disorder versus major depression. *Ann Clin Psychiatry*. 2005;17(2):77–81.

Henriksson MM, Aro HM, Marttunen MJ, et al. Mental disorders and comorbidity in suicide. *Am J Psychiatry*. 1993;150:935–940.

Jones R, Yates WR, Williams S, et al. Outcome for adjustment disorder with depressed mood: Comparison with other mood disorders. *J Affect Disord*. 1999;55:55–61.

Jones R, Yates WR, Zhou MH. Readmission rates for adjustment disorders: Comparison with other mood disorders. *J Affect Disord*. 2002;71:199–203.

Kovacs M, Gatsonis C, Pollock M, et al. A controlled prospective study of DSM-III adjustment disorder in childhood: Short-term prognosis and long-term predictive validity. *Arch Gen Psychiatry*. 1994;51: 535–541.

Kryzhanovskaya L, Canterbury R. Suicidal behavior in patients with adjustment disorders. *Crisis*. 2001; 22(3):125–131.

Looney JG, Gunderson EK. Transient situational disturbances: Course and outcome. *Am J Psychiatry*. 1978; 135:660–663.

Marttunen MJ, Aro HM, Henriksson MM, et al. Mental disorders in adolescent suicide. DSM-III-R axes I and II diagnoses in suicides among 13- to 19-year-olds in Finland. *Arch Gen Psychiatry*. 1991;48: 834–839.

Pelkonen M, Marttunen M, Henriksson M, et al. Suicidality in adjustment disorder: Clinical characteristics of adolescent outpatients. *Eur Child Adolesc Psychiatry*. 2005;14:174–180.

Portzky G, Audenaert K, van Heeringen K. Adjustment disorder and the course of the suicidal process in adolescents. *J Affect Disord*. 2005;87:265–270.

Rich CL, Sherman M, Fowler RC. San Diego Suicide Study: The adolescents. *Adolescence*. 1990;25: 855–865.

Rijsdijk FV, Snieder H, Ormel J, et al. Genetic and environmental influences on psychological distress in the population: General health questionnaire analyses in UK twins. *Psychol Med*. 2003;33:793–801.

Schaffer D, Gould MS, Fisher P, et al. Psychiatric diagnosis in child and adolescent suicide. *Arch Gen Psychiatry*. 1996;53:339–348.

Snyder S, Strain JJ, Wolf D. Differentiating major depression from adjustment disorder with depressed mood in the medical setting. *Gen Hosp Psychiatry*. 1990;12:159–165.

Strain JJ, Smith GC, Hammer JS, et al. Adjustment disorder: A multisite study of its utilization and interventions in the consultation-liaison psychiatric setting. *Gen Hosp Psychiatry*. 1998;20:139–149.

Vaillant GE. Theoretical hierarchy of adaptive ego mechanisms: A 30-year follow-up of 30 men selected for psychological health. *Arch Gen Psychiatry*. 1971;24:107–118.

van der Klink JJ, van Dijk FJ. Dutch practice guidelines for managing adjustment disorders in occupational and primary health care. *Scand J Work Environ Health*. 2003;29(6):478–487.

Woolston JL. Theoretical considerations of the adjustment disorders. *J Am Acad Child Adolesc Psychiatry*. 1988;27(3):280–287.

CHAPTER 20

Nutan Atre Vaidya

Personality Disorders

Personality consists of long-standing, relatively stable behaviors termed *traits*. Traits are habitual patterns of behavior that result in individual differences in personality. Personality traits are expressions of brain systems and interact with the environment. An individual's personality traits are highly heritable (approximately 50% to 60%) and inherited independently of one another (Bouchard, 1994; Widiger and Frances, 1994). Therefore, personality is the combination of long-standing, stable, habitual patterns of behavior that characterize an individual, interact with environmental factors, and are highly heritable. Human personality traits are normally distributed; that is, they can be represented by a bell-shaped curve, which means personality traits in the majority of the population are distributed within 1.5 standard deviations (SD) from the mean.

Individuals whose combinations of personality traits are at the extremes of the distribution (i.e., >1.5 SD from the mean) are statistically deviant or abnormal. Although this does not imply that they are deviant or abnormal because of neuropathology, it does mean that because they are behaviorally deviant, they are more likely to have problems interacting with others. Individuals with difficulties due to a deviant personality are said to have a personality disorder.

THE *DIAGNOSTIC AND STATISTICAL MANUAL OF MENTAL DISORDERS'* PERSONALITY DISORDER SYSTEM

The standard definition of a personality disorder, from the *Diagnostic and Statistical Manual of Mental Disorders,* Fourth Edition, Text Revision (DSM-IV-TR) (American Psychiatric Association, 2000), is "inflexible, maladaptive long-standing behaviors that begin early in life and lead to interpersonal distress affecting several areas of one's life."

General Information About Personality Disorders

Although DSM-IV-TR describes 11 personality disorders with unique sets of problems, all personality disorders share general features. The following generalizations facilitate understanding and management of patients with personality disorders.

Personality disorders are hard to treat. Personality patterns are "set" before age 35 and therefore are less amenable to change after age 35. Psychotherapies (e.g., cognitive, interpersonal) report successes, but studies demonstrate that the effect is small and primarily predicted by the patient's perception of his or her relationship with the therapist. The better the perception

---

Clinical Characteristics of Personality Disorder

- Personality traits are inflexible and maladaptive and cause clinically significant functional impairment or distress.
- Inner experiences and behaviors deviate markedly from cultural expectations.
- Inflexible and pervasive maladaptive behaviors are stable and long lasting, begin in childhood or adolescence, and do not result from another mental disorder.

of the relationship, the more likely the patient's behavior patterns will change (Verheul and Herbrink, 2007).

Personality disorders run in families. In families with antisocial personality (ASP) disorder, the occurrence of antisocial, histrionic, or narcissistic personality disorder is 10 times as frequent as that for families in the general population. The risk is increased for personality disorder in the first-degree relatives of patients with personality disorders, but the familial aggregation is nonspecific (Coid, 1999). Therefore, although more relatives than expected in the general population will have a personality disorder in the same cluster, the specific personality disorder will vary. Personality disorders are often comorbid with nonpsychotic disorders. Of patients who have one personality disorder diagnosis, 40% to 60% also meet criteria for a second or third. This is not the same as having "multiple personalities." Having a second or third personality disorder means meeting criteria for more than one disorder, while having only one personality. Of individuals with anxiety disorders, nonmelancholic depressions, eating disorders, and adjustment disorders, 40% to 60% have a preexisting personality disorder (Oldham et al., 1995).

Personality disorders are medical diagnoses, and approximately 10% of persons in general populations have them (Oldham, 1994). Physicians can influence a particular patient's condition and treatments by educating family members about how to help the patient. Knowing about the patient's personality can guide that influence. Personality dimensions predict the likelihood that a person will smoke, abuse alcohol, or use street drugs and engage in high-risk or criminal behaviors, as well as the treatments that might work best for treating nonmelancholic depressions and anxiety disorders and encouraging smoking cessation and abstinence from alcohol or street drugs (Cloninger et al., 1994).

Specific Information About Personality Disorders

DSM-IV-TR divides personality disorders into three clusters: A, B, and C (Grant et al., 2004; Tyrer et al., 1991).

Cluster A

Cluster A includes odd-eccentric personalities (see Table 20-1). Patients in this category are awkward in thinking and have reduced interest in forming relationships. Patients with *paranoid personalities* are often individuals who show a lifelong pattern of suspiciousness. They do not easily trust other people and often hold grudges for a long time. These individuals will often write long letters to multiple organizations complaining about the unfair treatment they perceive that they have received. Patients with *schizoid personality disorder* are often loners who like to be alone. These patients are restricted in their affect as well as their relationships. They have few interests in life and usually are employed in positions where people contact is minimal. Patients with schizoid personality disorders are often low in all the Cloninger's temperament dimensions (described in subsequent text). Patients with *schizotypal personality disorder* (SPD) are similar to patients with schizoid personality disorder. In addition, they exhibit vague speech patterns and interest in unusual topics such as supernatural phenomena and extraterrestrials. They also experience various illusions. Among the first-degree relatives of

TABLE 20-1	Cluster A Personality Disorders
Disorder	**Description**
Paranoid (<1% of the general population)	Mistrustful, suspicious, unforgiving, grudge-bearing, tending to perceive threats
Schizoid (<1%)	Detached and restricted in range of emotional expression; has a paucity of interests, activities, and friends
Schizotypal (3%)	Schizoid traits plus vague in speech, problems with perception (illusions), and having odd beliefs and experiences (e.g., extrasensory perception [ESP], sensing spirits, other paranormal phenomena)

A CASE OF PARANOID PERSONALITY DISORDER

A 50-year-old married Vietnam veteran has always been careful about revealing anything about himself to others out of concern that they might deceive him. He refuses sincere efforts of help from acquaintances because he suspects their motives. He believes that the government is against him and trying to deny him service-connected disability. He suspects but is not sure if the government can get into his computer. He never reveals his identity to a caller without first questioning the caller about the nature of his or her business. He stores all his correspondence in a secret safe so that he could use it as evidence in case his disability payments are cut. He has never had delusions or hallucinations.

schizophrenics and persons with mood disorders, the risk for SPD is very high (Kendler and Walsh, 1995).

In addition to aggregating in the families of patients with schizophrenia and mood disorder, patients with schizoid and schizotypal personality disorders exhibit mild brain aberrations, also seen in some patients with schizophrenia (e.g., abnormal electroencephalogram [EEG] and evoked potential, attention, and cognitive problems) (Kendler and Walsh, 1995). Although still in the DSM personality disorder category because their behaviors are long-standing, habitual, and stable, schizoid and schizotypal disorders are most likely mild forms of illness related to the psychoses. The perceptual distortions and thinking problems of schizotypal patients may respond to low doses of neuroleptics or anticonvulsants.

There are no systematic data about paranoid personality. It is rare (<1% of the general population). There may be a familial relationship between paranoid personality disorder and delusional disorder. The risk for paranoid personality disorder is higher than expected in the relatives of patients with delusional disorder.

Cluster B

Cluster B includes dramatic-emotional personalities (see Table 20-2). As a group these individuals are sensation seeking and may act without thinking of consequences. Patients with *antisocial personality disorder* show a lifelong pattern of disregard for people, society, and the law. They lack remorse. Although this diagnosis cannot be given until age 18, these individuals exhibit aggression toward animals and people and a pattern of violating societal rules from childhood and may receive a diagnosis of conduct disorder. As adults, these individuals engage in criminal behaviors. They often become easily bored, abuse drugs and alcohol, and are promiscuous. They act irresponsibly and often fail to pay their debts and support their families. Patients with ASP disorder are often superficially charming and use people for their own pleasure or profit.

Patients with *narcissistic personality disorder* have a sense of entitlement and are in constant need of admiration. They believe they are special and that the world exists to serve them. They get

TABLE 20-2	Cluster B Personality Disorders
Disorder	**Description**
Antisocial (3% of males, 1% of females, 0 older than age 55)	Disregards and violates the rights of others, nonconforming to social and legal norms; deceitful, impulsive, aggressive, reckless, irresponsible, remorseless
Histrionic (2%–3%)	Excessively emotional and attention seeking; seductive, dramatic, and suggestible; emotionally unstable and shallow; vague in speech
Narcissistic (<1%)	Grandiose sense of self-importance; sense of entitlement and need for excessive admiration; interpersonally exploitative, lacks empathy
Borderline (2%)	Unstable relationships and self-image; outbursts of anger; impulsive; fearful of abandonment; suicidal; self-mutilating; intense, reactive, and unstable moods

angry if they do not receive special treatment. They often exaggerate their own accomplishments and fish for compliments. They respond to criticism either with cool indifference or severe anger. Patients with narcissistic personality disorder can be superficially charming but lack empathy and use people for their own benefit.

Patients with *histrionic personality disorder* show shallowness of emotions and language. Their emotions are often intense, and their language is highly impressionistic. They are also uncomfortable in situations where they are not the center of attention. Patients with histrionic personality are highly suggestible, often romanticize relationships, and can be highly seductive.

The key feature of *borderline personality disorder* is that patients display intense and labile moods, impulsivity, and recurrent suicidal behaviors and have a chronic sense of emptiness. Patients with borderline personality disorder also have a pattern of either idealizing or devaluating their relationships. In addition, they show frantic efforts to avoid real or perceived abandonment.

Of patients meeting criteria for antisocial personality, 90% are male, whereas of patients meeting criteria for histrionic personality, 90% are female. Antisocial and histrionic personality disorders co-occur in the same families, with male relatives most commonly being antisocial and abusers of alcohol and street drugs and female relatives most commonly histrionic. Approximately 25% of patients with one disorder also meet criteria for both disorders (Lilienfeld et al., 1986).

Patients with cluster B disorders are also at greater risk than the general population for somatization disorder; conversion disorder; drug and alcohol abuse; criminality (some antisocial patients); sexually transmitted diseases (including acquired immunodeficiency syndrome [AIDS]); and childhood conduct disorder, including the triad of bed-wetting, fire setting, and cruelty to animals (Goodwin and Guze, 1996; Simonoff et al., 2004). In persons younger than age 55, the morbid risk for cluster B disorders is approximately 6%. In persons older than age 55 this risk is approximately 2%, with antisocial becoming very rare. This is explained by early death due to high-risk behaviors and "mellowing out" with age. Some patients respond to lithium, monoamine oxidase inhibitors (MAOIs), and anticonvulsants. First-degree relatives have an increased risk for mood disorders (Goodwin and Guze, 1996).

Borderline personality is heterogeneous, with many such persons experiencing early-onset and chronic and less episodic mood disorders. Biologic markers and treatment studies support this view. Abnormal dexamethasone suppression is found in 50% to 60% of patients, and 30% have mildly abnormal EEGs. Up to 50% of patients meeting criteria for borderline personality disorder also meet criteria for bipolar II disorder or cyclothymia. For patients who have a diagnosis of borderline personality disorder, the largest subgroup is a variant of mood disorder. Other diagnoses to consider in the differential diagnosis of borderline personality disorder are other cluster B disorders, drug abuse, epilepsy, and head injury syndromes. Patients have traits of high behavioral activation (novelty seeking) and low behavioral inhibition (harm avoidance) that encourage taking high risks, resulting in brain dysfunction from illicit drug use or traumatic brain injury (TBI). These conditions in turn exaggerate their other personality traits of impulsiveness and aggressiveness, resulting in a combination of state and trait behaviors. The end result is that treatments for traits (cognitive and dialectic behavior therapy) may be unsuccessful in these cases.

Cluster C

Cluster C includes anxious-fearful personalities (see Table 20-3) (Grant et al., 2004). Patients with cluster C disorder have behavioral traits of high harm avoidance and low novelty seeking. Those with avoidant and dependent personality disorder also exhibit high reward dependence.

A CASE OF BORDERLINE PERSONALITY DISORDER

A 28-year-old woman is referred to a clinic for anger management. She has a long history of recurrent major depression and polysubstance abuse (e.g., alcohol, cocaine). She has experienced intense mood swings all of her life. She has not been able to sustain relationships and jobs because of her inability to control her rage. She was referred because of her recurrent suicide attempts, irritability, and difficulty getting along with her therapist. When she first started seeing the therapist, she liked her very much but became upset when the therapist refused to give out her personal phone number.

TABLE 20-3   Cluster C Personality Disorders

Disorder	Description
Avoidant	Socially inhibited; hypersensitive to criticism; feeling inadequate; avoiding interpersonal contact and risks; viewing self as inept, inferior, and unappealing
Dependent	Submissive and clinging; fearing separation; indecisive; unassertive; low self-confidence; follower
Obsessive-compulsive	Preoccupied with orderliness; perfectionistic; preoccupied with mental and interpersonal control; inflexible, stubborn; decreased openness and efficiency; miserly, hoarding; cannot delegate, overly conscientious, scrupulous, workaholic

Patients with *avoidant personality disorder* are individuals who crave social interactions but avoid them for fear of rejection, criticism, or disapproval. These individuals are highly sensitive to criticism and often have low self-esteem. They see themselves as inferior to others and avoid new situations. Patients with *dependent personality disorder* see themselves as inept and show an overreliance on others. They allow significant others to make all major decisions for them. They often do not show disagreements because they are afraid that others would not like them. These individuals are often followers and will not initiate any task or project on their own. Patients with *obsessive-compulsive personalities* are perfectionists. However, often they are not able to finish tasks on time because of their excessive attention to details. They have a need for following rules, regulations, and symmetry and are inflexible. They have highly moralistic, ethical views and are usually overly conscientious and stubborn and may lack a sense of humor. They are devoted to their work and often fail to delegate tasks.

Patients with a cluster C personality disorder have a greater risk than the general population for several axis I disorders, including anxiety disorder, nonmelancholic depression, eating disorders, adjustment disorders, and benzodiazepine abuse. One third of patients with obsessive-compulsive personality disorder (OCPD) also have obsessive-compulsive disorder (OCD). OCPD is differentiated from OCD by the absence of clear obsessions. Avoidant personality disorder and social phobia also have some overlap (Reichborn-Kjennerud et al., 2007). Avoidant personality disorder can be differentiated from social phobia by the presence (in the former) of additional symptoms such as feelings of inadequacy and low self-esteem. The obsessive-compulsive and avoidant personality is frequently comorbid in depressive disorders; however, antidepressant treatment with selective serotonin reuptake inhibitors (SSRIs) reduces the number of patients meeting the criteria, which suggests that, at least in some patients with avoidant traits, presence of depression leads to a diagnosis of personality disorder (Fava et al., 2002).

Dependent personality is more frequently diagnosed in women. It is likely that in some women, behaviors that conform to gender role stereotypes, such as allowing one's husband to make important decisions regarding the household, may contribute toward this diagnosis. In such cases clear evidence of personal distress and social impairment is essential. Patients with cluster

A CASE OF AVOIDANT PERSONALITY DISORDER

A 39-year-old woman is referred by her primary care physician. She has had two previous major depressive episodes that required treatment, but she says she now frequently feels "down" and anxious. She says she is a shy, overly cautious person, a "worry-wart," who is generally pessimistic about events or situations in her life. She says she is afraid of her own shadow and unable to assert herself, even when she knows she is right. She has few friends and trouble making new ones. She also states that people think she is good-hearted. She thinks she is a loving person (she likes to be demonstrative with close friends and family and craves affection), but she has difficulty establishing relationships because of her shyness. She is afraid to approach people for fear of being rejected.

A CASE OF OBSESSIVE-COMPULSIVE PERSONALITY DISORDER

A 44-year-old married teacher is the hardest worker at her school. She tries to tutor many students at the same time and has trouble turning down new students. She is too much of a perfectionist to delegate work to her teaching assistant. Her colleagues complain that she pays too much attention to details. Departmental secretaries have trouble working for her because she is too critical of their mistakes, rigid, and controlling. She works 12 to 14 hours a day and comes home late and tired. Because of this, her husband is annoyed at her for not paying any attention to him. She is bright and articulate and loves her husband but has trouble expressing her emotions to him. She has been this way since high school.

C personality disorders tend to have family members who also meet criteria for these disorders, although the aggregation is not specific in type, only to the cluster.

PERSONALITY DISORDER DUE TO GENERAL MEDICAL CONDITIONS

Several general medical and neurologic conditions are likely to affect an individual's personality by altering the central nervous system and its response to environmental cues (Cummings and Mega, 2003). Table 20-4 lists the conditions most likely to alter personality.

Personality Changes Associated with Seizure Disorder

Up to 60% of patients with epilepsy are reported to have permanent changes in personality after several decades of illness. The "adhesive" or "viscous" personality is characterized by perseveration, stubbornness, a narrow field of interest and attention, loss of humor (humorless sobriety), circumstantial and cliché-filled speech, and a pedantic, dry manner (Bear and Fedio, 1977). Patients with this personality seem compelled to begin a conversation, exhaust the topic regardless of previous iterations, and are reluctant to stop. They lose sight of the "big picture" or the concept of their topic or theme and focus on minutiae. They "stick" to the topic and to the person to whom they are speaking.

Patients with chronic manic-depressive illness may have similar personality changes, but these are less severe in expression. These patients also are circumstantial and adhesive and may keep copious notes of their medical treatments and illness experiences. They write excessively and keep detailed diaries. They may focus attention on esoteric philosophic or theologic topics beyond their training and understanding but they are compelled to talk about them (pseudoprofundity). Patients with chronic limbic system disease or alcoholism may become moody and irritable, quarrelsome, spiteful, suspicious, and malicious. They may hold grudges, vigorously protest mild or imagined slights, and become litigious. They can become the "neighborhood cranks."

TABLE 20-4	Conditions and Personality Changes	
Condition	**Personality Change**
Epilepsy	Adhesive or paranoid (like DSM cluster A subtype)
Head injury	Irritable and coarsening
Stroke	Avolitional or disinhibited frontal lobe syndromes
Drug abuse	Avolitional, irritable/paranoid, viscous/adhesive
Bipolar mood disorder	Adhesive
Degenerative brain disease	Avolitional or disinhibited frontal lobe syndromes

Personality Changes Following Injury or Disease

Traumatic Brain Injury

Personality changes are common following moderate to severe TBI, particularly when frontal lobe circuitry is involved. Lateral orbital prefrontal injury leads to irritability and episodic dyscontrol and unplanned violence. These patients are emotionally labile, restless, and impulsive. They often lack insight and have self-destructive and unrealistic plans. They are often overly talkative and exuberant and can be childishly self-centered and insensitive toward others. Patients with dorsolateral prefrontal injury lack spontaneity, initiative, drive, ambition, and interests. Their mood is often dysphoric, and they are sluggish and socially isolated. In children, TBI elicits personality changes associated with attention-deficits and hyperactivity. One of the earliest documented cases of severe brain injury is that of Phineas Gage (1823–1860), who suffered major personality changes after brain trauma (Ratiu and Talos, 2004).

Gage was foreman of a crew of railroad construction workers. On the day of his accident, he was preparing for an explosion by compacting a bore with explosive powder using a tamping iron. A spark from the tamping iron ignited the powder, causing the iron to be propelled at high speed straight through Gage's skull. It entered under his left cheek bone and exited through the top of his head. It is unclear if Gage lost consciousness, but he was conscious and able to walk within minutes of the accident.

After a few days, Gage's brain became infected with a "fungus," and he lapsed into a semicomatose state. Two weeks after the accident, his physician, Harlow, drained an abscess under Gage's scalp. Gage was reported to be leading a normal life within a year. According to Harlow, Gage retained "full possession of his reason" after the accident, but Gage's wife and other people close to him soon began to notice dramatic changes in his personality. His contractors, who regarded him as the most efficient and capable foreman before his injury, considered the change in his mind so marked that they could not give him his place again. He was fitful, irreverent, and often used profane language (a change from his previous pattern). He also showed little deference for his fellow workers and was obstinate, yet capricious and vacillating. He was impatient, especially if his needs were not met. He would make many future plans, which he would then abandon in favor of other plans that he thought were more feasible. In this regard, his mind was radically changed, so that his friends and acquaintances said he was "no longer Gage."

Therefore, the damage to Gage's frontal cortex had resulted in a complete loss of social inhibitions, which often led to inappropriate behavior. In effect, the tamping iron had performed a frontal lobotomy on Gage, but the exact nature of the damage incurred to his brain has been a subject of debate ever since the accident occurred. This is because the damage can only be inferred from the path of the tamping iron through Gage's skull, which in turn can only be inferred from the damage to the skull.

Stroke

Akin to TBI, stroke can also result in changes in personality, particularly after large or multiple strokes in anterior brain regions. These changes are the same as those seen following TBI.

"Frontal Lobe" Personality

Persons with neurodegenerative diseases, such as frontal lobe disease, commonly exhibit personality changes characterized by disinhibition or apathy. They may become irritable, insensitive to others' feelings, neglectful of appearance, or lack social graces. In addition, they may be inappropriately jocular, indifferent, or placid and minimize difficulties, as well as act in an impulsive, unpredictable, impatient, rule-breaking, demanding, aggressive, or pseudopsychopathic manner. They may have reduced interests. They might also become more pleasant and sentimental.

NEUROIMAGING IN PERSONALITY DISORDERS

Borderline, schizotypal, and antisocial remain the best-studied personality disorders. The structural and functional imaging findings are consistent with patients' behavioral abnormalities (McCloskey et al., 2005).

Schizotypal Personality Disorder

Patients with SPD show brain changes that are somewhat different from those of patients with schizophrenia. Although temporal volume reductions appear to be common to both SPD and schizophrenia, compared with schizophrenia, SPD shows preservation of frontal lobe volume (Siever and Davis, 2004; Kurachi, 2003a,b). Similarly, long insular cortex, which connects to the temporal regions, is reduced in both patients with SPD and patients with schizophrenia, but short insular cortex, which has close connections with frontal cortex, is preserved in patients with SPD. The size of the pulvinar, which projects to temporal lobe structures, is reduced in SPD as well as in schizophrenia, while the size of the dorsomedial nucleus of the thalamus, associated with the prefrontal region, is decreased only in schizophrenia (Byne et al., 2001). These findings suggest that although the two disorders share vulnerability to psychosis, patients with SPD have preserved frontal lobe function.

Antisocial Personality Disorder

Neuroimaging studies suggest that patients with ASP disorder have abnormalities of frontosubcortical systems, such as decreased brain perfusion in large areas of the right prefrontal and temporal lobe (Goethals et al., 2005). Magnetic resonance imaging (MRI) studies have documented reduced volumes of the frontal lobes and the hippocampus in ASP disorder (Laakso et al., 2001; Raine et al., 2000). Other areas, such as the amygdala and basal ganglia, parahippocampal gyrus, and anterior superior temporal gyrus, also show abnormalities (Bassarath, 2001). The relevant functional anatomy includes limbic and paralimbic structures and can be called the *paralimbic system* (Kiehl, 2006).

Borderline Personality Disorder

Several imaging studies have looked at patients with borderline personality disorder (McCloskey et al., 2005; Skodol et al., 2002a,b). Most of these reveal limbic and frontal dysfunction. Structural imaging studies show reduced volume in the hippocampus and amygdala and loss of frontal gray matter volume. Functional imaging studies show decreased brain perfusion in the right prefrontal and temporal lobe and increased activity in the amygdala in response to emotions. These changes are associated with impulsive and aggressive behavior, which reflects failure of frontal inhibition and limbic excitability (Skodol et al., 2002a,b).

APPROACHES TO PERSONALITY AND PERSONALITY DISORDERS

Diagnostic and Statistical Manual "Categorical" Approach

Almost all medical diagnosis is categorical; for example, a patient either has hypertension or does not, or has a depression or does not. The choices are a category of sickness versus wellness with no middle ground. Personality, however, represents a combination of behavioral traits that are dimensional, not categorical (Oldham, 2005; Widiger and Frances, 1994). The dimension is the bell-shaped curve, and an individual can be anywhere on that curve for each personality dimension. There is no clear point where a person is high or low on a dimension.

Superimposing a categorical diagnostic structure on a biologically dimensional entity creates several problems. For example, 40% to 50% of patients meet criteria for more than one personality disorder, which is biologically improbable because people have only one personality. Studies have shown that some patients meet criteria for a personality disorder 1 year but not the next, contradicting the concept of stable trait behavior. This is observed more frequently with cluster B personality disorders. DSM criteria are not very clear about what is considered "significant" cognitive, affective, or interpersonal dysfunction, or how inflexible "inflexible" is.

Patients can get into the same category for different reasons. For example, a pattern of criminality and remorselessness and a pattern of nonconforming and impulsive behaviors can result in two markedly different persons being diagnosed as having ASP disorder. There are also conceptual disagreements among and within categories. For example, is borderline personality an illness or a pattern of traits? In making categorical diagnosis, important information is lost. Often clinicians consider only those behaviors that meet criteria. None of these predict other behaviors or treatment response.

Dimensional Approach

Rather than placing persons into personality categories (e.g., an individual either does or does not meet criteria for antisocial personality), the dimensional approach is based on the definition of normal personality. The "dimension" is the traits that comprise personality (John, 1990). Traits can be measured. On the basis of that measurement, an individual can be placed on the bell-shaped curve. Therefore, deviance (i.e., abnormality) becomes relative. There are many points of deviance at the extremes. The dimensional approach is theoretically consistent; it does not confuse state (e.g., depression) and trait (e.g., high harm avoidance).

Researchers agree on the general dimensional structure of personality (Siever and Davis, 2004; Widiger and Mullins-Sweat, 2005). Dimensional personality measurements have good reliability. An individual's measures are stable over time, avoid the artificial boundaries of the categories, and explain the within-category heterogeneity and co-occurring personality diagnoses of DSM. Dimensions can predict DSM categories and therefore can be useful in clinical diagnosis.

Dimensions predict other behaviors. For example, novelty seeking explains 60% of the variance of problem drinking, smoking, and drug abuse.

Dimensions predict treatment response. For example, dimensions can be used to guide pharmacologic treatment of associated nonmelancholic depressions (e.g., using serotonin reuptake inhibiting drugs to treat depression in patients with high harm avoidance) and guide psychotherapy and management (e.g., high reward dependence can be reinforced to help modify other behaviors) (Cloninger et al., 1994).

Dimensional Personality Models

Eysenck, Tellegen, and Costa developed reliable and valid dimensional personality models (Widiger and Mullins-Sweat, 2005).

Three-factor models

The earlier models proposed by Eysenck and Tellegen are each composed of three factors. Eysenck's model includes the dimensions of neuroticism, extraversion, and psychoticism. Tellegen's model includes positive affectivity, negative affectivity, and constraints. Eysenck's neuroticism and Tellegen's negative affectivity measure the same dimension of anxiety, irritability, and poor frustration tolerance. Extraversion and positive affectivity refer to social desirability. Persons with these traits tend to be sociable, talkative, optimistic, and fun loving.

Five-factor model

The five-factor model (FFM) by Costa and Widiger (1994) expanded on the three-factor model. These dimensions, which are also called the *big five*, include the following.

Neuroticism (N), included in the three-factor model, refers to a chronic level of adjustment problems and includes poor frustration tolerance, anxiety, anger, hostility, impulsivity, depression, and vulnerability.

Extraversion (E), also in the three-factor model, refers to the quantity and intensity of preferred interpersonal attachment, activity level, need for stimulation, and capacity for joy. Persons low on extraversion tend to be reserved, soft, aloof, independent, and quiet. They are not unhappy people, but they are not as exuberant as extroverts.

Openness to experience (O) involves active seeking and appreciation of experiences. Open individuals are curious, imaginative, and willing to entertain novel ideas and unconventional values.

Agreeableness (A), like E, is an interpersonal dimension and refers to interactions that an individual prefers, ranging from cooperation to antagonism. People high in agreeableness are softhearted, good natured, trusting, helpful, forgiving, and altruistic. They are eager to help others.

Conscientious (C) assesses degree of organization, persistence, control, and motivation in goal-directed behaviors. People high in C are organized, self-directed, punctual, reliable, hardworking, scrupulous, ambitious, and persevering.

Cloninger's model

Cloninger's model is consistent with the basic construct of personality accepted by most personality researchers (Cloninger et al., 1993; Svrakic et al., 1993). It also has the advantage of being empirically supported by data in behavioral genetics, neurochemistry, neurophysiology, learning theory, and behavioral descriptive analysis. Four temperament and three character, behavioral, and attitudinal dimensions are inherited independently from one another. Their interaction and the ensuing behaviors represent the individual's personality. Each person has some amount of each dimension. All possible combinations of various dimension strengths account for individual differences in personality. Character dimensions are more environmentally influenced than temperament and may be more accessible to change.

The four temperament dimensions are tendencies to behave in a certain way under certain circumstances. A person with high harm avoidance will fear new situations or unknown objects and become inhibited. He or she will be shy with new people. If punished or not rewarded, the person will stop and try to "blend into the woodwork." Persons with high novelty seeking will be curious about new situations, and the riskier the situation, the greater the "buzz" they get. If punished, they actively leave or attack. If not rewarded, they become bored and leave. Persons with high reward dependence want to please others and social institutions that provide rewards. They do this by continuing behaviors that previously got them rewards and conforming to the reward system. People who are high in persistence usually stay at a task longer than others. They often do not require immediate gratification or praise.

The three character dimensions of Cloninger's model represent tendencies to behave in a certain way or to have certain attitudes under certain circumstances. Persons high on self-directedness are purposeful and resourceful and take responsibility for their own lives. Persons low on self-directedness are unreliable, ineffective, and dependent and are likely to have a personality disorder. Persons high on cooperativeness are empathic, helpful, and compassionate. Persons low on cooperativeness are intolerant and vengeful. Persons very high on cooperativeness may "live for others." Persons very low on cooperativeness may be antisocial. Both very high and very low cooperativeness indicate a personality disorder. Persons high on self-transcendence are philosophic and can be unconventional. Persons low on self-transcendence are often unimaginative and conventional.

TREATMENT OF PERSONALITY DISORDERS

Treatment of personality disorder is complex. Patients often come to the psychiatrist's attention due to comorbid axis I disorders or behavioral problems in general medical/surgical wards. The literature is replete with contradictory findings about the efficacy of one treatment modality over another. The setting and modality of treatment depend on the severity of the personality disorder (McMain and Pos, 2007; Mercer, 2007; Paris, 2007). Severe personality disorder may require a more intense, structured setting and benefit from more cognitive behavioral, interpersonal, and supportive therapy, whereas milder personality disorders can be treated in outpatient settings by more psychodynamic or analytic therapies (Gunderson et al., 2005). The role of psychopharmacologic interventions is often limited to treating comorbid axis I disorders, but certain personality disorders, such as schizoid, schizotypal, and avoidant, may benefit from psychopharmacologic intervention. Table 20-5 lists some general rules for treating personality disorder.

TABLE 20-5 Some General Rules in Treating Personality Disorder
Be very clear about the goals and outcomes of the treatment
Take into account the severity of pathology and comorbid axis I disorders in the treatment setting and modality
Form a working alliance with patients (i.e., the ability to work collaboratively toward the same goal)
Set a structure and limits to the therapeutic process and focus on the patients' needs, not necessarily their wants
Remember that not all patients are capable of introspection and self-analysis
Clinicians often experience emotionally difficult interpersonal interactions with patients who have a personality disorder; be aware that the clinician's negative feelings for a patient can interfere with patient care

Inpatient Settings

Cluster B disorders, such as borderline personality and ASP disorders, often come to psychiatrists' attention because of the disruptive nature of the psychopathology, as well as axis I pathology, including depression and substance abuse. These patients can be demanding and argumentative. They often refuse the routine and may misinterpret the health care provider.

Patients with ASP disorder usually learn to "work the system" and may threaten to go to the supervisor or initiate a lawsuit. In the hospital, these patients require a clear understanding of the rules and structure of the ward. They should be treated firmly and empathically. Psychodynamically oriented, introspective therapies have not been shown to be effective in these patients (McMain and Pos, 2007). Because of their superficial charm, they can easily identify and manipulate the naïve health care provider.

Because of the heterogeneity of the diagnosis, many patients with borderline personality disorder need to be carefully reevaluated to ensure that the psychiatrist is not missing another axis I diagnosis (Davis and Akiskal, 1986). Patients should receive an adequate trial of medications to control bipolar mood disorder, major depression, and epilepsy (Mercer, 2007). Dialectical behavioral therapy is a form of cognitive behavioral therapy that has been shown to reduce hospitalizations and suicidal symptoms (Linehan et al., 2006).

Outpatient Settings

There are three levels of outpatient settings for treating personality disorders: partial or day hospitalization, intensive outpatient therapy, and office-based outpatient therapy. Partial hospitalization requires the patient to go to a day hospital program. The structure of this is similar to that of an inpatient program, except that the patient is not on a locked unit and, therefore, has to be willing to commit and adhere to treatment.

Intensive outpatient therapy is often multimodal. In addition to one-on-one therapy, the patient is often required to attend group therapy. The goal here is not just stabilization but also socialization. As with inpatient therapy, patients with borderline personality disorder often need partial hospitalization and/or intensive outpatient therapies.

The goal of outpatient therapy is often personal growth and reduction of psychological distress. Several different types of therapies are described in the literature, such as cognitive behavioral, interpersonal, and psychodynamic. There is no clear evidence that one is superior to another. The most consistent predictor of a good outcome is the patient's relationship with the therapist.

Generally less severe personality disorders, such as obsessive-compulsive, high functioning histrionic and narcissistic, and avoidant and dependent personality disorders, are well suited for psychodynamically oriented outpatient therapies.

Psychopharmacologic Treatments

Personality disorders that are comorbid with axis I disorders need psychopharmacologic treatment for the axis I disorder. Usually, for most personality disorders, pharmacotherapy is short term and limited to crisis management. In some cases, such as borderline personality disorder, long-term treatment may also be required. In the overall treatment of personality disorder, pharmacotherapy has a small role compared with a supportive therapeutic interaction between physician and patient (Mercer, 2007). Most of the pharmacologic research is limited to treatment of borderline personality disorder. The treatment of other personality disorders in the absence of an axis I diagnosis is not well studied.

Psychotropic drugs have been shown to help patients with personality disorders that are closely related to axis I disorders (e.g., SPD and schizophrenia, avoidant personality disorder and generalized social phobia, borderline personality disorder and affective disorders). In addition, medications influence certain psychopathological symptom clusters present in various disorders (e.g., cognitive-perceptual organization, impulsivity/aggression, affective instability, anxiety/inhibition) (Mercer, 2007). The effects of medications on impulsive aggressiveness are supported, evident early, and independent of the effects on mood, including depression.

ACKNOWLEDGMENTS

The author acknowledges Dr. Michael Alan Taylor for his contribution to parts of this chapter and Dr. Frederick S. Sierles for his helpful comments.

Clinical Pearls

- Persons with anxious-fearful personality are prone to nonmelancholic depression, anxiety, obsessive-compulsive disorders, eating disorders, and sedative-hypnotic substance abuse.
- More than 50% to 60% of patients seen in psychiatric clinics may have a personality disorder.
- Personality traits develop in the formative years and are habitual, characteristic of the person, and mostly unchanging. A dramatic personality change after ages 30 to 35 almost always means brain disease.
- Most patients show worsening of their personality traits during stress or illness; it is therefore advisable to defer the diagnosis of personality disorder on an inpatient unit until a longitudinal history of personality profile is available.
- Many patients with borderline personality disorders may have an undiagnosed bipolar mood disorder.
- Self-mutilation is not essential for the diagnosis of borderline personality disorder, and everyone who self-mutilates does not automatically have borderline personality disorder.
- Paranoid personality disorder is rare and not well studied. It may be associated with delusional disorder.
- Antisocial and histrionic personality disorders co-occur in the same families at a rate higher than that seen in the general population.
- Of patients meeting criteria for antisocial personality disorder, 90% are male.

Self-Assessment Questions and Answers

20-1. A 42-year-old single man had a lifelong pattern of being socially isolated. He lives alone and has no friends. He works as a filing clerk in a library, where he does not have to interact much with coworkers or patrons. His coworkers and neighbors perceive him as odd, distant, cooperative, and polite. He cooks for himself. He has unusual, quirky thoughts. For example, for 2 days he wondered about the washing instructions on a pair of jeans he just purchased: Did "wash before wearing" mean the jeans should be washed before wearing the first time, or did they need, for some reason, to be washed each time before he wore them? Often he thought about witchcraft and wondered if he should visit Salem, Massachusetts, where, in the 17th century, alleged witches were tried and those found guilty were burned at the stake. He decided not to go because that would mean interacting with Salem residents. Sometimes he had illusions of witches in shadows near his house. He was never psychotic. Of the following, which is the most likely diagnosis?

A. Avoidant personality disorder
B. Borderline personality disorder
C. Paranoid personality disorder
D. Schizoid personality disorder
E. Schizotypal personality disorder

His lifelong pattern of social isolation and interpersonal difficulties places him in cluster A (odd and eccentric type). He does not exhibit any paranoid ideation, so paranoid personality is not likely. Patients with schizoid personality do not have a pattern of unusual thoughts or perceptual illusion as this patient is exhibiting. Therefore, schizotypal personality is the most likely. *Answer: E*

20-2. A 34-year-old divorced cocaine dealer has been arrested >15 times and in the past has served 4 years in a federal prison. He routinely abuses cocaine, alcohol, and opiates. As a child he frequently ran away from home and stayed at a friend's place. He was suspended from school several times for bullying children and taking their lunch money. During his evaluation he is calm and tells the doctor about his run-ins with the law. He also coldly says that he threatened to kill anyone who would testify against him. He has had several girlfriends and has fathered a few children but has no contact with them. Which of the below is the most likely diagnosis?

A. Antisocial personality disorder
B. Borderline personality disorder
C. Narcissistic personality disorder
D. Paranoid personality disorder
E. Schizoid personality disorder

20-3. For which of these disorders are his female relatives at greater risk?

A. Anxiety disorder
B. Depression
C. Dissociative amnestic disorder
D. Paranoid personality disorder
E. Somatization disorder

A pattern of conduct problems since childhood, criminal behavior as an adult, lack of social responsibility, and complete disregard for law, as evidenced by his calm demeanor and failure to support his children, all point toward a diagnosis of antisocial personality (ASP) disorder. Although drug use is seen in other disorders and can account for prison sentences, patients who abuse drugs and do not have antisocial personality do not exhibit the pattern evidenced here. Female relatives of patients with ASP disorders are also at greater risk than the general population for somatization disorder. *Answers: A, E*

20-4. A 55-year-old right-handed married woman is a clinically and academically successful dermatologist. She is an articulate and well-organized lecturer and seminar leader, as well as a skillful journal article writer and editor. She is well liked, hard working, effective, and respected professionally. She has had no neuropsychiatric illnesses. However, she is much better at doing one task at a time than multitasking. She solves problems based on logic and experience rather than intuition or creativity. Compared with her colleagues, she has more trouble understanding the humor and meanings of cartoons. In medical school, she received a C in her surgery clerkship and would have failed if her supervisors had not appreciated her hard work and sincerity. Which of the following best characterizes her?

A. She has obsessive-compulsive personality disorder.
B. She has narcissistic personality disorder.
C. She has histrionic personality traits.
D. She does not have a personality disorder.
E. There is not enough information to diagnose her as having a personality disorder.

An individual must have inflexible personality traits and either subjective or observable distress to be diagnosed with a personality disorder. The above vignette, although rich in its description, does not comment about any habitual pattern of behaviors nor does it mention that this individual is distressed by her personality traits. There is no evidence that her behavior is markedly different from the norm. *Answer: E*

20-5. A 37-year-old woman has a 2-month history of sad and irritable mood, fatigue, appetite and sleep abnormalities, weight loss, self-pity, trouble concentrating, reduced enjoyment of usual activities, and recurrent suicidal ideation with no suicide plans. In the past, she attempted suicide by cutting her wrists. She has had similar episodes at least five times since age 20, and each time she recovered fully with treatment. She never had a hypomanic or manic episode. Her condition cannot be explained by a general medical or neurologic disorder or psychoactive substance abuse. She has had difficulty forming and maintaining relationships and jobs since her late teens. Which of the following is the most likely diagnosis?

A. Bipolar I disorder
B. Borderline personality disorder
C. Dysthymic disorder
D. Major depressive disorder
E. Mood disorder due to multiple sclerosis

Absence of a manic episode and general medical or neurologic disorder rule out choices A and E. Her symptoms are severe enough to warrant hospitalization; therefore, she does not have dysthymic disorder. Although she has had interpersonal difficulty, suicidal attempts, and irritability that have onset since age 20, these symptoms have always occurred during a mood episode. Patients with personality disorder often have personality problems even in the absence of a mood episode and often have mood swings that cannot be identified as a mood episode. She meets the criteria for a major depressive episode. *Answer: D*

References

American Psychiatric Association. *Diagnostic and statistical manual of mental disorders*, 4th ed., text revision. Washington, DC: American Psychiatric Association; 2000.

Bassarath L. Neuroimaging studies of antisocial behaviour. *Can J Psychiatry*. 2001;46:728–732.

Bear DM, Fedio P. Quantitative analysis of interictal behavior in temporal lobe epilepsy. *Arch Neurol*. 1977;34:454–467.

Bouchard TJ. Genes, environment, and personality. *Science*. 1994;264:1700–1701.

Byne W, Buchsbaum MS, Kemether E, et al. Magnetic resonance imaging of the thalamic mediodorsal nucleus and pulvinar in schizophrenia and schizotypal personality disorder. *Arch Gen Psychiatry*. 2001;58:133–140.

Coid JW. Aetiological risk factors for personality disorders. *Br J Psychiatry*. 1999;174:530–538.

Costa PT Jr, Widiger TA. Introduction: Personality disorders and the five-factor model of personality. In: Costa PT, Widiger TA, eds. *Personality disorders and the five-factor model of personality*. Washington, DC: American Psychological Association; 1994.

Cloninger CR, Przybeck TR, Svrakic DM, et al. *The temperament and character inventory (TCI): A guide to its development and use*. St. Louis: Washington University, Center for Psychobiology of Personality; 1994.

Cloninger CR, Svrakic DM, Przybeck TR. A psychobiological model of temperament and character. *Arch Gen Psychiatry*. 1993;50:975–990.

Cummings JL, Mega MS. *Neuropsychiatry and behavioral neuroscience*. New York: Oxford University Press; 2003:256.

Davis GC, Akiskal HS. Descriptive, biological, and theoretical aspects of borderline personality disorder. *Hosp Comm Psychiatry*. 1986;37:685–692.

Fava M, Farabaugh AH, Sickinger AH, et al. Personality disorders and depression. *Psychol Med*. 2002;32:1049–1057.

Goethals I, Audenaert K, Jacobs F, et al. Brain perfusion SPECT in impulsivity-related personality disorders. *Behav Brain Res*. 2005;157:187–192.

Goodwin DW, Guze SB. *Psychiatric diagnosis*, 5th ed. New York: Oxford University Press; 1996.

Grant BF, Hasin DS, Stinson FS, et al. Prevalence, correlates, and disability of personality disorders in the United States: Results from the national epidemiologic survey on alcohol and related conditions. *J Clin Psychiatry*. 2004;65:948–958.

Gunderson JG, Gratz KL, Neuhaus E, et al. Levels of care in treatment. In: Oldham JM, Skodol AE, Bender DS, eds. *The American psychiatric publishing textbook of personality disorders*. Washington, DC: American Psychiatric Publishing; 2005.

John OP. The "Big Five" factor taxonomy: Dimensions of personality in the natural language and in questionnaires. In: Pervin LA, ed. *Handbook of personality*. New York: Guilford Press; 1990.

Kendler KS, Walsh D. Schizotypal personality disorder in parents and the risk for schizophrenia in siblings. *Schizophr Bull*. 1995;21:47–52.

Kiehl KA. A cognitive neuroscience perspective on psychopathy: Evidence for paralimbic system dysfunction. *Psychiatry Res*. 2006;142:107–128.

Kurachi M. Pathogenesis of schizophrenia: Part I. Symptomatology, cognitive characteristics and brain morphology. *Psychiatry Clin Neurosci*. 2003a;57:3–8.

Kurachi M. Pathogenesis of schizophrenia: Part II. Temporo-frontal two-step hypothesis. *Psychiatry Clin Neurosci*. 2003b;57:9–15.

Laakso MP, Vaurio O, Koivisto E, et al. Psychopathy and the posterior hippocampus. *Behav Brain Res*. 2001;118:193–197.

Lilienfeld SO, Van Valkenburg C, Larntz K, et al. The relationship of histrionic personality disorder to antisocial personality and somatization disorders. *Am J Psychiatry*. 1986;143:718–722.

Linehan MM, Comtois KA, Murray AM, et al. Two-year randomized controlled trial and follow-up of dialectical behavior therapy versus therapy by experts for suicidal behaviors and borderline personality disorder. *Arch Gen Psychiatry*. 2006;63:757–766.

McCloskey MS, Luan Phan K, Coccaro EF. Neuroimaging and personality disorders. *Curr Psychiatry Rep*. 2005;7:65–72.

McMain S, Pos AE. Advances in psychotherapy of personality disorders: A research update. *Curr Psychiatry Rep*. 2007;9:46–52.

Mercer D. Medications in the treatment of borderline personality disorder 2006. *Curr Psychiatry Rep.* 2007;9:53–62.

Oldham JM. Personality disorders: Current perspectives. *JAMA.* 1994;272:1770–1776.

Oldham JM. Personality disorders: Recent history and future directions. In: Oldham JM, Skodol AE, Bender DS, eds. *The American psychiatric publishing textbook of personality disorders.* Washington, DC: American Psychiatric Publishing; 2005.

Oldham JM, Skodol AE, Kellman HD, et al. Comorbidity of axis I and axis II disorders. *Am J Psychiatry.* 1995;152:571–578.

Paris J. Intermittent psychotherapy: An alternative to continuous long-term treatment for patients with personality disorders. *J Psychiatr Pract.* 2007;13:153–158.

Raine A, Lencz T, Bihrle S, et al. Reduced prefrontal gray matter volume and reduced autonomic activity in antisocial personality disorder. *Arch Gen Psychiatry.* 2000;57:119–127.

Ratiu P, Talos IF. Images in clinical medicine. The tale of Phineas Gage, digitally remastered. *N Engl J Med.* 2004;351:e21.

Reichborn-Kjennerud T, Czajkowski N, Torgersen S, et al. The relationship between avoidant personality disorder and social phobia: A population-based twin study. *Am J Psychiatry.* 2007;164:1722–1728.

Siever LJ, Davis KL. The pathophysiology of schizophrenia disorders: Perspectives from the spectrum. *Am J Psychiatry.* 2004;161:398–413.

Simonoff E, Elander J, Holmshaw J, et al. Predictors of antisocial personality: Continuities from childhood to adult life. *Br J Psychiatry.* 2004;184:118–127.

Skodol AE, Gunderson JG, Pfohl B, et al. The borderline diagnosis I: Psychopathology, comorbidity, and personality structure. *Biol Psychiatry.* 2002a;51:936–950.

Skodol AE, Siever LJ, Livesley WJ, et al. The borderline diagnosis II: Biology, genetics, and clinical course. *Biol Psychiatry.* 2002b;51:951–963.

Svrakic DM, Whitehead C, Przybeck TR, et al. Differential diagnosis of personality disorders by the seven-factor model of temperament and character. *Arch Gen Psychiatry.* 1993;50:991–999.

Tyrer P, Casey P, Ferguson B. Personality disorder in perspective. *Br J Psychiatry.* 1991;159:463–471.

Verheul R, Herbrink M. The efficacy of various modalities of psychotherapy for personality disorders: A systematic review of the evidence and clinical recommendations. *Int Rev Psychiatry.* 2007;19:25–38.

Widiger TA, Frances AJ. Toward a dimensional model for the personality disorders. In: Costa PT, Widiger TA, eds. *Personality disorders and the five-factor model of personality.* Washington, DC: American Psychological Association; 1994.

Widiger TA, Mullins-Sweat, SN. Categorical and dimensional models of personality disorders. In: Oldham JM, Skodol AE, Bender DS, eds. *The American psychiatric publishing textbook of personality disorders.* Washington, DC: American Psychiatric Publishing; 2005.

Therapeutic Interventions for Mental Illness

21

Mark J. Gorman, Steven A. Safren,
Pamela R. Handelsman, and Bruce J. Masek

Behavioral Medicine Strategies

This chapter overviews behavioral medicine as practiced in an outpatient or general hospital setting. The chapter begins by defining behavioral medicine and then discusses interventions to instill motivation for change, because many patients need to change their behavior to enhance their health and well-being or reduce the behavioral, psychological, or biomedical effects of illness. The chapter then describes the most frequent behavioral medicine interventions, which range across illnesses and problems, and focuses on cognitive behavioral strategies. Finally, specific examples of intervention for particular medical conditions are provided.

DEFINITION OF BEHAVIORAL MEDICINE

Behavioral medicine is defined as "the field concerned with the development of behavioral science knowledge and techniques relevant to the understanding of physical health and illness and the application of this knowledge and techniques to prevention, diagnosis, treatment, and rehabilitation. Psychosis, neurosis, and substance abuse are included only insofar as they contribute to physical disorders as an end point" (Schwartz and Weiss, 1978). Patients who seek behavioral medicine treatment are at risk for developing a medical or mental health problem, already have a medical problem and need assistance with self-care strategies to manage it, or already have a medical problem, need assistance with self-care strategies to manage it, and have a comorbid psychiatric disorder or other mental health concerns.

At the start of treatment, patients are commonly asked to monitor the severity of their medical symptom, focusing on antecedent events associated with a change in severity, and the consequences their symptoms have on daily functioning. During treatment, patients continually observe the utility of strategies for self-management. The vast majority of behavioral medicine practitioners are clinical psychologists with specialized training that facilitates a close working relationship with other health care providers, particularly physicians and surgeons, to help patients better manage their illness or cope with its consequences (Masek and Scharff, 2004).

BEHAVIORAL MEDICINE AND SELF-CARE

One way in which behavioral medicine interventions can increase adherence to self-care behaviors is to address why patients do not optimally respond to their existing medical treatment. Failure to adhere to recommendations can occur for a variety of reasons, including complications from the medical illness itself. Patients have competing life demands that interfere with behavioral aspects of self-care. They are influenced by a variety of social psychological variables, including perceived self-efficacy, norms about health behavior, and benefits and barriers to engaging in self-care behavior; motivational issues; absence of sufficient behavioral skills; and lack of knowledge or understanding of the importance of self-care. The interplay of medical illness and psychiatric comorbidity can also affect adherence. Models of self-care attempt to account for the complex relationship between the patient and the health care system (Shumaker et al., 1998). Many behavioral medicine interventions are based on models derived from social psychological theory and cognitive behavioral research.

Teaching patients about adherence strategies for complex medical treatments is one of the roles of behavioral medicine practitioners and includes helping patients learn how to initiate the behavioral changes necessary to implement the recommended medical treatment. Patients may be facing a brief or chronic treatment and/or recovery phase and often are dealing with the crisis of a new diagnosis and learning to manage their new lifestyle (medications, physical activity, nutrition, and sleep). In the hospital, acute symptoms (e.g., medical symptoms and shock) are primarily treated by the patient's physician and medical staff, and behavioral medicine practitioners may help the patient with support or brief services based on crisis management. In chronic illness, patients are primarily treated as outpatients by their entire medical team. These patients often have difficulty adjusting to cost and side effects of new medications and self-care behaviors (e.g., poor medication adherence, poor self-monitoring of blood sugar).

Patients with medical illness may also experience comorbid psychiatric illness, most commonly depression and anxiety. Evidence suggests that depression is significantly higher in individuals with medical illness than those without, with most of the studies being conducted in patients with human immunodeficiency virus (HIV), diabetes, heart disease, and cancer (Anderson et al., 2001; Dew et al., 1997; Egede et al., 2002; Frasure-Smith et al., 1995; Januzzi et al., 2000; Pirl and Roth, 1999; Spiegel and Giese-Davis, 2003). Comorbid depression and medical illness are particularly challenging because patients with depression are three times more likely to not adhere to medical treatment (DiMatteo et al., 2000).

MOTIVATION AND CHANGE

Motivation is an essential, but not sufficient, human factor predictive of success in effecting adaptive and permanent behavior change. One important consideration for health care and mental health care providers who assist patients in making behavioral change is the patient's willingness to change. Prochaska et al. (1992) have articulated this phenomenon through their transtheoretic model of change, which posits that achieving health behavior goals depends on the stages through which people pass in their attempt to bring about successful and maintained behavior change. Prochaska et al. have identified five stages of change: precontemplation, contemplation, preparation (or determination), action, and maintenance. These are split into lower, middle, and upper stages of change, based upon the extent to which the individual has taken steps toward change (see Table 21-1). Motivational interventions need to correspond to the relevant stage of change and typically focus on resolving patients' ambivalence about change and

TABLE 21-1 Motivation and Change		
Stage of Change		**Therapy Focus**
The lower stages of change	Precontemplative	Encourage self-exploration
	Contemplative	Resolve ambivalence
The middle stages of change	Preparation (or determination)	Problem solving
		Validate skills
		Identify social support
	Action	Self-efficacy
		Social support
		Overcome barriers to making behavioral change
		Begin focus on long-term benefits
The higher stages of change	Maintenance	Follow-up support
		Reinforce internal rewards
		Relapse prevention
After a relapse		Evaluate triggers to relapse
		Reassess motivation and barriers to making behavioral change
		Strengthen coping skills

bringing them to the next level. This technique is called *motivational interviewing* (MI) (Miller and Rollnick, 2002) and is described in more detail in the subsequent text.

Lower Stages of Change

In the precontemplation stage of change, an individual has neither the intention to change nor the awareness of a problem and hence is not ready to initiate change behaviors. During treatment, the health care provider would encourage self-exploration instead of action.

In the contemplation stage, the individual has become aware of his or her problem and is seriously considering overcoming it, yet has not made a commitment to action. The patient feels ambivalent about making behavioral changes. Interventions targeting motivation would examine the pros and cons of change while encouraging behavioral outcome expectations.

In these lower stages of change, the patient has not yet taken any action and may question why he or she should change. Treatment may focus on resolving the ambivalence.

Middle Stages of Change

In the preparation (or determination) stage of change, the individual already intends to take action and usually has unsuccessfully taken action within the past year or more. An individual at this stage is prepared for action but has not yet made an effective effort to reduce problematic behaviors. Behavioral medicine therefore focuses on problem solving (including removing obstacles to change), validating skills, identifying social support, and taking initial steps toward change. The action stage sees the individual modifying his or her experience, behavior, or environment to eliminate problematic behaviors. Accordingly, interventions focus on self-efficacy, social support, and overcoming barriers, all with an emphasis on long-term benefits.

Higher Stages of Change

In the higher stages of change, the patient has initiated health behavior change for the short term, and the focus shifts to long-term maintenance of new skills. In the maintenance phase, the individual is working to prevent relapse and extend gains made during the action stage. Behavioral medicine interventions focus on reinforcing internal rewards and planning for follow-up support and coping with any lapse or relapse into previous behaviors.

After the patient has achieved the maintenance stage, he or she may terminate treatment or relapse to previous behavior. After a relapse, therapy focuses on evaluating the triggers to relapse, reassessing motivation and barriers, and strengthening coping skills.

COMMON BEHAVIORAL MEDICINE TREATMENT STRATEGIES AND COGNITIVE BEHAVIORAL THERAPY

Behavioral medicine treatment strategies are generally short term (4 to 20 sessions) and focus on setting goals and monitoring progress toward them. Patients who may benefit from behavioral medicine intervention may have a chronic illness and a comorbid psychiatric disorder (e.g., HIV and depression), a subclinical psychiatric disorder (e.g., increased anxiety or depressive symptoms), or no psychiatric diagnosis but need help with self-care (e.g., diabetes, obesity, smoking cessation, problematic drinking, and substance abuse).

Behavioral medicine practitioners are skilled in implementing behavior change techniques, which are the basis of cognitive behavioral therapy (CBT) (see Chapter 23 for further discussion of CBT). Behavioral medicine strategies are both didactic (psychoeducation) and Socratic (psychotherapy). Fisher and Fisher (1992) posit that information alone is not enough to facilitate health-related behavioral change in patients with HIV; patients also require motivation and behavioral skills. Accordingly, behavioral medicine treatment strategies tend to incorporate both MI and CBT. Specific treatment strategies are discussed later.

Psychoeducation

As a foundation for further intervention techniques, the patient and therapist review the set of problems, information about the diagnosis, and the patient's self-care behavior. During a psychoeducation and/or feedback session, the therapist and patient conclude whether a behavioral medicine intervention is recommended and determine the costs and benefits of the treatment.

The therapist may further analyze the presenting problem, such as the connection between the patient's mood and adherence to self-care behaviors, providing information about how mood can negatively affect medical adherence; the therapist may also discuss the patient's symptoms and the CBT model of mood (cognitive–behavioral–physiological).

Motivational Interviewing

MI is a "client-centered directive method for enhancing intrinsic motivation to change by exploring and resolving ambivalence" (Miller and Rollnick, 2002). MI's goal is to bring an individual from an earlier stage of change (e.g., precontemplation or contemplation) to one in which the individual actually makes changes (e.g., preparation or action). Therapy works to resolve and explore the patient's ambivalence about making changes. A key component involves articulating and weighing the pros and cons of changing and not changing (see Table 21-2). To maximize motivation, it is important to acknowledge and validate both the pros of the status quo and the cons of change. Advising or directly persuading a patient to change typically does not have as strong an effect. Instead, the therapist works to develop a partnership with the patient and provides an atmosphere conducive to drawing out the patient's internal motivation to change (Miller and Rollnick, 2002).

Basic principles of MI include expressing empathy, developing discrepancy, rolling with resistance, and supporting self-efficacy. The therapist expresses empathy through reflective listening to understand and accept the patient's perspective, without judging the patient. The therapist then develops discrepancy by helping the patient understand the difference between stated goals and current behavior. Patients who successfully verbalize the discrepancy may then be motivated toward the necessary behaviors to bring about changes. The patient may become resistant to making changes, but instead of opposing the patient's resistance, the therapist asks for new takes on the situation and helps the patient develop answers to difficult circumstances. Finally, the therapist helps support the patient's belief that he or she can change and, in fact, is responsible for making the behavioral change required (Miller and Rollnick, 2002).

Activity Scheduling and Pacing

Patients with a medical illness often develop depression, which makes them three times more likely to not adhere to medical treatment (DiMatteo et al., 2000). A key component of depression is a drop in the frequency of pleasurable activities. Therefore, an important behavioral medicine technique is to work on pacing the patient's activities and to make sure that, despite a medical condition, the patient can continue to make informed decisions about how and when to maximize his or her ability to participate in enjoyable activities. Accordingly, monitoring activities, mood, and physical symptoms can make mood and physical symptoms more predictable and, consequently, more controllable.

TABLE 21-2 Sample Pros and Cons of Change		
	Pros	**Cons**
Changing Working to increase physical activity	Makes me feel better and less stressed Makes me stronger and more flexible Helps me manage my blood pressure and blood sugar Helps my cardiovascular health Increases my self-esteem	I will be more tired It may cause more pain, particularly muscle pain I will have less time for alternative activities, like spending time with my family I would have to get up even earlier in the morning to fit it in
Not changing Keeping things the way they are	I will stay comfortable I do not have to work hard or put effort into physical activity	My illness or disease may worsen I will be at an increased risk for a multitude of other diseases I will still have a really hard time playing ball with my daughter

Tools such as a positive events checklist (Blanchard and Hickling, 2006; Linehan, 1993; Safren et al., 2007a; Safren et al., 2007b) can be used to help individuals identify pleasurable events and increase involvement in these activities. Pacing then involves learning how to maximize activities when symptoms are less severe and maximize rest when symptoms are greater. Individuals learn their limits and patterns of behavior through self-monitoring.

Cognitive Restructuring

Cognitive restructuring is a traditional CBT technique in which patients learn how to complete a thought record to identify thoughts and cognitive distortions (Safren et al., 2007a; Safren et al., 2000b). Using the CBT model of the interrelatedness of mood, behavior, and cognition, patients will be able to challenge negative thoughts or beliefs about their illness or disability and/or associated mood symptoms. Accordingly, the idea is for patients to learn to think more realistically (or utilize adaptive thinking) both generally and specifically to help them participate in activity scheduling.

Mindfulness

Mindfulness is a key component of newer acceptance-based psychotherapies and particularly applies to coping with medical illnesses. Some medical stressors are real, uncontrollable, and life threatening (such as a terminal illness). In these situations, strategies such as cognitive restructuring need to be administered with caution, because some negative thoughts may actually be realistic.

"Mindfulness means paying attention in a particular way: on purpose, in the present moment, and nonjudgmentally" (Kabat-Zinn, 1994). It entails bringing the individual's awareness of his or her thoughts, feelings, and actions into the present moment and has been utilized with patients with a wide variety of illnesses, including heart disease, cancer, bipolar disorder, chronic pain, and anxiety disorders (Carlson et al., 2007; Williams et al., 2008; Kabat-Zinn et al., 1985, 1992; Tacon et al., 2003).

Problem Solving

Some evidence suggests that when confronted with a medical illness, individuals have greater difficulty solving problems. Hence, behavioral medicine practitioners help patients relearn effective problem solving. Typical steps involve orienting the individual to the problem, generating alternative behavioral responses, reviewing decision-making practices, and implementing the chosen solution(s) (D'Zurilla, 1986; D'Zurilla and Sheedy, 1991; Nezu et al., 1989, 1998). Problem-solving techniques are broken down into five components: articulate the problem, list all possible solutions, list the pros and cons of each solution, rate each solution, and implement the best option. With respect to the fifth step, the therapist assists the patient with identifying overwhelming tasks and breaking them down into manageable steps.

Relaxation and Stress Management

Relaxation and stress management interventions (e.g., diaphragmatic breathing, biofeedback, progressive muscle relaxation [PMR], and clinical hypnosis) work to control somatic symptoms of stress for patients with conditions such as cancer, high blood pressure, pain, irritable bowel syndrome, epilepsy, insomnia, myofascial pain, or headache. The patient is generally given recorded instructions of multiple relaxation techniques and encouraged to practice one or more daily, with emphasis on using subtle, brief versions in stressful situations (Cameron et al., 2007; Elkins et al., 2007; Flory et al., 2007; Hudacek, 2007; Kohen and Zajac, 2007; McGrady et al., 1986; Montgomery et al., 2007; Morgenthaler et al., 2006; Puskarich et al., 1992; Shaw et al., 1991).

Diaphragmatic Breathing

During diaphragmatic breathing exercises, patients are taught to focus on and bring awareness to their breathing state (shallow or deep) and to take deep, relaxing breaths from their diaphragm. Diaphragmatic breathing (or deep breathing) helps patients ground themselves and relax in times of stress and directly cope with symptoms.

Biofeedback

Biofeedback uses electronic sensors and computer technology to teach patients to control various physiological signals that are thought to play a role in maintaining their symptoms.

Heart rate, skeletal muscle activity, blood pressure, surface skin temperature, respiration, and galvanic skin response are the most common signals used in biofeedback training. For example, a patient may learn to reduce facial muscle activity by watching a continuous analog representation of the electromyographic (EMG) activity on a monitor, recorded from the frontalis muscle region. Patients may also be taught to monitor and raise the temperature of their hands, referred to as thermal biofeedback, as a useful intervention for migraine headaches.

Progressive Muscle Relaxation

During PMR training, patients are taught to systematically relax muscle groups throughout their bodies to reduce tension and anxiety. Patients learn to alternate between a tense and relaxed state, which results in an overall reduction in body tension. PMR is helpful in teaching patients how to relax in situations that may cause stress or pain.

Clinical Hypnosis

Clinical hypnosis is a procedure used to help patients attain a state of calm and relaxation and to facilitate therapy for headaches, chronic illness, pain, acute distress during medical procedures, cancer, and depression (Kohen and Zajac, 2007; Elkins et al., 2007; Flory et al., 2007; Hudacek, 2007; Montgomery et al., 2007).

Self-Monitoring

A common technique to aid behavioral modification is to teach patients to keep a daily log of the desired action (e.g., number of pills prescribed vs. those taken for the day, amount of exercise or sleep, and nutrition). Therapists and patients then work together to understand the functional analysis of the problems better, learn about antecedents and consequences, and further shape healthy behavior with the goal of gradually increasing it. Self-monitoring is the hallmark of lifestyle interventions.

Self-Regulation Interventions

Many patients who have difficulty adhering to their health care provider's recommendations also have difficulty with self-regulation behaviors. Assisting with medical adherence is a key component of behavioral medicine interventions. Providers can assist with adherence in several ways, such as MI, described in preceding text.

"Life-Steps," an intervention developed at Massachusetts General Hospital and Fenway Community Health, is a protocol designed for patients to increase their adherence to self-care behaviors (Safren et al., 1999). It has successfully assisted patients with HIV (Safren et al., 2001) and is part of a more intensive intervention that targets adherence and depression in medical illness (Safren et al., 2007a; Safren et al., 2007b). It is a single session that includes elements of CBT, problem solving, and MI (D'Zurilla, 1986; Miller and Rollnick, 1991) and targets psychoeducational motivation for adherence, getting to appointments, obtaining medications, coping with side effects, communicating with treatment providers, formulating a daily medication schedule, storing medications, cues for pill taking (cue control strategies), guided imagery (review of successful adherence in response to daily cues), responding to slips in adherence, and procedure review and phone follow-up.

Sleep Hygiene

Sleep loss has been associated with a host of medical comorbidities such as cardiovascular disease, stroke, obesity, depression, diabetes, and impaired immune function (Irwin et al., 1994; Plante, 2006; Riemann et al., 2001; Spiegel et al., 2005). Therapists work with patients to address environmental, cognitive, and behavioral components through stimulus control, CBT, paradoxical intention, biofeedback, and relaxation techniques (Edinger et al., 2005; Morgenthaler et al., 2006). Specific interventions include sleep restriction (i.e., restricting time in bed), eliminating naps during the day, setting a bedtime and awake time, and conditioning the bedroom with sleep (e.g., not spending >15 minutes in bed awake). The bedroom environment is also a key part of sleep hygiene; the patient learns to keep the room at a steady temperature (fluctuations may disrupt sleep state) and dark (e.g., eliminating illuminated wall clocks, putting

TABLE 21-3   Illnesses and Treatment Techniques

Condition	Major Behavioral Issues	Common Interventions
Asthma	Medication adherence Trigger avoidance Anxiety Self-monitoring symptoms (e.g., lung functioning)	Adherence training Problem solving Stress reduction Cognitive restructuring Self-monitoring
Cancer (medical illness comorbid with anxiety)	Self-care Navigating medical system Anxiety	Adherence training Cognitive restructuring Stress reduction Mindfulness Exposure-based therapies
Cardiac disease (e.g., coronary artery disease)	Medication adherence Lifestyle change[a] Anxiety Depression	Adherence training Self-monitoring Cognitive restructuring Problem solving Activity scheduling Stress management
Chronic illness (e.g., tuberculosis, epilepsy, end-stage renal disease) or organ transplant	Self-care Depression Medication adherence Lifestyle change Navigating medical system	Adherence training Cognitive restructuring Activity scheduling Problem solving
Diabetes mellitus	Blood glucose monitoring Medication adherence Keeping appointments Depression Lifestyle change	Adherence training Self-monitoring Cognitive restructuring Activity scheduling
Hepatitis C (e.g., interferon therapy)	Medication adherence Depression	Adherence training Cognitive restructuring
HIV/acquired immunodeficiency syndrome (AIDS)	Navigating medical system Medication adherence Depression	Adherence training Cognitive restructuring Activity scheduling
Hypertension	Lifestyle change Medication adherence Depression	Adherence training Activity scheduling Self-monitoring Problem solving Cognitive restructuring
Obesity	Lifestyle change Depression Anxiety Continuous positive airway pressure (CPAP) compliance	Self-monitoring Adherence training Cognitive restructuring Activity scheduling Stress reduction Sleep hygiene
Pain	Anxiety Depression	Activity scheduling Adherence training Sleep hygiene Problem solving

[a]For example, nutrition, physical activity.

shades on windows, and using a sleep mask). Because sleeping is associated with a decline in core body temperature from a state of warmth, patients are taught tips to increase their core body temperature by exercising a few hours before bed or taking a warm bath 20 minutes before bed. Finally, patients are taught to reduce or eliminate stimulants (caffeine and nicotine) and depressants (alcohol), because they may disrupt the sleep cycle, and encouraged to self-monitor all sleep behaviors (e.g., napping, bedtime, and number and duration of awakenings) to review and make behavioral changes as needed.

BEHAVIORAL MEDICINE INTERVENTIONS COMBINED WITH PSYCHIATRIC ILLNESS

Behavioral medicine therapists typically see patients struggling to cope with or adhere to a medical illness regimen in the context of a psychiatric disorder. There are few current, specific protocols for such an approach; however, most behavioral medicine therapists utilize an integration of CBT for the particular disorder and behavioral medicine techniques.

Massachusetts General Hospital developed one such treatment program (Safren et al., 1999), which incorporates CBT for depression. It is modular and includes psychoeducation about CBT and MI (one session); adherence training (Life-Steps) (one session); activity scheduling (one session); cognitive restructuring (three sessions); problem solving (three sessions); relaxation training and diaphragmatic breathing (one session); and a review with discussion of maintenance and relapse prevention. This intervention has been successfully tested in patients with HIV, revealing increased adherence and decreased depression in two open phase studies (Safren et al., 2004; Soroudi et al., 2008) and one randomized controlled trial (Safren et al., 2009). Currently it is being tested in HIV-infected methadone patients and individuals with depression and diabetes.

CONCLUSION

Making necessary behavioral changes is integral to treatment for many medical conditions. This chapter reviewed behavioral medicine as it can be practiced in an outpatient or general hospital setting. Behavioral medicine practitioners are vital contributors to the welfare of the patient, whether through MI, cognitive behavioral strategies to promote treatment adherence, newer acceptance-based psychotherapies, and integrating the treatment of a psychiatric disorder such as depression with improving or maintaining the self-care behaviors needed to manage a medical illness. Specific examples of treatment interventions are provided in Table 21-3. By integrating behavioral medicine treatment into clinical care, practitioners can help their patients manage chronic illness.

Clinical Pearls

- Depression is significantly higher in individuals with medical illness than those without, and patients with depression are three times more likely to not adhere to medical treatment.
- Information alone is not enough to facilitate health-related behavioral change: patients also require motivation and behavioral skills.
- The goal of motivational interviewing is to bring patients from a lower stage of change to one in which they actually make changes (e.g., preparation or action).
- In the lower stages of change (precontemplative and contemplative), treatment may focus on resolving ambivalence about change.
- Directing a patient to change through persuasion or giving advice typically does not have as strong an effect.
- Most people know how to relax or solve problems, but they do not spend the necessary time focusing on putting these changes into place. Therapy can help patients remove barriers to make desired behavioral changes.

Self-Assessment Questions and Answers

21-1. A 45-year-old obese father of three sees a physician for his diabetes. The physician refers him to a behavioral medicine program for help with weight loss. The patient has a history of unsuccessful attempts at losing weight that he ultimately gives up because of his family's hectic schedule. He usually ends up eating in his car or at his children's sporting events. In which stage(s) of change is he?
   A. Contemplative stage
   B. Determination stage
   C. Maintenance stage
   D. Contemplative stage and preparation stage
   E. Determination stage and preparation stage

21-2. What kind of intervention would be appropriate to move him to the next stage?
   A. Behavioral modification
   B. Planning for coping with relapse
   C. Problem solving
   D. Reinforcing internal rewards
   E. Resolving ambivalence about taking action

   The man is in the middle stage of change, specifically the determination–preparation stage. He intends to take action and has a history of failed attempts. He is prepared but has not been successful in reducing problematic behaviors. An effective method would be to help him with problem solving to eat healthy and increase physical activity. He has already resolved any ambivalence about changing his behavior. Employing behavioral modification occurs in the next stage of change. Planning for relapse and reinforcing internal rewards are for people who have already changed behavior and are maintaining it (Prochaska et al., 1992). *Answers: E, C*

21-3. At a regular visit with her therapist, a 35-year-old woman with breast cancer reports having a higher level of anxiety than before her diagnosis, which is interfering with her care. Which of the following would be an appropriate intervention?
   A. Activity scheduling
   B. Mindfulness

   C. Problem solving
   D. Self-monitoring
   E. Sleep hygiene

   Mindfulness is an effective method in reducing anxiety and coping with a diagnosis. Self-monitoring, activity scheduling, and problem solving would not be appropriate because cancer treatments are largely out of the patient's hands and often cause fatigue. Therefore, a psychiatrist would not encourage more activity. Sleep hygiene is not necessary because she is not losing sleep (Carlson et al., 2007). *Answer: B*

21-4. Which of the following is a basic principle of motivational interviewing?
   A. Challenging thoughts
   B. Confronting resistance
   C. Developing discrepancy
   D. Discouraging self-efficacy
   E. Expressing frustration

   Challenging thoughts is a technique used in CBT as part of cognitive restructuring. MI is a separate tool that includes expressing empathy, developing discrepancy, rolling with resistance, and supporting self-efficacy (Miller and Rollnick, 2002; Safren et al., 2007a; Safren et al., 2007b). *Answer: C*

21-5. Brian, a 25-year-old graduate student, is having trouble sleeping. He finds that he is tired, but when he gets into bed, he lies awake for hours before finally falling asleep. What recommendation for sleep hygiene may help him sleep?
   A. Count backward from 1000.
   B. Drink a glass of warm milk.
   C. Leave the bedroom curtains open to keep the body in tune with the outdoors.
   D. Start restricting the amount of time spent awake in bed.
   E. Take an over-the-counter antihistamine.

   Drinking warm milk and counting backward are old wives' tales and would work against sleep restriction, a useful part of sleep hygiene. Bedroom shades are encouraged, because the room is best kept dark. Although taking an antihistamine would help Brian fall asleep, this is not a good permanent solution. *Answer: D*

References

Anderson RJ, Freedland KE, Clouse RE, et al. The prevalence of comorbid depression in adults with diabetes: A meta-analysis. *Diabetes Care.* 2001;24:1069–1078.

Blanchard EB, Hickling EJ. *Overcoming the trauma of your motor vehicle accident: A cognitive behavioral treatment program workbook.* New York: Oxford University Press; 2006.

Cameron LD, Booth RJ, Schlatter M, et al. Changes in emotion regulation and psychological adjustment following use of a group psychosocial support program for women recently diagnosed with breast cancer. *Psychooncology*. 2007;16:171–180.

Carlson LE, Speca M, Faris P, et al. One year pre-post intervention follow-up of psychological, immune, endocrine and blood pressure outcomes of mindfulness-based stress reduction (MBSR) in breast and prostate cancer outpatients. *Brain Behav Immun*. 2007;21:1038–1049.

Dew MA, Becker JT, Sanchez J, et al. Prevalence and predictors of depressive, anxiety and substance use disorders in HIV-infected and uninfected men: A longitudinal evaluation. *Psychol Med*. 1997;27:395–409.

DiMatteo MR, Lepper HS, Groghan TW. Depression is a risk factor for noncompliance with medical treatment: Meta-analysis of the effects of anxiety and depression on patient adherence. *Arch Intern Med*. 2000;160(14):2101–2107.

D'Zurilla TJ. *Problem solving therapy: A social competence approach to clinical interventions*. New York: Springer; 1986.

D'Zurilla TJ, Sheedy CF. Relation between social problem-solving ability and subsequent level of psychological stress in college students. *J Pers Soc Psychol*. 1991;61:841–846.

Edinger JD, Wohlgemuth WK, Krystal AD, et al. Behavioral insomnia therapy for fibromyalgia patients: A randomized clinical trial. *Arch Intern Med*. 2005;165(21):2527–2535.

Egede LE, Zheng D, Simpson K. Comorbid depression is associated with increased health care use and expenditures in individuals with diabetes. *Diabetes Care*. 2002;25:464–470.

Elkins G, Jensen MP, Patterson DR. Hypnotherapy for the management of chronic pain. *Int J Clin Exp Hypn*. 2007;55:275–287.

Fisher JD, Fisher WA. Changing AIDS-risk behavior. *Psychol Bull*. 1992;111:455–474.

Flory N, Martinez Salazar GM, Lang EV. Hypnosis for acute distress management during medical procedures. *Int J Clin Exp Hypn*. 2007;55:303–317.

Frasure-Smith N, Lesperance F, Talajic M. Depression and 18-month prognosis after myocardial infarction. *Circulation*. 1995;91:999–1005.

Hudacek KD. A review of the effects of hypnosis on the immune system in breast cancer patients: A brief communication. *Int J Clin Exp Hypn*. 2007;55:411–425.

Irwin M, Mascovich A, Gillin JC. Partial sleep deprivation reduced natural killer cell activity in humans. *Psychosom Med*. 1994;56:493–498.

Januzzi JL, Stern TA, Pasternick RC, et al. The influence of anxiety and depression on outcomes of patients with coronary artery disease. *Arch Intern Med*. 2000;160:1913–1921.

Kabat-Zinn J. *Wherever you go, there you are: Mindfulness meditation in everyday life*. New York: Hyperion; 1994.

Kabat-Zinn J, Lipworth L, Burney R. The clinical use of mindfulness meditation for the self-regulation of chronic pain. *J Behav Med*. 1985;8:163–190.

Kabat-Zinn J, Massion AO, Kristeller J, et al. Effectiveness of a meditation-based stress reduction program in the treatment of anxiety disorders. *Am J Psychiatry*. 1992;149:936–943.

Kohen DP, Zajac R. Self-hypnosis training for headaches in children and adolescents. *J Pediatr*. 2007;150:635–639.

Linehan M. *Skills training manual for treating borderline personality disorder*. New York: Guilford Press; 1993.

Masek BM, Scharff L. Behavioral medicine. In: Stern T, Fricchione G, Cassem N, et al., eds. *Massachusetts general hospital handbook of general hospital psychiatry*. Boston: Elsevier Science; 2004.

McGrady A, Woerner M, Argueta Bernal GA, et al. Effect of biofeedback-assisted relaxation on blood pressure and cortisol levels in normotensives and hypertensives. *J Behav Med*. 1986;10:301–310.

Miller WR, Rollnick S. *Motivational interviewing: Preparing people to change addictive behavior*. New York: Guilford Press; 1991.

Miller WR, Rollnick S. *Motivational interviewing: Preparing people for change*, 2nd ed. New York: Guilford Press; 2002.

Montgomery GH, Bovbjerg DH, Schnur JB, et al. A randomized clinical trial of a brief hypnosis intervention to control side effects in breast surgery patients. *J Natl Cancer Inst*. 2007;99:1304–1312.

Morgenthaler T, Kramer M, Alessi C, et al. Practice parameters for the psychological and behavioral treatment of insomnia: An update. An American Academy of sleep medicine report. *Sleep*. 2006;29:1415–1419.

Nezu AM, Nezu CM, Friedman SH, et al. *Helping cancer patients cope: A problem-solving approach*. Washington, DC: American Psychological Association; 1998.

Nezu AM, Nezu CM, Perri MG. *Problem-solving therapy for depression: Theory, research, and clinical guidelines*. England: John Wiley and Sons; 1989.

Pirl WF, Roth AJ. Diagnosis and treatment of depression in cancer patients. *Oncology (Huntingt)*. 1999;13: 1293–1301.

Plante GE. Sleep and vascular disorders. *Metabolism*. 2006;55:S45–S49.

Prochaska JO, DiClemente CO, Norcross JC. In search of how people change: Applications to addictive behaviors. *Am Psychol*. 1992;47:1102–1114.

Puskarich CA, Whitman S, Dell J, et al. Controlled examination of effects of progressive relaxation training on seizure reduction. *Epilepsia*. 1992;33:675–680.

Riemann D, Berger M, Voderholzer U. Sleep and depression—results from psychobiological studies: An overview. *Biol Psychol*. 2001;57(1-3):67–103.

Safren S, Gonzalez J, Soroudi N. *CBT for depression and adherence in individuals with chronic illness: Client workbook (Treatments that Work)*. New York: Oxford Press; 2007a.

Safren S, Gonzalez J, Soroudi N. *CBT for depression and adherence in individuals with chronic illness: Therapist guide (Treatments that Work)*. New York: Oxford Press; 2007b.

Safren SA, Hendriksen ES, Mayer KH, et al. Cognitive behavioral therapy for HIV medication adherence and depression. *Cogn Behav Pract*. 2004;11:415–423.

Safren SA, O'Cleirigh C, Tan J, et al. A randomized controlled trial of cognitive behavioral therapy for adherence and depression (CBT AD) in HIV infected individuals. *Health Psychol*. 2009;28:1–10.

Safren SA, Otto MW, Worth J. Life-steps: Applying cognitive-behavioral therapy to patient adherence to HIV medication treatment. *Cogn Behav Pract*. 1999;6:332–341.

Safren SA, Otto MW, Worth JL, et al. Two strategies to increase adherence to HIV antiretroviral medication: Life-steps and medication monitoring. *Behav Res Ther*. 2001;39(10):1151–1162.

Schwartz GE, Weiss SM. Yale conference on behavioral medicine: A proposed definition and statement of goals. *J Behav Med*. 1978;1:3–12.

Shaw G, Srivastava ED, Sadlier M, et al. Stress management for irritable bowel syndrome: A controlled trial. *Digestion*. 1991;50:36–42.

Shumaker SA, Schron EB, Ockene JK, et al. *The handbook of health behavior change*, 2nd ed. New York: Springer; 1998.

Soroudi N, Perez GK, Gonzalez JS, et al. CBT for medication adherence and depression (CBT-AD) in HIV-infected individuals receiving methadone maintenance therapy. *Cogn Behav Pract*. 2008;15:93–106.

Spiegel D, Giese-Davis J. Depression and cancer: Mechanisms and disease progression. *Biol Psychiatry*. 2003;54:269–282.

Spiegel K, Knutson K, Leproult R, et al. Sleep loss: A novel risk factor for insulin resistance and Type 2 diabetes. *J Appl Physiol*. 2005;99:2008–2019.

Tacon AM, McComb J, Caldera Y, et al. Mindfulness meditation, anxiety reduction, and heart disease: A pilot study. *Fam Community Health*. 2003;26:25–33.

Williams JMG, Alatiq Y, Crane C, et al. Mindfulness-based Cognitive Therapy (MBCT) in bipolar disorder: Preliminary evaluation of immediate effects on between-episode functioning. *J Affect Disord*. 2008;107(1-3):275–279.

22

Minninder J. Sandhu, Steven J. Garlow, and Charles B. Nemeroff

Psychopharmacological Therapies

Psychopharmacology is the field of pharmacology specifically focused on psychoactive agents, that is, substances that impact mental processes, including emotional, behavioral, cognitive, sensorial, and other domains. Throughout history, almost every culture has sought ways to alter consciousness and influence the mind by experimenting with plants and herbal remedies. With the advent of the scientific revolution, the use of traditional herbal remedies fell out of favor with the mainstream medical establishment. The latter half of the 20th century celebrated the inception of a new era of medicine, including psychiatry, in which an upsurge of research led to the discovery and testing of many new drugs. The formal use of psychiatric drugs to restore mental health was implemented in Western medicine in the 1950s, when a number of new classes of drugs were discovered, notably, barbiturates, lithium, antipsychotics, and antidepressants. For the first time in history, psychiatric diseases began to be viewed as medical problems requiring medical solutions.

Most of the original psychiatric drugs were discovered serendipitously. However, after careful study, researchers developed a deeper level of understanding of both brain functioning and the mechanism of action of this first generation of psychopharmacological agents. The breakthrough finding was the discovery of the nature of chemical neurotransmission, recognizing that neurons within particular brain regions contained and utilized different neurotransmitters. The brain began to be viewed as a stable, organized, dynamic set of neural circuits. Antipsychotic drugs were discovered to block certain dopamine (DA) receptors, and this property was correlated with therapeutic efficacy. The now well-known DA hypothesis of schizophrenia was proposed and led to further understanding of psychotic illnesses. Mood disorders were suggested to be due to alterations in monoaminergic neurotransmission. This theory, known as the *monoamine hypothesis*, provided the theoretical framework for the development of the monoamine oxidase inhibitors (MAOIs) and the tricyclic antidepressants (TCAs).

Today, these theories are considered too simplistic to precisely explain the mechanism of action of antipsychotics and antidepressants. Despite several decades of investigation, the mechanism(s) of various centrally acting drugs remains unclear. Nonetheless, our understanding of psychopharmacology and the biology of the underlying psychiatric disorders has grown exponentially. Although a cure for many mental illnesses is still beyond our reach, it is clear that the treatment of mental illness has evolved dramatically in the last half century. The future development of psychopharmacology depends on continued research into the pathophysiology of psychiatric disease.

BASIC PHARMACOLOGY: PHARMACOKINETICS AND PHARMACODYNAMICS

Pharmacology is the study of how exogenously administered agents interact with and alter the functions of biological systems. Related to the practice of medicine, this is the study of how agents with medicinal properties (drugs, medicines, pharmaceuticals) interact with human beings. Inevitably, pharmaceutical agents have both positive and negative effects, and one of the essential roles of a physician is to understand the properties of medications and balance therapeutic benefits against potential adverse impacts, with the ultimate goal of improving the condition of the patient.

Pharmacokinetics formally refers to the time course of a drug in the body, sometimes described as "what the body does to the drug." The concentration of the drug at any moment in the body is dependent on its pharmacokinetic properties. *Pharmacodynamics* refers to the biochemical and physiological impact of a pharmaceutical agent on an organism, sometimes described as "what the drug does to the body." The specific targets to which a drug binds and the biochemical, physiological, and behavioral consequences of that interaction are defined through the pharmacodynamic properties of that agent. Understanding pharmacokinetics, pharmacodynamics, and the interaction of both is essential to the effective practice of psychiatry. Therapeutic benefit, adverse events, and drug–drug interactions can be understood by the interaction of pharmacokinetic and pharmacodynamic properties of medications.

The pharmacokinetic properties of a drug are dependent on a series of interrelated biochemical and physiological reactions, which can be remembered by the acronym LADME: **l**iberation of the active agent from the administered form, **a**bsorption into the circulatory system, **d**istribution into the various body compartments, **m**etabolic transformation, and **e**xcretion from the body. Although these are discrete processes, they occur simultaneously, such that the pharmacokinetic profile of a drug is a composite of all five processes.

The *volume of distribution* of a drug is the total bodily fluid in which the drug is dissolved, that is, the total amount of drug in the body (generally reflected in the dose) divided by its serum concentration. Drugs that have low lipid solubility, and hence stay in the aqueous compartments, have a lower volume of distribution than agents that are highly lipid soluble. *Clearance* of a drug is defined as the volume of plasma or other bodily fluid from which a drug is irreversibly eliminated in a given unit of time. Elimination *half-life* (signified with $t_{1/2}$) is the time it takes for the concentration of a drug to be reduced by 50%. This variable is important in determining dosing regimens for medications. After a single dose of an agent, 94% will be eliminated after four half-lives have elapsed. In a practical sense, steady state concentrations of a drug will be obtained with repeated doses administered at the half-life interval over four to five half-lives, if the dose is held constant. *Bioavailability* refers to the amount of the active drug that ultimately makes it to the site of action. Practically this refers to the amount of active drug that reaches the circulatory system. A wide range of factors, some intrinsic to the formulation of the medication and some to physiological and biochemical characteristics of individual patients, influence the bioavailability of a drug. Many pharmaceutical agents bind to soluble proteins in the circulatory system, in particular, to albumin and α-1-acid glycoprotein. The specificity and strength of drug–protein interactions are described through pharmacodynamic variables, and the interaction of both pharmacological processes affects the use of specific agents. Protein binding influences bioavailability in that only the drug that is free in the serum is available to interact with the therapeutic targets and, in the case of psychopharmacological agents, to cross the blood–brain barrier (BBB) into the central nervous system (CNS). Some drugs compete for the same protein binding sites and can have significant influence on the functional blood level of each other.

Central to the elimination of many pharmaceutical agents from the body is the metabolic processing by hepatic enzymes. The hepatic drug metabolizing enzymes are part of the heme-containing cytochrome P450 (CYP450) super family of proteins. The CYP450 enzymes are central to oxidative metabolism of exogenously administered drugs and toxins and of endogenous compounds. The most abundant CYP450 in the liver and gastrointestinal (GI) tract is the CYP3A4 isozyme that utilizes a very wide range of pharmaceutical compounds, including many important psychotherapeutic medications, as substrates. The CYP2D6 isozyme also participates in the metabolism of many psychopharmacological agents. Table 22-1 lists some relevant substrates, inhibitors, and inducers of the CYP450 system.

The term *hepatic enzyme* is a misnomer, because many of these proteins also reside in the mucosal lining of the intestine and actively metabolize drugs during absorption from the GI tract, although 70% of this activity is from CYP3A4. *First-pass metabolism* refers to the process wherein an orally administered drug that is absorbed from the GI tract is metabolized by the CYP450 enzymes in the gut wall and liver, before entering the general circulatory system. This affects the bioavailability of the compound because it reduces the amount reaching the circulation, but, depending on the agent, may generate pharmacologically active metabolites.

Compounds that alter the activity of the CYP450 enzymes can have a dramatic effect on bioavailability. Some agents, known as *enzyme inducers*, induce the synthesis of additional CYP450 enzyme, which causes a decrease in the concentration of compounds metabolized by

TABLE 22-1 Psychiatric Medications That Are Substrates of Various CYP450 Enzymes			
CYP450	**Substrates**	**Inhibitors**	**Inducers**
CYP1A2	Clozapine, haloperidol, imipramine, tacrine	Ciprofloxacin, fluvoxamine	Carbon containing combustion products (tobacco, marijuana smoke, charcoal cooked meats), cruciferous vegetables, omeprazole
CYP2C9	Amitriptyline, metoclopramide, phenytoin, propranolol	Sulfaphenazole	Rifampin
CYP2C19	Amitriptyline, clomipramine, imipramine, diazepam, desmethyldiazepam, moclobemide	Omeprazole	Rifampin
CYP2D6	Amitriptyline, desipramine, haloperidol, imipramine, nortriptyline, paroxetine, risperidone, thiorodazine, venlafaxine, pindolol, propranolol	Fluoxetine, paroxetine, quinidine, sertraline	
CYP3A4	Alprazolam, amitriptyline, bupropion, carbamazepine, clonazepam, codeine, desmethyldiazepam, diazepam, fluoxetine, haloperidol, imipramine, midazolam, nefazodone, sertraline, trazodone, triazolam, venlafaxine, zolpidem	Fluoxetine, fluvoxamine, ketoconazole, naringenin (grapefruit), nefazodone, sertraline	

This list is not comprehensive for all potential interactions by other classes of medications.

the induced isozyme. Some drugs and other substances are *inhibitors* of CYP450 enzymes, which cause increased concentrations of drugs that are the substrates of the inhibited enzyme.

Genetic differences in expression and activity of CYP450 enzymes have been described that affect the bioavailability of compounds on an individual basis. Various diagnostic tests are being developed to measure these genetic differences and form the basis of the emerging field of "individually tailored pharmacotherapy," wherein medications and dosages are chosen on the basis of the predicted drug metabolizing profile of an individual patient.

The dose–response relationship between drug and effect depends on many different parameters, including the chemical characteristics of the agent and the biochemical and physiological milieu of the individual patient. The sum of the specific interactions between a pharmaceutical compound and all the targets with which it interacts in the body will determine its therapeutic action as well as its side effect and adverse outcomes profile. The serum concentration of a medication in which 50% of some particular response has been realized is referred to as the EC_{50}. The difference between therapeutic EC_{50} and toxic EC_{50} values is known as the *therapeutic window* for that drug. The wider the gap between these values, the safer the drug will be in clinical practice. Ideally the serum concentration for therapeutic EC_{50} would be several orders of magnitude removed from the EC_{50} for a limiting toxicity.

ANTIPSYCHOTIC DRUGS

The first antipsychotic medication, chlorpromazine, a phenothiazine derivative, was discovered serendipitously while researchers were searching for new antimalarial drugs. After chlorpromazine was shown to be effective as an antipsychotic medication, other phenothiazine derivatives, including haloperidol and thiothixene, were synthesized. Shortly after antipsychotic use became prevalent, psychiatrists began to notice in their patients signs of what are now known as *extrapyramidal symptoms* or *EPS*. This tendency of antipsychotics to mimic neurologic illness led to the use of the term *neuroleptic*. In the 1990s, several atypical, or second-generation, antipsychotics were launched onto the market. Because these new medications advertised equal efficacy but significantly less EPS than the classic antipsychotics (also known as *typical*, or *first-generation*), they soon came into favor. Since the 1990s, the use of typical antipsychotics has drastically declined because they have been largely replaced by the atypical antipsychotics. Whether these newer agents are truly more efficacious or have significantly lower side effect burdens than first-generation antipsychotics remains an active topic of scientific debate.

Antipsychotic medications treat psychotic symptoms, which may include hallucinations, delusions, disorganized speech, and disorganized or catatonic behavior. The aforementioned symptoms are generally categorized as positive symptoms of psychosis. Negative symptoms comprise restriction of affect, emotional withdrawal, apathy, anhedonia, lack of motivation, and impaired abstraction. Antipsychotic medications are relatively ineffective in treating negative symptoms, though the second-generation antipsychotics may be somewhat superior in this regard.

The primary indications for antipsychotic medications are schizophrenia, schizoaffective disorder, psychotic depression, and mania as well as acute agitation related to any of these diagnoses. Additionally, antipsychotics are clearly effective in treating psychotic symptoms that result from other etiologies, including substance-induced psychoses, delirium, dementia, and other medical/neurologic causes of psychosis. In recent years, it has also become apparent that antipsychotics are efficacious in various phases of bipolar disorder, including nonpsychotic mania, and many second-generation antipsychotics have gained U.S. Food and Drug Administration (FDA) approval for bipolar illness (Geodon, 2005; Seroquel, 2005; Symbyax, 2007). There is accumulating evidence that all of the second-generation antipsychotics are effective in converting patients with unipolar major depression who are antidepressant nonresponders into responders.

Dysfunction of DA containing neurocircuits is critically related to the biological basis of primary psychotic illness (e.g., schizophrenia). There are four major dopaminergic pathways in the brain. One such pathway, the mesolimbic, projects from the ventral tegmental area of the brain stem to the limbic areas of the brain. Hyperactivity, or an increase in DA neurotransmission, in this pathway produces positive symptoms of psychosis (Stahl, 2002). All known antipsychotic drugs treat positive symptoms by blocking DA receptors, particularly D_2 receptors.

Unfortunately, antipsychotic medications cannot preferentially block the mesolimbic pathway; instead, they block all four of the brain's dopaminergic pathways to some extent. A DA deficit in the mesocortical pathway has been posited to worsen negative symptoms and, possibly, the cognitive impairment seen in psychotic illnesses (Stahl, 2002). Deficiencies in the nigrostriatal pathway cause movement disorders, most notably Parkinson disease (PD); consequently, a blockade of DA receptors in this pathway, which occurs with all antipsychotic medications, can cause difficulties that mimic primary movement disorders (Stahl, 2002). The fourth and final DA pathway is the hypothalamic tuberoinfundibular tract (Stahl, 2002). DA in this pathway normally inhibits prolactin release; when the DA receptors on the anterior pituitary are blocked (as with antipsychotic medications), hyperprolactinemia can result. The essential mechanism of action of all antipsychotic medications thus far developed is primarily mediated through DA receptor antagonism, more specifically, DA D_2 receptor blockade in the mesolimbic pathway. Decades ago, the emergence of EPS was believed to signal adequacy of antipsychotic dose. However, researchers later discovered that EPS emerges with blockade of 80% or more of D_2 receptors in the nigrostriatal pathway; only 65% to 70% D_2 receptor occupancy is needed for maximal antipsychotic response (Wilkaitis et al., 2004). In addition, D_2 blockade in the mesocortical pathway apparently contributes to the cognitive blunting seen in patients treated with these agents.

Typical Antipsychotics (First Generation)

The first class of typical antipsychotics was the phenothiazines, which share a structural similarity. This class includes chlorpromazine (Thorazine), thioridazine (Mellaril), mesoridazine (Serentil), fluphenazine (Prolixin), perphenazine (Trilafon), and trifluoperazine (Stelazine). The thioxanthenes are a second class of typical antipsychotics, comprising chlorprothixene (Taractan) and thiothixene (Navane). Haloperidol belongs to a third class known as the *butyrophenones*. The only FDA-approved agent within the dibenzoxapine class is loxapine, which is somewhat unique among the typical antipsychotics in that it is structurally most like clozapine and, pharmacologically, blocks both DA and serotonin (5-HT) receptors. Molindone (Moban), the only member of the dihydroindoles, is unique in that it is not associated with any weight gain or seizure risk, unlike other typical antipsychotics.

Typical antipsychotics are primarily indicated for the treatment of schizophrenia and schizoaffective disorder and are still currently used for these disorders. This class of medications is best utilized in treating positive symptoms of psychosis; its major disadvantages are the inability to improve negative symptoms and the propensity to cause EPS and tardive dyskinesia (TD). Pimozide is a typical antipsychotic that is the only drug which is FDA approved for treatment of the tics of Tourette syndrome. Some lower-potency antipsychotics such as chlorpromazine are occasionally used for the treatment of nausea as well as intractable hiccups (Wilkaitis et al., 2004).

One of the greatest problems in the treatment of schizophrenia is medication nonadherence and consequent repeated psychotic relapse. In community and outpatient settings, 70% to 80% of patients are either partially or totally nonadherent (Weiden, 1997). In an effort to manage this problem, depot (long-acting) antipsychotic preparations were created with the hope of improved adherence (Nasrallah, 2007). There is considerable evidence that depot medications do, in fact, reduce the risk of relapse (Schooler, 2003). Currently, haloperidol and fluphenazine are the only *typical* antipsychotics available in a depot form. Fluphenazine decanoate must be administered every 2 weeks, whereas haloperidol decanoate, due to its longer half-life, may be given every 4 weeks. Use of these long-acting preparations should always be preceded by a trial of the oral formulation to determine therapeutic benefit and tolerability (Wilkaitis et al., 2004).

Typical antipsychotics are all considered equally effective, but they differ in potency and side effects. Drug potency refers to the milligram equivalence of drugs. Therefore, although haloperidol is more potent than chlorpromazine (2 mg haloperidol = 100 mg chlorpromazine), at therapeutically equivalent doses they are equally effective. As a rule, among the first-generation antipsychotics, the high-potency antipsychotic drugs (haloperidol, thiothixene, fluphenazine) have a high propensity for EPS and low levels of sedation and autonomic side effects. Conversely, low-potency antipsychotic drugs (chlorpromazine, thioridazine) tend to be sedating and produce autonomic side effects but have a lower propensity for EPS. Those antipsychotic drugs with intermediate potency (perphenazine) have a side effect profile intermediate between that of these two classes of antipsychotic drugs.

In addition to their effects on DA receptors, typical antipsychotics act on many other neurotransmitter receptors, which accounts for many of the side effects associated with this group of medications. Typical antipsychotics are antagonists at muscarinic cholinergic receptors, α-adrenergic receptors, and histamine (H_1) receptors. Anticholinergic side effects include dry mouth, blurred vision, nausea, constipation, urinary retention, cognitive impairment/confusion, prolonged QRS interval, and open-angle glaucoma crisis. α-adrenergic side effects include orthostatic hypotension, dizziness, QRS or QTc prolongation, reflex tachycardia, incontinence, and sedation. Cardiac dysrhythmias (such as torsades de pointes) and sudden death can result from the prolongation of QRS and QTc intervals, with thioridazine having been most associated with this adverse event. A baseline electrocardiogram (ECG) is recommended before treatment with thioridazine, mesoridazine, or pimozide (American Psychiatric Association, 2004). Of note, mesoridazine, chlorpromazine, and thioridazine are the most potent α_1 receptor antagonists of the antipsychotic drugs. Finally, antihistaminic side effects include sedation and weight gain (see Table 22-2).

Other side effects of typical antipsychotics include an increased seizure risk because these agents have been shown to lower seizure threshold. Some typical antipsychotics are associated with sexual side effects in both men and women, including erectile dysfunction and anorgasmia. Thioridazine may produce painful retrograde ejaculation, in which semen is ejected into the bladder. This typical antipsychotic is also associated with a pigmentary retinopathy that can lead to blindness. Many patients treated with typical antipsychotics become more sensitive to the effects of sunlight, which can lead to severe sunburn. Hyperprolactinemia commonly occurs with typical antipsychotics because of D_2 receptor blockade in the anterior pituitary. Elevated prolactin levels are associated with galactorrhea, gynecomastia, amenorrhea, infertility, and sexual dysfunction.

Most of the typical antipsychotics are metabolized in the liver by the CYP450 enzymes 2D6 and 3A4. This becomes clinically relevant when these medications are administered in conjunction with 2D6 or 3A4 inhibitors.

TABLE 22-2 Histaminic α-Adrenergic Muscarinic (HAM) Side Effects

Histaminic	α-Adrenergic	Muscarinic
Sedation	Orthostasis	Dry mouth
Weight gain	Reflex tachycardia	Blurred vision
	QTc prolongation	Constipation
	Drowsiness	Urinary retention
		Confusion

(Wilkaitis et al., 2004.)

Extrapyramidal Symptoms

EPS refers to a set of adverse reactions that are induced by antipsychotic medications. The four main subcategories of EPS include akathisia, acute dystonias, parkinsonism, and TD. The mechanism of acute dystonias and parkinsonian symptoms is secondary to blockade of D_2 receptors in the striatum that results in a relative increase in cholinergic activity (Glazer, 2000). One way to maintain the DA/ACh balance is to coadminister an anticholinergic medication (e.g., benztropine) along with the typical antipsychotic.

With the potential exceptions of high doses of risperidone and paliperidone, atypical antipsychotics have decreased risk of EPS compared with typical antipsychotics (Glazer, 2000). Patients who develop acute EPS are at a higher risk of later developing TD, which can be irreversible (Kane et al., 1986).

Akathisia is a subjective feeling of inner restlessness along with restless movements, usually in the legs or feet. This side effect typically arises early in treatment with high-potency agents. Patients who experience akathisia will often pace continuously or be unable to sit still. Severe akathisia can be particularly disconcerting for patients, who may feel anxious or irritable as a result. Akathisia frequently goes unnoticed by clinicians or is misdiagnosed as anxiety or agitation, which can result in the antipsychotic dose being increased. Consequently, akathisia is a major cause of antipsychotic drug nonadherence. Treatment options include decreasing the antipsychotic dosage or adding a centrally acting β-adrenergic antagonist, such as propranolol 10 to 20 mg three times daily (Minagar and Kelley, 2004).

Acute dystonias are involuntary muscular spasms and abnormal postures affecting mainly the musculature of the head and neck but sometimes the trunk and lower extremities. Common dystonias include torticollis (abnormal positioning of the neck), trismus (tonic contraction of muscles of mastication, otherwise known as *lockjaw*), dysphagia (impaired swallowing), enlarged or protruded tongue, oculogyric crisis (sustained deviations of the eyes, typically upward), and blepharospasm (abnormal tic or twitch of eyelid). A laryngeal dystonia can affect speech, swallowing, and breathing, which can be potentially life threatening (Schneider et al., 2006). Acute dystonias tend to appear within the first few days of antipsychotic treatment or following a rapid dose increase (Ayd, 1961; Remington and Kapur, 1996; Barnes and Spence, 2000). Younger patients, particularly men younger than 30 years, tend to be at higher risk of developing acute dystonia. This side effect may occur in up to 10% of patients. Treatment should be initiated immediately, with either an intramuscular (IM) anticholinergic (benztropine, trihexiphenidyl) or antihistaminic medication (diphenhydramine). Drugs given to reverse a dystonic reaction can wear off after several hours. Given the long half-lives of some antipsychotic medications, prolonged treatment with anticholinergics is often essential for several days.

Parkinsonism consists of resting tremor ("pill-rolling"), muscular (cogwheel) rigidity, bradykinesia, and stooped posture. Bradykinesia can include a slowing of movement (shuffling gait), a decrease in spontaneous movement (decreased arm swing), or masked facies. The features of this medication-induced disorder are similar to the idiopathic variant, PD. This motor disturbance affects approximately 30% of patients who are chronically treated with first-generation antipsychotics. The onset of this side effect is gradual and may not appear for weeks after initiation of antipsychotic drug therapy. Risk factors for antipsychotic-induced parkinsonism include increasing age, higher dosages, a history of parkinsonism, and underlying basal ganglia damage. As with acute dystonias, anticholinergic medications are the treatment of choice and usually effective. Additional treatment recommendations include lowering the dose of antipsychotic medication or switching antipsychotics entirely (Stanilla and Simpson, 2004). Unfortunately, the chronic use of anticholinergic agents is associated with cognitive dysfunction in patients with schizophrenia.

TD is an irreversible syndrome of involuntary movements caused by long-term administration of antipsychotic medications. This syndrome was first described in the 1950s, shortly after the advent of these agents. The mechanism of this disorder is thought to be related to upregulation of D_2 receptors as a consequence of long-term D_2 blockade (Stahl, 2002). The most common form of TD involves spastic/dyskinetic movements of the mouth, face, tongue, trunk, and extremities. Orofacial tardive can manifest as grimacing, facial tics, lip smacking, chewing, sucking, puckering, and worm-like movements of the tongue. Involvement of the trunk, limbs, fingers, and toes may occur as choreoathetoid movements described as slow and writhing in nature.

Although there is still some debate, most studies have shown that the newer second-generation antipsychotic medications carry a significantly lower risk of TD compared with first-generation antipsychotics (Kane, 2006). The literature estimates the risk of TD with typical antipsychotics as 3% to 5% per year of exposure (Kane et al., 1982). Risk factors for TD include older age, female gender, mood disorders, and neurologic disorders. Early occurring EPS are a significant risk factor for TD (Kane, 2006). It is important to note that although the risk may be lower, atypical antipsychotics can still cause TD, just as they can cause acute EPS.

As with most EPS, treatment options for TD include minimizing the antipsychotic dose or switching to a potentially lower-risk agent (Kane, 2006). This clinically significant side effect necessitates regular screening and monitoring for symptoms as well as review of whether antipsychotic medications continue to be indicated in each patient. The current American Psychiatric Association (APA) guidelines suggest that clinicians complete an Abnormal Involuntary Movement Scale (AIMS) every 3 to 6 months on any patient taking any antipsychotic medication. More importantly, the risks and benefits of continuing antipsychotic medication should be discussed in detail with both the patient and his or her family. There is some evidence that patients with TD may improve when treated with clozapine. Moreover, a recent placebo-controlled, double-blind study revealed the efficacy of vitamin B_6 in the treatment of TD (Lerner et al., 2007).

Neuroleptic Malignant Syndrome

Neuroleptic malignant syndrome (NMS) is a rare, but potentially fatal, condition that is associated with the administration of antipsychotic medications. Approximately 80% of cases occur within the first 2 weeks of initiation of antipsychotic treatment (Janicek et al., 1993). Clinical manifestations of NMS are fever, muscular rigidity, altered mental status, and autonomic dysfunction (irregular pulse or blood pressure, orthostatic hypotension, tachycardia, diaphoresis, cardiac dysrhythmia). Laboratory abnormalities in NMS include elevated creatine phosphokinase (CPK), elevated white blood cell (WBC) count, myoglobinuria, and acute renal failure (Pelonero et al., 1998; Geodon, 2005). This is a relatively rare condition that can be severe and life threatening.

Although high-potency typical antipsychotics are generally the offending agents in NMS, all antipsychotic medications are capable of inducing this syndrome. In fact, even certain nonantipsychotic DA D_2 receptor antagonists, such as metoclopramide and amoxapine, have been implicated as causative agents (Pelonero et al., 1998), the latter due to a metabolic conversion of the parent compound to loxapine, a typical antipsychotic. Risk factors that predispose to the development of NMS include dehydration, high doses of antipsychotics, rapid rate of antipsychotic dose escalation, concomitant use of lithium, depot antipsychotic preparations, and prolonged use of physical restraints (Pelonero et al., 1998).

NMS has a very broad differential diagnosis, and therefore, it is extremely important to consider other etiologies with similar clinical presentations. Certain CNS infections, such as meningitis, encephalitis, brain abscess, and neurosyphilis, can mimic NMS; as a result, a lumbar puncture and electroencephalogram (EEG) are often essential components of the diagnostic workup. If a structural lesion is suspected, a computed tomography or magnetic resonance imaging scan of the brain is indicated. Hyperthyroidism, hypocalcemic tetany, or hypomagnesemic tetany can easily be ruled out by appropriate laboratory tests. Malignant hyperthermia has an identical clinical presentation but is associated with the administration of halogenated inhalation anesthetic agents and succinylcholine. Heatstroke can be mistaken for NMS, but a careful physical examination will usually reveal the absence of rigidity (Pelonero et al., 1998). When in doubt, it is always advisable to discontinue any antipsychotic medications when NMS is being considered in the differential diagnosis.

Most cases of NMS can be adequately treated with supportive management alone. First and foremost, all antipsychotic medications should be immediately discontinued. Lithium and any anticholinergic medications should be discontinued. Close monitoring is indicated, preferably in an intensive care unit. CPK levels, electrolytes, and renal function should be closely monitored. Supportive treatment may include antipyretics, a cooling blanket, intravenous fluids, oxygen, aspiration precautions, and intubation and ventilator support if necessary. Subcutaneous heparin is also recommended for deep venous thrombosis (DVT)/pulmonary embolism (PE) prophylaxis. Lastly, physical therapy and nutritional support are important aspects of supportive management. If the patient's condition fails to improve or if it worsens within 1 to 3 days, it is appropriate to consider pharmacologic treatment. Although there is no established pharmacotherapy of choice in the treatment of NMS, dantrolene, a muscle relaxant, is often used on the basis of its efficacy in malignant hyperthermia. It can be administered intravenously 1 to 10 mg/kg body weight or orally 50 to 600 mg daily (Pelonero et al., 1998). Another effective pharmacological agent for NMS is the DA receptor agonist bromocriptine (Lazarus et al., 1989).

The mortality rate for NMS is significantly lower than it was in previous years, mostly due to better and earlier detection of the syndrome. Most patients recover from NMS without any lasting physical or cognitive impairments. However, studies show that the mortality rate is still between 8% and 11% (Pelonero et al., 1998). Death typically occurs secondary to complications of rigidity and immobilization. Causes of death from NMS include dysrhythmias, aspiration pneumonia, renal failure, or pulmonary failure (Pelonero et al., 1998; Wilkaitis et al., 2004).

Reconsideration of antipsychotic therapy in a patient who has had NMS is still controversial and problematic. Medications in other classes, such as mood stabilizers and benzodiazepines, as well as electroconvulsive therapy (ECT) should initially be considered. However, after careful evaluation, if an antipsychotic medication is found to be essential to the treatment regimen, rechallenge can be undertaken with appropriate informed consent. Studies indicate that choosing an antipsychotic with lower D_2 potency (i.e., atypical antipsychotics) and slow dose titration may decrease the risk of NMS recurrence (Lazarus et al., 1989). In addition, allowing for complete recovery from NMS, a minimum of 2 weeks, before reintroduction of antipsychotics is strongly advised (Rosebush et al., 1989).

Atypical Antipsychotics (Second Generation)

The introduction of second-generation, or atypical, antipsychotics brought the promise of a newer, safer, and possibly more effective class of antipsychotic medication. Clozapine is the prototype for this class; the term *atypical* is derived from clozapine's strong antipsychotic efficacy combined with its virtual lack of EPS (Factor, 2002). Atypicality has also been thought to denote increased efficacy on the negative symptoms of schizophrenia (Factor, 2002), though the magnitude of this effect compared with the older drugs remains a matter of intense debate. Pharmacologically, this class occupies a lower percentage of D_2 receptors and is a very potent antagonist of the serotonin 5-HT$_2$ class of receptors (Lieberman et al., 2005). The 5-HT$_2$ blockade is believed to balance the effect of DA receptor blockade, resulting in less EPS (Marder and Wirshing, 2004). Alternatively, the lack of EPS with second-generation antipsychotics may be related to their fast dissociation from D_2 receptors (Marder and Wirshing, 2004). Aripiprazole is unique among atypical antipsychotics in acting as a partial agonist at the D_2 receptor (Abilify, 2006) and has been conceptualized as a DA system stabilizer.

Risperidone, the second atypical antipsychotic on the market, was approved in the United States in 1994. Risperidone is approved for use in the treatment of schizophrenia in adults and adolescents aged 13 to 17 years; the short-term treatment of acute manic or mixed episodes associated with bipolar I disorder, either as monotherapy or in combination with lithium or valproate in adults; or as monotherapy in children and adolescents aged 10 to 17 years (Risperdal, 2007). It also recently received an indication for the treatment of irritability associated with autistic disorder in children and adolescents aged 5 to 16 years. Risperidone has a high affinity for 5-HT$_2$ receptors and a high 5-HT$_2$/D$_2$ ratio, characteristic of atypicality (Factor, 2002). It also has moderate potency at D$_2$ receptors and, at higher doses, is pharmacologically more similar to typical agents. Only at doses <6 mg per day does this drug function as an atypical agent (Factor, 2002). Risperdal Consta is the first depot (long-acting) atypical antipsychotic to be released. The pharmacokinetic profile of Risperdal Consta necessitates that it be administered every 2 weeks.

The FDA approved olanzapine in 1997 for treatment of schizophrenia. This drug is now also indicated as monotherapy for an acute manic or mixed episode in bipolar disorder, combination therapy with lithium or valproate for acute mania, and maintenance therapy in bipolar disorder (if the patient responded to olanzapine during the acute episode). In addition, a combination of fluoxetine and olanzapine (Symbyax) was approved for the treatment of bipolar depression in 2004. Olanzapine is chemically related to clozapine and therefore has a similar affinity profile (high 5-HT$_2$/D$_2$ ratio). It is well absorbed orally and reaches its peak concentrations within 6 hours, with a half-life of 21 to 54 hours (Zyprexa, 2007). Its absorption is unaffected by food, and dosing adjustments are not needed in renal or hepatic impairment. The recommended starting dose for schizophrenia is 5 to 10 mg once daily, with a target daily dose of 10 mg and a maximum daily dose of 20 mg. For bipolar disorder, the recommended starting daily dose is 10 to 15 mg.

Quetiapine, the fourth medication in this class, was approved for schizophrenia in 1997 and subsequently received FDA approval for the treatment of mania associated with bipolar disorder. Recently quetiapine became the only atypical antipsychotic approved as monotherapy for the treatment of bipolar depression. The efficacy of quetiapine for depression is thought to be mediated by the norepinephrine (NE) reuptake blockade produced by its major metabolite (Jensen et al., 2007). Like other atypical antipsychotic agents, quetiapine has been shown in patients with unipolar depression to convert selective serotonin reuptake inhibitor (SSRI) nonresponders to responders. Quetiapine is thought to act somewhat selectively in the mesolimbic system and, like other second-generation antipsychotics, exhibits a high 5-HT$_2$/D$_2$ ratio (Factor, 2002). Quetiapine has a low propensity for EPS, rendering it a good choice for treating psychosis in PD (Factor, 2002). The drug is mainly metabolized hepatically, and its half-life is approximately 6 hours (Seroquel, 2005). Drug–drug interactions are minimal. When used in schizophrenia, quetiapine is often initiated at doses of 25 mg twice daily and titrated over several days to a recommended dose range of 150 to 750 mg daily. When used in bipolar mania, quetiapine can be titrated more rapidly, with a target dose range of 400 to 800 mg daily (Seroquel, 2005). In May 2007, the FDA approved an extended-release (ER) formulation of quetiapine marketed as Seroquel XR, for the once-daily treatment of schizophrenia. However, both forms of quetiapine are commonly used as single nighttime doses.

Ziprasidone, approved in 2001, is currently FDA approved for the treatment of schizophrenia and bipolar disorder (acute manic or mixed episodes with or without psychotic features) (Geodon, 2005). The FDA recommends a starting dose of 20 mg twice daily with food for schizophrenia, but in clinical practice, higher doses are often initially used. Efficacy in schizophrenia was demonstrated at a dose range of 20 to 100 mg twice daily. Initial dosage in bipolar mania is usually 40 mg twice daily with food, and then titration upward can occur as early as day 2. Efficacy in bipolar mania was demonstrated at 80 to 160 mg daily in divided doses (Geodon, 2005). Elimination of ziprasidone is mostly through hepatic metabolism with an average half-life of approximately 7 hours. Most antipsychotic medications can be given with or without food; however, absorption of ziprasidone is increased up to twofold if taken with food and is absolutely essential to maximize efficacy (Geodon, 2005). No dosage adjustments are necessary for either hepatic or renal impairment.

Aripiprazole, approved in 2002, is currently FDA approved for schizophrenia and bipolar disorder (acute manic or mixed episodes with or without psychotic features). Aripiprazole is the first atypical antipsychotic agent to gain FDA approval in converting patients with unipolar depression who are SSRI nonresponders into responders. The effective dose range for schizophrenia is 10 to 30 mg daily with a starting dose of 10 to 15 mg daily, while the starting dose for bipolar disorder is 30 mg daily (Abilify, 2006).

Paliperidone, the newest of the atypical antipsychotics, was approved by the FDA in 2006 for acute and maintenance treatment of schizophrenia. Paliperidone is the major active metabolite of risperidone, 9-hydroxy risperidone; not surprisingly, the two agents are quite similar (Invega,

2007). The key difference between these two medications is the delivery system. Paliperidone is the only antipsychotic drug that is virtually completely renally excreted and not metabolized by the liver. The dose range is 3 to 12 mg once per day, with a recommended daily dose of 6 mg (Invega, 2007). Its metabolism is unaffected by food and its half-life is approximately 23 hours. Because of its renal excretion, paliperidone does not appear to have significant drug–drug interactions, as does risperidone, and is not a substrate or inhibitor of any CYP450 isoenzyme (Invega, 2007). However, its dose should be reduced in moderate to severe renal impairment.

Three of the atypical antipsychotics are available in IM form for the short-term treatment of agitation associated with schizophrenia or mania in the emergency department setting or on an inpatient psychiatric unit. These medications provide clinicians with alternatives to haloperidol and chlorpromazine as agents to be utilized in the treatment of acute agitation. As would be expected, the primary advantage to these newer IM agents compared with the older typical antipsychotics is a lower rate of EPS. Ziprasidone mesylate is indicated for agitation associated with schizophrenia and available in a single-dose vial for IM administration, with each milliliter containing 20 mg of the drug (Geodon, 2005). The recommended dose of ziprasidone injection is 10 to 20 mg IM as needed up to a maximum of 40 mg per day. Peak concentrations occur approximately 60 minutes after administration, and the half-life ranges from 2 to 5 hours, though the beneficial effects are usually observed within 15 minutes of injection (Geodon, 2005). Aripiprazole for injection is indicated for agitation associated with schizophrenia and mania and available in single-dose vials of 9.75 mg for IM administration, with a recommended dose range of 5.25 to 15 mg per injection as needed, up to 30 mg per day (Abilify, 2006). Olanzapine IM is indicated for agitation associated with schizophrenia and mania, and each vial contains 10 mg of olanzapine, with a dose range of 2.5 to 10 mg IM. The recommended dose of olanzapine injection is 10 mg as needed, up to a maximum of 30 mg per day. Olanzapine IM is rapidly absorbed within 15 to 45 minutes (Zyprexa, 2007).

Clozapine was first introduced to the market in 1972 but was quickly withdrawn due to numerous reports of fatal agranulocytosis. It was not available in the United States until 1990, when it was conclusively shown to be effective in patients with treatment-refractory schizophrenia. Clozapine was the first antipsychotic agent to exhibit efficacy without causing EPS; this concept challenged the prevailing "neuroleptic dogma" that EPS were a necessary feature of an antipsychotic drug. It is still unclear specifically which pharmacological properties of clozapine account for its superior efficacy. As with all antipsychotics, clozapine is a D_2 receptor antagonist, but it occupies a much lower percentage of receptors (Factor, 2002), which underlies its lack of EPS. Clozapine, as well as certain other atypical antipsychotics, has been posited to bind less tightly to DA receptors, a concept known as *fast dissociation* (Marder and Wirshing, 2004). This may also contribute to lower EPS liability. Yet another explanation for its low EPS is its preferential blockade of DA receptors in the mesolimbic pathway, as opposed to the nigrostriatal pathway (Factor, 2002). The effectiveness of clozapine may also be linked to high-affinity blockade of $5\text{-}HT_2$ and $5\text{-}HT_3$ receptors, as well as D_4 receptor blockade (Factor, 2002).

Several niche treatment domains exist for which clozapine is particularly well suited. Although it is not considered a first-line agent because of the risk of agranulocytosis, it is the treatment of choice for treatment-refractory positive symptoms in schizophrenia (Lehman et al., 2004). According to APA guidelines, a trial of clozapine should be considered in any patient who has failed two antipsychotics, at least one of which was an atypical agent (American Psychiatric Association, 2004). Clozapine has been shown to be useful in refractory cases of schizoaffective disorder and psychotic mood disorders (McElroy et al., 1991). In addition, it has proven efficacy in managing persistent suicidal ideation unresponsive to other treatments, particularly in psychotic disorders (American Psychiatric Association, 2004). Indeed it is the only antipsychotic shown to reduce suicidality (Meltzer et al., 2003). Clozapine is the preferred agent for schizophrenic patients who exhibit hostile and aggressive behaviors (Marder and Wirshing, 2004). Furthermore, like other antipsychotics, clozapine has been shown to be effective in the treatment of acute mania and especially effective in refractory, rapid-cycling bipolar patients.

Initial dosing is usually 12.5 mg once or twice daily and should be slowly titrated up to an effective dose range of 300 to 600 mg per day (Clozaril, 2005). Some patients may require doses up to 900 mg to achieve a response. Doses may be divided to minimize dose-dependent side effects, or administered at bedtime. In 2004, clozapine also became available in an orally disintegrating tablet, marketed as FazaClo (Waknine, 2007). Monitoring plasma concentrations of clozapine may be clinically useful. Studies have found that patients are more likely to respond when clozapine plasma levels are ≥ 350 ng per mL (Miller, 1996). Clozapine has an elimination half-life of 12 hours. It is primarily metabolized by the CYP450 1A2 isoenzyme, and therefore plasma concentrations can be substantially elevated with concomitant use of the SSRI fluvoxamine, a potent 1A2 inhibitor.

Side Effects of Atypical Antipsychotics

Frequent side effects of atypical antipsychotic drugs, in general, include somnolence, dry mouth, orthostatic hypotension, and EPS, though very significant differences exist among the members of the class regarding the propensity for each of these and other side effects. Orthostatic hypotension is thought to be mediated by antagonism of the α-adrenergic receptor and tends to be more of an issue with quetiapine and clozapine (Clozaril, 2005). Tachycardia is also a common side effect of clozapine, and a rare, but potentially fatal, myocarditis and cardiomyopathy can also occur (Clozaril, 2005). Anticholinergic effects, due to affinity for the muscarinic cholinergic receptor, likely account for side effects such as dry mouth, blurred vision, and constipation; somnolence and weight gain are secondary to the antihistaminic properties of atypical antipsychotics. Of this class, aripiprazole and ziprasidone are the least sedating agents. Clozapine is specifically associated with the problematic side effect of sialorrhea, excessive salivation (Clozaril, 2005). All atypical antipsychotics, but particularly clozapine, should be used cautiously in patients with seizure disorders. Clozapine carries a dose-dependent risk of seizures; at doses <300 mg per day, the risk is just 1%, whereas between 300 and 600 mg per day, the risk is 2.7%, and >600 mg per day, the risk jumps to 4.4% (Devinsky et al., 1991).

The atypical antipsychotic class has been associated with an increased risk of developing the metabolic syndrome, with some of these drugs carrying a higher risk than others. The metabolic syndrome is a cluster of features including abdominal obesity, dyslipidemia, hypertension, and insulin resistance. This syndrome is of immense clinical significance because it is linked to increased cardiovascular risk. Several atypical antipsychotics have been associated with worsening of lipid profiles. The highest risk for lipid changes occurs with olanzapine and clozapine (Lieberman et al., 2005; McEvoy et al., 2006). A meta-analysis comparing weight gain in various typical and atypical agents found clozapine to have the greatest potential to induce weight gain, with the average being 4.45 kg, followed by olanzapine (Allison et al., 1999). Quetiapine and risperidone also cause moderate weight gain (an average of 0.5 lb per month) with 16% and 14% of patients gaining $\geq 7\%$ of their baseline weight. In contrast, ziprasidone appears to be weight neutral (Lieberman et al., 2005). Aripiprazole appears to be weight neutral, and while there is insufficient data to fully evaluate paliperidone, given its similarity to risperidone the expectation is that both agents will have similar weight-gain profiles (see Table 22-3).

TABLE 22-3 Side Effect Profile of Atypical Antipsychotics					
Name	Effective Dose (mg)	Prolactin Elevation	Weight Gain	Glucose and Lipid Changes	EPS
Olanzapine (Zyprexa)	10–30	0	+++	+++	0
Clozapine (Clozaril)	150–600	0	+++	+++	0
Risperidone (Risperdal)	2–8	+++	++	++	+
Quetiapine (Seroquel)	300–800	0	++	++	0
Ziprasidone (Geodon)	120–200	+	0	0	0
Aripiprazole (Abilify)	10–30	0	0	0	0
Paliperidone (Invega)	6–12	+++	[a]	[a]	+

EPS, extrapyramidal symptoms.
[a]Insufficient data on paliperidone.
(Adapted from American Psychiatric Association, 2004; Geodon, 2005; Seroquel, 2005; Abilify, 2006; Risperdal, 2007; Zyprexa, 2007.)

TABLE 22-4 **Monitoring for Patients Taking Atypical Antipsychotics**

Baseline Monitoring	Continued Monitoring
Measure baseline height, weight, and BMI	Measure BMI at every visit for 6 mo, quarterly thereafter
Check fasting blood sugar and Hb$_{A1c}$	Check Hb$_{A1c}$ after 4 mo, then annually
Check fasting lipid panel	Check lipid panel every 5 yr (if normal)
Check prolactin level if clinically indicated	Check liver function, renal function, and electrolytes annually
Obtain ECG with ziprasidone if cardiac risk factors are present	Eye examination every 6 mo with quetiapine
Eye examination with quetiapine	

BMI, body mass index; ECG, electrocardiogram.
(American Psychiatric Association, 2004; Seroquel, 2005.)

Hyperglycemia, sometimes associated with ketoacidosis, hyperosmolar coma, or even death, has been reported in patients treated with atypical antipsychotics (Clozaril, 2005; Geodon, 2005; Seroquel, 2005; Abilify, 2006; Invega, 2007; Risperdal, 2007; Zyprexa, 2007). Given the many confounders, the true relationship between atypical antipsychotics and hyperglycemia-related adverse events is not completely understood. Nonetheless, all patients on atypical antipsychotics should be warned about these risks. In addition, patients with an established diagnosis of diabetes should be monitored regularly for worsening glucose regulation. The current APA guidelines for all patients treated with atypical antipsychotics suggest measuring fasting blood glucose at baseline and monitoring hemoglobin A1C (Hb$_{A1c}$) and random blood glucose every 6 months, thereafter (American Psychiatric Association, 2004). A fasting lipid panel and height, weight, and body mass index (BMI) at baseline and at regular intervals should also be measured (see Table 22-4).

Similar to typical antipsychotics, some of the atypicals are associated with hyperprolactinemia. Prolactin increase occurs as a result of DA receptor blockade in the anterior pituitary, blocking the effects of DA released in the tuberoinfundibular pathway (Stahl, 2002; Zyprexa, 2007). Many studies have shown that of the second-generation antipsychotics, risperidone is the most likely to cause changes in prolactin levels (Lieberman et al., 2005). Given that paliperidone is 9-hydroxy risperidone, the major active metabolite of risperidone, it is predictable that similar increases in prolactin levels occur with this agent. The remaining drugs in this class have little to no effect on prolactin levels. It is advisable that clinicians screen their patients for symptoms of hyperprolactinemia such as gynecomastia and galactorrhea on a regular basis.

All antipsychotic medications, typical and atypical, are capable of producing EPS. However, high-potency typical agents clearly have a higher propensity for causing EPS than atypical agents. Among the atypical antipsychotics, however, certain drugs are associated with an increased risk of EPS. At higher doses, both risperidone and paliperidone tend to act pharmacologically more like high-potency typical antipsychotics in this regard. The remaining atypical antipsychotics all have a low propensity to produce treatment-emergent EPS (Daniel et al., 2004; Lieberman, 2004; Seroquel, 2005; Zyprexa, 2007). Clozapine is known for its virtual lack of EPS. This makes it a particularly useful agent in low doses for psychotic patients with PD.

One side effect of concern specific to ziprasidone is a dose-related prolongation of the QTc interval; it is therefore contraindicated in patients with a history of QTc prolongation, recent acute myocardial infarction (MI), or uncompensated heart failure. In addition, ziprasidone should not be given in combination with other drugs that prolong the QTc interval (Geodon, 2005). Certain electrolyte abnormalities (hypokalemia, hypomagnesemia) can increase the risk of QTc prolongation and arrhythmias; therefore, patients with cardiac risk factors should have baseline serum potassium, serum magnesium, and ECG checked before initiation of ziprasidone treatment (American Psychiatric Association, 2004). Ziprasidone should be discontinued in patients who have a persistent QTc >500 msec (Geodon, 2005). However, the recently completed 18,000-patient Zodiac study revealed no significant cardiac side effects of ziprasidone (Strom et al., 2008).

The development of cataracts was observed in dogs after treatment with quetiapine. Lens changes have been detected in some patients on chronic quetiapine therapy, but the causal relationship has not been established. Current recommendations suggest a baseline eye examination, as well as eye examinations every 6 months, for patients on quetiapine (Seroquel, 2005).

Clozapine is associated with a 1.3% risk of agranulocytosis (Clozaril, 2005). Agranulocytosis, defined as an absolute neutrophil count (ANC) <500 per mm^3, can prove fatal if not recognized early in treatment, which is why monitoring is so stringent (Clozaril, 2005). Patients receiving clozapine must undergo a baseline WBC count and ANC before initiation of therapy, as well as repeated evaluations during treatment that continues for at least 4 weeks after therapy discontinuation. The WBC count and ANC should be performed weekly for the first 6 months of therapy; at that point, if WBC count is ≥3,500 cells per mm^3 and ANC is ≥2,000 cells per mm^3, monitoring can be performed every 2 weeks for the next 6 months. Patients who have maintained satisfactory counts for 1 year of continuous therapy can be evaluated once monthly thereafter (Waknine, 2007). Rechallenge with clozapine is not recommended in patients who have experienced moderate-to-severe leukopenia, that is, WBC <3,000 (Clozaril, 2005).

All the atypical antipsychotics have a boxed warning for increased mortality in elderly patients with dementia-related psychosis (Geodon, 2005; Seroquel, 2005; Invega, 2007; Risperdal, 2007; Zyprexa, 2007). This warning was based on several trials showing that the use of atypical antipsychotic drugs (risperidone, olanzapine, aripiprazole, and quetiapine were specifically tested) was associated with an increased risk of mortality compared to placebo (4.5% vs. 2.6%). These deaths were mostly of a cardiovascular or infectious nature. This 1.6- to 1.7-fold increase in mortality risk appears to be a class effect because it was linked to all four atypical antipsychotics tested (Waknine, 2007). Despite this warning, atypical antipsychotics are still frequently used in dementia-related psychosis because there are no better alternatives to treat this condition in demented patients, and moreover, the increased risk is quite low. As a general rule, all antipsychotics should be prescribed at reduced dosages in elderly patients, after a careful discussion of risks and benefits.

ANTIDEPRESSANT MEDICATIONS

The first TCA was developed in the 1950s. A derivative of chlorpromazine, it was originally tested as a novel antipsychotic agent. Instead, this drug, imipramine, was found to be an effective antidepressant and became the first of a generation of drugs used in the treatment of depression. Partly based on the mechanism of action of imipramine and other early TCAs, the monoamine hypothesis of depression was developed. Depression was posited to be a neurochemical disorder caused by a functional deficiency of monoamine neurotransmitters such as serotonin, NE, and/or DA. Many antidepressant drugs do, in fact, block the uptake of NE, serotonin, or both into the presynaptic terminals, thereby increasing the concentration of these neurotransmitters in the synaptic cleft. These effects occur acutely, yet the antidepressants are not effective for 3 to 5 weeks after initiating treatment. Moreover, a significant proportion of depressed patients (20% to 40%) do not respond to conventional antidepressants. Until there is a greater understanding of the precise pathophysiology of depression, the precise mechanism of action of antidepressants will likely remain obscure.

In contrast to the older antidepressant classes such as TCAs and MAOIs, the newer classes generally have more favorable side effect profiles. Furthermore, there is virtually no toxicity in overdose with the newer antidepressants, making them safer for patients at risk for suicide. A major advantage of the SSRIs is their superior therapeutic index.

Historically the primary indication for use of an antidepressant medication was for the treatment of major depressive disorder. However, in recent years, antidepressants have been proven effective for many other psychiatric syndromes, including panic disorder, posttraumatic stress disorder (PTSD), generalized anxiety disorder (GAD), obsessive-compulsive disorder (OCD), social anxiety disorder (SAD), and premenstrual dysphoric disorder (PMDD). Some antidepressants are also effective in the treatment of migraine headaches, chronic pain syndromes, enuresis, bulimia nervosa, and other conditions.

Choosing an Antidepressant

The psychiatric history, current symptoms, comorbid medical and psychiatric disorders, and mental status of depressed patients are major factors in the choice of an appropriate pharmacological agent. In addition, before initiating an antidepressant, it is critical that the clinician has thoroughly inquired as to a history of manic or hypomanic episodes. Treating bipolar depression with an antidepressant alone can substantially increase the risk of inducing a manic or mixed episode (Effexor, 2006). If mania/hypomania occurs while a patient is receiving an antidepressant, it should be discontinued, and a diagnosis of underlying bipolar disorder should be thoroughly investigated. If the hypomania is severe or if mania develops, a mood stabilizer should be initiated. Patients with bipolar disorder may experience more frequent mood cycling and treatment resistance when treated chronically with antidepressants (Ghaemi, 2003).

Many factors go into choosing the most appropriate antidepressant for an individual patient, including the patient's history of previous treatment response, response of first-degree family relatives, side effect profile of the medication, medical status of the patient, and risk of suicide by overdose. In addition, the presence of psychosis or atypical symptoms gives the clinician important information about depression subtype that will help guide the choice of treatment regimen. If the patient has psychotic features, this warrants the addition of an antipsychotic to the antidepressant regimen or treatment with ECT. Multiple studies have established that psychotic depression clearly responds better to treatment with a combination of antidepressant and antipsychotic medications than with either alone (American Psychiatric Association, 2000). If the patient has atypical depression, characterized by hypersomnia, hyperphagia, and other symptoms, an MAOI may be the treatment of choice.

An adequate trial of antidepressant medication consists of treatment with therapeutic doses of the drug (see Table 22-5) for a minimum of 6 to 8 weeks. At the end of this period, a patient can be determined to have a full response, a partial response, or no response. In the past, the goal of psychiatric treatment was often measured as response, defined as a 50% or more reduction in symptoms. However, in recent years, it has become clear that the goal of treatment needs to be more than just response, but full remission (Depression Guideline Panel, 1993). Remission is often defined as the virtual absence of symptoms, or a Hamilton Depression Rating Scale score of ≤ 7. Numerous studies have reported that major depressive disorder often necessitates more than one medication or combination medication/psychotherapy to achieve remission (Rush et al., 2006). In these situations, it is common to add a second antidepressant medication, or an adjunctive medication that is not in itself an antidepressant, to enhance the efficacy of the first (Fava et al., 2003). Patients who do not remit after an adequate therapeutic trial of an antidepressant are often defined as treatment resistant, or treatment refractory. Factors that can contribute to treatment resistance include nonadherence, occult substance use, axis II

TABLE 22-5 **Pharmacokinetics of Selective Serotonin Reuptake Inhibitors (SSRIs)**

Name	Parent Half-Life ($t_{1/2}$) (hr)	Active Metabolite	Effective Dose Range (mg)
Fluoxetine (Prozac)	24–72	Norfluoxetine	20–80
Paroxetine (Paxil)	15–20	None	10–50
Sertraline (Zoloft)	26–32	Desmethylsertraline	50–200
Fluvoxamine (Luvox)	15	None	50–300
Citalopram (Celexa)	33–35	None	10–40
Escitalopram (Lexapro)	27–32	None	10–20

(Rosenbaum and Tollefson, 2004; Celexa, 2007; Lexapro, 2007; Paxil, 2007; Zoloft, 2007.)

comorbidity, occult general medical conditions, and inadequate dose or duration of the initial medication trial (Rush and Thase, 1997). One important strategy to employ in depression, particularly in treatment-resistant patients, is to optimize the current medication dose and be sure the patient has, in fact, completed a therapeutic trial of adequate duration (Rush and Thase, 1997). The current standard of care in the treatment of depression supports the continuation of antidepressant therapy for at least 6 to 9 months following the acute treatment response (Keller et al., 1998). After the maintenance phase of treatment, antidepressants can be gradually tapered and discontinued. However, several studies have demonstrated that antidepressants extend the time in remission in high-risk populations (Rush and Thase, 1997; Keller et al., 1998). This evidence supports a multiyear, possibly lifelong, maintenance phase treatment for the chronically and recurrent depressed patient (Rush and Thase, 1997). Discontinuation of antidepressant therapy early in the course has been associated with a 25% relapse rate within 2 months (Keller et al., 1998). From 2001 to 2004, a major National Institutes of Health (NIH)–sponsored effectiveness study, the Sequenced Treatment Alternatives to Relieve Depression (STAR*D), was completed, in which outpatients with major depressive disorder were all initially treated with citalopram, a prototype SSRI (Trivedi et al., 2006). Even when treated at a therapeutic dose (average 41.8 mg per day) for a full 12 weeks, only approximately one third of patients achieved remission. This supports the notion that in the real world, many patients need to be switched from one antidepressant to another or need a second agent added to achieve remission. According to the results of the trial, there was equal efficacy regardless of whether a patient was switched within an antidepressant class or switched to another class, that is, SSRI to SNRI (Rush and Thase, 1997). The STAR*D study also compared various medications as augmenting agents or combination treatments for depression, demonstrating that adding bupropion or buspirone were equally effective in achieving remission in major depression (Trivedi et al., 2006).

Selective Serotonin Reuptake Inhibitors

The synthesis of the first SSRI, fluoxetine, in 1972, marked the inception of an exciting new era in the field of psychiatry. Currently, SSRIs are considered first-line antidepressant treatment for both depression and anxiety disorders. The International Consensus Group on Depression and Anxiety recommends SSRIs as first-line treatment for social phobia and panic disorder (Ballenger et al., 1998a, b).

SSRIs have many similarities by virtue of the shared property of blocking serotonin uptake; however, each of them possesses unique secondary pharmacodynamic and pharmacokinetic properties. SSRIs act primarily by inhibiting the reuptake of serotonin, which increases the concentration of serotonin in the synaptic cleft, leading to enhanced serotonergic neurotransmission. Of the SSRIs, paroxetine is the most potent inhibitor of the serotonin transporter (Herr and Nemeroff, 2004). Compared to TCAs, most SSRIs do not significantly inhibit NE or DA reuptake. However, sertraline is a relatively potent inhibitor of DA uptake (Shim and Yonkers, 2004), and paroxetine is a relatively potent NE reuptake inhibitor (Herr and Nemeroff, 2004). Unlike TCAs, SSRIs have little to no effect on histaminergic, α-adrenergic, or muscarinic receptors, resulting in a very favorable side effect profile (Rosenbaum and Tollefson, 2004). As with all antidepressants, there is a well-established 2- to 4-week lag time before the therapeutic effects of SSRIs become evident. These drugs must therefore produce their benefits beyond simply acutely inhibiting monoamine reuptake (Fairbanks and Gorman, 2004). After chronic administration, SSRIs normalize both 5-HT_{1a} and 5-HT_2 receptor density by down-regulation of binding sites (Rosenbaum and Tollefson, 2004). Desensitization of 5-HT autoreceptors also occurs, permitting serotonergic neurons to reestablish a normal firing rate (Rosenbaum and Tollefson, 2004). Increased hippocampal neurogenesis, another effect observed after chronic antidepressant treatment, may mediate the behavioral effects of these drugs (Table 22-5).

In general, the SSRIs appear to be equally efficacious, and in addition, SSRIs have been shown to possess similar efficacy as the TCAs (Rickels and Schweizer, 1990; Frazer, 1997; Hirschfeld, 1999). It is important to note that patients may experience improvement in their energy level while still experiencing the hopelessness that characterizes depression. Such patients may be at increased risk of suicide during this time and should be monitored closely.

In addition to their utility in the treatment of depression, SSRIs are effective in various anxiety disorders. In OCD, higher doses of antidepressants and longer treatment periods are often necessary to achieve a response. In contrast, in panic disorder, SSRIs should be initiated at lower than usual dosages (e.g., fluoxetine 10 mg) because these patients are usually sensitive to the anxiogenic side effects of these drugs early in treatment. Titration to usual antidepressant dosages is required for optimal response. The APA (2006) practice guidelines are based on substantial evidence in support of maintenance treatment of panic disorder for 6 to 12 months after remission is attained. Many patients will relapse when medication is discontinued, and they may require prolonged treatment. Among individuals with panic disorder, the lifetime prevalence rate of major depression is 50% to 60% (Lesser et al., 1989). Not surprisingly, SSRIs are an ideal treatment for patients with comorbid anxiety and depressive symptoms.

Fluoxetine has FDA indications for the treatment of adult and pediatric major depression, adult and pediatric OCD, bulimia nervosa, and panic disorder. Fluoxetine is efficacious both in the acute treatment of a major depressive episode and prevention of relapse (Prozac, 2007). It is available in capsules, oral solution, and a delayed-release, once weekly formulation. The recommended starting dose for both depression and OCD is 20 mg daily with an effective dose range of 20 to 80 mg. In depressed children and adolescents 10 to 20 mg is recommended; up to 60 mg daily is recommended for treatment of OCD, however. In bulimia nervosa, 60 mg daily was found to be an effective dose. Lower and less frequent dosing is recommended in patients with hepatic impairment. Fluoxetine is extensively metabolized in the liver to its active metabolite norfluoxetine (Prozac, 2007). The half-life of fluoxetine is 24 to 72 hours but increases to 4 to 6 days after chronic administration; the half-life of norfluoxetine is 4 to 16 days. Because of its long half-life, a washout period of 4 to 5 weeks is necessary for fluoxetine.

Sertraline was initially approved for the treatment of major depressive disorder in 1992. Over the years, sertraline has also been approved for treatment of adult and pediatric OCD, panic disorder, PTSD, SAD, and PMDD. The recommended starting daily dose for depression, PMDD, and OCD is 50 mg, with an effective dose range of 50 to 200 mg daily (Zoloft, 2007). For the remaining anxiety disorders (panic disorder, SAD, PTSD), a lower starting daily dose of 25 mg is suggested. The half-life of sertraline is 26 to 32 hours, but the half-life of its active metabolite, N-desmethylsertraline, is 62 to 104 hours. Liver impairment extends the half-life threefold; therefore, the use of sertraline in patients with liver disease should be approached with caution.

Paroxetine was the third SSRI approved by the FDA. It has been approved for the treatment of major depression, panic disorder, OCD, SAD, GAD, and PTSD. Studies have also found paroxetine to be efficacious in depression associated with medical illness, including rheumatoid arthritis, irritable bowel syndrome, ischemic heart disease, and interferon-α–induced depression (Herr and Nemeroff, 2004). A controlled-release formulation is now available and reported to have improved tolerability (Herr and Nemeroff, 2004). The recommend starting daily dose of the controlled-release formulation is 25 mg, with or without food, with an effective dose range of 25 to 62.5 mg daily. As with other antidepressants, a lower starting dose (e.g., 12.5 mg daily) should be used in panic disorder and SAD. Patients with hepatic or renal impairment should be treated with lower doses.

Fluvoxamine has been available in Europe since 1983 and is FDA approved in the United States only for the treatment of adult, adolescent, and childhood OCD. Although all the SSRIs have efficacy in the treatment of OCD, fluvoxamine has arguably been the most extensively studied. There is also evidence to support its use in other anxiety disorders, as well as depression. Fluvoxamine is as effective as TCAs and other SSRIs in the treatment of depression (Fairbanks and Gorman, 2004). The recommended starting dose in OCD is 50 mg per day, with an effective daily dose of 100 to 300 mg in divided doses. OCD symptoms typically respond after 6 to 10 weeks of treatment. Fluvoxamine is metabolized in the liver, and its absorption is not affected by food. Fluvoxamine has a relatively short half-life and no active metabolites. Nonlinear pharmacokinetics emerge when dosages exceed 100 mg per day, but blood levels of fluvoxamine are typically not informative in optimizing clinical treatment (Fairbanks and Gorman, 2004).

The FDA approved citalopram in 1998 for acute and maintenance treatment of major depressive disorder. Citalopram is a racemic mixture (50/50 of the S and R enantiomers); the inhibition of serotonin reuptake is primarily due to the S-enantiomer (Celexa, 2007). This SSRI has minimal impact on other brain transporters' receptors. The recommended starting dose of citalopram is 20 mg per day, with an effective dose range of 20 to 60 mg daily. Dosing is once daily, with or without food. A reduced dosage of 20 mg daily is recommended in elderly and hepatically impaired patients. Its half-life is 35 hours, and it has no active metabolite. In the NIH funded STAR*D trial, the remission rate in the open arm of the study after up to 14 weeks of treatment with citalopram was only 28%.

Escitalopram, the newest member of the SSRI class, is currently approved for the treatment of GAD and acute and maintenance treatment in major depressive disorder. Escitalopram is the purified S-enantiomer of citalopram, making these two medications structurally very similar. However, escitalopram is at least 100-fold more potent than the R-enantiomer (Lexapro, 2007). Like citalopram, escitalopram is considered an especially "clean" drug in that it is very selective for blocking serotonin reuptake, has negligible effects on other neurotransmitter systems, and has minimal drug–drug interactions. Its absorption is unaffected by food, and its half-life is 27 to 32 hours. The recommended starting dose of escitalopram is 10 mg per day with an effective dose range of 10 to 20 mg daily. A reduced dosage of 10 mg daily is recommended in the elderly and patients with hepatic impairment.

SSRIs share a common side effect profile and are generally well tolerated, much more so than TCAs (Rosenbaum and Tollefson, 2004). Anxiety, agitation, headache, and insomnia are very common with the SSRIs, particularly with fluoxetine. GI side effects, including nausea, anorexia, and diarrhea, are also quite common, though these typically resolve within a few days. Sertraline causes higher rates of diarrhea, paroxetine constipation, and fluvoxamine headache and GI distress when compared to other SSRIs. The high affinity of paroxetine for the muscarinic cholinergic receptor is responsible for its propensity to cause dry mouth, blurred vision, and constipation (Herr and Nemeroff, 2004). However, in comparison to TCAs, paroxetine still produces markedly fewer anticholinergic effects (Boyer and Blumhardt, 1992). Paroxetine, compared with other SSRIs, tends to have higher rates of somnolence and weight gain. Rarely, SSRIs have been associated with hyponatremia and the syndrome of inappropriate antidiuretic hormone (SIADH) secretion.

Sexual dysfunction has been associated with almost every class of antidepressants, including the SSRIs. Sexual dysfunction is reported in up to 20% of patients, but underreporting of this symptom is very common. Not surprisingly, this side effect tends to impede medication adherence. Sexual side effects can include impotence, delayed ejaculation, anorgasmia, and decreased interest and enjoyment of sexual activities for both men and women. In a prospective multicenter study, paroxetine was shown to generate more delay in orgasm or ejaculation and more impotence than other SSRIs (Montejo-Gonzalez et al., 1997).

When SSRI treatment is abruptly stopped, patients may develop a discontinuation syndrome that consists of irritability, agitation, dizziness, nausea, sensory abnormalities, headache, and insomnia (Celexa, 2007; Lexapro, 2007; Prozac, 2007; Zoloft, 2007). This syndrome tends to occur with SSRIs with shorter half-lives whereas the relatively long half-life of fluoxetine confers some protection against these symptoms. Paroxetine is notorious for being the most liable to cause discontinuation symptoms, likely secondary to its short half-life and lack of an active metabolite (Herr and Nemeroff, 2004). Sertraline and fluvoxamine occasionally cause these symptoms whereas longer half-life agents such as fluoxetine are not associated with a discontinuation syndrome (Herr and Nemeroff, 2004). Slow tapering of short half-life agents is advised to avoid this withdrawal syndrome. Patients should be informed of the potential for this syndrome when discontinuing treatment with an SSRI.

Drug–drug interactions are significant for paroxetine, fluoxetine, and fluvoxamine. Various CYP450 enzymes metabolize citalopram and escitalopram, and these agents are not inhibitors of any of these enzymes, which minimize significant drug–drug interactions. Metabolism of paroxetine and fluoxetine is dependent on the P450-CYP-2D6 enzyme, and both agents are 2D6 inhibitors, as is sertraline at higher doses. This causes increased levels of other drugs that are metabolized by the 2D6 enzyme. For example, these drugs elevate plasma levels of thioridazine, which can lead to QTc prolongation and increase levels of risperidone, which can result in EPS (Paxil, 2007; Prozac, 2007). Moreover, both fluoxetine and paroxetine increase blood levels of TCAs and antiarrhythmics such as propafenone and flecainide (Rosenbaum and Tollefson, 2004; Prozac, 2007). Fluvoxamine, on the other hand, is a moderate inhibitor of P450 enzymes 2C19 and 3A4 and a potent inhibitor of 1A2. Clinically relevant drug–drug interactions for fluvoxamine include the following 1A2 substrates: caffeine, clozapine, propranolol, tacrine, tertiary-amine TCAs, theophylline, and warfarin (Fairbanks and Gorman, 2004).

All of the newer antidepressants (SSRIs, SNRIs, bupropion, mirtazapine, trazodone, nefazodone), with the exception of paroxetine, are classified as a pregnancy category C. Paroxetine was recently reclassified as a pregnancy category D after evidence emerged that first-trimester exposure to paroxetine is linked to an increased risk of cardiovascular malformations (primarily atrial septal defects [ASDs] and ventricular septal defects [VSDs]) (Paxil, 2007). The data suggest that paroxetine has a higher risk compared with other SSRIs. This is somewhat surprising given the limited passage of paroxetine across the placental barrier. Nevertheless, women who become pregnant while taking paroxetine should generally be tapered off and switched to another SSRI. An additional study reported a class effect of SSRI use during pregnancy. This study found that infants exposed to SSRIs *in utero* might have an increased risk for persistent pulmonary hypertension of the newborn (Celexa, 2007; Lexapro, 2007; Paxil, 2007; Prozac, 2007; Zoloft, 2007). The risk of this condition appears to be sixfold higher for infants exposed to SSRIs after the 20th week of gestation, but the absolute rate is very low. As with any medication during pregnancy, an appropriate discussion of the risks and benefits of treatment versus nontreatment should occur between clinician and patient before a therapeutic decision is made.

Members of the SSRI class should never be used in conjunction with MAOIs or within 14 days of discontinuing therapy with an MAOI because of the risk of serotonin syndrome. Because of the long half-life of fluoxetine, a 5-week-longer washout period is required before initiation of MAOI treatment.

Serotonin Syndrome

The serotonin syndrome is a consequence of excess serotonergic activity at serotonin receptors and is thought to be a result of stimulation of the 5-HT_{1a} and 5-HT_{2a} receptors (Bijl, 2004). This drug-induced syndrome is characterized by neurologic, autonomic, and neuromuscular changes. Diagnosis is based entirely on clinical symptoms that can range from very mild to fatal, though the latter is extremely rare. The diagnosis requires three of the following symptoms: confusion, agitation, fever or hyperthermia, diaphoresis, shivering, diarrhea, myoclonus, hypertonia/hyperreflexia, and tremor (Bijl, 2004; Rapaport, 2007). Other associated symptoms include insomnia, restlessness, tachycardia, tachypnea, dyspnea, hypotension or hypertension, flushing, incoordination, mydriasis, and ataxia. Most cases are caused by a combination of two or more serotonergic drugs, most commonly an MAOI and an SSRI or TCA (Rapaport, 2007). This syndrome can also occur, though rarely, with concomitant administration of an SSRI or SNRI with tramadol, lithium, triptans, or St. John's Wort (Prozac, 2007). Serotonin syndrome typically develops after a dose increase, a second agent is added, or an overdose (Bijl, 2004). It has also been implicated in cases where patients used the street drug 3,4-methylenedioxy-*N*-methylamphetamine (MDMA, or ecstasy) (Green et al., 1995). The differential diagnosis for serotonin syndrome includes NMS, carcinoid syndrome, thyroid storm, pheochromocytoma, and other causes of agitated delirium (Bijl, 2004). Clonus, hyperreflexia, and flushing are the most specific signs of serotonin syndrome and useful in differentiating it from other diagnoses (Bijl, 2004).

The treatment of choice for serotonin syndrome is discontinuation of all serotonergic medications. More often than not, the syndrome will be self-limited and improve solely on the basis of the offending drug(s) being stopped. Typically, mild cases resolve within 72 hours. However, moderate to severe cases may require hospitalization, and patients with hyperthermia will require intensive care management (Bijl, 2004; Rapaport, 2007). Preventively, providers should tread carefully when combining serotonergic medications; they should also be aware that when discontinuing a serotonergic agent with a long half-life, it may require an extended washout period before starting a new medication (Bijl, 2004). A standard recommendation is to wait at least five times the half-life of the antidepressant (or its metabolite) before administering the next serotonergic agent (Rosenbaum and Tollefson, 2004).

Bupropion

Bupropion was introduced in the United States in 1989 as an "atypical" antidepressant. Its mechanism of action remains obscure, but it clearly does not act pharmacodynamically like any other antidepressant. Bupropion is indicated for the treatment of major depressive disorder, seasonal affective disorder, and for smoking cessation, marketed under the name Zyban.

Bupropion has also demonstrated efficacy in attention-deficit/hyperactivity disorder (ADHD) in children and adults, possibly as a second-line agent to atomoxetine and psychostimulants.

Bupropion is available in three formulations: the immediate-release form; the sustained-release form (Wellbutrin SR), which allows for twice daily dosing; and the ER form (Wellbutrin XL), which allows for once daily dosing. The starting dose of the SR formulation is 150 mg per day for 3 days, then 150 mg twice daily, with the latter dose scheduled before 5:00 PM. Dosing any later than this may interfere with sleep continuity (Ghaemi, 2003). Target dosing for the SR and XL formulations is 300 mg daily (Wellbutrin, 2007). The same dosing schedule applies to smoking cessation, in which case a "quit date" should be set 1 to 2 weeks after beginning treatment (Hudziak and Rettew, 2004). The liver metabolizes bupropion, primarily by the CYP450 2D6 isoenzyme; as a result, caution should be used with coadministration of other drugs that are inhibitors of this enzyme. In addition, lower doses are recommended in both hepatic and renal impairment (Wellbutrin, 2007).

Multiple head-to-head trials have compared the efficacy of bupropion with SSRIs and TCAs, all of which have found comparable antidepressant efficacy with similar remission rates (Hudziak and Rettew, 2004; Stahl et al., 2004; Thase et al., 2005). In addition to being used as a first-line antidepressant, bupropion is commonly prescribed as an augmentation agent, combined with other antidepressants in patients who are nonresponders. Bupropion SR was shown to be effective as combination medication in the treatment of depression in the STAR*D trial at an average dose of 267.5 mg daily and was slightly superior to buspirone in efficacy and tolerability (Trivedi et al., 2006).

Bupropion has a favorable side effect profile, including a low rate of sedation and weight-neutrality. In fact, some studies have found bupropion to be helpful as an adjunct for weight loss, particularly in obese individuals (Stahl et al., 2004). Bupropion also carries the lowest risk of sexual dysfunction of all the antidepressants, with the possible exception of mirtazapine (Stahl et al., 2004). There is some evidence that bupropion can ameliorate the sexual dysfunction caused by SSRIs and SNRIs (Stahl et al., 2004). The most common side effects that occur with bupropion are insomnia, dry mouth, and nausea (Stahl, 2002; Wellbutrin, 2007). Bupropion can be anxiogenic and activating (Wellbutrin, 2007), making it a less preferred choice in particularly anxious patients. Also noteworthy, bupropion decreases seizure threshold, carrying a significant seizure incidence of 0.4% with the immediate-release formulation and a more acceptable 0.1% rate with the sustained-release formulations (Wellbutrin, 2007). Seizure risk appears to be much higher in doses >450 mg daily. Because of the seizure risk, bupropion is contraindicated in patients with seizure disorders or eating disorders.

All antidepressants carry the risk of inducing mania in patients with bipolar disorder. However, bupropion is less likely than most other antidepressants to switch patients into mania (Hudziak and Rettew, 2004); as such, bupropion is often considered the preferred antidepressant in bipolar depression.

Serotonin-Norepinephrine Reuptake Inhibitors

Venlafaxine (Effexor), a serotonin-norepinephrine reuptake inhibitor (SNRI), was approved in 1994 for the treatment of depression, with an ER formulation approved in 1997 for once-daily dosing. Duloxetine (Cymbalta), the second medication of this class, was approved in 2001. The mechanism of action of both venlafaxine and duloxetine is inhibition of serotonin and NE reuptake in the CNS, similar to many TCAs, such as imipramine. At lower doses (<100 mg per day), venlafaxine tends to block mainly 5-HT reuptake, whereas at doses >150 mg per day, it begins to block NE reuptake (Owens et al., 1997). Therefore, venlafaxine at low doses is essentially an SSRI. Duloxetine, in contrast, is relatively more potent, inhibiting NE reuptake across the dose range (Greden, 2004).

Venlafaxine is FDA approved for the treatment of major depressive disorder, GAD, SAD, and panic disorder. Although duloxetine shares only two of these indications, major depressive disorder and GAD, it has an additional unique FDA approval for the management of diabetic peripheral neuropathic pain (DPNP) and pending approval for the treatment of fibromyalgia. In depression and GAD trials, venlafaxine was shown to be effective both during the acute treatment phase and in maintenance for up to 6 months. The recommended starting dose of venlafaxine is 75 mg daily (once daily with XR formulation and twice daily with the immediate-release formulation) (Effexor,

2006). Maximum daily dosing is 375 mg with immediate-release venlafaxine and 225 mg with ER venlafaxine, though in practice higher doses of the XR are often prescribed. The recommended starting dosing of duloxetine in major depression is 20 mg twice daily with titration up to a target dose of 60 mg daily (it can be given once or twice daily) (Cymbalta, 2007). Similar target dosing is recommended for both GAD and DPNP. The ER formulation of venlafaxine provides a slower rate of absorption than the immediate-release form but the same extent of absorption. Venlafaxine undergoes extensive hepatic metabolism to its active metabolite O-desmethylvenlafaxine, which was recently approved by the FDA as an antidepressant, but has a low potential for drug–drug interactions (Thase and Sloan, 2004). Duloxetine is also primarily metabolized in the liver by both cytochrome enzymes 1A2 and 2D6. Although venlafaxine requires dosage adjustment in patients with liver and renal disease (Effexor, 2006), duloxetine is not recommended for patients with any hepatic impairment or severe renal impairment (Cymbalta, 2007).

Like the SSRIs, both venlafaxine and duloxetine are generally well tolerated. The most common side effects are nausea, dizziness, and somnolence (Effexor, 2006; Cymbalta, 2007), with nausea typically being the most problematic (Thase and Sloan, 2004). Venlafaxine can cause a dose-related increase in blood pressure that is sustained in some patients. This increase is mild and appears to occur only in doses >100 mg daily. Venlafaxine is most like the TCAs in having considerable liability for death in overdose (Buckley and McManus, 2002) and adverse cardiac effects, including reduced heart rate variability, which is a risk factor for MI. Duloxetine can also cause a very mild blood pressure increase, but the mean systolic blood pressure increase in studies was only 2 mm Hg (Cymbalta, 2007). This side effect may be particularly relevant in patients with preexisting hypertension. Blood pressure should be measured before initiating treatment and periodically throughout treatment (Effexor, 2006, Cymbalta, 2007). As with all serotonergic antidepressants, both drugs are associated with sexual side effects, including decreased libido, anorgasmia, and abnormal ejaculation (Cymbalta, 2007). Venlafaxine and duloxetine both appear to be weight neutral.

Abrupt withdrawal of venlafaxine and duloxetine can result in discontinuation symptoms (Effexor, 2006, Cymbalta, 2007). This is likely a serotonin withdrawal syndrome, which consists of symptoms such as electric shock–like sensations in the upper extremities, nausea, fatigue, dizziness, headache, insomnia, and anxiety (Ghaemi, 2003; Thase and Sloan, 2004). For this reason, it is preferable to slowly taper these medications before discontinuation. As with all serotonergic agents, neither of these medications should be used in conjunction with MAOIs or within 14 days of discontinuing treatment with an MAOI because of the risk of the serotonin syndrome (Effexor, 2006).

Mirtazapine

Mirtazapine (Remeron) is a structurally unique antidepressant that was introduced in the United States in 1996. Its mechanism of action is likely through enhancement of both noradrenergic and serotonergic neurotransmission (Hirschfeld, 1999; Remeron, 2007). Its specific pharmacological actions include potent antagonism at 5-HT$_2$, 5-HT$_3$, and α_2 adrenergic receptors (Remeron, 2007). Mirtazapine is indicated for the treatment of major depressive disorder and has been shown to be effective in maintenance studies for up to 40 weeks (Remeron, 2007). Several studies have found mirtazapine to be equally effective and as well tolerated as the SSRIs (Flores and Schatzberg, 2004). There is considerable evidence that the addition of mirtazapine in patients who failed to respond to an SSRI is a successful combination strategy (Carpenter et al., 2002). Finally, there is some evidence that mirtazapine may be useful in the treatment of dysthymia, PTSD, chronic pain, and nausea in cancer patients; however, further study is needed to corroborate these preliminary findings (Flores and Schatzberg, 2004).

Mirtazapine is available in tablets and orally disintegrating tablets. Dosing should begin at 15 mg per day, preferably in the evening, with an effective dose range of 15 to 45 mg per day. The mean half-life is between 20 and 40 hours. Clearance of mirtazapine is decreased in both hepatic and renal impairment. Mirtazapine has a high affinity for histamine receptors, a likely explanation for its most prominent side effects: sedation, increased appetite, and weight gain, the latter a major drawback to the medication. Somnolence has been reported to occur in >50% of patients treated with mirtazapine (Remeron, 2007). Mirtazapine can also cause dizziness and orthostasis in some patients. Advantageous aspects of its side effect profile compared to that of SSRIs include a lower rate of sexual dysfunction and a lack of GI side effects, likely due to blockade of $5-HT_2$ and $5-HT_3$ receptors, respectively (Ghaemi, 2003).

Trazodone and Nefazodone

Trazodone (Desyrel) was introduced in the United States in the 1980s and its chemical derivative, nefazodone (Serzone), followed a few years later. Trazodone has mixed effects on the serotonin system; it acts as a weak, but selective, serotonin reuptake inhibitor, but its primary mechanism of antidepressant action is as an antagonist at postsynaptic $5-HT_2$ receptors. Its active metabolite, *m*-chlorophenylpiperazine (*m*-CPP), is also a potent serotonin receptor agonist (Golden et al., 2004). Trazodone has minimal effects on NE or DA neurons. Nefazodone shares the effect on postsynaptic $5-HT_2$ receptors and weakly inhibits 5-HT and NE reuptake (Bremner, 1995; Serzone, 2002). The two drugs share m-CPP as an active metabolite, but nefazodone has two other active metabolites.

Trazodone and nefazodone are indicated for the treatment of major depressive disorder. In head-to-head trials, nefazodone has performed comparably to the SSRIs, specifically fluoxetine, sertraline, and paroxetine, in the treatment of depression (Hirschfeld, 1999). Both of these medications are relatively sedating antidepressants, making them a preferable choice in depressed patients with significant insomnia. Low doses of trazodone, such as 50 to 100 mg, are commonly used to treat insomnia (Wagner et al., 1998). Controlled trials have confirmed the efficacy of low-dose trazodone in treating insomnia related to other antidepressants (Nierenberg et al., 1994). However, much higher doses of trazodone are generally required to achieve an antidepressant effect.

The suggested initial dose of trazodone for major depression is 150 mg per day in divided doses, with a maximum recommended dose of 400 mg per day in outpatients and 600 mg per day in inpatients with severe depression (Desyrel, 2003). When being prescribed as a sleep aid, low doses of up to 150 mg nightly are sufficient. Nefazodone should be initiated at 200 mg per day in divided doses, with an effective dose range of 300 to 600 mg per day (American Psychiatric Association, 2000; Serzone, 2002). Lower doses are suggested in elderly patients. For both drugs, the dose should be gradually increased to minimize side effects, principally sedation. As with other antidepressants, it may take up to 2 to 4 weeks for a therapeutic effect to be evident (Desyrel, 2003). Both these medications are extensively hepatically metabolized, and nefazodone has several drug–drug interactions. One major advantage to nefazodone is its low rates of sexual dysfunction (Ghaemi, 2003). Both trazodone and nefazodone are potent α_1 adrenoreceptor antagonists, associated with orthostatic hypotension and sedation. Because orthostasis can predispose to falls, both agents are less favorable as treatment in geriatric populations (Golden et al., 2004). Nefazodone may also be associated with nausea and visual disturbances (Serzone, 2002). One potentially serious side effect of trazodone is priapism. Although this is rare (approximately 1/6,000 male patients), it may require surgical intervention and can lead to permanent impairment of erectile function (Ghaemi, 2003). Patients with prolonged erections should immediately discontinue this medication and consult a physician (Desyrel, 2003).

Nefazodone is being prescribed less and less frequently because it now carries a boxed warning for life-threatening liver failure. The reported rate of liver failure resulting in death or transplant is 1 case per 250,000 to 300,000 patient-years of nefazodone treatment (Serzone, 2002). Although there is no way to predict which patients will develop liver failure, this drug should not be initiated in anyone who has acute liver disease or elevated transaminases at baseline. Owing to this warning, the APA (American Psychiatric Association, 2005) suggests careful consideration of the risks before initiating treatment with nefazodone, and it should no longer be considered a first-line agent.

Tricyclic Antidepressants

First employed in the 1950s, the TCAs were the first class of drugs to be extensively used in the treatment of depression. In fact, TCAs were considered the gold standard of antidepressant treatment for decades, until newer, more tolerable antidepressants came onto the market. Their unavoidable side effect profile and a lethal overdose potential are the biggest disadvantages to the TCA class. Several studies have found that newer generation antidepressants are better tolerated than TCAs (Hirschfeld, 1999). In addition, TCAs have the propensity of inducing mania in patients with bipolar disorder (Ghaemi, 2003).

The TCAs are believed to act primarily by blocking the presynaptic reuptake of 5-HT and NE, thereby increasing the availability of these neurotransmitters at postsynaptic receptor sites. Tertiary amines such as amitriptyline and imipramine appear to be equally potent as NE and 5-HT reuptake inhibitors. Of the group, clomipramine is the most potent of its class in blocking 5-HT reuptake. In contrast, secondary amines such as desipramine, nortriptyline, and protriptyline are relatively selective NE reuptake inhibitors (Frazer, 1997).

All of the TCAs are FDA approved for major depressive disorder except clomipramine, which is approved for OCD. Imipramine is additionally approved for use in children with nocturnal enuresis. Beyond these FDA-approved uses, TCAs have been utilized successfully for a wide variety of other conditions as well, including panic disorder, ADHD, chronic pain, migraine prophylaxis, and insomnia. The structurally unique tetracyclic antidepressant, amoxapine, is the only drug of this class that has both antipsychotic and antidepressant effects because it is metabolized into the antipsychotic drug loxapine (Nelson, 2004). The efficacy of the TCAs has been well established in many studies over the last 50 years. A recent systematic review of 194 randomized clinical trials (RCTs) demonstrated that amitriptyline is at least as efficacious as newer antidepressants, though its burden of side effects is greater (Guaiana et al., 2003). Some data also suggested that TCAs may be particularly well suited for patients with severe depression with melancholia (Guaiana et al., 2003). Clomipramine was the first agent studied extensively for the treatment of OCD and was found to be clearly superior to the other TCAs and the MAOIs.

Four of the TCAs have been found to have a demonstrable relationship between their plasma levels and response (Nelson, 2004). For imipramine, drug levels >200 ng per mL were found to be more effective than lower levels. Similarly, desipramine levels >125 ng per mL were found to be more effective. Therapeutic levels for nortriptyline are slightly different, as a curvilinear relationship defines a therapeutic window with plasma levels between 50 and 150 ng per mL. Plasma concentrations of protriptyline are also associated with therapeutic efficacy. TCA blood levels can be used as a guide for treatment and as an indication of toxicity.

Hepatic metabolism is the primary method of clearance for these drugs. Of note, desipramine and nortriptyline are hydroxylated through the CYP450 2D6 pathway. This is of clinical significance because this isoenzyme exhibits genetic variability, with some patients being poor metabolizers and others very rapid metabolizers (Nelson, 2004). Moreover, drugs that inhibit the 2D6 isoenzyme, such as paroxetine, fluoxetine, chlorpromazine, and perphenazine, increase plasma levels of desipramine and nortriptyline, potentially resulting in toxicity. Drug–drug interactions can also occur with MAOIs and quinidine. Most of the TCAs have half-lives of approximately 24 hours; therefore, these drugs can typically be dosed once daily. The more sedating members of the class should always be given at bedtime to minimize daytime somnolence.

Given the structural similarities between TCAs and typical antipsychotics, it is not surprising that these two classes share several features of their side effect profile (Table 22-4). TCAs are antihistaminergic and therefore produce sedation, increased appetite, and weight gain. Tertiary amines are the most potent antagonists at histamine H_1 receptors; doxepin is the prototype and therefore the most sedating. Orthostatic hypotension due to blockade of α_1 adrenoreceptors can occur with all TCAs. This can be especially hazardous in elderly patients, because it may increase risk of falls and hip fracture. Nortriptyline has been found to cause less orthostatic hypotension than other members of the TCA class. TCAs also block muscarinic receptors, causing side effects such as dry mouth, blurred vision, urinary retention, and constipation (Hirschfeld, 1999). Amitriptyline is one of the most potent antagonists among the TCAs at muscarinic receptors and therefore has severe anticholinergic side effects (Nelson, 2004). Because of the anticholinergic effects, patients with prostatic hypertrophy and narrow angle glaucoma must be treated conservatively with this class of drugs. In addition, anticholinergic action in the elderly can contribute to confusion and delirium (Nelson, 2004). All TCAs are associated with a dose-dependent seizure risk. Maprotiline, a tetracyclic compound, has been associated with seizures in both therapeutic and toxic doses, especially at doses >200 mg per day.

Cardiovascular side effects of TCAs are among the most concerning side effects of this class. Tachycardia tends to occur with all TCAs and is often persistent. TCAs possess quinidine-like properties that delay conduction. They therefore should not be used in patients with preexisting heart block, or markedly prolonged QRS or QTc intervals. Indeed, TCAs can lead to second-degree or third-degree heart block—a life-threatening condition. There is also evidence that due to quinidine-like effects as well as reduced heart rate variability, TCAs increase the risk of sudden death following MI. Clearly, TCAs should be avoided in the elderly and in patients with cardiac disease.

An overdose of 10 times the total daily dose of a TCA can be lethal, rendering the therapeutic index of these drugs universally low. That means that less than a 2-week supply taken in overdose has a risk of fatality. Death typically occurs from cardiac arrhythmia, though seizures and CNS depression can also occur. Because the risk of suicide is very high in depressed patients, deliberate overdose with antidepressant drugs is a common occurrence. Steps to minimize this risk in patients treated with TCAs include dispensing only a week's supply of medication at a time and monitoring blood levels for adherence (to detect potential medication hoarding in preparation for an overdose).

Monoamine Oxidase Inhibitors

MAOIs were first identified as antidepressants in the 1950s when iproniazid, an MAOI used for the treatment of tuberculosis, was noted to have mood-elevating properties. The MAOIs have a unique mechanism of action. The enzyme monoamine oxidase (MAO) inactivates epinephrine, NE, 5-HT, DA, and tyramine through oxidative deamination. MAOIs block this enzyme, thereby increasing the concentration of these neurotransmitters in the brain. There are two MAO isoenzymes, designated MAO-A and MAO-B. MAO-A acts on epinephrine, NE, and 5-HT, and MAO-B preferentially affects phenylethylamine, tyramine, and benzylamine. DA is metabolized by both isoenzymes. Inhibition of MAO-A is associated with antidepressant activity (Frazer, 1997).

MAOIs are indicated in the treatment of major depressive disorder, dysthymia, panic disorder, bulimia, and PD. Studies have shown that MAOIs are more effective than other classes of antidepressants in treating the atypical subtype of depression (Quitkin et al., 1990). Atypical depression is characterized by reversed neurovegetative symptoms (increased sleep and appetite), mood reactivity, prominent anxiety, and a sense of fatigue known as *leaden paralysis*, or an extreme heaviness in the arms and legs (Liebowitz et al., 1988).

Currently available MAOIs are either hydrazine or nonhydrazine derivatives. The hydrazine derivatives, phenelzine (Nardil) and isocarboxazid (Marplan), are related to the original MAOI iproniazid. The nonhydrazine derivatives include tranylcypromine (Parnate) and selegiline (Eldepryl oral, Emsam transdermal patch). Moclobemide, the only reversible MAO-A, is not available in the United States. Tranylcypromine is structurally similar to amphetamines and appears to have a mild stimulant-like effect on the brain. Previously, selegiline was known for its use in the adjunctive treatment of PD. At low doses, it is an irreversible MAO-B inhibitor, and it slows progression in PD by an unknown mechanism. However, selegiline becomes nonselective at higher doses and inhibits both MAO-A and B. In 2006, a new transdermal form of selegiline marketed as Emsam was approved for use in major depression in the United States. Recent placebo-controlled trials have shown transdermal selegiline to be an effective treatment of major depression for preventing relapse of depression for up to 1 year (Amsterdam and Bodkin, 2006). The dosing options for this patch are 6, 9, or 12 mg daily. Dietary precautions are not necessary with the 6-mg patch (Emsam, 2007).

MAOIs have fallen out of favor as a result of concerns over dietary restrictions and the potentially serious side effect of hypertensive crisis. In patients treated with an MAOI, intestinal MAO is inactivated, preventing the metabolism of tyramine. When tyramine is ingested, it is not metabolized and instead enters the systemic circulation. The result can be a hypertensive crisis, sometimes called the *cheese reaction* because tyramine is present in higher concentrations in aged cheese. In fact, multiple foods and beverages contain tyramine and cannot be ingested by MAOI-treated patients. MAO-B is not involved in the intestinal tyramine metabolism; therefore, dietary interactions do not occur with selective MAO-B inhibitors, such as oral selegiline, at low doses. However, at higher doses (10 mg per day), dietary interactions may occur. With the transdermal formulation, selegiline is directly absorbed into the systemic circulation, bypassing the GI tract. This allows the drug to be delivered to the brain while leaving enough functional MAO-A in the GI tract to metabolize dietary tyramine (Amsterdam and Bodkin, 2006). As a result, there are no dietary restrictions with the 6 mg dose; however, data are limited regarding the 9 and 12 mg formulations, so restrictions are indicated at these doses.

Drug–drug interactions are also critically important with MAOI use. MAOIs cannot be combined with multiple other medications, including meperidine, dextromethorphan, tryptophan, SSRIs, SNRIs, TCAs, buspirone, psychostimulants, illicit drugs, tramadol, pseudoephedrine (in over-the-counter cold medicine), and Novocain (a local anesthetic). Certain combinations can precipitate a potentially fatal hypertensive crisis, while others can induce the serotonin syndrome (Rapaport, 2007). Patients taking MAOIs should be encouraged to consult with their physician before adding any new prescription or over-the-counter medication to their regimen.

MAO must be newly synthesized after MAOI treatment in order for the activity of the enzyme to be reestablished. This means that the risks of drug and food interactions with irreversible MAOIs will persist for 10 to 14 days after discontinuation of these drugs. This time period must therefore elapse before initiating other antidepressants or allowing the prohibited drugs or foods that may interact with the MAOIs. All the currently marketed MAOIs, with the exception of selegiline, are *nonselective* in that they inhibit both MAO-A and MAO-B. To date, there have been no reports of any hypertensive crisis in patients receiving transdermal selegiline (Goodnick, 2007).

A mild tyramine reaction may include sweating, palpitations, and headache. A more serious, potentially fatal, reaction manifests as a hypertensive crisis, with severe occipital headache, hypertension, neck stiffness, dilated pupils, and possible intracerebral hemorrhage. The reaction typically develops within 20 to 60 minutes after ingestion of the prohibited food item or drug. Patients treated with an MAOI who experience a severe or even moderately painful occipital headache, should immediately seek medical attention. Treatment of the hypertensive crisis usually is comprised of an α-adrenergic antagonist, such as intravenous phentolamine, and other measures to quickly reduce blood pressure. Patients should be advised to carry an identification card that notifies emergency medical personnel that they are currently taking MAOIs.

The most frequent side effects with MAOIs are orthostatic hypotension, headache, dry mouth, constipation, blurred vision, urinary hesitancy, nausea, peripheral edema, insomnia, and weakness (Krishnan, 2004). As with all classes of antidepressants, sexual dysfunction is a common complaint with MAOIs. Phenelzine is particularly prone to cause orthostatic hypotension, often a reason for discontinuation. Weight gain tends to occur more frequently with phenelzine and isocarboxid (hydrazine derivatives). Tranylcypromine is more likely to cause increased agitation and insomnia because of its stimulant-like effect. Transdermal selegiline appears to be well tolerated, with its most common side effects being headache, insomnia, mild orthostasis, and application site reactions (Amsterdam and Bodkin, 2006; Goodnick, 2007). Transdermal selegiline does not appear to be associated with sexual dysfunction or weight gain (Amsterdam and Bodkin, 2006; Goodnick, 2007).

According to the APA (American Psychiatric Association, 2000), this class of medications should be used in the context of treatment-refractory depression, when patients do not respond to other treatment choices. This class has become one of the last options in the treatment algorithm for depression because of the potentially lethal dietary and drug–drug interactions.

Antidepressants and Suicide-Related Behaviors

In 2004, a public health advisory, also known as a *boxed warning*, was issued on all classes of antidepressant medications (Effexor, 2006; Cymbalta, 2007; Prozac, 2007; Remeron, 2007; Wellbutrin, 2007) suggesting that antidepressants may increase the risk of suicidal thinking and behavior in children, adolescents, and young adults being treated for depression. These studies did not find an increased risk in adults beyond age 24 and, in fact, found a risk reduction in adults older than 65 years. Of note, there were *no* completed suicides in any of the 24 trials studied. It is important to appreciate the fact that suicidal thoughts and behaviors are an integral part of the syndrome of major depression. The preponderance of evidence strongly suggests that antidepressant use reduces suicide burden, and in fact, there has been a sudden and dramatic increase in adolescent suicides since the warning was issued, directly in parallel to the decrease in use of antidepressants in this age-group (Gibbons et al., 2007b; Nemeroff et al., 2007). Analysis of treatment utilization patterns reveals that the highest numbers of suicide attempts occur in the month before initiation of antidepressant or psychotherapy and decrease as treatment proceeds (Gibbons et al., 2007a; Simon and Savarino, 2007). One interpretation of these results is that the emergence of suicide ideation or attempts is the event that leads people with depression to seek treatment. Currently, the FDA recommends close monitoring of patients on antidepressants for potential clinical worsening or emergence of suicidal thoughts or behaviors. It also advises weighing the risks and benefits of antidepressant treatment versus no treatment, considering the burden of morbidity and potential mortality inherent in major depression when prescribing for younger patients.

MOOD STABILIZERS

Bipolar disorder, previously referred to as *manic-depressive illness*, is a chronic, severe mental illness characterized by recurrent pathological mood episodes, including manic, hypomanic, mixed, or depressive. An acute manic episode is defined as a distinct period of persistently elevated or irritable mood in conjunction with decreased need for sleep, increase in goal-directed activity, increased talkativeness, flight of ideas, grandiosity, and reckless behavior. Although treating the acute manic episode is of paramount importance, it is also essential to improve interepisode functioning by treating depressive episodes and preventing subsequent cycling into mania or depression, thereby maintaining the euthymic state.

The true definition of a *mood stabilizer* is still debated, but the most conservative definition refers to a medication that is efficacious in two of three phases of bipolar illness, one of which must be prophylaxis (Ghaemi, 2003). In bipolar disorder, *prophylaxis* means prevention of cycling into pathological mood states or extending the duration of euthymic periods. According to this definition, lithium, lamotrigine, olanzapine, and aripiprazole meet the criteria of mood stabilizer. Olanzapine was the first atypical antipsychotic to meet the definition of mood stabilizer and is FDA approved for use in maintenance treatment of bipolar disorder, if the patient responded to olanzapine during the preceding acute episode. Aripiprazole has also received FDA approval as maintenance therapy in bipolar disorder for patients who responded to this drug in the preceding acute episode. However, all of the atypical antipsychotics are commonly used in the treatment of bipolar disorder, particularly in acute mania. Olanzapine, risperidone, quetiapine, ziprasidone, and aripiprazole are FDA approved for acute mania in bipolar disorder, and clozapine is clearly effective as well. Paliperidone has not yet been studied for this condition, but given its similarity to risperidone, the expectation is that it will also have efficacy as an antimanic agent. Similar to the typical antipsychotic agents that preceded them, the atypical antipsychotics are a valuable addition to the treatment armamentarium for bipolar disorder, especially for acute mania. The current APA guidelines (2002) recommend treatment of severe manic or mixed episodes with lithium or valproate plus an atypical antipsychotic, while less ill patients can be treated with lithium, valproate, or atypical antipsychotic monotherapy.

Lithium

Lithium salts were first promoted in 1859 as a treatment for gout, and it was not until 1949 that Cade (1949) described the efficacy of lithium in patients with acute mania. Lithium (Lithobid, Eskalith) was approved by the FDA in 1970 for acute mania in bipolar disorder and then later for prophylaxis of bipolar disorder (Price and Heninger, 1994). Lithium is considered the gold standard in the treatment of bipolar disorder. Patients with classic features of grandiose mania tend to respond more favorably to lithium (Kleindienst and Greil, 2003) than patients with psychotic, dysphoric, mixed (Swann et al., 1997), or rapid-cycling features (Bowden, 1995). Lithium is an efficacious maintenance treatment that is better at preventing manic than depressive episodes. Lithium can also be used to augment the effects of antidepressants in refractory, or treatment-resistant, depression (Price and Heninger, 1994), though its efficacy in this role in the STAR*D trial was not impressive.

The precise pharmacological mechanism of action of lithium as a mood stabilizer remains obscure. Several theories have arisen involving inositol depletion, inhibition of glycogen synthase kinase-3 (GSK-3), and ultimately an effect on various neurotransmitter systems (serotonin, NE, glutamate, γ-aminobutyric acid [GABA]) (Freeman et al., 2004). Lithium carbonate is available as a tablet and lithium citrate as a liquid formulation. Peak plasma concentrations occur rapidly, only 1 to 2 hours after an oral dose. Slow-release preparations absorb more slowly and have lower peak plasma concentrations, lessening the GI side effects (Price and Heninger, 1994). For acute mania, the starting dose of lithium is 1,200 to 1,800 mg daily, and for maintenance treatment of bipolar disorder, a dose of 900 to 1,500 mg daily is recommended. Treatment should be initiated with twice or thrice daily dosing to minimize dose-related side effects, though lithium can be administered in 1 or 2 doses later in treatment (Price and Heninger, 1994). Lithium has a narrow therapeutic index, thereby requiring monitoring of serum levels. The target blood level in acute mania and maintenance of bipolar disorder is 0.5 to 1.2 mEq per L. In contrast, lithium is often prescribed in lower doses (i.e., 600 to 900 mg) when used as an adjunct for unipolar depression (Bauer and Döpfmer, 1999), though plasma levels of 0.8 mEq per L are recommended. To obtain an accurate lithium level, blood should be sampled approximately 12 hours after the last lithium dose. Given its plasma half-life of 20 to 24 hours, it takes approximately 5 days to achieve steady state (Keck and McElroy, 2002).

Lithium can cause a wide variety of bothersome side effects, which is often the reason that patients discontinue this medication. Side effects include cognitive dulling, sedation, weight gain, GI distress, fine tremor, renal tubular damage, sinus bradycardia, sinus node dysfunction, hypothyroidism, and sexual dysfunction (Freeman et al., 2004). Diabetes insipidus, associated with polyuria and polydipsia, occurs in approximately 10% of patients on long-term treatment (Bendz and Aurell, 1999). Elderly patients and those with multiple medical comorbidities tend to be more sensitive to the side effects of lithium. Before lithium is initiated, patients should undergo baseline laboratory tests, including thyroid and renal function tests, and an ECG for all patients older than 40 years (American Psychiatric Association, 2002). Treatment guidelines recommend that renal function is monitored every 2 to 3 months and thyroid function tested once or twice during the first 6 months of treatment. After 6 months, these laboratory tests should be repeated every 6 to 12 months.

Lithium toxicity usually becomes symptomatic when plasma levels rise >1.5 mEq per L (American Psychiatric Association, 2002). Symptoms include marked tremor, nausea, diarrhea, vertigo, confusion, and increased deep tendon reflexes. When plasma levels increase beyond 2.0 mEq per L, patients can experience seizures, coma, and permanent neurologic damage. Treatment is mostly supportive, though hemodialysis may be necessary in severe cases. Of note, concurrent use of nonsteroidal anti-inflammatory drugs (NSAIDs) increases the risk of lithium toxicity. Thiazide diuretics and angiotensin-converting enzyme inhibitors (ACE-I) also increase lithium levels. Permanent renal damage is associated with repeated episodes of lithium levels >1.5 mEq per L.

Lithium is teratogenic and purportedly associated with an increased, albeit low, risk for Ebstein anomaly, a dysplastic tricuspid valve fetal malformation. First-trimester lithium exposure is linked to a 0.05% to 0.10% prevalence of Ebstein anomaly, signifying a relative risk of 10 to 20 compared with the general population (Cohen and Rosenbaum, 1998). Despite this risk, lithium is still preferable for use during pregnancy when compared with the other, more highly teratogenic, mood stabilizers.

Valproic Acid/Divalproex Sodium

Valproate is an anticonvulsant that has been available in the United States since the 1970s but was not approved for bipolar mania until 1995. There are three formulations of this medication available, including valproic acid, sodium valproate, and divalproex sodium (Depakote, Depakene, Depakote ER). Divalproex sodium is comprised of 50% sodium valproate and 50% valproic acid. Once in the GI tract, all of these forms dissociate into the same active ingredient and are clinically interchangeable. For the purposes of this discussion, all forms will be referred to as valproate. Valproate is indicated for the treatment of acute manic episodes associated with bipolar disorder; in addition, it is approved for prophylactic treatment of migraine headache, complex partial seizures, and absence seizures (Depakote, 2006). Its mechanism of therapeutic action remains obscure.

Many studies have shown valproate to be a safe and effective treatment for acute manic episodes (Bowden et al., 1994). It can be particularly useful for patients who are lithium nonresponders and/or cannot tolerate lithium due to side effects. Several studies have shown that valproate or carbamazepine may be more effective in patients with certain subtypes of bipolar disorder, including rapid-cycling, mixed, or dysphoric mania (Bowden et al., 1994; Bowden, 1995; Swann et al., 1997), and in patients with bipolar disorder with comorbid substance use (Bowden, 2004). In addition, valproate is often used in conjunction with other mood stabilizers or antipsychotics to improve the treatment response. Although not specifically FDA approved for this use, valproate is commonly continued as prophylactic long-term treatment for bipolar disorder.

Valproate is available in delayed-release tablets and sprinkles as well as an ER formulation, allowing for once-daily dosing. Its half-life is 9 to 16 hours. The initial dosing recommendation in acute mania is 750 mg daily in divided doses (delayed-release formulation) or 25 mg/kg/day (ER formulation) (Depakote, 2006). Dosing should be reduced in elderly patients. Several studies have found that in acute mania, valproate treatment can be initiated safely with oral loading doses of 20 to 30 mg/kg/day to induce a more rapid response (Allen et al., 2006). The maximum recommended dosage is 60 mg/kg/day. The APA practice guidelines suggest a broad therapeutic range for trough valproate serum concentrations of 50 to 125 μg per mL. However, a recent study revealed that higher valproate serum levels are associated with greater efficacy in the treatment of acute mania, with the optimal level being >94 μg per ml (Allen et al., 2006).

Valproate is primarily metabolized by hepatic glucuronidation. This has important implications for clinical practice; specifically valproate is contraindicated in patients with moderate to severe liver disease. In addition, agents that induce hepatic enzymes affect its metabolism. For example, enzyme inducers such as carbamazepine or phenobarbital will result in a marked increase in valproate clearance. Unlike other anticonvulsants, valproate inhibits drug oxidation, thereby increasing serum concentrations of many other drugs, including TCAs, phenobarbital, phenytoin, and lamotrigine.

Valproate is generally well tolerated by patients. The most common side effects observed are nausea, vomiting, somnolence, dizziness, hair loss, and weight gain (Depakote, 2006). Patients should be warned that valproate carries a risk of asymptomatic thrombocytopenia, for which regular monitoring of platelet counts is necessary. Valproate also carries a risk of hyperammonemia, but ammonia levels need only be checked when clinically indicated. Valproate can cause a benign elevation of hepatic transaminases; however, it has also been associated with a potentially fatal, idiosyncratic hepatotoxicity, for which it carries a boxed warning. Three analyses of valproate-associated hepatic fatalities have been published to date, all of which concur that this rare reaction is more likely to occur in children younger than 2 years, patients with developmental delay, patients with metabolic disorders, and those receiving valproate as polypharmacy (Bryant and Dreifuss, 1996). This hepatotoxicity tends to occur more commonly in the first 6 months of treatment. It is recommended to monitor liver function tests in all patients on valproate at baseline, frequently over the first 6 months of treatment, and every 6 months thereafter (Depakote, 2006). Additionally, rare cases of life-threatening pancreatitis have been reported in patients taking valproate, prompting a second boxed warning. Patients should be warned of the symptoms of pancreatitis (nausea, vomiting, abdominal pain) and made aware of this potential risk.

Lastly, valproate is a well-documented teratogen; therefore, it is classified as category D for use during pregnancy. It is associated with a fourfold increased risk of congenital malformations, especially with first-trimester exposure. Before implementing valproate therapy in women of childbearing age, a pregnancy test is essential. Women of childbearing age should be strongly encouraged to use an effective form of contraception while being treated with valproate. This should be part of the informed consent process before initiating treatment with valproate. Given these serious risks, the benefit–risk analysis of continuing valproate treatment during pregnancy should be carefully reviewed with the patient who becomes pregnant. Because neural tube defects are the most commonly observed abnormality, folic acid supplementation should be recommended to women treated with valproate who are considering pregnancy (Depakote, 2006).

Carbamazepine

Carbamazepine (Tegretol, Tegretol XR, Equetro, Carbatrol) is an anticonvulsant that was only recently FDA approved for the treatment of acute manic or mixed symptoms in bipolar I disorder. It is also approved for use in generalized tonic-clonic seizures, partial seizures with complex symptomatology, mixed seizure patterns, and pain associated with trigeminal neuralgia. The mechanism of action of this drug in bipolar disorder remains unclear.

The efficacy of carbamazepine in acute mania has not been established in trials longer than 3 weeks (Equetro, 2007). Prophylactic lithium was superior to carbamazepine in bipolar disorder (Denicoff et al., 1997). In this same study, the combination of carbamazepine and lithium was more effective than either agent alone (Denicoff et al., 1997). Unfortunately, concomitant use of lithium and carbamazepine is also associated with an increased risk of neurotoxic side effects (Equetro, 2007).

Carbamazepine is usually initially prescribed at a daily dose of 200 to 600 mg, in three to four divided doses. The ER formulation is available in capsules and started at 200 mg twice daily with a daily increase in dose up to a maximum daily dosage of 1,600 mg. Therapeutic serum levels of carbamazepine have not been specifically established for bipolar disorder, but the range of 4 to 12 μg per mL used in epilepsy is generally accepted. Blood levels should be monitored approximately every 6 months.

The CYP450-3A4 isoenzyme primarily metabolizes carbamazepine. This drug is a potent inducer of the P450-3A4 isoenzyme, which decreases levels of many other medications. In addition, carbamazepine induces its own metabolism, a phenomenon known as *autoinduction*, which results in a fluctuating half-life. When coadministered with carbamazepine, drugs that are CYP450-3A4 inhibitors increase plasma carbamazepine concentrations. Conversely, drugs that induce activity of this enzyme, such as rifampin, phenobarbital, phenytoin, theophylline, and carbamazepine, all decrease plasma carbamazepine levels.

Carbamazepine is associated with many dose-related side effects, including diplopia, somnolence, nausea, vomiting, weight gain, dizziness, and ataxia. Benign rash is a common side effect of carbamazepine, with some studies estimating the incidence to be 3%, while others have estimated this incidence to be as high as 20% (Denicoff et al., 1997). However, severe dermatologic reactions such as toxic epidermal necrolysis (TEN) and Stevens-Johnson syndrome (SJS) can also occur. These reactions are very rare, but potentially fatal. Carbamazepine is also linked to hyponatremia and thrombocytopenia, the former a particular concern in the elderly. A boxed warning has been issued for rare, idiosyncratic reactions such as agranulocytosis and aplastic anemia. Studies have found that carbamazepine is linked to a fivefold to eightfold increased risk of developing these reactions. Baseline liver function tests, renal function tests, and hematologic profile are all recommended, with close monitoring during the first 2 months of treatment and every 3 months thereafter (American Psychiatric Association, 2002).

Carbamazepine is a category D drug for use during pregnancy (Equetro, 2007). It is associated with an increased risk of congenital malformations, particularly spina bifida. A pregnancy test should be obtained before initiating carbamazepine treatment in women with childbearing potential. Women of childbearing age should be strongly encouraged to use an effective form of contraception if carbamazepine is prescribed. This should be part of the informed consent process before initiating carbamazepine treatment. Of note, carbamazepine increases the metabolism of oral contraceptives through hepatic enzyme induction, which can lead to unintended conception. Therefore, oral contraceptives cannot be relied upon in carbamazepine-treated women. Folic acid supplementation is also recommended for women treated with carbamazepine who are considering pregnancy.

Lamotrigine

Lamotrigine (Lamictal) is an anticonvulsant drug of the phenlytriazine class, not chemically related to any other antiepileptic (Lamictal, 2007). In 2003, lamotrigine received FDA approval for maintenance treatment of bipolar I disorder to delay the time to occurrence of mood episodes (depression, mania, hypomania, mixed episodes). Data suggest that lamotrigine is an effective maintenance treatment for bipolar disorder, particularly for prophylaxis of depression (Calabrese et al., 2003). Lamotrigine has also been found to be particularly helpful in preventing mood episodes in rapid-cycling or type II bipolar disorder (American Psychiatric Association, 2002). Unlike valproate and carbamazepine, lamotrigine is not effective in acute mania. Lastly, there is some evidence, albeit conflicting, that lamotrigine may be effective in the treatment of bipolar depression.

The mechanism of action of this medication has not yet been established. One proposed mechanism suggests that lamotrigine inhibits voltage-sensitive sodium channels, thereby modulating presynaptic release of excitatory amino acids such as glutamate and aspartate (Lamictal, 2007). How this molecular mechanism translates into a therapeutic benefit in bipolar disorder is unclear, but it is assumed to be related to its anticonvulsant activity (Miller et al., 1986).

Lamotrigine is supplied in oral tablets as well as chewable dispersible tablets. Lamotrigine is absorbed quickly and completely after oral administration, with a $t_{1/2}$ of 27 hours and a bioavailability unaffected by food (Lamictal, 2007). Lamotrigine should be initiated at a dose of 25 mg daily for the first 2 weeks, 50 mg daily for the third and fourth week, 100 mg daily the fifth week, and finally to the target dose of 200 mg daily by the sixth week (Lamictal, 2007). This slow titration schedule is critical to decreasing the risk of SJS. Lamotrigine is metabolized primarily by glucuronic acid conjugation, which potentially results in many significant drug–drug interactions. Of note, valproate inhibits glucuronidation, which decreases the clearance of lamotrigine, almost doubling its elimination half-life (Lamictal, 2007). As a result of this interaction, if lamotrigine and valproate are concomitantly prescribed, the lamotrigine titration schedule must be slowed, such that it reaches 100 mg daily within 5 weeks, which is the target dose in this circumstance (Lamictal, 2007). Conversely, agents that induce hepatic enzymes (e.g., carbamazepine, phenytoin, phenobarbital, rifampin) increase the clearance of lamotrigine. Therefore, patients on these medications will need a faster titration schedule, ending with a higher target dose of up to 400 mg daily (Lamictal, 2007).

The most common side effects seen with lamotrigine are headache, rash, dizziness, diarrhea, and dream abnormalities (Lamictal, 2007). Rash is recognized as the most clinically significant side effect of which to be aware in lamotrigine-treated patients. The most common rash seen with lamotrigine is a benign maculopapular rash (Shelton and Calabrese, 2004). However, serious rash associated with hospitalization occurred in 0.08% of patients with mood disorders when lamotrigine was the initial monotherapy and in 0.13% of patients who received lamotrigine as adjunctive therapy (Lamictal, 2007). The incidence of these rashes included some cases of SJS and TEN, both of which can be fatal. SJS typically begins with symptoms of fever, sore throat, chills, headache, and malaise and classically involves various mucous membranes such as oral, nasal, eye, vaginal, or urethral membranes. Although no factors are completely predictive of risk of severe rash, several factors have been implicated in an increased risk of rash with lamotrigine. Evidence has shown that concomitant lamotrigine and valproate use increases the risk of serious, life-threatening rash in adults (Lamictal, 2007). Exceeding the recommended starting dose or escalating the dose faster than recommended may increase serious rash risk. Most cases of life-threatening rash have occurred in the first 8 weeks of treatment. Overall, it is impossible to predict which rashes will become serious or life threatening, and as a result, lamotrigine should be discontinued at the first sign of any type of rash (Lamictal, 2007).

ANXIOLYTIC MEDICATIONS

Anxiety disorders encompass a wide range of conditions including GAD, SAD, PTSD, and panic disorder. These disorders are very prevalent and also quite often comorbid with other psychiatric illnesses. In addition to the specified disorders, anxiety symptoms are very common in many psychiatric and medical conditions and in a wide variety of psychosocial circumstances.

Before the arrival of benzodiazepines in the 1960s, barbiturates were commonly used to treat anxiety disorders and insomnia. Potentially fatal respiratory depression can occur with these drugs at only mildly toxic dosages, and as a result, barbiturates were mostly replaced soon after the arrival of the safer benzodiazepines. Historically, benzodiazepines have had many uses in medicine, including anesthesia induction, as antispastic and muscle relaxants, and in seizure control. Furthermore, over the last 50 years, benzodiazepines have been the mainstay of treatment of anxiety disorders, including GAD, panic disorder, SAD, and PTSD. This class of medications is very commonly prescribed for intermittent and chronic insomnia. Because of the cross-tolerance of benzodiazepines and alcohol, benzodiazepines are the mainstay of treatment for alcohol withdrawal and detoxification. Benzodiazepines are commonly used for management of acute agitation, particularly in psychotic disorders and bipolar disorder, often in combination with antipsychotic agents.

Today, SSRIs and SNRIs are recognized as the definitive treatments for many anxiety disorders. Benzodiazepines are often relegated to an adjunctive role in treatment of anxiety disorders. For example, the APA (1998) guidelines for the treatment of panic disorder advocate SSRI therapy as first-line therapy and suggest benzodiazepine use for acute anxiety management rather than long-term treatment. Despite this recommendation, benzodiazepines continue to be very commonly prescribed for the treatment of panic disorder (Bruce et al., 2003). Clearly, this class of medications still has a great deal to offer as an effective and safe treatment for several psychiatric disorders.

Benzodiazepines

The first benzodiazepine, chlordiazepoxide, was patented in 1959. Since the 1960s, benzodi-azepines have been widely prescribed for a range of anxiety disorders by both psychiatrists and general practitioners. The widespread use of this class of medication is likely a function of its efficacy and rapid onset of anxiolytic effect (Stevens and Pollack, 2005). Structurally, drugs in this class have a similar 1,4-benzodiazepine ring system. Benzodiazepines share four main pharmacological properties: sedative, anxiolytic, anticonvulsant, and muscle relaxant. Because they can be associated with daytime somnolence, cognitive impairment, and abuse, there is considerable controversy surrounding their long-term use.

Benzodiazepine receptors are closely linked with the receptor for GABA, the major inhibitory neurotransmitter in the CNS. The $GABA_A$ receptor, often referred to as the GABA–benzodiazepine receptor complex, can be modulated by benzodiazepines, as well as by barbiturates and alcohol. Benzodiazepines bind to a different site on the receptor than GABA and potentiate the action of GABA on the receptor. This has been hypothesized to account for the anxiolytic effects of these drugs. $GABA_A$ receptors are widely distributed throughout the CNS, highly concentrated in the brain stem, thalamus, cerebellum, hippocampus, amygdala, and cortex; several of these areas have been implicated in the pathogenesis of anxiety (Roy-Byrne, 2005).

Two different types of benzodiazepine receptors have been associated with $GABA_A$ receptors. These benzodiazepine receptor subtypes are referred to as BZ_1 and BZ_2. Nonbenzodiazepine sedative-hypnotics (zolpidem) bind relatively specifically to the BZ_1 subtype, whereas the BZ_2 receptor has a low affinity for this class of compound. Benzodiazepines act nonselectively on both BZ_1 and BZ_2 receptor subtypes.

Benzodiazepines differ in pharmacological properties such as potency, half-life, and the presence of active metabolites. However, at equipotent doses, they are all equally effective (Stevens and Pollack, 2005), but these pharmacokinetic differences have a major impact on their clinical applications (see Table 22-6).

There is considerable evidence that benzodiazepines are effective in treatment of panic disorder. Two members of this class, alprazolam and clonazepam, are currently FDA approved for the treatment of panic disorder (American Psychiatric Association, 2006). Benzodiazepines are also effective in the treatment of GAD and social phobia. This class is notable for its rapid onset of symptom relief in anxious patients. Benzodiazepines are also useful as adjuncts in acute mania or psychosis and can be used for acute agitation in oral, intravenous, and IM forms. Many members of this class have been used for the treatment of insomnia as well. Currently, five traditional benzodiazepines have FDA approval for the treatment of insomnia: estazolam, flurazepam, quazepam, temazepam, and triazolam. In the 1980s, triazolam (Halcion) and temazepam (Restoril) were widely utilized as sleep aids, and flurazepam (Dalmane) was the most commonly prescribed sedative-hypnotic agent of the time. The use of triazolam became

TABLE 22-6	Pharmacokinetics of Benzodiazepines		
Name	**Half-Life ($t_{1/2}$) (hr)**	**Onset of Action**	**Common Uses**
Triazolam (Halcion)	<6	Fast	Insomnia, acute anxiety
Temazepam (Restoril)	8–20	Intermediate	Insomnia
Lorazepam (Ativan)	10–20	Intermediate	Acute anxiety, alcohol withdrawal, agitation
Alprazolam (Xanax)	10–15	Fast	Panic disorder
Clonazepam (Klonopin)	>24	Slow	Panic disorder, adjunct for mania/psychosis
Chlordiazepoxide (Librium)	>24	Intermediate	Alcohol withdrawal
Diazepam (Valium)	>24	Fast	All anxiety disorders
Flurazepam (Dalmane)	>48	Fast	Insomnia with daytime anxiety

(Raj and Sheehan, 2004.)

problematic because its short half-life contributed to the risk of rebound insomnia, early-morning awakening, memory impairment, and withdrawal symptoms (Raj and Sheehan, 2004). The metabolite of flurazepam has a very long elimination half-life, which results in daytime sedation and impaired motor performance. Accumulation of this metabolite in the body is especially problematic for elderly patients. As a result of these problems, many of these agents have fallen out of favor, having been replaced by newer and safer medications. Agents with rapid onset of action such as diazepam, alprazolam, or lorazepam are useful medications on an "as-needed" basis. Longer-acting agents, such as ER alprazolam and clonazepam, may be better choices for long-term daily treatment. Advantages of the ER formulation over traditional alprazolam include less frequent dosing (Raj and Sheehan, 2004), reduced likelihood of rebound anxiety, and decreased abuse potential (Stevens and Pollack, 2005). For highly anxious patients, benzodiazepines prescribed concurrently with an antidepressant can often bring much needed relief and reduce the side effects of the antidepressant. The benzodiazepine can then be tapered and discontinued in 3 to 4 weeks after the therapeutic effect of the antidepressant is evident. Unfortunately, discontinuation of benzodiazepines can be difficult in some patients after physiologic dependence has developed.

When benzodiazepines are taken for an extended period of time, tolerance may develop to certain of the therapeutic effects. This is more of an issue for the sedative-hypnotic effects than for the anxiolytic effects. It is important to distinguish this normal physiologic dependence, a predictable adaptation of the body, from addiction, which is characterized by compulsive drug-seeking behavior and a loss of control (O'Brien, 2005). Patients abusing these medications are typically seeking euphoric effects whereas individuals with anxiety disorders are seeking relief from their anxiety. Although the prevalence of benzodiazepine abuse is relatively low, it has been shown that individuals who abuse multiple substances are more likely to abuse benzodiazepines (Stevens and Pollack, 2005). Therefore, benzodiazepines are relatively contraindicated in patients with a history of substance abuse (American Psychiatric Association, 1998). It is imperative that abuse potential be weighed against the potentially beneficial therapeutic effects of benzodiazepines.

If these medications are abruptly discontinued, particularly those with a short half-life, withdrawal symptoms often occur, which can include tachycardia, increased blood pressure, tremor, muscle cramps, rebound anxiety/panic attacks, insomnia, memory impairment, confusion, and perceptual disturbances. In its most severe form, symptoms can progress to seizures, delirium, and even death. These withdrawal symptoms may begin the day after discontinuing benzodiazepines and rarely can persist for days to weeks. Withdrawal tends to be worse with shorter half-life benzodiazepines (Rickels et al., 1990) after long duration of treatment and higher doses (O'Brien, 2005; Rosenbaum, 2005). For patients treated with benzodiazepines for any considerable length of time, a gradual taper is strongly recommended. The dose should be decreased by approximately 5% to 10% weekly; clinicians should anticipate that the last few decrements in dose would be the most difficult for the patient to discontinue. Switching to a longer-acting benzodiazepine such as clonazepam may help prevent or lessen withdrawal symptoms (O'Brien, 2005).

Side effects of benzodiazepines include residual daytime sedation, rebound insomnia, psychomotor impairment (Raj and Sheehan, 2004), and anterograde amnesia (Wagner et al., 1998). Anterograde amnesia is a well-documented phenomenon that occurs most frequently with short half-life agents including triazolam, alprazolam, and lorazepam (Raj and Sheehan, 2004). There is some evidence that long-term benzodiazepine use may lead to cognitive impairment, which can persist after the drug is discontinued (Stevens and Pollack, 2005). Psychomotor impairment can be dangerous for any patient, but benzodiazepines are specifically associated with a significantly increased risk of falls and subsequent hip fractures in the elderly (Allain et al., 2005). To minimize this risk, clinicians should assess patients for underlying balance and gait abnormalities, avoid concomitant use of other benzodiazepines and CNS depressants, and use lower doses in this population (Allain et al., 2005). It is also advisable to choose a benzodiazepine with a shorter half-life for elderly patients (Raj and Sheehan, 2004). In general, all patients should be advised to avoid alcohol or other sedatives when being treated with benzodiazepines because of their potentially harmful additive effects (Van Steveninck et al., 1996).

The liver metabolizes benzodiazepines through microsomal oxidation or glucuronide conjugation. Age, hepatic disease, and drugs such as estrogens, cimetidine, and MAOIs affect the oxidative pathway. Therefore, benzodiazepines that are conjugated (e.g., temazepam, oxazepam, lorazepam) are safer in the elderly and patients with hepatic disease (Raj and Sheehan, 2004). Another important drug–drug interaction is between benzodiazepines and digoxin. Benzodiazepines tend to increase digoxin levels, with a subsequently higher chance of digoxin toxicity.

There is a possibility of teratogenic effects with benzodiazepines (Raj and Sheehan, 2004). Some studies have found an increased risk of facial clefts and skeletal anomalies following first or second trimester exposure to benzodiazepines, and consequently this class is category C for use in pregnancy. There is more compelling evidence of neonatal CNS depression and withdrawal symptoms due to third trimester benzodiazepine exposure. As a result, it is recommended that women should be tapered off these medications before conception. However, patients should be advised to not abruptly discontinue benzodiazepine use during pregnancy because this could precipitate a withdrawal seizure (in mother and fetus) and miscarriage.

Benzodiazepines can suppress respiratory drive and are therefore contraindicated in patients with sleep apnea and chronic obstructive pulmonary disease (COPD). In overdose, these drugs can result in dangerous respiratory depression, particularly when combined with other sedating drugs or alcohol. A safe and effective benzodiazepine antagonist, flumazenil, is now available. It can be used in an emergency setting to reverse the effects of benzodiazepine overdose; however, supportive medical management is often still necessary.

Buspirone (Buspar)

Buspirone, a member of the azapirone class, is a unique anxiolytic drug approved by the FDA for the treatment of GAD in 1986. Its anxiolytic action is mediated by agonist activity at the 5-HT_{1a} receptor. Acutely, buspirone decreases serotonin release in the dorsal raphe nucleus. With chronic exposure, these receptors become desensitized, and serotonergic activity is actually increased (Suranyi-Cadotte et al., 1990). This delayed effect is believed to account for the slow onset of therapeutic action when buspirone is administered clinically. As with antidepressants, the therapeutic effects of buspirone take several weeks to become apparent. The effective dose range is 30 to 90 mg daily, and because of its short half-life, it is administered twice or three times daily. It has a relatively benign side effect profile, which includes dizziness, headache, and nausea.

In recent years, buspirone has been prescribed less by psychiatrists than general practitioners, perhaps due to skepticism regarding its efficacy. A systematic review of 36 RCTs was conducted to evaluate the effectiveness of buspirone in GAD (Chessick et al., 2006). Clearly buspirone is an effective treatment for patients with GAD compared with placebo. This same study suggested that benzodiazepines might be superior in efficacy to buspirone in these patients. Of note, patients formerly treated with benzodiazepines tend not to respond as favorably to buspirone as benzodiazepine-naive patients (Chessick et al., 2006).

Buspirone has also been found to have some utility in the treatment of major depression, typically as an adjunctive medication. It is thought to enhance the activity of SSRIs through the 5-HT_{1a} receptors (Redrobe and Bourin, 1998). In the STAR*D trial, buspirone, at an average daily dose of 40.9 mg, was shown to be as effective as bupropion as an adjunct to citalopram for major depression (Trivedi et al., 2006). Unlike benzodiazepines and other sedative-hypnotics, buspirone lacks sedative, muscle relaxant, and anticonvulsant effects. This pharmacological profile offers several advantages for an antianxiety medication, including lack of tolerance, withdrawal symptoms, or abuse liability. Given these advantages, buspirone is regarded as a particularly safe choice for patients with comorbid alcohol dependence and anxiety. It is also reasonable to consider buspirone as a second-line agent for GAD in patients who cannot tolerate SSRIs. Unlike the SSRIs and benzodiazepines, buspirone is not effective in the treatment of panic disorder, OCD, or PTSD.

INSOMNIA MEDICATIONS

Insomnia is a significant public health problem, affecting up to 40% of the general population at some point in their lives (Walsh and Engelhardt, 1992; Elie et al., 1999). Sleep disturbances can include difficulty falling asleep, frequent awakenings, and early-morning awakening (Wagner et al., 1998). Acute insomnia refers to a sleep disturbance lasting less than a month, typically more easily treatable, as opposed to chronic insomnia, which lasts more than a month and can be very difficult to treat. Sleep disturbances, both acute and chronic, can often be a sign of underlying medical or psychiatric illness. It is imperative that the clinician performs a thorough evaluation of any patient with insomnia (see also Chapter 20). If a thorough assessment finds no underlying explanation for a patient's insomnia, treatment options can be considered, such as sedative-hypnotics and cognitive behavioral therapy (CBT).

When it is determined that drug therapy is warranted, it is reasonable to treat acute insomnia with a 7- to 10-day course of pharmacotherapy (Wagner et al., 1998). In chronic insomnia, there are no specific guidelines for duration of treatment other than to base the decision on the patient's response to therapy and the tolerability of the medication (Wagner et al., 1998).

Several options are available when choosing a pharmacological intervention for insomnia. Benzodiazepine sedative-hypnotics are often used. Four nonbenzodiazepine sedative-hypnotic agents are FDA approved for use in the United States. Three of the four agents, zolpidem, zaleplon, and eszopiclone, also known as the Z drugs, are schedule IV controlled substances. The Z drugs share some pharmacological properties with benzodiazepines; accordingly, they also carry the potential for a withdrawal syndrome when abruptly discontinued and rebound insomnia after discontinuation. In addition, these three sedative-hypnotics carry some intrinsic abuse potential. When combined with alcohol, benzodiazepines, narcotics, antihistamines, or any other CNS depressant, these medications can have additive CNS-depressant effects (Sonata, 2003; Ambien, 2007; Lunesta, 2007). However, because of their more selective mechanism of action, these sedative-hypnotics induce fewer side effects than the classic benzodiazepine sedative-hypnotics. In addition, these medications are much less likely to cause falls in the elderly, compared with benzodiazepines (Allain et al., 2005). Ramelteon, the last sleep-inducing agent discussed in this section, represents a first-in-class agent, distinct from benzodiazepines and all other sedative-hypnotics.

Zolpidem

Zolpidem (Ambien) is an imidazopyridine hypnotic that was approved for the treatment of insomnia in 1993. It is specifically indicated for the short-term treatment of insomnia characterized by difficulty with sleep initiation (Ambien, 2007). In 2005 an extended release formulation, marketed as Ambien CR, became available, with the specific indication for treatment of insomnia characterized by difficulty with sleep onset and/or maintenance. In contrast to benzodiazepines, which nonselectively bind both benzodiazepine receptor subtypes of the $GABA_A$ receptor complex, zolpidem binds the BZ_1 receptor subtype preferentially (Ambien, 2007). The BZ_1 receptor subtype is thought to be responsible for sedation. The result of this selectivity is that zolpidem has sedative effects with minimal muscle relaxant, anxiolytic, or anticonvulsant effects (Wagner et al., 1998; Ambien, 2007).

Zolpidem has been shown to improve sleep latency and total sleep time (Wagner et al., 1998). It is available in 5 and 10 mg tablets with a recommended dose of 10 mg immediately before bedtime. The ER oral tablets are available in 6.25 and 12.5 mg tablets with a recommended dose of 12.5 mg just before bedtime. Elderly patients or patients with hepatic impairment should be prescribed a lower dose of 5 mg of immediate release or 6.25 mg of the ER formulation. Zolpidem has a rapid onset of action and a half-life of 1.5 to 2.4 hours (Wagner et al., 1998).

The most common side effects seen with zolpidem are daytime drowsiness, dizziness, headache, and GI distress (Wagner et al., 1998; Ambien, 2007). Side effects appear to be dose related. Zolpidem does appear to increase the risk of falls in the elderly, though not to the extent of the benzodiazepine class. One trial showed 1.5% of patients older than 60 reported falls while taking zolpidem (Ambien, 2007). In addition, confusion and anterograde amnesia have been reported in patients treated with zolpidem and tend to be more frequent in the elderly. Rebound insomnia on the day after zolpidem discontinuation is another potential adverse event.

Zolpidem, as with other Z drugs, is pharmacologically similar to benzodiazepines and has abuse potential. It should be used cautiously in patients with a history of drug or alcohol addiction. In addition, patients should be explicitly warned not to combine this medication with alcohol.

Zaleplon

Zaleplon (Sonata) is a sedative-hypnotic of the pyrazolopyrimidine class approved in 1999 by the FDA for the short-term treatment of insomnia (Sonata, 2003). Like zolpidem, zaleplon acts on the GABA–benzodiazepine receptor complex. Specifically, zaleplon binds to the BZ_1 receptor of the $GABA_A$ receptor complex. Zaleplon has been shown in clinical trials to decrease the time to sleep onset, but not necessarily to affect duration of sleep or number of sleep awakenings.

Zaleplon is available in 5 and 10 mg tablets. The recommended dosage for most healthy adults is 10 mg at bedtime, with a daily maximum dosage of 20 mg. A lower dosage of 5 mg at bedtime is recommended for elderly patients and patients with mild to moderate hepatic impairment. Because of its rapid absorption (within 1 hour of ingestion), it is essential that patients take this medication immediately before going to bed or after they have gone to bed and experienced sleep difficulty. A high-fat or heavy meal reduces absorption of zaleplon and its effect on sleep (Sonata, 2003). Zaleplon is partially metabolized by CYP450-3A4 and therefore can be affected by coadministration of a 3A4 inducer (e.g., rifampin, phenytoin, carbamazepine, phenobarbital) or 3A4 inhibitor (e.g., erythromycin, ketoconazole, cimetidine). Side effects include next-day amnesia, headache, somnolence, and rebound insomnia, particularly on the first night after discontinuation.

Eszopiclone

Eszopiclone (Lunesta) is a sedative-hypnotic agent of the cyclopyrrolone class indicated for the treatment of acute and chronic insomnia. Eszopiclone, released in 2005, is the S-isomer of the nonbenzodiazepine hypnotic zopiclone, available in Europe and South America. Eszopiclone acts on the BZ_1 receptor of the GABA–benzodiazepine receptor complex in a similar manner as with zolpidem and zaleplon. The effectiveness of eszopiclone in reducing sleep latency and improving sleep maintenance was established in five controlled trials of 6 months' duration (Lunesta, 2007). Eszopiclone is rapidly absorbed with a time to peak concentration of 1 hour and a $t_{1/2}$ of 6 hours. Because of its rapid absorption, patients should take this medication immediately before going to bed. The effects of eszopiclone on sleep onset may be reduced if it is taken with or after a high-fat meal. The recommended dose is 2 to 3 mg but should be reduced to 1 to 2 mg in elderly patients and those with severe hepatic impairment. CYP450-3A4 is a major metabolic pathway for eszopiclone, so 3A4 inhibitors and inducers can affect metabolism of the drug. The side effect profile of eszopiclone is very similar to that of the other Z sedative-hypnotics and commonly includes dry mouth, dizziness, and unpleasant taste. Side effects appear to be dose related; therefore, treating with the lowest effective dose is advised. Mild memory impairment or amnesia emerged with the 3 mg dose, but only in 1.3% of patients. The sedative effect of this medication appears to wear off completely by 5 hours after the dose, diminishing the likelihood of next-day sedation.

Ramelteon

Ramelteon (Rozarem) received FDA approval in 2005 for insomnia characterized by difficulty with sleep onset. It is a selective melatonin receptor agonist and thought to target melatonin MT_1 and MT_2 receptors, which are believed to be involved in the regulation of circadian rhythm and, in turn, the sleep–wake cycle (Kato et al., 2005; Rozarem, 2006). Studies have shown it to be more potent and selective for MT_1 receptors, thereby allowing it to better induce sleep onset. Unlike benzodiazepines and other sedative-hypnotics, ramelteon has no affinity for the GABA–receptor complex, hence its absence of abuse liability (Miyamoto et al., 2003; Rozarem, 2006). In addition, unlike other sedative-hypnotics, ramelteon appears to produce no next-day residual or "hangover" effects. The recommended dose is 8 mg nightly, to be taken within 30 minutes of bedtime. Ramelteon should be avoided in patients with severe liver disease and in patients taking fluvoxamine, because it is metabolized by CYP450-1A2 enzymes. The most common side effects are somnolence, dizziness, nausea, and fatigue (Rozarem, 2006).

ADDICTION MEDICATIONS

Substance use disorders are a significant public health problem with medical, social, and economic consequences. A number of agents currently are approved for treatment of substance use disorders, but it is essential that all pharmacological agents be used in conjunction with comprehensive psychosocial treatments.

Disulfiram

In 1951, disulfiram (Antabuse) became the first medication approved by the FDA for treatment of alcoholism. When combined with alcohol, this drug creates a physical reaction so unpleasant that it becomes an aversive stimulus to drinking alcohol. Disulfiram inhibits aldehyde dehydrogenase, a key enzyme needed to metabolize alcohol. By blocking this enzyme, acetaldehyde accumulates, producing an unpleasant disulfiram–ethanol reaction, which includes facial flushing, sweating, and headache, that occurs immediately after drinking (Suh et al., 2006). At a moderate level of intensity, the reaction can also include nausea, tachycardia, palpitations, hyperventilation, hypotension, and dyspnea. Severe disulfiram–ethanol reactions can rarely progress to cardiovascular collapse and death (Suh et al., 2006).

The FDA-recommended maintenance dose of disulfiram is 250 mg daily, with a range of 125 to 500 mg (maximum daily dose). Disulfiram is a safe, well-tolerated medication that can be used as an adjunct to the treatment of alcoholism to prevent alcohol use and relapse (Suh et al., 2006), providing patients do not stop taking it and subsequently relapse on alcohol.

Naltrexone

Naltrexone (Revia) has historically been used in the treatment of opioid addiction. However, in 1994, it was also approved for the treatment of alcohol dependence, making it only the second medication approved for this disorder. Naltrexone is an opioid receptor antagonist with highest affinity for the μ opioid receptor. In opioid addiction, naltrexone completely blocks the euphoric effects of opioids. When alcohol is consumed, release of endorphin is hypothesized to occur in the CNS, triggering reinforcement that tempts an alcoholic to drink more (Addiction Treatment Forum, 2002). Naltrexone, by blocking opioid receptors, impedes the reinforcing effects of alcohol (Addiction Treatment Forum, 2002). Naltrexone has been found to significantly reduce alcohol relapses and alcohol craving (Addiction Treatment Forum, 2002). Naltrexone, unlike disulfiram, does not react aversively with alcohol. It is available in tablet form as well as an ER injectable suspension (Vivitrol), which is administered once per month (Vivitrol, 2006) with the intent of improving adherence to treatment. The recommended dose for alcohol-dependent patients is 50 mg daily (Revia, 1998), with some patients treated with higher doses of 100 to 150 mg daily (Addiction Treatment Forum, 2002). Similar dosing has been utilized in opioid dependence, and it is critical that these patients be opioid-free for 7 to 10 days before treatment initiation to avoid acute opioid withdrawal. In alcohol dependence, treatment for at least 6 months is recommended (1997), though evidence has emerged that the benefits of naltrexone treatment may start to diminish once the medication is discontinued (Addiction Treatment Forum, 2002). Naltrexone undergoes first-pass metabolism in the liver and is contraindicated in acute hepatitis or liver failure (Revia, 1998). Periodic laboratory monitoring of liver enzymes is recommended. The most common side effects are nausea, vomiting, headache, and dizziness.

Acamprosate

Acamprosate (Campral) is the newest addition to the class of drugs approved for alcohol dependence. It was FDA approved in 2004 for the maintenance of abstinence from alcohol. Acamprosate is believed to act as a glutamate receptor modulator (Campral, 2006), decreasing glutamate activity and increasing GABA transmission, thereby theoretically reducing the protracted withdrawal symptoms that often lead to relapse (Suh et al., 2006). The starting and maintenance dose is 666 mg tablets three times daily, which can be taken with or without meals. Of note, acamprosate does not eliminate or diminish acute withdrawal symptoms. The most common adverse events are asthenia, diarrhea, flatulence, nausea, and pruritis. Acamprosate is contraindicated in patients with severe renal impairment (Campral, 2006).

Methadone

Since the 1960s, methadone maintenance therapy has been the mainstay of pharmacotherapy for opioid dependence. Although the use of one opiate in the treatment for addiction of another remains somewhat controversial, many obvious benefits are associated with methadone. The use of methadone has been proven to decrease criminal behavior associated with narcotic addiction and to improve the social and occupational circumstances of previous opioid addicts. In addition, reducing risk for various medical consequences of heroin dependence (e.g., hepatitis, endocarditis, human immunodeficiency virus [HIV]/acquired immunodeficiency syndrome [AIDS]) is a major advantage of methadone maintenance therapy in heroin-dependent patients. In the United States, methadone is available only in government-approved clinics, which adhere to strict state and federal guidelines. Most clinics prescribe doses between 30 and 100 mg daily.

Levo-α-acetylmethadol

Levo-α-acetylmethadol (LAAM) is a long-acting opioid agonist used as an alternative to methadone in the treatment of opiate dependence. It has two active metabolites, nor-LAAM and dinor-LAAM, both of which are more potent opioid receptor agonists than LAAM itself. In contrast to methadone, which requires once-daily dosing, the prolonged half-lives of these metabolites (62 and 162 hours, respectively) allow for dosing three times per week. As with methadone, LAAM is prescribed in certain clinics that are closely regulated by government agencies. Because of potential QTc prolongation, all patients starting LAAM maintenance therapy should have a baseline ECG and a follow-up ECG at 4 months.

Buprenorphine

Buprenorphine (Subutex) monotherapy and buprenorphine/naloxone (Suboxone) combination were both approved in 2002 for the treatment of opiate dependence. Methadone and LAAM are full agonists, but buprenorphine is a partial agonist at the μ opioid receptor. At low doses buprenorphine produces sufficient agonist effect to enable addicted individuals to discontinue the abuse of opioids without suffering withdrawal symptoms (Substance Abuse Health and Services Administration [SAMHSA], 2007). The agonist effects of buprenorphine increase linearly until they reach a plateau and no longer increase with higher doses—this is known as the *ceiling effect*. As a result, buprenorphine carries a lower risk of abuse, addiction, and side effects compared with full opioid agonists such as methadone and LAAM. Buprenorphine appears to be as effective as methadone in detoxification from heroin dependence (Bickel et al., 1988). It is available as a sublingual tablet, in 2 mg and 8 mg strengths. Suboxone, also a sublingual tablet, comes in two dosage forms: 2 mg buprenorphine/0.5 mg naloxone and 8 mg buprenorphine/2 mg naloxone. This combination product is designed to decrease the potential for abuse by injection.

The major advantage of buprenorphine is that it is the only medication that meets federal requirements to be prescribed from physician offices rather than a separate opiate treatment clinic. Physicians who choose to prescribe buprenorphine must obtain special certification from the government.

COGNITIVE ENHANCERS

Cognitive enhancers target the diseases that affect cognition, particularly memory loss associated with dementia. Four agents are FDA approved to treat cognitive impairment in Alzheimer disease (AD). It has long been recognized that one of the cardinal neurochemical pathology findings of AD is degeneration of the cholinergic system in the brain (Sunderland et al., 2004). There is also considerable evidence that the cholinergic system is integral to normal memory formation. These theoretical underpinnings formed the basis for the development of acetylcholinesterase (AChE) inhibitors as treatments for the memory loss of AD. Three of the four drugs approved for treatment of AD fall into this category and appear to be equally efficacious, though very few comparison studies have been conducted (Sunderland et al., 2004). They enhance cholinergic function by blocking the enzyme responsible for hydrolysis of acetylcholine (ACh), thereby increasing the concentration of ACh in the synaptic cleft. The fourth agent, memantine, is also approved for the treatment of AD but has a distinct mechanism of action. Unfortunately, none of these medications alter the course of the underlying disease process.

Donepezil

Donepezil (Aricept) is approved for the treatment of mild, moderate, or severe AD. It was shown to improve cognitive performance in patients with AD, but this improvement was not sustained after the drug was discontinued (Aricept, 2006). Donepezil is a reversible and noncompetitive inhibitor of AChE, resulting in an increased amount of ACh. This is the common mechanism of action among the AChE inhibitors. Unlike its predecessors, donepezil is relatively selective for CNS AChE, with minimal peripheral activity (Sunderland et al., 2004). Among this class of drugs, donepezil has the longest duration of action ($t_{1/2} = 70$ hr) and therefore can be dosed once daily (Aricept, 2006). The recommended daily dose is 5 to 10 mg per day in mild-moderate AD and 10 mg per day in severe AD. Donepezil is generally well tolerated and has minimal side effects, though it can induce dose-dependent nausea, vomiting, and diarrhea (Aricept, 2006). Donepezil does not have any major drug–drug interactions.

Rivastigmine

Rivastigmine (Exelon) is a reversible inhibitor of AChE that is approved for the treatment of dementia associated with AD and PD. Rivastigmine has an intermediate duration of action of approximately 10 hours, requiring twice daily dosing. The recommended target dosage in AD is 6 to 12 mg per day divided in two doses. Treatment in AD is initiated at 1.5 mg twice a day and increased every 2 weeks to 3 mg twice daily, 4.5 mg twice daily, and finally to the target dose of 6 mg twice daily. The recommended dose range for dementia associated with PD is 3 to 12 mg daily, divided into two doses. Treatment is initiated at 1.5 mg twice daily, and this dose is maintained for 4 weeks before increasing it. Dose titration in PD should occur at 4-week intervals to the maximum dose of 6 mg twice a day. Rivastigmine should be taken with meals. A transdermal patch delivery system has been developed. Treatment should be initiated with one 4.6-mg patch applied to the skin every 24 hours. If this initial dose is tolerated, after 4 weeks the dose can be increased to one 9.5-mg patch applied to the skin every 24 hours. Some studies have found rivastigmine to have more GI side effects compared to donepezil.

Galantamine

Galantamine (Reminyl, Razadyne ER) is approved for the treatment of mild to moderate AD. It is a reversible, competitive AChE inhibitor that also has muscle relaxant properties (Sunderland et al., 2004). Galantamine also potentiates the nicotinic receptor response to ACh. Galantamine has been shown to improve cognitive performance in both AD and vascular dementia. Galantamine has a half-life of 7 hours and is dosed twice daily; however, an ER formulation is available, which allows for once-daily dosing (Razadyne, 2007). As with the other drugs in this class, the most common side effects are nausea, vomiting, and diarrhea; it has some other side effects also, including blurred vision, hypersalivation, and ECG changes (Sunderland et al., 2004). Galantamine is metabolized by P450 enzymes 2D6 and 3A4 and is not recommended for patients with severe hepatic or renal impairment (Razadyne, 2007).

Memantine

Memantine (Namenda) is the only non-AChE inhibitor drug approved for the treatment of moderate to severe AD. Patients treated with memantine showed significant improvement in two domains: cognitive and day-to-day functions. Day-to-day function was assessed by an inventory of activities of daily living. Memantine acts primarily as an *N*-methyl-D-aspartate (NMDA) receptor antagonist. Persistent activation of NMDA receptors due to the excitatory action of glutamate is one hypothesized contributor to the pathophysiology of AD (Sunderland et al., 2004; Namenda, 2007). Memantine is an antagonist at 5-HT$_3$ and nicotinic cholinergic receptors. Memantine should be initiated at 5 mg daily with an effective dose of 20 mg daily. It has a half-life of 60 to 80 hours. Patients with severe renal impairment should be prescribed lower doses. Memantine is not metabolized by the P450 system and has minimal drug–drug interactions (Namenda, 2007). There is some evidence that the combination of memantine and an AChE inhibitor (mainly donepezil) is a safe and well-tolerated combination in dementia treatment (Hartmann and Mobius, 2003).

PSYCHOSTIMULANTS AND ATOMOXETINE

Amphetamines have played a role in psychopharmacology since the 1800s. They are best known for their efficacy in ADHD in children. Stimulants have also been explored in the treatment of narcolepsy and as adjunctive treatment for depression, particularly in the medically ill.

Methylphenidate is a racemic mixture approved for the treatment of ADHD and narcolepsy. It is available in various formulations under several different trade names, including Ritalin, Ritalin SR, Focalin, Concerta, and Metadate-CD (Ballas et al., 2004). Methylphenidate is both an NE and DA reuptake inhibitor, and it causes release of these monoamines as well. It is classified as a schedule II drug because of its abuse liability. Methylphenidate has a short half-life of only 3 hours, which is why several ER formulations have been developed. Methylphenidate has a side effect profile representative of most stimulants, including insomnia, anxiety, and anorexia. It can also cause dose-dependent increases in blood pressure and heart rate (Ballas et al., 2004); as a result, checking vital signs at baseline and regularly after medication initiation is recommended.

Atomoxetine (Strattera) is the first and only nonstimulant medication approved by the FDA for the treatment of ADHD in children, adolescents, and adults. Its mechanism is through selective NE reuptake inhibition, a completely different mode of action from the stimulants. It is likely effective because it increases DA availability in the prefrontal cortex. Several clinical trials have shown atomoxetine to be efficacious in treating hyperactivity and inattention (Strattera, 2007). Target daily dosing for children under 70 kg is 1.2 mg per kg, whereas for children over 70 kg and adults, dosing is 80 to 100 mg daily (Strattera, 2007). Atomoxetine is generally well tolerated, with its most common side effects being anorexia, nausea, vomiting, dizziness, and mood swings (Strattera, 2007). Atomoxetine is primarily metabolized by CYP450-2D6. It should not be prescribed with an MAOI or within 2 weeks of discontinuing an MAOI. This drug is also contraindicated in patients with underlying cardiac disease. Of note, atomoxetine, similar to all antidepressants, has a boxed warning for increased risk of suicidal ideation in children and adolescents; therefore, it is imperative that children started on this medication are monitored closely.

Clinical Pearls

- Match medications to the specific diagnosis and not to the symptoms. As an example, insomnia due to major depressive disorder is most definitively treated with antidepressants and not sleep-promoting agents.
- Conduct a thorough diagnostic assessment, including past experiences with medications, family history, and response of family members to medication, before initiating a new agent.
- Engage in an ongoing dialog of informed consent and shared decision making with patients about the use of psychotropic medications, focused on the risks of the disease untreated versus the potential benefits of the treatment versus the treatment's potential risks. The first-order risk that defines treatment imperative is the risk of the disease.
- Balance therapeutic benefit of a medication to the patient with tolerability and safety.
- Many medical illnesses and conditions can present with symptoms identical to those of mental illnesses. Conduct a thorough medical evaluation before initiating treatment with psychotropic medications to rule out medical conditions that would require very different treatment intervention.
- An adequate dose and duration trial of a medication is critical to determining whether an agent is beneficial to a patient. Develop an understanding of the parameters of this concept for specific medications in specific disorders.
- Endeavor to use as few different medications as possible, based on the diagnosis; one is better than two and two is better than three different agents. Pick one and optimize its dose before introducing a second agent.
- Allow sufficient time for a therapeutic response to develop for an adequate dose of a single agent before introducing a second or third agent.

continued

- Ask about treatment adherence when assessing lack of response to an otherwise appropriate medication choice. The most common reason for lack of response (or relapse) is lack of adherence to treatment.
- Always ask about medication allergies and other previous adverse medication reactions before initiating therapy.
- Test for pregnancy in women of childbearing potential before initiating psychopharmacological agents, being especially diligent before initiating mood-stabilizing medications.
- Have a frank discussion on the need for adequate methods of contraception in women of childbearing potential being treated with mood-stabilizing medications.
- Measure metabolic parameters (weight, BMI, blood pressure, fasting glucose, lipid panel) on all patients with mental illness, both at baseline and periodically throughout the course of treatment, regardless of treatment. Some medications have a greater liability for metabolic consequences than others, but recognize that the mentally ill are a highly vulnerable population for these disorders.
- New does not equal better in terms of efficacy, tolerability, or safety of psychotropic medications. Some older medications, such as lithium, are still the definitive standard in treatment of mental illnesses.
- Practice evidence-based medicine to the extent possible in any given clinical situation, utilizing the informational hierarchy of publication quality to guide treatment decisions.

Self-Assessment Questions and Answers

22-1. Before initiating treatment with a psychotropic agent, the psychiatrist should:

A. Tell the patient that this medication is perfectly safe and without potential adverse outcomes.

B. Remind the patient that the physician has many years of training and experience and knows what is best for the patient.

C. Engage in a thorough and ongoing discussion of the consequences of the disease, potential benefits of treatment, and potential risks of the medication.

D. Tell the patient that, in the physician's experience, this medication cures "100%" of those who take it.

The process of shared decision making between treatment provider and patient is central to all medical practice, including psychiatry. Informed consent and risk–benefit decision making is an ongoing process that should be revisited regularly in the course of treatment. The first-order risk is of the disease untreated; the consequences of the disease state establish the treatment imperative. Mental illnesses are chronic, progressive, and potentially lethal and should be approached with this in mind when making treatment decisions. *Answer: C*

22-2. True or False: Factors that impact the bioavailability of oral medications include the health and function of the patient's

GI tract, the chemical and physical formulation of the medication, the activity of the CYP450 enzymes in the liver and GI tract, and concomitant use of other medications.

A. True

B. False

Bioavailability is a broad concept that includes characteristics of the medication and of the individual patient. Ultimately the amount of active medication that reaches its molecular target is the bioavailability for that individual patient and is impacted by the factors listed and potentially many more. *Answer: A*

22-3. A patient presents with complaints of sleep disturbance, feeling "stressed out" and anxious, difficulty concentrating; reports being "easily distracted," with low motivation, and just not enjoying life. The appropriate next step is to:

A. Advise the patient that this is normal, of course the patient feels this way, anybody would in his or her circumstances and the patient will get over it.

B. Initiate treatment with a psychostimulant, such as methylphenidate, and an anxiolytic, such as alprazolam, to give the patient more energy, improve concentration, and calm his or her nerves.

C. Conduct a thorough diagnostic interview and medical evaluation before deciding on a treatment course.

D. Begin treatment with a second-generation antipsychotic because that is the community standard in this circumstance.

The first step is to establish the correct diagnosis and then direct treatment specifically at that disease condition. The full evaluation would include medical and psychiatric assessment and then develop a treatment plan for the resulting disease entity. Always strive to target medications at the underlying disease as opposed to merely treating symptoms. Utilizing one medication is preferable to multiple agents if at all possible. *Answer: C*

22-4. A patient takes a deliberate overdose of a medication with a 24-hour elimination half-life. Most (>90%) of the medication will have been eliminated from the patient's system in:

A. Two days; the first half will be eliminated in the first 24 hours and the second half in the next 24 hours.

B. After 4 to 5 days, approximately 94% will have been eliminated.

C. Most of the medication will be gone in the first 24 hours.

D. Elimination of 90% of this medication could take as much as 2 weeks.

For agents with first-order elimination kinetics, approximately 94% will be eliminated in four to five half-lives. In this case, the agent has a 24-hour half-life, so the blood level will drop down to approximately 5% of the original level by 5 days. *Answer: B*

References

Abilify (aripiprazole) [package insert]. L. Bristol-Myers Squibb Company. Otsuka Pharmaceutical Co., Tokyo, Japan., Bristol-Myers Squibb Company. 2006.

Allain H, Bentue-Ferrer D, Polard E, et al. Postural instability and consequent falls and hip fractures associated with the use of hypnotics in the elderly: A comparative review. *Drugs Aging*. 2005;22(9): 749–765.

Allen MH, Hirschfeld RM, Wozniak PJ, et al. Linear relationship of valproate serum concentration to response and optimal serum levels for acute mania. *Am J Psychiatry*. 2006;163(2):272–275.

Allison DB, Mentore JL, Heo M, et al. Antipsychotic-induced weight gain: A comprehensive research synthesis. *Am J Psychiatry*. 1999;156:1686–1696.

Ambien (zolpidem tartrate) [package insert]. U. S. L. B. Sanofi-Aventis, NJ. Bridgewater, NJ, Sanofi-Aventis, U.S. L.L.C. 2007.

American Psychiatric Association. *Practice guideline for the treatment of patients with panic disorder*. Arlington: American Psychiatric Association; 1998:1–60.

American Psychiatric Association. *Practice guideline for treatment of patients with major depressive disorder*. Arlington: American Psychiatric Association; 2000:1–78.

American Psychiatric Association. Practice guideline for the treatment of patients with bipolar disorder. *Am J Psychiatry*. 2002;159(Suppl 4):1–50.

American Psychiatric Association. *Practice guidelines for the treatment of patients with schizophrenia*. Arlington: American Psychiatric Association; 2004:1–184.

American Psychiatric Association. *Guideline watch: Practice guideline for the treatment of patients with major depressive disorder*. Arlington: American Psychiatric Association; 2005.

American Psychiatric Association. *Guideline watch: Practice guideline for the treatment of patients with panic disorder*. Arlington: American Psychiatric Association; 2006.

Amsterdam JD, Bodkin JA. Selegiline transdermal system in the prevention of relapse of major depressive disorder: A 52-week, double-blind, placebo-substitution, parallel-group clinical trial. *J Clin Psychopharmacol*. 2006;26(6):579–586.

Aricept (donepezil) [package insert]. New York, NY, Eisai Inc. 2006.

Ayd FJ. A survey of drug-induced extrapyramidal reactions. *JAMA*. 1961;175:1054–1060.

Ballas CA, Evans DL, Dinges DF. Psychostimulants in psychiatry: Amphetamine, methylphenidate, and modafinil. In: Schatzberg AF, Nemeroff CB, eds. *Textbook of psychopharmacology*, 3rd ed. Arlington: American Psychiatric Publishing; 2004.

Ballenger JC, Davidson JRT, Lecrubier Y, et al. Consensus statement on social anxiety disorder from the International Consensus Group on Depression and Anxiety. *J Clin Psychiatry*. 1998a; 59(Suppl 17):54–60.

Ballenger JC, Davidson JRT, Lecrubier Y, et al. Consensus statement on panic disorder from the International Consensus Group on Depression and Anxiety. *J Clin Psychiatry*. 1998b;59(Suppl 8):47–54.

Barnes T, Spence S. *Movement disorders associated with antipsychotic drugs: Clinical and biological implications*. New York: Oxford University Press; 2000.

Bauer M, Döpfmer S. Lithium augmentation in treatment-resistant depression: Meta-analysis of placebo-controlled studies. *J Clin Psychopharmacol*. 1999;19:427–434.

Bendz H, Aurell M. Drug-induced diabetes insipidus: Incidence, prevention and management. *Drug Saf*. 1999;21:449–456.

Bickel WE, Stitzer ML, Bigelow GE, et al. A clinical trial of buprenorphine: Comparison with methadone in the detoxification of heroin addicts. *Clin Pharmacol Ther*. 1988;43:72–78.

Bijl D. The serotonin syndrome. *Neth J Med*. 2004;62(9):309–313.

Bowden CL. Predictors of response to divalproex and lithium. *J Clin Psychiatry*. 1995;56:25–30.

Bowden CL. Valproate. In: Schatzberg AF, Nemeroff CB, eds. *Textbook of psychopharmacology*, 3rd ed. Arlington: American Psychiatric Publishing; 2004:567–579.

Bowden CL, Brugger AM, Swann AC, et al. Efficacy of divalproex versus lithium and placebo in the treatment of mania. *JAMA*. 1994;271(12):918–924.

Boyer WF, Blumhardt CL. The safety profile of paroxetine. *J Clin Psychiatry*. 1992;52:61–66.

Bremner JD. A double-blind comparison of Org 3770, amitriptyline, and placebo in major depression. *J Clin Psychiatry*. 1995;56:519–525.

Bruce SE, Vasile RG, Goisman RM, et al. Are benzodiazepines still the medication of choice for patients with panic disorder with or without agoraphobia? *Am J Psychiatry*. 2003;160(8):1432–1438.

Bryant AEI, Dreifuss FE. Valproic acid hepatic fatalities, III, US experience since 1986. *Neurology*. 1996;46(2):465–469.

Buckley NA, McManus PR. Fatal toxicity of serotoninergic and other antidepressant drugs: Analysis of United Kingdom mortality data. *Br Med J*. 2002;325:1332–1333.

Cade JF. Lithium salts in the treatment of psychotic excitement. *Med J Aust*. 1949;36:349–352.

Calabrese JR, Bowden CL, Sachs G, et al. A placebo-controlled 18-month trial of lamotrigine and lithium maintenance treatment in recently depressed patients with bipolar I disorder. *J Clin Psychiatry*. 2003;64(9):1013–1024.

Campral (acamprosate) [package insert]. I. Forest Pharmaceuticals. 2006.

Carpenter LL, Yasmin S, Price LH, et al. A double-blind, placebo-controlled study of antidepressant augmentation with mirtazapine. *Biol Psychiatry*. 2002;51(2):183–188.

Celexa (citalopram) [package insert]. St. Louis, MO, Forest Pharmaceuticals, Inc. 2007.

Chessick CA, Allen MH, Thase M, et al. Azapirone for generalized anxiety disorder *Cochrane Database Syst Rev*. 2006;3:CD006115.

Clozaril (clozapine) [package insert]. East Hanover, NJ, Novartis Pharmaceuticals Corporation. 2005.

Cohen LS, Rosenbaum JF. Psychotropic use during pregnancy: Weighing the risks. *J Clin Psychiatry*. 1998;59:18–28.

Cymbalta (duloxetine hydrochloride) [package insert]. E. L. & Company. Indianapolis, IN, Eli Lilly and Company. 2007.

Daniel DG, Copeland LF, Tamminga C, et al. Ziprasidone. In: Schatzberg AF, Nemeroff CB, eds. *Textbook of clinical psychopharmacology*, 3rd ed. Arlington: American Psychiatric Publishing; 2004:507–518.

Denicoff KD, Smith-Jackson EE, Disney ER, et al. Comparative prophylactic efficacy of lithium, carbamazepine, and the combination in bipolar disorder. *J Clin Psychiatry*. 1997;58:470–478.

Depakote (sodium valproate) [package insert]. Barceloneta, PR, Abbott Pharmaceuticals, Ltd. 2006.

Depression Guideline Panel. Depression in primary care. *Clinical practice guideline*, Number 5, Publication No 93-0551. Rockville: Public Health Service, Agency for Health Care Policy and Research; 1993.

Desyrel (trazodone) [package insert]. Princeton, NJ, Bristol-Myers Squibb Company. 2003.

Devinsky O, Honigfeld G, Patin J. Clozapine-related seizures. *Neurology*. 1991;41(3):369–371.

Effexor (venlafaxine) [package insert]. W. P. Inc. Philadelphia, PA, Wyeth Pharmaceutical, Inc. 2006.

Elie R, Ruther E, Farr I, et al. Sleep latency is shortened during 4 weeks of treatment with zaleplon, a novel nonbenzodiazepine hypnotic. *J Clin Psychiatry*. 1999;60(8):536–543.

Emsam (selegiline transdermal system) [package insert]. Princeton, NJ, Bristol-Myers Squibb Company. 2007.

Equetro (carbamazepine) [package insert]. I. P. Validus Pharmaceuticals, NJ. Parsippany, NJ, Validus Pharmaceuticals, Inc. 2007.

Factor SA. Pharmacology of atypical antipsychotics. *Clin Neuropharmacol*. 2002;25(3):153–157.

Fairbanks JM, Gorman JM. Fluvoxamine. In: Schatzberg AF, Nemeroff CB, eds. *Textbook of psychopharmacology*, 3rd ed. Arlington: American Psychiatric Publishing; 2004.

Fava M, Rush AJ, Trivedi M, et al. Background and rationale for the sequenced treatment alternatives to relieve depression (STAR*D) study. *Psychiatr Clin North Am*. 2003;26:457–494.

Flores BH, Schatzberg AF. Mirtazapine. In: Schatzberg AF, Nemeroff CB, eds. *Textbook of psychopharmacology*, 3rd ed. Arlington: American Psychiatric Publishing; 2004:341–347.

Frazer A. Pharmacology of antidepressants. *J Clin Psychopharmacol*. 1997;17(2 Suppl 1):2S–18S.

Freeman MP, Wiegand C, Gelenberg AJ. Lithium. In: Schatzberg AF, Nemeroff CB, eds. *Textbook of psychopharmacology*, 3rd ed. Arlington: American Psychiatric Publishing; 2004:547–565.

Geodon (ziprasidone) [package insert]. Division of Pfizer, Inc. NY, NY. New York, NY, Division of Pfizer, Inc. 2005.

Ghaemi SN. *Mood disorders*. Philadelphia: Lippincott Williams & Wilkins; 2003.

Gibbons RD, Brown CH, Hur K, et al. Relationship between antidepressants and suicide attempts: An analysis of the Veterans Health Administration data sets. *Am J Psychiatry*. 2007a;164(7):1044–1049.

Gibbons RD, Brown CH, Hur K, et al. Early evidence on the effects of regulators' suicidality warnings on SSRI prescriptions and suicide in children and adolescents. *Am J Psychiatry*. 2007b;164:1356–1363.

Glazer WM. Extrapyramidal side effects, tardive dyskinesia, and the concept of atypicality. *J Clin Psychiatry*. 2000;61(Suppl 3):16–21.

Golden RN, Dawkins K, Nicholas L. Trazodone and nefazadone. In: Schatzberg AF, Nemeroff CB, eds. *Textbook of psychopharmacology*, 3rd ed. Arlington: American Psychiatric Publishing; 2004:315–325.

Goodnick PJ. Seligiline transdermal system in depression. *Expert Opin Pharmacother*. 2007;8(1):59–64.

Greden JF. Duloxetine and milnacipran. In: Schatzberg AF, Nemeroff CB, eds. *Textbook of psychopharmacology*, 3rd ed. Arlington: American Psychiatric Publishing; 2004:361–370.

Green AR, Cross AJ, Goddwin GM. Review of the pharmacology and clinical pharmacology of 3,4-methylenedioxymethaphamine (MDMA or 'Ecstasy'). *Psychopharmacology (Berl)*. 1995;119:247–260.

Guaiana G, Barbui C, Hotopf M. Amitriptyline versus other types of pharmacotherapy for depression. *Cochrane Database Syst Rev*. 2003;2:CD004186.

Hartmann S, Mobius HJ. Tolerability of memantine in combination with cholinesterase inhibitors in dementia therapy. *Int Clin Psychopharmacol*. 2003;18(2):81–85.

Herr KD, Nemeroff CB. Paroxetine. In: Schatzberg AF, Nemeroff CB, eds. *Textbook of psychopharmacology*, 3rd ed. Arlington: American Psychiatric Publishing; 2004.

Hirschfeld RM. Efficacy of SSRIs and newer antidepressants in severe depression: Comparison with TCAs. *J Clin Psychiatry*. 1999;60(5):326–335.

Hudziak JJ, Rettew DC. In: Schatzberg AF, Nemeroff CB, eds. *Textbook of psychopharmacology*, 3rd ed. Arlington: American Psychiatric Publishing; 2004:327–339.

Invega (paliperidone) [package insert]. L. P. Janssen. Titusville, NJ, Janssen, L.P. 2007.

Janicek P, Davis JM, Preskorn SH, et al. *Principles and practice of psychopharmacotherapy*. Baltimore: Williams & Wilkins; 1993.

Jensen NH, Rodriguez RM, Caron MG, et al. N-Desalkylquetiapine, a potent norepinephrine reuptake inhibitor and partial 5-HT1A agonist, as a putative medicator of quetiapine's antidepressant activity. *Neuropharmacology*. 2007:1–10 [online].

Kane JM. Tardive dyskinesia circa 2006. *Am J Psychiatry*. 2006;163(8):1316–1318.

Kane J, Woerner M, Borenstein M. Integrating incidence and prevalence of tardive dyskinesia. *Psychopharmacol Bull*. 1986;22:254–258.

Kane JM, Woerner M, Weinhold P, et al. A prospective study of tardive dyskinesia development: Preliminary results. *J Clin Psychopharmacol*. 1982;22:345–349.

Kato K, Hirai K, Nishiyama K, et al. Neurochemical properties of ramelteon (TAK-375), a selective MT1/MT2 receptor agonist. *Neuropharmacology*. 2005;48(2):301–310.

Keck PJ, McElroy S. Clinical pharmacodynamics and pharmacokinetics of anti-manic and mood-stabilizing medications. *J Clin Psychiatry*. 2002;63(Suppl 4):3–11.

Keller MB, Kocsis JH, Thase ME, et al. Maintenance phase efficacy of sertraline for chronic depression. *JAMA*. 1998;280(19):1665–1672.

Kleindienst N, Greil W. Lithium in the long-term treatment of bipolar disorders. *Eur Arch Psychiatry Clin Neurosci*. 2003;253:120–125.

Krishnan, KRR. Monoamine oxidase inhibitors. In: Schatzberg AF, Nemeroff CB, eds. *Textbook of psychopharmacology*, 3rd ed. Arlington: American Psychiatric Publishing; 2004:303–314.

Lamictal (lamotrigine) [package insert]. Research Triangle Park, NC, GlaxoSmithKline. 2007.

Lazarus A, Mann SC, Caroff SN. *The neuroleptic malignant syndrome and related conditions*. Washington, DC: American Psychiatric Press; 1989.

Leavitt SB. Addiction Treatment Forum. *Evidence for the efficacy of naltrexone in the treatment of alcohol dependence (Alcoholism)*. Mundelein: Clinco Communications Inc; 2002:1–8.

Lehman AF, Kreyenbuhl J, Buchanan RW, et al. The schizophrenia patient outcomes research team (PORT): Updated treatment recommendations 2003. *Schizophr Bull*. 2004;30:193–217.

Lerner V, Miodownik C, Kaptsan A, et al. Vitamin B6 treatment for tardive dyskinesia: A randomized, double-blind, placebo-controlled, crossover study. *J Clin Psychiatry*. 2007;68(11):1648–1654.

Lesser IM, Rubin RT, Pecknold JC, et al. Secondary depression in panic disorder and agoraphobia, II: Dimensions of depression symptomatology and their response to treatment. *J Affect Disord*. 1989;16: 49–58.

Lexapro (escitalopram oxalate) [package insert]. St. Louis, MO, Forest Pharmaceuticals, Inc. 2007.

Lieberman JA. Aripiprazole. In: Schatzberg AF, Nemeroff, CB, eds. *Textbook of psychopharmacology*, 3rd ed. Arlington: American Psychiatric Publishing; 2004:487–494.

Lieberman JA, Stroup ST, McEvoy JP, et al. Effectiveness of antipsychotic drugs in patients with chronic schizophrenia. *N Engl J Med*. 2005;353(12):1209–1223.

Liebowitz MR, Quitkin FM, Stewart JW, et al. Antidepressant specificity in atypical depression. *Arch Gen Psychiatry*. 1988;45:129–137.

Lunesta (eszopiclone) [package insert]. S. Inc. Marlborough, MA, Sepracor. 2007.

Marder SR, Wirshing DA. Clozapine. In: Schatzberg AF, Nemeroff CB, eds. *Textbook of psychopharmacology*, 3rd ed. Arlington: American Psychiatric Publishing; 2004:443–456.

McElroy SL, Dessain EC, Pope HG Jr, et al. Clozapine in the treatment of psychotic mood disorders, schizoaffective disorder, and schizophrenia. *J Clin Psychiatry*. 1991;52(10):411–414.

McEvoy J, Lieberman J, Stroup TS, et al. Effectiveness of clozapine versus olanzapine, quetiapine, and risperidone in patients with chronic schizophrenia who did not respond to prior atypical antipsychotic treatment. *Am J Psychiatry*. 2006;163:600–610.

Meltzer HY, Alphs L, Green A, et al. Clozapine treatment for suicidality in schizophrenia: International Suicide Prevention Trial (InterSePT). *Arch Gen Psychiatry*. 2003;60:182–191.

Miller DD. The clinical use of clozapine plasma concentrations in the management of treatment-refractory schizophrenia. *Ann Clin Psychiatry*. 1996;8(2):99–109.

Miller AA, Wheatley P, Sawyer DA, et al. Pharmacological studies on lamotrigine, a novel antiepileptic drug: Anticonvulsant profile in mice and rats. *Epilepsia*. 1986;27:483–489.

Minagar A, Kelley RE. Movement disorders. *Prim Care*. 2004;31(1):111–127.

Miyamoto M, Nishikawa H, Ohta H, et al. Behavioral pharmacology of TAK-375 in small animals. *Ann Neurol*. 2003;54(Suppl 7):S46.

Montejo-Gonzalez A, Liorca G, Izquierdo JA, et al. SSRI-induced sexual dysfunction: Fluoxetine, paroxetine, sertraline, and fluvoxamine in a prospective, multicenter, and descriptive clinical study of 344 patients. *J Sex Marital Ther*. 1997;23(3):176–194.

Naltrexone: An option for alcohol-dependent patients? *Drugs Ther Perspect* 1997;10(1):5–8.

Namenda (memantine) [package insert]. St, Louis, MO, Forest Pharmaceuticals, Inc. 2007.

Nasrallah HA. The case for long-acting antipsychotic agents in the post-CATIE era. *Acta Psychiatr Scand*. 2007;115:260–267.

National Institutes of Mental Health. *Abnormal involuntary movement scale*. Washington, DC: 2000.

Nelson JC. Tricyclic and tetracyclic drugs. In: Schatzberg AF, Nemeroff, CB eds. *Textbook of psychopharmacology*, 3rd ed. Arlington: American Psychiatric Publishing; 2004.

Nemeroff CB, Kalali A, Keller MB, et al. Impact of publicity concerning pediatric suicidality on physician practice patterns in the United States. *Arch Gen Psychiatry*. 2007;64:46–472.

Nierenberg A, Adler LA, Peselow E, et al. Trazodone for antidepressant-associated insomnia. *Am J Psychiatry*. 1994;151:1069–1072.

O'Brien CP. Benzodiazepine use, abuse, and dependence. *J Clin Psychiatry*. 2005;66(Suppl 2):28–33.

Owens MJ, Morgan WN, Plott S, et al. Neurotransmitter receptor and transporter binding profile of antidepressants and their metabolites. *J Pharmacol Exp Ther*. 1997;283(3):1305–1322.

Paxil (paroxetine hydrochloride) [package insert]. Research Triangle Park, NC, GlaxoSmithKline. 2007.

Pelonero AL, Levenson JL, et al. Neuroleptic malignant syndrome: A review. *Psychiatr Serv*. 1998;49:1163–1172.

Price L, Heninger G. Lithium in the treatment of mood disorders. *N Engl J Med*. 1994;331:591–598.

Prozac (fluoxetine capsules) [package insert]. Indianapolis, IN, Eli Lilly and Company. 2007.

Quitkin FM, McGrath PJ, Stewart JW, et al. Atypical depression, panic attacks, and response to imipramine and phenelzine: A replication. *Arch Gen Psychiatry*. 1990;47:935–941.

Raj A, Sheehan D. Benzodiazepines. In: Schatzberg AF, Nemeroff CB, eds. *Textbook of psychopharmacology*, 3rd ed. Arlington: American Psychiatric Publishing; 2004:371–385.

Rapaport MH. Dietary restrictions and drug interactions with monoamine oxidase inhibitors: The state of the art. *J Clin Psychiatry*. 2007;68(Suppl 8):42–46.

Razadyne (galantamine HBr) [package insert]. Titusville, NJ, Ortho-McNeil Neurologics, Inc. 2007.

Redrobe JP, Bourin M. Dose-dependent influence of buspirone on the activities of selective serotonin reuptake inhibitors in the mouse forced swimming test. *Psychopharmacology (Berl)*. 1998;138:198–206.

Remeron (mirtazapine orally disintegrating tablets) [package insert]. I. R. Organon USA, NJ. Roseland, NJ, Organon USA, Inc. 2007.

Remington G, Kapur S. Neuroleptic-induced extrapyramidal symptoms and the role of combined serotonin/dopamine antagonist (monograph). *J Clin Psychiatry*. 1996;14:14–24.

Revia (naltrexone hydrochloride tablets) [package insert]. Wilmington, DE, Dupont Pharma. 1998.

Rickels K, Schweizer E. Clinical overview of serotonin reuptake inhibitors. *J Clin Psychiatry*. 1990;51:9–12.

Rickels K, Schweizer E, Case WG, et al. Long-term therapeutic use of benzodiazepines, Part 1: Effects of abrupt discontinuation. *Arch Gen Psychiatry*. 1990;(47):899–907.

Risperdal (risperidone) [package insert]. Titusville, NJ, Janssen, L.P. 2007.

Rosebush P, Stewart T, Gelenberg AJ. Twenty neuroleptic rechallenges after neuroleptic malignant syndrome in 15 patients. *J Clin Psychiatry*. 1989;50:295–298.

Rosenbaum JF. Attitudes towards benzodiazepines over the years. *J Clin Psychiatry*. 2005;66(suppl 2):4–8.

Rosenbaum JF, Tollefson GD. Fluoxetine. In: Schatzberg AF, Nemeroff CB, eds. *Textbook of psychopharmacology*, 3rd ed. Arlington: American Psychiatric Publishing; 2004:231–246.

Roy-Byrne PP. The GABA-benzodiazepine receptor complex: Structure, function, and role in anxiety. *J Clin Psychiatry*. 2005;66(Suppl 2):14–20.

Rozarem (ramelteon) [package insert]. Deerfield, IL, Takeda Pharmaceuticals America, Inc. 2006.

Rush AJ, Thase ME. Strategies and tactics in the treatment of chronic depression. *J Clin Psychiatry*. 1997;58(Suppl 13):14–22.

Rush AJ, Trivedi MH, Wisniewski SR, et al. Bupropion-SR, sertraline, or venlafaxine-XR after failure of SSRIs for depression. *N Engl J Med*. 2006;354:1231–1242.

SAMHSA. *About buprenorphine therapy*. 2007.

Schneider S, Aggarwal A, Bhatt M, et al. Severe tongue protrusion dystonia. *Neurology*. 2006;67:940–943.

Schooler NR. Relapse and rehospitalization: Comparing oral and depot antipsychotics. *J Clin Psychiatry*. 2003;64(Suppl 16):14–17.

Seroquel (quetiapine fumarate) [package insert]. Wilmington, DE, AstraZenica Pharmaceuticals, LP. 2005.

Serzone (nefazadone HCl) [package insert]. Princeton, NJ, Bristol-Myers Squibb Company. 2002.

Shelton, MD, Calabrese JR. Lamotrigine. Schatzberg AF, Nemeroff CB, eds. *Textbook of psychopharmacology*, 3rd ed. Arlington: American Psychiatric Publishing; 2004:615–626.

Shim, J, Yonkers KA. Sertraline. In: Schatzberg AF, Nemeroff CB, eds. *Textbook of psychopharmacology*, 3rd ed. Arlington: American Psychiatric Publishing; 2004:247–257.

Shulman KI, Walker SE, MacKenzie S, et al. Dietary restriction, tyramine, and the use of monoamine oxidase inhibitors. *J Clin Psychopharmacol*. 1989;9(6):397–402.

Simon GE, Savarino J. Suicide attempts among patients starting depression treatment with medications or psychotherapy. *Am J Psychiatry*. 2007;164:1029–1034.

Sonata (zaleplon) [package insert]. Philadelphia, PA, Wyeth Pharmaceuticals, Inc. 2003.

Stahl SM. *Essential psychopharmacology of antipsychotics and mood stabilizers*. Cambridge: Cambridge University Press; 2002.

Stahl SM, Pradko JF, Haight BR, et al. A review of the neuropharmacology of bupropion, a dual norepinephrine and dopamine reuptake inhibitor. *Prim Care companion J Clin Psychiatry*. 2004;6(4): 159–166.

Stanilla JK, Simpson GM. Drugs to treat extrapyramidal side effects. In: Schatzberg AF, Nemeroff CB, eds. *Textbook of psychopharmacology*, 3rd ed. Arlington: American Psychiatric Publishing; 2004:519–544.

Stevens JC, Pollack MH. Benzodiazepines in clinical practice: Consideration of their long-term use and alternative agents. *J Clin Psychiatry*. 2005;66(Suppl 2):21–27.

Strattera (atomoxetine HCl) [package insert]. Indianapolis, IN, Eli Lilly and Company. 2007.

Strom BL, Faich GA, Reynolds RF, et al. The Ziprasidone Observational Study of Cardiac Outcomes (ZODIAC): Design and baseline subject characteristics. *J Clin Psychiatry*. 2008;69(1):114–121.

Suh JJ, Pettinati H, Kampman KM, et al. The status of disulfiram: A half of a century later. *J Clin Psychopharmacol*. 2006;26(3):290–302.

Sunderland T, Mirza N, Linker G, et al. Cognitive enhancers. In: Schatzberg AF, Nemeroff CB, eds. *Textbook of psychopharmacology*, 3rd ed. Arlington: American Psychiatric Publishing; 2004.

Suranyi-Cadotte BE, Bodnoff SR, Welner SA, et al. Antidepressant-anxiolytic interactions: Involvement of the benzodiazepine-GABA and serotonin systems. *Prog Neuropsychopharmacol Biol Psychiatry*. 1990;14(5):633–654.

Swann AC, Bowden CL, Morris D, et al. Depression during mania. Treatment response to lithium or divalproex. *Arch Gen Psychiatry*. 1997;54:37–42.

Symbyax (olanzapine and fluoxetine HCl capsules) [package insert]. Indianapolis, IN, Eli Lilly and Company. 2007.

Thase ME, Haight BR, Richard N, et al. Remission rates following antidepressant therapy with bupropion or selective serotonin reuptake inhibitors: A meta-analysis of original data from 7 randomized controlled trials. *J Clin Psychiatry*. 2005;66(8):974–981.

Thase ME, Sloan DM. Venlafaxine. In: Schatzberg AF, Nemeroff CB, eds. *Textbook of psychopharmacology*, 3rd ed. Arlington: American Psychiatric Publishing; 2004:349–360.

Trivedi MH, Fava M, Wisniewski SR, et al. Medication augmentation after the failure of SSRIs for depression. *N Engl J Med*. 2006;354(12):1243–1252.

Trivedi MH, Rush AJ, Wisniewski S, et al. Evaluation of outcomes with citalopram for depression using measurement-based care in STAR*D: Implications for clinical practice. *Am J Psychiatry*. 2006;163(1):28–40.

Van Steveninck AL, Gieschke R, Schoemaker RC, et al. Pharmacokinetic and pharmacodynamic interactions of bretazenil and diazepam with alcohol. *Br J Clin Pharmacol*. 1996;41:565–573.

Vivitrol (naltrexone for extended-release injectable suspension) [package insert]. I. C. Alkermes, MA. Cambridge, MA, Alkermes, Inc. 2006.

Wagner J, Wagner ML, Hening WA. Beyond benzodiazepines: Alternative pharmacologic agents for the treatment of insomnia. *Ann Pharmacother*. 1998;32:680–691.

Waknine Y. FDA Approvals: Fazaclo, Seroquel XR, Doxil. Medscape Medical News. 2007.

Walsh JK, Engelhardt CL. Trends in the pharmacologic treatment of insomnia. *J Clin Psychiatry*. 1992;53(Suppl 12):S10–S17.

Weiden P, Zygmunt A. Medication noncompliance in schizophrenia. Part I. Assessment. *J Pract Psychiatry Behav Health*. 1997;3:106–110.

Wellbutrin (bupropion hydrochloride extended-release tablets) [package insert]. Research Triangle Park, NC, GlaxoSmithKline. 2007.

Wilkaitis J, Mulvihill T, Nasrallah HA. Classic antipsychotic medications. In: Schatzberg AF, Nemeroff CB, eds. *Textbook of psychopharmacology*, 3rd ed. Arlington: American Psychiatric Publishing; 2004:425–441.

Zoloft (sertraline hydrochloride) [package insert]. New York, NY, Division of Pfizer, Inc. 2007.

Zyprexa (olanzapine) [package insert]. Indianapolis, IN, Eli Lilly and Company. 2007.

Psychotherapies

Psychotherapy is the "talking cure," treatment directed at changing behavior through verbal exchange. By using words to create understanding, guidance, and support, the psychotherapist leads the patient to new experiences and new learning. The psychotherapist seeks to eliminate symptoms of illness and increase the patient's productivity and enjoyment of life. The brain is the target organ of psychotherapy. Behavior, thoughts, and emotions are brain activities at the neuroanatomical, neurochemical, and neurophysiological levels. The psychotherapies aim to alter this brain "patterning" and function. In contrast, psychopathology frequently limits a patient's ability to see and experience options and choices. Patients' behaviors, thoughts, and feelings are constricted by their psychiatric illness, leading them to see only some options and experience a limited range of feelings. Therapists treating patients with psychotherapy increase patients' insight into their lives and their range of behavioral options and decrease painful constricting symptoms.

Psychotherapeutic approaches to psychopathology vary widely and reflect different concepts and theories of mental life, personality development, abnormal behavior, and the role of environmental and biological determinants. Psychotherapy is both cost effective and efficacious (Lazar, 1998). Recent studies show that patients receiving psychotherapy achieve significant benefits when compared with controls. Experience indicates that the most successful strategy is often an *integrated* approach to treatment, combining medications with psychological therapy. Different patients benefit from different types of psychotherapy, just as they may benefit from different types of psychotropic medications. Because of this, the medically trained psychiatrist can provide the most comprehensive evaluation for combining medication with psychotherapeutic treatment. The psychiatrist can use combined medication and psychotherapeutic treatments and is trained to recognize and manage the potential interactions of these two treatments. The psychiatrist also is alert to changes in the patient's medical status that can be a cause of or a result of psychiatric illness. Patients with significant medical illness as part of their health history (e.g., migraine, ulcers, human immunodeficiency virus [HIV], cardiac disease, cancer, and psychosomatic illnesses) are best treated by the psychiatrist who, as a physician and skilled psychotherapist, is knowledgeable of these disorders and their effects on feelings, behaviors, and life adjustment. Additionally, the psychiatrist can evaluate the possible effects of medications on patients' presenting mental status. Often, the seriously depressed or psychotic patient is more comfortable with a psychiatrist who is trained in managing life-and-death issues, chronic illness, and the medical side effects of medication. Sometimes, psychiatrists may work with nonphysician therapists (e.g., psychologists or social workers) as part of the mental health team. In these situations, the psychiatrist prescribes the medication and provides some psychotherapeutic interventions. The nonphysician therapist then meets more frequently with the patient and provides most of the psychotherapy. Good communication among the psychiatrist, the nonphysician therapist, and any other physicians involved in a patient's care is essential to the successful management of psychiatric illness.

The major psychotherapies are reviewed in the following sections. An understanding of these techniques and their concepts is important to the treatment armamentarium of inpatient, outpatient, and consultation–liaison psychiatric practices, as well as general medical practice.

PSYCHOANALYTIC PSYCHOTHERAPIES
Psychoanalysis

Although psychoanalysis is not the most common of the psychotherapies, many of its concepts and techniques form the basis of other psychotherapy techniques. Psychoanalysis was originally developed by Sigmund Freud in the late 19th century. Freud found that his patients' life difficulties were related to unrecognized (unconscious) conflicts that arise in childhood and continue into adult life. Such conflicts are typically between libidinal (sexual and/or emotional) and aggressive wishes and the fear of loss, condemnation, retaliation, the constraints of reality, or the opposition of other incompatible wishes. "Libidinal wishes" are best thought of as longings for gratification, including pleasure, safety, power, and recognition. It is important to keep in mind that in psychoanalytic thinking, sexual pleasure refers to the broad concept of bodily pleasure, the state of excitement and pleasure experienced by various bodily sensations beginning in infancy. Aggressive wishes may either be primary destructive impulses or arise in reaction to perceived frustration, deprivation, or attack. Such conflicts may give rise to a variety of manifestations in adulthood, including anxiety, depression, and somatic symptoms, as well as work, social, or sexual inhibitions and maladaptive ways of relating to other people. These conflicts, historically termed *neurotic*, cause distress to an individual but do not prevent rational thought.

The goal of psychoanalysis is to understand the patient's childhood conflicts (the "infantile neurosis") and their manifestations in adult life. This goal is accomplished through identifying and reexperiencing these conflicts in relation to the analyst (the "transference neurosis"). This is a major undertaking that requires a great deal of the patient to sustain the treatment. Psychoanalytic patients must be able to access their fantasy lives in an active and experiencing manner and be able to "leave it behind" at the end of a session. Psychoanalysis is frequently criticized for being used to treat reasonably healthy people; however, all medical treatments require certain innate capacities of the patient (e.g., an intact immune system for successful antibiotic therapy) for the patient to use the treatment successfully and not be injured by it. Generally, healthy people may also have painful neurotic conflicts that interfere with both their work and personal lives and, therefore, require treatment.

Psychoanalysis focuses on the recovery of childhood experiences as they are recreated in the relationship with the analyst (Sandler et al., 1973). This recreation in the doctor–patient relationship of the conflicted relationship with a childhood figure is called the *transference neurosis* (see Table 23-1). In the therapeutic relationship with the analyst, the emotional conflicts and trauma from the past are relived. The feelings and conflicts that were part of the relationship with major childhood figures, most frequently the parents, are "transferred" to the analyst. When the transference neurosis is present, the patient emotionally experiences and reacts to the analyst in

TABLE 23-1	Psychoanalysis
Goal	Resolution of symptoms and major reworking of personality structures related to childhood conflicts
Patient selection criteria	No psychotic potential Able to use understanding High ego strength Able to experience and observe intense emotional states Psychiatric problem derived from childhood conflicts
Techniques	Focus on fantasies and the transference Free association Couch Interpretation of defenses and transference Frequent meetings Neutrality of the analyst
Duration	3–6 yr

TABLE 23-2	Common Terms in Psychoanalysis or Psychoanalytically Oriented Psychotherapy
Defense mechanisms	A psychological strategy that individuals use to protect themselves from painful awareness of feelings or memories that can provoke overwhelming anxiety
Neurosis	The experience of internal conflict that causes subjective distress but does not prevent rational thought
Free association	A core technique in psychoanalysis, the reporting of all things that come to mind
Transference	Re-creation in the doctor–patient relationship of feelings and conflicts that were part of the patient's relationships with major figures during childhood development, most frequently the parents
Countertransference	The clinician's transference response to the patient

a very real manner, as if the analyst were the significant figure from the past (see Table 23-2). Frequently, this experience is accompanied by other elements of the past being experienced in the patient's life. Countertransference, the analyst's transference response to the patient, is increased by life stress and unresolved conflicts in the analyst. It can appear as either identification with or a reaction to the patient's conscious and unconscious fantasies, feelings, and behaviors (Racker, 1968). Specifically, in concordant countertransference, the physician experiences and empathizes with the patient's emotional experience and perception of reality. In complementary countertransference, the physician experiences and empathizes with the emotional experience and perception of reality of an important figure from the patient's life. Understanding one's countertransference reactions can allow a psychotherapist to recognize subtle aspects of the transference relationship and understand the patient's experience better.

Psychoanalytic treatment attempts to arrange a therapeutic situation in which the patient's observing capacity (ability to see oneself) can be used to analyze the transference neurosis. Transference reactions do occur not only in psychoanalysis but also throughout life and, in particular, are a frequent accompaniment of the doctor–patient relationship in the medical setting. However, psychoanalysis is unique in its efforts to establish a setting in which the transference, when it appears, can be analyzed and worked through in an intense manner to facilitate recovery from psychiatric illness by understanding patterns of feelings, fantasies, and interpersonal behaviors.

Modern psychoanalysis requires four to five sessions a week (45 to 50 minutes per session), continued, on average, for 3 to 6 years. This frequency of sessions is necessary for patients to develop sufficient trust to explore their inner life and subjective experience. Likewise, given the number of events that occur daily in one's lifetime, the frequent meetings are necessary for the patient to be able to explore fantasies, dreams, and reactions to the analytic situation instead of focusing only on daily reality-based crises and stresses. Individuals who are in severe crisis and are, therefore, focused on the crises in their life are generally not candidates for psychoanalysis. If major crises do occur during analysis, formal analysis may be temporarily suspended for a more supportive psychotherapeutic approach. In general, psychoanalytic patients are encouraged to use a recumbent position on the couch to facilitate their ability to freely associate and verbalize their thoughts and feelings. In addition, the analyst usually sits out of the patient's view to assist the process of free association.

Free association, the reporting of all thoughts that come to mind, is a core technique in psychoanalytic treatment. It is difficult to attain, and much of the work of psychoanalysis is based on identifying those times when free association breaks down (the occurrence of a defense, clinically experienced by the analyst as "resistance"). When the patient is easily able to free associate, the neurotic conflicts have been largely removed and termination of treatment is near.

Early in treatment, the analyst establishes a therapeutic alliance with the patient, which allows for a reality-based consideration of the demands of the treatment and a working collaboration between the analyst and analysand (patient) directed toward understanding the patient. The analyst points out the defenses the patient uses. Defenses or defense mechanisms are psychological

AN EVALUATION FOR PSYCHOTHERAPY

A 35-year-old man was referred for evaluation due to ongoing conflicts at work. He described a successful career in which he had changed work groups several times because he had become "disillusioned" with his supervisor, who he believed was "not bright enough" and was controlling him and demeaning him for his success. After each episode he felt depressed, lost 10 lb, and had difficulty sleeping. He had previously been treated with antidepressants with no response and had two courses of supportive psychotherapy. His father, who completed eighth grade, had a small tobacco farm. His mother, a high school graduate, worked at the local grocery store. She had developed breast cancer when he was age 5. Although he respected his father for working hard, he never believed that he shared his father's interests and often thought his father envied his successes in school. When asked about his bosses with whom he had argued, he said they "seemed like farmers" and "never knew what it meant to actually think." The psychiatrist considered that the patient experienced repeated depressions related to experiences of conflict with his bosses that were similar to the conflict he felt with his father and said at the end of the evaluation, "I wonder if you ever thought that some of the arguments you had with your bosses were like the ones you had with your father?" The patient said yes, he had noticed that, and in fact, his wife has told him, "You are fighting with your father again." The psychiatrist discussed psychoanalysis with the patient as one approach to the treatment, given the evidence of childhood patterns reappearing in adult relations and of lack of successful treatment with antidepressants and supportive therapy.

strategies individuals use to reduce anxiety and protect themselves from the painful awareness of conflicts, disturbing feelings, and memories. Healthy individuals use a variety of defense mechanisms at different times throughout their development. Defenses become pathologic only when they lead to maladaptive behaviors or psychiatric illness. Dreams, slips of the tongue, and symptoms provide avenues to the understanding of unconscious motivations, feelings, and ideas.

The specific treatment effects of psychoanalysis result from the progressive understanding of defensive patterns and, most important, the feelings, cognitions, and behaviors that are transferred to the analyst from patterns of relationships with significant individuals in the patient's past. In the context of the arousal associated with reexperiencing these figures from the past and simultaneously understanding the experience, behavioral change occurs. Interpretation is an important technical procedure in this process. An interpretation links the patient's current experience with the analyst to an experience with a significant childhood figure during development. The therapist works to understand and not to direct or take sides with the patient's wishes, fears, or superego (rules and directions that are applied to the self that derive from childhood).

Medications have historically been infrequently used in psychoanalysis, although integrating psychoanalytic treatment with medication, particularly for mild to moderate mood disorders, has become increasingly common (Glick and Roose, 2006; Lebovitz, 2004). In these cases, medication is used to stabilize moods so that psychoanalysis can be directed toward aiding the change in behaviors that may have been learned over a long time and may be interfering with the return of good psychosocial functioning.

The assessment of a patient for psychoanalysis must include diagnostic considerations, as well as an evaluation of the patient's ability to make use of the psychoanalytic situation for behavioral change. A patient's ability to use psychoanalysis depends on the patient's psychological mindedness; the availability of supports in the real environment to sustain the psychoanalysis, which can be felt as quite depriving; and the patient's ability to experience and simultaneously observe highly charged emotional states. Because of the frequency of the sessions and the duration of the treatment, the cost of psychoanalysis can be prohibitive; however, low-fee training clinics frequently make treatment available to patients who could not otherwise afford it. Psychoanalysis has been useful in the treatment of obsessional disorders, conversion disorders, anxiety disorders, dysthymic disorders, and moderately severe personality disorders (Leichsenring, 2005). Individuals with chaotic life settings and an inability to establish long-term, close relationships are usually not good candidates for psychoanalysis. In the present cost-effective climate, psychoanalysis is more frequently recommended after a course of brief psychotherapy has proved either ineffective or insufficient. Little empirical research is available on the efficacy of psychoanalysis compared with other psychotherapies. In general, those patients who can use understanding, introspection, and self-observation to modify their behavior find the treatment beneficial and productive.

Intensive (Long-Term) Psychoanalytically Oriented Psychotherapy

Psychoanalytically oriented psychotherapy—also known as *psychoanalytic psychotherapy, psychodynamic psychotherapy,* and *explorative psychotherapy*—is a psychotherapeutic procedure that recognizes the concepts of transference and resistance in the psychotherapy setting (Bruch, 1974; Reichmann, 1950). Both long-term and brief psychodynamic psychotherapy are possible. Psychoanalytic psychotherapy is usually more focused than is the extensive reworking of personality undertaken in psychoanalysis. In addition, psychoanalytic psychotherapy is somewhat more "here and now" oriented, with less attempt to reconstruct the developmental origins of conflicts completely.

The psychoanalytic techniques of interpretation and clarification (comments made by the psychiatrist to elucidate a reference or statement a patient makes in therapy) are central to psychoanalytic psychotherapy. Psychoanalytic psychotherapy makes more use of supportive techniques—such as suggestion, reality testing, education, and confrontation—than does psychoanalysis. This allows for its application to a broader range of patients, including those with the potential for severe regression (the experience of feelings, thoughts, and actions from childhood).

Patients in long-term psychoanalytic psychotherapy are usually seen one, two, or three times a week. Patient and therapist meet in face-to-face encounters with free association encouraged. Psychoanalytic psychotherapy may extend for several months to several years, at times being as long as psychoanalysis. The length is determined by the number of focal problem areas undertaken in the treatment. Medications can be used in psychoanalytic psychotherapy and may provide another means of titrating the level of regression a patient may experience.

The same patients who are treated in psychoanalysis can be treated in psychoanalytic psychotherapy (see Table 23-3). The psychosocial problems and internal conflicts of patients who cannot be treated in psychoanalysis, such as those with major depression, schizophrenia, and borderline personality disorder, can be addressed in long-term psychoanalytic psychotherapy. In long-term psychoanalytic psychotherapy, the regressive tendencies of such patients can be controlled with greater support, medication, and reality feedback through their face-to-face encounter with the therapist. Historically, there have been few empirical data available on the efficacy of psychoanalytically oriented psychotherapy, although it has been highly valued by many clinicians and patients. Recent review of 23 randomized controlled trials of manual-guided psychodynamic psychotherapy applied in specific psychiatric illnesses has shown evidence that psychodynamic psychotherapy is superior to control conditions (treatment as usual or wait list) and as effective as already established therapies such as cognitive behavioral therapy (CBT) (Leichsenring and Leibing, 2007). Studies have supported the importance of

TABLE 23-3	Psychoanalytically Oriented Psychotherapy
Goal	Understanding conflict area and particular defense mechanisms used More "here and now" than psychoanalysis
Patient selection criteria	Similar to psychoanalysis Also includes personality disorders with psychotic potential (borderline, narcissistic) Some major depressions and schizophrenia may be helped when combined with medication during periods of remission for the treatment of psychosocial features
Techniques	Face to face—sitting up Free association Interpretation and clarification Some supportive techniques Medication as adjunct
Duration	Months to years

working with the transference to create behavioral change (Luborsky and Crits-Christoph, 1990).

Interpersonal psychotherapy (IPT) (Klerman et al., 1984) has many psychodynamic principles and has been shown to be effective in studies using combined psychotherapy and medication interventions (Weissman, 2007). A time-limited therapy, IPT was initially developed for patients with depression but has been adapted and shows some promise for treatment of other disorders (e.g., bipolar affective disorder [BPAD], bulimia nervosa). IPT is based on the concept that depression occurs in the context of social and interpersonal events. Interpersonal behavior is emphasized as the cause of depression as well as the method of cure. There are three major parts of depression: symptoms, social and interpersonal context, and personality. IPT therapists do not try to treat personality. They recognize that many behaviors that appear enduring and lifelong in the course of an interpersonal crisis may, in fact, be a reflection of the depression itself.

Focal problem areas are grief (complicated bereavement), interpersonal role dispute, interpersonal role transition, and interpersonal deficits. Patients are taught to realistically evaluate their interactions with others and become aware of their own behaviors that may contribute to or worsen their mood. In IPT, the therapist often gives direct advice and helps the patient with decision making. The focus is on the here and now. Supportive, flexible, and empathic, the psychiatrist helps clarify areas of conflict and pays little or no attention to transference. The goal of IPT is to help the patient understand the interpersonal context in which the depressive symptoms arose and how these relate to the current social and personal context. By coping with current problems, the patient develops self-reliance. Symptoms then improve through the process of clarification, understanding, and handling these interpersonal and environmental stressors.

Brief Psychodynamic Psychotherapy

An increased demand for psychotherapy following World War II led to the development of briefer forms of psychotherapy. In addition, the community mental health movement and, more recently, the increasing cost of mental health care and managed care have stimulated efforts to find briefer forms of psychotherapy. Brief psychotherapy is a necessary, efficacious, and central part of the psychiatrist's armamentarium (Crits-Christoph, 1992; Leichsenring et al., 2004).

The goals of brief psychotherapy are described by most authors as facilitation of health-seeking behaviors and the mitigation of obstacles to normal growth. From this perspective, brief psychotherapy focuses on the patient's continuous development throughout adult life in the context of conflicts relating to environment, interpersonal relationships, biological health, and developmental stages. This picture of brief psychotherapy supports modest goals and the avoidance of "perfectionism" by the therapist.

Although many of the selection criteria emphasized in the literature of brief psychotherapy are common to all kinds of psychodynamic psychotherapy, certain unique criteria are required because of the brief duration of treatment (see Table 23-4). Patients in brief psychodynamic psychotherapy must be able to engage quickly with the therapist and terminate therapy in a short period. The necessity of greater independent action by the patient mandates high levels of emotional strength, motivation, and responsiveness to interpretation. The importance of rapidly establishing the therapeutic alliance underlies a substantial number of the selection and exclusion criteria.

Some exclusion criteria for brief psychotherapy were developed by Malan (1975), such as a history of serious suicidal attempts, drug addiction, long-term hospitalization, more than one course of electroconvulsive therapy (ECT), chronic alcoholism, severe chronic obsessional symptoms, severe chronic phobic symptoms, or gross destructive or self-destructive behavior. Patients who are unavailable for therapeutic contact or need prolonged work to generate motivation, penetrate rigid defenses, deal with complex or deep-seated issues, or resolve intense transference reactions are also not likely to benefit from brief psychotherapy and may have negative side effects.

The importance of focusing on a circumscribed area of current conflict in brief psychotherapy is mentioned by nearly all authors (Davanloo, 1980; Malan, 1975; Mann, 1973; Sifneos, 1972). They also emphasize the importance of the evaluation sessions to determine the focus of treatment. The formulation of the focus to the patient may be, for example, in terms of the patient's conscious fears and pain, but it is important for the therapist to construct the psychodynamic focus at a

TABLE 23-4	Brief Psychodynamic Psychotherapy
Goal	Clarify and resolve focal area of conflict that interferes with current functioning
Patient selection criteria	High ego strength High motivation Can identify focal issue Can form strong interpersonal relationships, including with the therapist, in a brief time Good response to trial interpretations
Techniques	Face to face Interpretation of defenses and transference Setting the time limit at the start of therapy Focus on patient reactions to limited duration of treatment
Duration	12–40 sessions; usually 20 sessions or less

deeper level to understand the work being done. Maintaining the focus is the primary task of the therapist. This enables the therapist to deal with complicated personality structures in a brief period of time. Resistance is limited through "benign neglect" of potentially troublesome but nonfocal areas of personality. The elaboration of techniques of establishing and maintaining the focus of treatment is critical to all brief individual psychodynamic psychotherapies.

Transference interpretations (i.e., making comments that link the patient's reactions to the therapist to feelings for significant individuals from the patient's past) are generally accepted as important in brief psychotherapy; however, the manner and rapidity in which transference is addressed vary considerably.

There is remarkable agreement on the duration of brief psychotherapy. Although the duration ranges from 5 to 40 sessions, authors generally favor 10 to 20 sessions. The duration of treatment is critically related to maintaining the focus within the brief psychotherapy. When treatment extends beyond 20 sessions, therapists frequently find themselves enmeshed in a broad character analysis without a focal conflict. Change after 20 sessions may be quite slow. Clinical experience generally supports the idea that brief individual psychodynamic psychotherapy should be between 10 and 20 sessions unless the therapist is willing to proceed to long-term treatment of >40 or 50 sessions.

Cognitive Psychotherapy

Cognitive psychotherapy is a method of brief psychotherapy developed over the last three decades by Aaron T. Beck and his colleagues at the University of Pennsylvania, primarily for the treatment of mild and moderate depressions and for patients with low self-esteem (Beck, 1976; Rush and Beck, 1988). It is based on the theoretic assumption that environmental events trigger cognitive processes and that these thoughts give an event personal meaning that leads to affective arousal. It is similar to behavior therapy in that it aims at the direct removal of symptoms rather than the resolution of underlying conflicts, as in the psychodynamic psychotherapies; however, unlike traditional behavioral approaches, the subjective experience of the patient is a major focus of the work. Cognitive therapists view the patient's conscious thoughts as central to producing and perpetuating symptoms such as depression, anxiety, phobias, and somatization (the tendency to convert psychological or psychosocial stress into a physical complaint). Both the content of thoughts and thought processes are seen as disordered in people with such symptoms. Therapy is directed toward identifying and altering these cognitive distortions.

The cognitive therapist sees the interpretations that depressed persons make about life as different from those of nondepressed individuals. Depressed people tend to make negative interpretations of the world, themselves, and the future (the negative cognitive triad) (see Table 23-5). Depressed individuals interpret events as reflecting defeat, deprivation, or disparagement and see their lives as filled with obstacles and burdens. They view themselves as unworthy, deficient, undesirable, or worthless, and they see the future as bringing a continuation of the miseries

TABLE 23-5	**Common Terms in Cognitive Therapy**
Negative cognitive triad	Negative interpretations that depressed individuals make about the world, themselves, and the future
Automatic thoughts	Arise spontaneously or in response to stimuli, have emotional validity The individual may be made fully conscious of these if attention is directed to them
Schemas	Assumptions about self and the world, typically out of the realm of consciousness of the individual

of the present. These evaluations are the result of the negative biases inherent in depressive thinking and applied regardless of the objective nature of the individual's circumstances. Other psychiatric conditions have their own characteristic cognitive patterns that determine the nature of the symptoms. The "thinking" distortions in depression include arbitrary inferences about an event, selective use of details to reach a conclusion, overgeneralization, overestimating negative and underestimating positive aspects of a situation, and the tendency to label events according to one's emotional response rather than the facts.

Such cognitions (verbal thoughts) often feel involuntary and automatic. This kind of thinking is so automatic in response to many situations, and the resultant cognitions so fleeting, that people may often be virtually unaware of them. Such automatic thoughts differ from unconscious thoughts in that they can easily be made fully conscious if attention is directed to them. A large portion of the work of cognitive psychotherapy is to train patients to observe and record their automatic thoughts.

Cognitive theory postulates a chronic state of depression-proneness that may precede the actual illness and remain after the symptoms have abated. Depression-prone individuals have relatively permanent depressive cognitive structures ("cognitive schemas") that determine how new stimuli are perceived and conceptualized. Typical schemas of depression include "I am stupid," or "I cannot exist without the love of a strong person." Unlike automatic thoughts, patients are not typically—and cannot easily become—aware of such underlying general assumptions. These must be deduced from many specific examples of distorted thinking. Schemas such as "I am stupid" may lie dormant much of the time, only to be reactivated by a specific event, such as difficulty in accomplishing a task. These enduring self-concepts and attitudes are assumed to have been learned in childhood on the basis of the child's experiences and the reactions of important family members. Once formed, such attitudes can be self-perpetuating.

A CASE OF COGNITIVE BEHAVIORAL THERAPY

The man described earlier decides not to enter psychoanalysis but instead pursues CBT. He learns to identify some of his negative thoughts about himself, the world, and the future and records events, thoughts, and emotions as a way of self-monitoring and increasing his awareness. Initially, he focuses on his relationship with his boss and feelings of anger that have led him in the past to leave jobs and become increasingly depressed. He describes his boss as being unable to give him a detailed explanation of a new policy change. He immediately thinks, "What an idiot! He does not know a thing about this business." The patient states, "I was so mad that I was ready to quit, again." He is asked to rate the believability of his thought about his boss on a scale of 1 to 100. He gives it a 75. The psychiatrist asks him to think of rational alternatives that rebut these negative thoughts. He observes that his boss went to a reputable university and had adjusted to many previous changes at work without difficulty. The psychiatrist asks him to identify his new affect based on these observations, and he then describes feeling "sort of irritated." Further processing allows him to see that he can experience uncomfortable thoughts and emotions and evaluate them rationally so that they do not lead to behaviors that ultimately cause him increased dysphoria (such as walking out on the job).

Just as depressive thoughts can be triggered by events, episodes of depressive illness may, from the cognitive perspective, be triggered by sufficient stress. Such stresses may be specific to the individual and his or her particular sensitivities developed in childhood. Alternatively, sufficient degrees of nonspecific stress may precipitate depression in vulnerable individuals. Experiences of loss, a setback in a major goal, a rejection, or an insolvable dilemma are especially common precipitants of depression. The onset of medical illness, with its attendant limitations and associated meanings, is also seen as likely to trigger depression in many people.

Researchers have accumulated considerable evidence that depressed individuals do indeed manifest negative biases in their views of themselves, their experiences, and the future (Ciesla and Roberts, 2007). In addition, they have attitudes (schemas) that distinguish them from nondepressed study participants, as well as distortions in logic and information processing. It is less clear whether all depressed people show the thinking distortions that Beck has described. Much of the cognitive depression research has been criticized because the studies have been on nonpatient populations, such as student volunteers, with relatively mild degrees of depression. These individuals may be very different from actual psychiatric patients. Whether cognitive distortions are a predisposing factor to depression is also unclear. Researchers have found that most distorted thinking disappears when depression is successfully treated, even with antidepressant medication. The findings suggest that these distortions are a symptom of depression rather than an enduring trait of depression-prone people. Response-styles theory postulates that rumination represents a trait vulnerable to depression. Recent evidence has suggested that rumination predicts changes in depression more strongly among individuals with high levels of negative cognition (Ciesla and Roberts, 2007). Clearly, further research is needed to test the causality of cognitive factors in depression.

Technique of cognitive psychotherapy

Cognitive psychotherapy is a directive, time-limited, multidimensional psychological treatment. The patient and therapist together discover the irrational beliefs and illogical thinking patterns associated with the patient's depressive affects (see Table 23-6). They then devise methods by which patients themselves can test the validity of their thinking. The therapist helps patients to become aware of their irrational beliefs and distorted thinking ("automatic thoughts").

Cognitive psychotherapy was developed for unipolar, nonpsychotic, mild to moderately depressed outpatients. The presence of bipolar illness, delusions or hallucinations, or extremely severe depression is a contraindication for cognitive psychotherapy as the sole or primary treatment modality. However, CBT has been used successfully as adjunctive therapy in the treatment of BPAD and treatment-refractory psychosis (Turkington et al., 2008). Other contraindications include the presence of underlying medical illness or medications that may be causing the depression, the presence of a neurologically based mental disorder, or an ongoing problem of substance abuse. In addition, cognitive psychotherapy may not be indicated as the sole form of treatment for major or "endogenous" depression (which may be accompanied by endocrine, sleep, or other biological abnormalities in which antidepressant medication or ECT is needed) or

TABLE 23-6	Cognitive Psychotherapy
Goal	Identify and alter cognitive distortions
Patient selection criteria	Unipolar, nonpsychotic depressed outpatients May be used as adjunctive treatment in treatment-resistant psychosis Relative contraindications include delusions, hallucinations, severe depression, severe cognitive impairment, ongoing substance abuse, enmeshed family system
Techniques	Behavioral assignments Reading material Taught to recognize negatively biased automatic thoughts Identify patients' schemas, beliefs, attitudes
Duration	Time limited: 15–25 sessions

for patients enmeshed in family systems that maintain a fixed view of themselves as helpless and dependent. Cognitive psychotherapy may be useful in patients who refuse to take, fail to respond to, or are unable to tolerate medication, as well as those who prefer a psychological approach in the hope of greater long-term benefits.

Cognitive psychotherapy is generally conducted over a period of 15 to 25 weeks in once-weekly meetings. With more severely depressed patients, two or three meetings per week are recommended for the first several weeks. Although cognitive psychotherapy was developed and is usually administered as an individual treatment, its principles have also been successfully applied to group settings.

A course of cognitive psychotherapy proceeds in a succession of regular stages. The first stage is devoted to introducing the patient to the procedures and rationale of the therapy, setting goals for the treatment, and establishing a therapeutic alliance. The therapist may assign reading material on the cognitive theory of depression. In the next stage, the therapist begins to demonstrate to the patient that cognitions and emotions are connected. Patients are taught to become more aware of their negatively biased automatic thoughts and to recognize, both during and outside of the psychotherapy hours, that negative affects are generally preceded by such thoughts. Behavioral assignments may be used. For example, in cognitive response prevention, the patient is given homework to act in a way that is inconsistent with his or her schema, which is meant to trigger automatic thoughts that the patient can challenge. That is, if the schema is "If I am not perfect, I will be unloved," the patient is encouraged to complete a task in a less-than-perfect manner and then challenge or prevent the automatic thoughts about being unworthy or unloved.

In the next phase, which normally comprises most of the work, the emphasis shifts to a detailed exploration of the patient's cognitions and their role in perpetuating depressive feelings. In the final stage of psychotherapy, patients will have had a great deal of experience in recognizing their habitual thought patterns, testing their validity, and modifying them when appropriate, with the result of substantial symptomatic relief. Psychotherapy then focuses on the attitudes and assumptions that underlie the patient's negatively biased thinking. For example, the patient might assume, "If I am nice, bad things will not happen to me." A logically equivalent assumption would then be, "If bad things happen to me, it is my fault because I am not nice." Target symptoms that might be the focus of a session include intense sadness, pervasive self-criticism, passivity and avoidance, sleep disturbance, or other affective, motivational, or cognitive manifestations of depression. The therapist repeatedly formulates the patient's beliefs and attitudes as testable hypotheses and helps the patient devise and implement ways of verifying them. The therapist maintains an inquiring attitude toward the patient's reactions to the therapist and the therapeutic procedures. Such reactions are explored for evidence of misunderstanding and distortion, which are then addressed in the same way as the patient's other cognitions.

A great variety of different techniques are used by cognitive therapists to break the cycle of negative evaluations and dysfunctional behaviors. Behavioral methods are often useful in the beginning of psychotherapy, particularly when the patient is severely depressed. Activity scheduling, mastery and pleasure exercises, graded task assignments, cognitive rehearsal, and role-playing may all be used.

More cognitively oriented methods are applied in the middle and late stages of psychotherapy as psychotherapy progresses. The therapist and patient explore the patient's inner life in a spirit of adventure. Patients become more observant of their peculiar construction of reality and usually focus more on actual events and their meanings. The fundamental cognitive technique is teaching patients to observe, record, and validate their cognitions.

Efficacy of cognitive psychotherapy

In contrast to most other psychotherapies, there is a substantial literature on the efficacy of cognitive psychotherapy. Cognitive psychotherapy has been shown to be more effective than no psychotherapy in treating both depressed volunteers and psychiatric patients with diagnoses of depression. In addition to depression, CBT has been shown to be effective in the treatment of various anxiety disorders, including panic disorder, generalized anxiety disorder, post-traumatic stress disorder, obsessive-compulsive disorder, social phobia, and eating disorders (Bandelow et al., 2007). It has shown efficacy in adult as well as child and adolescent populations.

TABLE 23-7	Supportive Psychotherapy
Goal	Maintain or reestablish best level of functioning
Patient selection criteria	Very healthy individuals exposed to stressful life circumstances (e.g., adjustment disorder) Individual with serious illness, ego deficits, (e.g., schizophrenia, major depression with psychosis) Individuals with medical illness
Techniques	Available, predictable therapist No or limited interpretation of transference Support intellectualization Therapist acts as a guide/mentor Medication frequently used Supportive techniques: suggestion, reinforcement, advice, teaching, reality testing, cognitive restructuring, reassurance Active stance Discuss alternative behaviors, social/interpersonal skills
Duration	Brief (days to weeks) to very long term (years)

Supportive Psychotherapy

Supportive psychotherapy aims to help patients maintain or reestablish the best level of functioning, given the limitations of their illness, personality, native ability, and life circumstances (see Table 23-7). In general, this goal distinguishes supportive psychotherapy from the change-oriented psychotherapies, which aim to reverse primary disease processes and symptoms or restructure personality.

The line between supportive and "change-oriented" psychotherapy, however, is frequently not so clear. The situation is somewhat analogous to the medical treatment of viral versus bacterial infections. Treatment of the former is basically supportive in that it aims to maintain normal bodily functions (e.g., fever reduction, control of cerebral edema, dietary compensation for liver failure) in the face of infection, while in the latter, the aim is to eliminate the infection. In addition to the supportive aspects of treating bacterial infections, however, antibiotic treatment itself is supportive in the sense that it works as an adjunct to the body's natural immune system, without which it is relatively ineffective. There are supportive elements, however, in all effective forms of psychotherapy, and the terms *supportive* and *change oriented* merely describe the balance of efforts in a particular case. The skilled psychiatrist is able to move along this spectrum based on the goals of the treatment and the level of functioning and needs of the patient at any given moment.

Patients who are generally very healthy and well adapted but who have become impaired in response to stressful life circumstances, as well as those who have serious illnesses that cannot be cured, can receive supportive psychotherapy. Supportive psychotherapy may be brief or long term. The "healthy" individual, when faced with overwhelming stress or crises (particularly in the face of traumas or disasters), may seek help and be a candidate for supportive psychotherapy. The relatively healthy candidate for supportive psychotherapy is a well-adapted individual (with good social supports and interpersonal relationships, flexible defenses, and good reality testing) who is in acute crisis. This individual continues to show evidence of well-planned behaviors and a healthy perspective on the crisis. The person makes use of social supports, does not withdraw, and anticipates resolution of the crisis. Although the patient is functioning below his or her usual level, this patient remains hopeful about the future and makes use of resources available for problem solving, respite, and growth. The patient uses supportive psychotherapy to reconstitute more rapidly, avoid errors in judgment by "talking out loud," relieve minor symptomatology, and grow as an individual by learning about the world.

The more typical candidate for supportive psychotherapy has significant deficits in ego functioning, including poor reality testing, impaired impulse control, and difficulties in interpersonal relations. Patients who have less ability to sublimate (divert energy from a negative impulse to a more socially and morally acceptable one) and are less introspective are frequently treated in supportive psychotherapy, where more directive techniques and environmental manipulation can be used.

Ego strength and the ability to form relationships may be more important than diagnosis in the selection of patients for supportive psychotherapy (Rockland, 1989; Werman, 1984). The ability of the patient to relate to the therapist; a past history of reasonable personal relationships, work history, and educational performance; and the use of leisure time for constructive activity and relaxation bear importantly on the treatment recommendation. Almost no information is known regarding which characteristics of the patient may predict a good result from supportive psychotherapy rather than merely a poor response to the change-oriented psychotherapies. Delineation of the minimum level of personal strengths needed to benefit from supportive individual psychotherapy is an important task for future research.

Technique of Supportive Psychotherapy

Psychoanalytic theory provides the major contributions to the theory of supportive psychotherapy. In-depth psychological understanding of patients in supportive psychotherapy is as necessary as in the change-oriented, explorative psychotherapies (Pine, 1986; Rockland, 1989; Werman, 1984). Understanding unconscious motivation, psychic conflict, the patient–therapist relationship, and the patient's use of defense mechanisms is essential to understanding the patient's strengths and vulnerabilities. This knowledge is critical to providing support as well as insight.

Therapists who are predictably available and safe (i.e., who accept the patient and put aside their own needs in the service of the treatment) assume some of the holding functions of the "good parent." In such a therapeutic situation, the patient is able to identify with and incorporate the well-functioning aspects of the therapist, such as the capacity for self-observation and the ability to tolerate ambivalence (Pine, 1986).

The containment of affect (feeling) and anxiety is an important supportive function. Patients in need of supportive psychotherapy typically fear the destructive power of their internal rage and envy. They are helped to modulate their emotional reactions by the reliable presence of the therapist and the therapeutic relationship that remains unchanged in the face of emotional onslaughts. Alexander (1946) described this as the "corrective emotional experience" in which the relationship between the patient and the therapist provides an opportunity for the therapist to display behavior that is different from the destructive or unproductive behavior of the patient's parent in the past. Although present thinking does not indicate that such a "correction" occurs at any biological level, the new and "better" relationship does offer a stabilizing influence and, for some, the chance to better understand what they missed.

The therapist fosters the supportive relationship by refraining from interpreting positive transference feelings and waiting until the intensity of feelings has abated before commenting about negative transference feelings. Interpretations of the negative transference are limited to those needed to ensure that the treatment is not disrupted. While maintaining a friendly stance toward the patient, the therapist respects the patient's need to establish a comfortable degree of distance. The therapist must not push for a more intimate or emotion-laden relationship than the patient can tolerate. The rapport with the patient, which the supportive psychotherapist tries to establish, differs from the therapeutic alliance of insight-oriented therapy. The doctor–patient relationship does not require the patient to observe and report on his or her own feelings and behavior to the same extent as in the change-oriented, explorative psychotherapies. The therapist acts more as a guide and a mentor.

There is virtually unanimous agreement among writers on supportive psychotherapy that fostering a good working relationship with the patient is the first priority. The therapist must be available in a regular and predictable manner. Rather than approach the patient as a "blank slate," the therapist actively demonstrates concern, involvement, sympathy, and a supportive attitude. The therapist serves as an auxiliary ego for the patient, helping to modulate among the primitive drives, morals, and reality. The auxiliary ego functions of the therapist can be seen in the therapist's use of suggestion, reinforcement, advice, teaching, reality testing, cognitive restructuring, and reassurance. In taking such an active stance, it is especially important for the therapist to guard against grandiosity and personal biases, so as not to become an "omnipotent decision maker." Rather, the therapist acts as "a strong, benign individual who is reasonably available when needed." To the extent that the patient develops the capacity to observe himself

TABLE 23-8	**Common Terms in Supportive Psychotherapy**
Auxiliary ego	Function of the therapist who helps the patient learn to modulate between primitive drives, morals, and reality
Supportive interpretation	Comment made by therapist to increase insight for patient It is not about the past but focused on the here and now and on what may frighten the patient in the present day

or herself, the psychotherapy may proceed beyond support and take on features of the explorative and change-oriented psychotherapies.

The defenses of denial and avoidance are handled by encouraging the patient to discuss alternative behaviors, goals, and interpretations of events. Reassurance has a variety of forms in supportive psychotherapy, including supporting an adaptive level of denial (such as patients may employ in coping with terminal illness); patients' experience of the therapist's empathic attitude; or the therapist's reality testing of patients' negatively biased evaluations of themselves or their situations. Reassuring a patient is not easy. It requires a clear understanding of what the patient fears. Overt expressions of interest and concern may be reassuring to a patient who fears rejection, but threatening to one who fears intrusion. Interpretations in supportive psychotherapy are limited to those that will decrease anxiety and strengthen (rather than loosen) defenses, particularly the defenses of intellectualization and rationalization (see Table 23-8).

The therapist's expressions of interest, advice giving, and facilitation of ventilation reinforce desired behaviors. Expressions of interest and solicitude are positively reinforcing. Advice can lead to behavioral change if it is specific and applies to frequent behaviors of the patient. Desired behaviors are rewarded by the therapist's approval and by social reinforcement. Venting of emotions is useful only if the therapist can help the patient safely contain and limit them, thereby extinguishing the anxiety response to emotional expression. Cognitive and behavioral psychotherapeutic interventions that strengthen the adaptive and defensive functions of the ego (e.g., realistic and logical thinking, social skills, and containment of affects such as anxiety) contribute to the supportive aspects of the psychotherapy.

Efficacy of Supportive Psychotherapy

Most data on the effectiveness of supportive psychotherapy come from studies in which supportive psychotherapy has been used as a control in testing the efficacy of other treatments. In such studies, the procedures used in supportive psychotherapy tend to be poorly specified, and no attempts are made to correlate individual supportive techniques with outcome. There are no studies in which supportive psychotherapy is compared with no treatment or minimal treatment. Despite its limitations, however, the research literature offers some evidence that supportive psychotherapy is an effective treatment, particularly when combined with medication, and at times, is even shown to be superior to pharmacotherapy alone (de Maat et al., 2008). This conclusion appears to be true in the treatment of depression, anxiety disorders, and schizophrenia.

Research indicates that supportive psychotherapy is an effective component of the treatment of patients with a variety of medical illnesses, including those with ulcerative colitis or myocardial infarction and cancer patients undergoing radiation treatment. In general, patients in supportive psychotherapy improve emotionally and have fewer days in the hospital, fewer complications, and more rapid recovery.

The evidence to date, although preliminary, suggests that supportive psychotherapy can be effective in both psychiatric and medical illnesses and is frequently more cost effective than more intensive psychotherapies for some disorders. More research is needed on the indications, contraindications, and techniques of supportive psychotherapy.

BEHAVIORAL THERAPY

Behavioral therapy (i.e., behavior modification) is based on the concept that all symptoms of a psychological nature are learned maladaptive patterns of behavior in response to environmental

TABLE 23-9	Behavioral Therapy (Behavioral Modification)
Goal	Eliminate involuntary disruptive behavior patterns and substitute appropriate behaviors
Patient selection criteria	Habit modification Targeted symptoms Phobias Some psychophysiological responses: headache, migraine, hypertension, Raynaud phenomenon Sexual dysfunction
Techniques	Systemic desensitization Implosion therapy and flooding Aversion therapy Biofeedback
Duration	Usually time limited

or internal stimuli. It does not concern itself with intrapsychic conflicts or reconstructing the patient's life story and the unconscious dynamics that are the focus of the psychodynamically oriented psychotherapies. Rather, it uses the concepts of learning theory to eliminate the involuntary, disruptive behavior patterns that constitute the essential features of psychopathology and substitutes highly adaptive and situation-appropriate patterns (Lazarus, 1971). Behavioral therapy has been useful in a wide range of disorders when specific behavioral symptoms can be targeted for change and this change is central to recovery. Eating disorders, chronic pain syndromes and illness behavior, phobias, sexual dysfunction, paraphilias, and conduct disorders of childhood are frequently treated with behavioral therapy techniques.

Techniques of Behavioral Therapy

A variety of techniques exist that permit the modification of undesirable and unwanted behaviors when applied by therapists skilled in their use (see Table 23-9). These approaches require careful history taking and behavioral analysis to identify the behaviors to be targeted for extinction or modification. Often, adjunctive techniques, such as the use of hypnosis and pharmacotherapy, are used to facilitate behavior modification but are not requisite for therapeutic success. Present-day behavioral therapists are usually alert to interpersonal and emotional aspects of psychiatric symptoms and the doctor–patient relationship. Psychodynamic, cognitive, and interpersonal techniques are frequently integrated into the therapy but are not seen as central to the therapeutic effect. Four of the more common behavioral techniques are described here (see Table 23-10).

TABLE 23-10	Common Terms in Behavioral Therapy
Systematic desensitization	Technique in which the patient is exposed to a progressive hierarchy of fear-inducing situations or objects
Flooding	Technique in which the patient is directly and immediately exposed to actual feared objects or situations, without gradual introduction
Implosion therapy	Technique in which the patient uses mental images as substitutes for the actual object or situation feared Exposure is immediate and without gradual introduction
Aversion therapy	Technique based on the principle of classical conditioning Pairs an aversive stimulus with the unwanted behavior
Progressive muscle relaxation	Stress management technique in which the patient learns to voluntarily relax certain muscle groups to decrease anxiety

Systematic Desensitization

Systematic desensitization refers to a technique whereby individuals are exposed to increasingly greater anxiety-provoking situations or objects, which is useful for the treatment of simple phobias, social phobia, generalized anxiety disorder, and panic disorder. The therapist first identifies a hierarchy of behaviors directed to approaching the phobic object or situation. Relaxation techniques are used to decrease anxiety at each stage of the hierarchy. The patient moves up to the next level of intensity when the stimulus no longer provokes intense anxiety. This particularly effective technique is useful in an office setting as well, because experience has demonstrated that the patient can confront the anxiety-provoking stimulus in his or her imagination with very much the same effects. Again, a hierarchy of increasingly anxious imaginary scenes is constructed. The patient visualizes each scene, reexperiences the anxiety associated with it, and then uses relaxation techniques to become gradually more comfortable with the fantasy. Patients move up the hierarchy of images until they are able to visualize fully the phobic object or situation without undue anxiety. Usually, this *in vitro* technique will be accompanied by *in vivo* practice exposures. Hypnotic procedures and the use of anxiolytic drugs are useful adjuncts in certain types of patients. There is some controversy regarding the mechanisms underlying the effect of systematic desensitization, for which various explanations have been suggested. It is possible, for example, that the graduated exposure to the anxiety-provoking situation represents nothing more than a sequential or progressive "flooding" technique (see section "Implosion Therapy and Flooding" in subsequent text). It is also possible that by exposing the individual to only small, and therefore more tolerable, amounts of anxiety, the individual is able to develop more appropriate and successful coping mechanisms. Other authors have suggested that the key to systematic desensitization lies in the suppression of anxiety, which is achieved by evoking a competitive physiological response such as progressive muscle relaxation.

Implosion Therapy and Flooding

Implosion therapy and flooding techniques vary only in the presentation of the anxiety-eliciting stimulus. Animal behaviorists discovered early on that avoidant behavior, which by its very nature can be expected to be highly resistant to extinction, could be extinguished rather rapidly by submitting the animal to a prolonged conditioned stimulus while restraining it and making the expression of the avoidant behavior impossible. In the therapeutic situation, the patient is directly exposed to the stressful stimulus until the anxiety subsides. This is in contrast to the graded exposure of systematic desensitization. In theory, each session should result in ever-decreasing intervals between exposure and cessation of anxiety. In implosion therapy, the patient uses mental images as substitutes for the actual feared object or situation, whereas in the flooding approach, the therapist conducts the procedure *in vivo*. Results appear to indicate that both approaches are equally effective. Some have questioned the ethics of submitting patients to such painful experiences, especially when other alternatives are available. A risk associated with this technique is the danger that the patient may refuse to submit to such an uncomfortable experience and may terminate the exposure before the abatement of the anxiety. This will result in a successful "escape" and therefore reinforce the phobic response.

Aversion Therapy

The aversion therapy treatment modality has its roots in classical conditioning. Controversial by its very nature, it has nevertheless found acceptance as a potentially useful avenue of therapy for a narrow range of disorders and unwanted habits. Perhaps the most common form of aversion therapy is the use of disulfiram (Antabuse) in alcoholics. This treatment approach is based on the fear of an extremely unpleasant, and indeed sometimes fatal, physiological response (the unconditioned stimulus) when someone who has been taking disulfiram then imbibes alcohol (which becomes the conditioned stimulus). In theory, the alcoholic patient on disulfiram therapy will avoid alcohol to avoid the alcohol-disulfiram reaction.

Mild aversive stimuli have also been used in smoking-cessation programs with variable results (Hajek and Stead, 2004). Because of safety considerations, and to ensure continued patient participation, aversive stimuli used under these conditions are often mild and may not constitute much more than having to hold the smoke in the oral cavity for a prolonged period of time or to smoke cigarettes rapidly.

Various aversive techniques have also been used in the treatment of sexual offenders, including such stimuli as mild electric shocks and unpleasant odors. Ethical considerations, understandable patient reluctance to participate in treatment, and pejorative associations by the general public with torture and other forms of maltreatment have resulted in rather limited applications for these techniques. In addition, their effectiveness has been more variable than that of other behavioral techniques (Mann, 2004).

Biofeedback

Biofeedback is not a type of behavioral therapy, *per se*, but, rather, a tool or technique that can be integrated with other operant procedures for the management of a number of psychophysiological disorders. Some of the conditions in which there is documented short-term efficacy for biofeedback are hypertension, migraine headaches, tension headaches, some cardiac arrhythmias, and Raynaud phenomenon (Karavidas et al., 2006; Linden and Mosley, 2006; Nestoriuc and Martin, 2007). This approach presumes that many pathological psychophysiological responses could be subject to modification if the individual could become aware of his or her existence and of positive changes incurred as a result of learned responses (Andrasik, 2007; Gaarder and Montgomery, 1977). For the conditioned response to be reinforced and for learning to take place, the patient must be aware that a response has taken place. Biofeedback techniques consist of measuring an individual's bodily responses (blood pressure, heart rate, galvanic skin response [sweating], and muscle tension) and conveying the information to the individual in real time to raise the patient's awareness of these physiologic changes. Biofeedback first burst on the scene amid great publicity and exaggerated claims regarding its efficacy. This was followed by an expected period of disenchantment and skepticism. Nevertheless, for selected patients, especially those suffering from psychophysiological disorders characterized by measurable vascular and neuromuscular changes, such as chronic tension headaches, this approach may be of some use either by itself or in conjunction with other therapies, including medication and formal psychotherapy. Biofeedback is often administered in clinics by technicians. There is a paucity of evidence, however, that for tension-related syndromes, such as chronic headache, it is any more effective than simple relaxation exercises (Trautmann et al., 2006).

Neurobiofeedback (also referred to as *neurofeedback* or *electroencephalogram [EEG] biofeedback*) is a somewhat controversial form of behavioral therapy aimed at developing skills for self-regulation of brain activity as measured by EEG and typically providing feedback to the patient through video, audio, or vibration. If the brain activity changes successfully, it is tied to a positive feedback or reward, and if there is a negative response, either negative or no feedback is given. This has been studied in some neuropsychiatric conditions, such as attention-deficit/hyperactivity disorder, tic disorder, and anxiety, with variable results. Further research is needed to clarify its efficacy and role in treatment (Heinrich et al., 2007).

Effectiveness of Behavioral Therapies

The behavioral approaches have proved to be of considerable value in the treatment of a wide spectrum of disorders, particularly phobias, muscle tension, and migraine headaches. They also may be considered as valuable adjunct techniques in the overall management of psychiatric and other medical conditions, such as headaches and eating disorders. Often, much time and effort are devoted to discussing the relative merits of behavioral techniques versus psychodynamic therapies. Elements from each approach play a significant factor in the other. Even in the most dynamically oriented therapy situation, the achievement of new insights, improvements in the quality of life, and the lessening of anxiety facilitate the progress toward wellness. Similarly, there has been little research into the nature of the relationship between the patient and the behavioral therapist. The degree to which conflicts between the behavioral therapist and the patient may re-create past relationships, how this is handled, and how this influences treatment progress are not well known.

GROUP THERAPIES

In its most basic form, group therapy can be described as the attainment of therapeutic goals through the skilled manipulation of group processes or mechanisms. The changes effected can be limited and situation specific, or they can be far reaching and foster personality development and

TABLE 23-11	Group Therapies
Goal	Alleviation of symptoms Change interpersonal relations Alter specific family/couple dynamics
Patient selection criteria	Vary greatly based on type of group Homogeneous groups target specific disorders Adolescents and patients with personality disorders may especially benefit Families and couples for whom the system needs change Contraindications: substantial suicide risk, sadomasochistic acting out in family/couple
Techniques	Directive/supportive group psychotherapy Psychodynamic/interpersonal group psychotherapy Psychoanalytic group psychotherapy Dialectical behavioral therapy Family therapy Couples therapy
Duration	Weeks to years; time limited and open ended

growth (Bion, 1961). Family and couples therapies are specific forms of group therapy directed to the family and the couple—usually the marital couple—in special group/interpersonal settings. In contrast to the individual therapies, the group therapies have direct access to the interpersonal processes of the patient with individuals of varying age and sex. Intrapsychic, interpersonal, communication, and system theories, as well as knowledge of family and couple development and roles, are used to elucidate various aspects of behavior and increase the patient's awareness. In addition, new behaviors can be tried in the group with the therapist present (Yalom, 1986). The different types of group therapy emphasize different theoretic perspectives and may have different group compositions (see Table 23-11). All groups provide members with support, a feeling of belonging, and a safe, secure environment where change can be effected and tried out first. The therapist uses the vast array of processes at work in a group to facilitate interaction among its members and to guide the work of the group toward the desired goal. Skill, training, and a keen understanding of group dynamics are required. Particular awareness of group fantasies, projections, scapegoating, and denial are part of most group therapy work. Frequently, cotherapists run the group. This often increases the ability to attend to the many processes occurring in the group and aids in the avoidance of countertransference pitfalls.

Group Psychotherapy

Group psychotherapists use a variety of techniques derived from knowledge of the dynamics and behavior of social groups to foster desired change in the individual members (Yalom, 1986). However, the theoretic framework supporting the various therapeutic modalities varies with the group's goals and purposes, type, and composition. A review of the literature reveals widely diverging definitions and classifications. Different approaches achieve a measure of fame and popularity, such as the so-called encounter groups, and then recede from the scene. In general, however, groups can be divided into three separate and distinct categories: directive, psychodynamic/interpersonal, and analytic. This classification is based largely on the degree to which the group fosters the exploration and evocation of repressed, unconscious material. As a result, each group type will vary widely in approach, techniques, composition, conceptual model, and defined goals. Group psychotherapy occurs in both inpatient and outpatient settings.

Directive/Supportive Group Psychotherapy

Directive/supportive psychotherapy groups usually have very specific, well-defined, and relatively limited goals. Good examples are Alcoholics Anonymous (AA) and Overeaters Anonymous (OA). The groups function within a very narrow set of guidelines defined by a specific philosophy, set of values, or religious orientation. In the case of AA, the members help each other achieve sobriety and cope with everyday problems of living by adhering to the Twelve Steps and entrusting their fate to a higher power. The group leader serves as a role model, stressing common sense, reality-oriented solutions to problems while using the group to apply peer pressure, enhance self-esteem, foster a feeling of togetherness and belonging, and provide a supportive and nurturing environment. Members usually share at least one major attribute in common (e.g., alcoholism), but in many other respects, the group is heterogeneous in composition. There may be a wide divergence in social background, education, personality types, and even the presence of major psychiatric disorders. Behavioral techniques often are applied in similar group situations to treat individuals with phobias while group support and encouragement are used to enhance efficacy.

Psychodynamic/Interpersonal Group Psychotherapy

Psychodynamic/IPT groups address the individual member's psychopathology, foster the development of insight, promote the development of better interpersonal and social skills, and, in general, promote improved coping skills for the here and now. Defenses are identified and challenged in an atmosphere of support and acceptance. Positive change is encouraged and reinforced. These groups may adhere to any of a wide variety of theoretic models or may be eclectic in their approach and incorporate aspects of these models into the system to fit the needs and characteristics of the group. However, they tend to focus on the individual's subjective experience and interpersonal behaviors. Psychodynamic concepts have been added to many group psychotherapies to focus on interpersonal relations and the "model" people carry from childhood.

Psychoanalytic Group Psychotherapy

Psychoanalytic group psychotherapy essentially uses the psychoanalytic approach, as applied in individual therapy. The therapist remains neutral and nondirective and thereby promotes a transference neurosis that can be analyzed. Defenses are identified and resistances interpreted. The group focuses on past experiences and repressed unconscious material as the underlying factors in psychopathology. The therapist attempts to identify individual transferences of the members, as well as shared group fantasies or assumptions.

In general, most patients who benefit from individual psychotherapy benefit from group psychotherapy. Empirical data are lacking, except for directive/supportive group psychotherapy approaches such as AA (Gossop et al., 2008). The differences and similarities in behavior change following group and individual psychotherapy are largely unknown. Although there is no hard evidence for the greater or lesser efficacy of either technique applied to appropriate patients, not all patients will do well in all groups, and some patients should not be considered for inclusion in a treatment group under any circumstances. Specifically, severely depressed and suicidal individuals should not be assigned to outpatient groups. Their emotional state will prevent them from becoming integrated into the group, and the lack of an initial, strong therapeutic relationship with a specific therapist may increase the risk of suicide. Such patients should be considered for individual and other more intensely supportive modalities and inpatient hospitalization when indicated. Patients who are manic tend to be disruptive to group process, and their impulsivity and lack of control prevent them from obtaining any real benefit from group work. Some types of personality disorders, such as explosive, narcissistic, borderline, and antisocial, may also present insurmountable difficulties for treatment with this modality. Patients with schizophrenia may do well in highly directive, structured groups with emphasis on reality testing and improving interpersonal coping skills. Group therapy can be used as an effective adjunct to either individual psychotherapy or psychotropic medications. Inpatient group psychotherapy is a very common treatment modality and differs from outpatient treatment because of the heterogeneity of the group and its frequent change in membership. Group psychotherapy may be particularly helpful with adolescents, who are highly sensitive to peer group support and influence.

Groups also provide a powerful arena in which individuals with personality disorders can become increasingly aware of their interpersonal problems. A specific form of manualized group therapy, dialectical behavioral therapy (DBT), was developed by Marsha Linehan in 1993 to treat borderline personality disorder, though it has also been used in the treatment of adolescent bipolar disorder (Goldstein et al., 2007), eating disorders, and substance abuse. It has both behavioral and cognitive aspects, with the central component being the concept of "mindfulness" (see Table 23-12). DBT requires both an individual and group setting. In the individual sessions,

TABLE 23-12	Common Terms in Dialectical Behavioral Therapy
Core mindfulness	Essential skills of observation, description, and participation that the patient learns to apply to life situations
Interpersonal effectiveness	Strategies the patient learns for coping with interpersonal conflict, including assertiveness training and problem solving
Distress tolerance	Techniques the patient learns to better accept, tolerate, and survive crises May include methods of distraction, self-soothing
Emotion regulation	Skills the patient learns to manage emotions May include identifying and labeling emotions or identifying obstacles to changing emotions

the patient and therapist focus on a hierarchy of issues that arise during the week. They work on issues of safety, suicidality, or self-injury, followed by issues that may interfere with the therapy, and finally they focus on ways to improve the patient's quality of life. The group meets once weekly for approximately 2 to 2.5 hours, during which time the patient learns specific skills in each of four areas: core mindfulness, emotion regulation, interpersonal effectiveness, and distress tolerance (Lynch et al., 2007).

Family Therapy

In family therapy, psychological symptoms are considered to be the pathological expression of disturbances in the social system of the family. For this discussion, "family" can include any members, ranging from the basic couple to children, grandparents, distant relatives, and even close friends of the family, in some cases. The essential feature is the relationship among the various members and how their behavior can affect the group as a whole and the individual family members. The theoretic models may run the whole gamut of therapeutic approaches, ranging from the psychoanalytic to the behavioral (Beels, 1988).

Most family therapists agree that family groups are extremely complex and dynamic systems with a definite hierarchical structure that is a result of cultural and societal proscribed roles, repetitive behavior patterns, and ingrained ways in which the family members have interrelated. Family structure can be seen as a self-regulating system with multiple control mechanisms designed to ensure some degree of a homeostatic equilibrium. The family system seeks stability and inherently resists change. When the system is subjected to internal or external stresses, the family may respond by "designating" one of its members as the "patient," and his or her "illness" may act as a safety valve to maintain system integrity. This same resistance to change will oppose any therapeutic efforts, of course, and may take the form of refusal to explore family issues by the other members of the family, missed appointments, no apparent therapeutic progress, and so forth. Some change does occur in any family as the passage of time thrusts on the system irresistible forces such as maturation of children, illness, death, old age, and personal growth and maturity. The family system may therefore be conceived as three dimensional: highly structured, homeostatic, but slowly evolving and changing its character over long periods of time (Fiore et al., 1994).

The clinical indications for family therapy are very broad. Psychopathology in any member of a family will undoubtedly influence family dynamics and *vice versa*. The treatment of children and adolescents frequently requires family therapy to deal with the environment that may be causing or sustaining the symptoms. Research indicates the particular value of family therapy in reducing relapse and rehospitalization rates in patients with schizophrenia (Glynn et al., 2007). Practical considerations such as geographic distance, economic situation, or refusal to participate can rule out family participation. When family members are being extremely destructive to the family unit or important familial relationships, family therapy should not be instituted or should be suspended for a brief time. The treatment of childhood disorders, eating disorders, alcoholism, and substance abuse generally requires a family therapy intervention.

Each clinician brings to the field his or her own conceptual framework, clinical experience, philosophical orientation, and training background. An orthodox psychoanalyst may conceive of family therapy as the individual treatment of the symptomatic member, while a social worker specializing in this form of treatment may include any or all members of the family in the sessions and use a highly directive approach, including didactic presentations and environmental manipulation. The focus of most family therapy is on current issues and achieving discrete changes toward an identifiable goal. Developmental conflicts, communication patterns, boundary management, flexibility, familial conflict resolution techniques, and roles accepted and proscribed by the system for each member are areas of therapeutic attention. Exploration of individual, unconscious material is usually avoided. When an individual psychotherapy is stalled, the use of family (or couples) therapy can help resolve environmental and family system variables that are inhibiting further individual progress. In such cases, a course of family (or couples) therapy can frequently reestablish the momentum of an individual treatment. Family therapy can be an important adjunct to inpatient treatment to facilitate discharge and psychosocial readjustment.

No single technique or procedure dominates family therapy. Therapists may see one or two members of the family, or they may see the entire group. The family may be seen together by a single therapist, individually by different therapists, or together by more than one therapist, or more than one family may be seen in special forms of multifamily group therapy. Similarly, the therapeutic techniques can range from inducing change by crisis to focusing on small aspects of how the family functions to create positive changes that the system can assimilate and incorporate over varying periods of time.

Couples Therapy

Couples therapy is the treatment of dysfunctional couples. In modern society, this includes both married and unmarried "dyads" and heterosexual as well as homosexual couples. It is very similar to, and, in fact, may be described as a form of, family therapy. The same theoretic concepts and treatment approaches described earlier apply. If the couple has an extreme sadomasochistic relationship, therapy may be blocked. During times when one partner is being overly destructive to the relationship or the other partner, the therapist may need to intervene directly. If destructive behavior cannot be limited in the treatment, a brief individual therapy with each partner may sufficiently resolve the tension to allow the couples therapy to continue. The goal of treatment may be to resolve conflict and to reconstruct the dyadic relationship or to facilitate disengagement in the least painful way possible.

SEXUAL DYSFUNCTION THERAPY

The term *sexual dysfunction therapy* encompasses the entire spectrum of accepted psychotherapies from the purely behavioral techniques to the psychodynamically oriented approaches. Treatment may be restricted to a single form of therapy or may consist of a combination of approaches. The focus, however, is the resolution of a specific sexual dysfunction, such as premature ejaculation, impotence, orgasmic dysfunction, or vaginismus (Masters and Johnson, 1970). Most sex therapists emphasize focusing on symptom relief with the use of behavior modification techniques, followed by attempts at resolution of underlying conflicts (which may represent the core of the disorder) by more traditional insight-oriented dynamic methods (see Table 23-13). In general, the brief focused therapies, whether used singly or in combination with other forms, seem to have a greater success rate with specific symptom relief than do the longer-term treatments. Overall, therapeutic approaches may include aspects of individual, psychodynamic, and behavioral therapy, as well as hypnosis, group therapy, and couples therapy. (For further discussion, see Chapter 15.)

The evaluation of sexual dysfunction should include a complete investigation of possible medical causes (see Chapter 15). A considerable number of physical illnesses, injuries, and congenital malformations can result in symptoms suggestive of a psychosexual disorder and, if not addressed, will render all other therapies useless (Kaplan, 1974). Similarly, medications can result in dysfunctional symptoms, causing great distress to the patient. Selective serotonin reuptake inhibitors, commonly used to treat depression and anxiety, are often associated with sexual dysfunction in otherwise normal men and women. In some situations, simple counseling and reassurance may suffice to calm the patient. Therefore, the role of careful history taking, a complete physical examination, and indicated laboratory testing cannot be overemphasized.

TABLE 23-13	Sexual Dysfunction Therapies
Goal	Resolution of specific sexual dysfunctions
Patient selection criteria	Couples Sexual dysfunction: impotence, premature ejaculation, vaginismus, orgasmic dysfunction Rule out medical causes
Techniques	Behavior modification techniques, including systematic desensitization, homework, education Psychodynamic approaches Hypnotherapy Group therapy Couples therapy as needed to address system dynamics
Duration	Weeks to months

SUMMARY

The psychotherapies are important components of the treatment plan for nearly all psychiatric illnesses. Both short- and long-term techniques are available. Which psychotherapy is most effective for which patient and with which therapist is less clear. Psychotherapy provides the patient with new problem-solving techniques. Some patients prefer one type of problem solving or can learn one type and not another.

How the outcomes from the different psychotherapies may differ and what this may mean for long-range health or relapse warrant further research. Increasingly, data indicate the effectiveness of the psychotherapies in reducing hospitalization rates and the use of other medical resources. Studies on the use of psychotherapy as an adjunct in the treatment of various physical illnesses also tend to indicate cost benefits in overall medical care dollars. The ability to use a range of psychotherapies is important in the treatment of psychiatric illness and in obtaining maximum benefit from medical case management and from the therapeutic effectiveness of the doctor–patient relationship.

For the nonpsychiatric physician, a referral for psychiatric assessment is essential when psychotherapy may be indicated. The psychiatric consultant can evaluate the interplay of biological, psychological, and social context variables that may be causing or maintaining illness in the patient. A comprehensive treatment plan and goals can then be formulated. Before referring a patient, the physician should educate the patient. Many patients will have the belief that the general population views psychiatric illness as fake or imaginary. They should be reassured that their distress and pain are real and that there is a wide array of possible treatments. Patients are best prepared when they can understand the role of medication in providing possible relief of symptoms and the role of the psychotherapies in learning new ways to handle the problems that may be precipitating their distress. For instance, the physician refers a patient to physical therapy to learn a new way to walk when the patient has developed a limp to compensate for chronic pain. (The limp may persist even after the pain is relieved by medication.) Similarly, the psychotherapies teach, through various means, new problem-solving techniques to relieve patterns of behaviors, feelings, and thoughts that are causing or maintaining impairment.

Finally, it should be emphasized that the best form of treatment is often integrated psychotherapy and pharmacotherapy. To withhold medication from patients who have clear and serious symptoms that are treatable with pharmacology and apparently biologically "loaded" disorders (e.g., a family history) because of a bias toward one sort of psychotherapy or another is unjustifiable on clinical grounds, if not overtly unethical. Hence, integrated psychotherapeutic *and* pharmacological treatment is often indicated and should be considered for every patient, regardless of the orientation of the psychotherapist. Psychiatrists or nonpsychiatric clinicians who are polarized one way or the other may offer a narrow range of treatment and overlook either a biological or psychological therapy that might potentially be dramatically effective for the patient. In making a referral for an initial evaluation, it is recommended that one consult a clinician who has a balanced, integrated approach. The success of a referral for psychiatric evaluation or psychotherapy is *critically* dependent on the attitude, confidence, and enthusiasm of the referring physician.

Clinical Pearls

- Integrated psychotherapeutic and psychopharmacologic treatment is often indicated in psychiatric illness. The risks and benefits of each treatment should be considered in every patient regardless of the orientation of the psychiatrist.
- Psychoanalytic psychotherapy focuses on understanding as the tool of change for defense mechanisms and interpersonal conflicts. Similar to psychoanalysis but less extensive and more focused on the present, it uses the techniques of clarification, interpretation, and free association, as well as the more supportive elements of education, reality testing, and confrontation.
- In cognitive psychotherapy, the patient's thoughts are central to producing and perpetuating symptoms such as depression and anxiety.
- In supportive psychotherapy, the psychiatrist fosters the therapeutic relationship by refraining from interpreting negative transference, except if it is likely to disrupt the treatment, and only interpreting positive transference when feelings are at their lowest.
- It is important to exhibit confidence and enthusiasm when making a referral for psychiatric evaluation or psychotherapy. Patients will detect ambivalence and skepticism on the physician's part about the need for such treatment. It is usually helpful to recommend a psychiatrist or other health professional who is known personally by the physician.
- Some patients may view a psychiatric referral as meaning the clinician is "dumping" them onto another doctor and as a rejection. Reassure patients that any psychiatric treatment will occur in parallel with their ongoing medical care.
- Have the name and telephone number of a referral source readily available to give to the patient. Alternatively, make the appointment for the psychiatric evaluation while the patient is still in the office.
- As with any medical consult, call the psychiatrist to explain personally the reason and need for the referral and what role you would like to continue to play in the patient's care.
- Schedule a follow-up appointment after the date of the psychiatric evaluation to check on the patient's reaction to the referral and response to initial treatment.

Self-Assessment Questions and Answers

23-1. The central component of dialectical behavioral therapy (DBT) is:

A. Automatic thought
B. Core mindfulness
C. Negative cognitive triad
D. Therapeutic alliance
E. Transference

The four components of DBT are core mindfulness, interpersonal effectiveness, distress tolerance, and emotional regulation. The central feature is core mindfulness, in which the patient learns skills of observation and description and applies these to life experiences to help manage crises and distress. In cognitive behavioral therapy, the negative cognitive triad is the set of negative views depressed patients have about themselves, the world, and the future. It also includes the concept of automatic thoughts, which are involuntary negative distortions that

have emotional validity. In psychoanalytic or psychoanalytically informed psychotherapy, transference refers to the re-creation of the feelings in the doctor–patient relationship that the patient experienced with an important figure from the past. Finally, the therapeutic alliance refers to the many aspects of the doctor–patient relationship during the course of psychotherapy. *Answer: B*

23-2. A 19-year-old woman with a history of anxiety and a genetic predisposition to panic disorder and depression is working with a psychiatrist to address her specific phobia of elevators. She has noted extreme anxiety and panic symptoms such as increased heart rate and feelings of doom whenever she approaches an elevator. Historically, she has been able to avoid elevators, always electing to take the stairs. She has not ridden one in years. However, she recently started attending college, and her dorm room is on the 11th floor. As part of her treatment, the psychiatrist instructs her to begin creating a hierarchy of increasingly anxious imaginary scenes. She pictures herself in multiple situations: walking to the elevator door, pushing the call button, watching the numbers approach her floor, and so on. Additionally, the psychiatrist begins to teach the patient about relaxation techniques. In behavioral therapy, this is an example of:

A. Aversion therapy
B. Flooding
C. Implosion therapy
D. Progressive muscle relaxation
E. Systematic desensitization

Systematic desensitization is a behavioral technique in which the patient constructs a hierarchy of increasingly anxiety-provoking situations. They may be first experienced *in vitro* (i.e., in the psychiatrist's office). The patient is taught relaxation techniques to manage stress. Following this, the exposure may be in person on a gradual basis. The key component to success is managing anxiety at each incremental stage, which is used as a lesson to the patient that she can manage the task without adverse outcome. Flooding and implosion therapy do not include gradual introduction to the fear. Flooding occurs *in vivo*, and in implosion therapy, the exposure is through mental images of the feared object or situation. Aversion therapy is based on classical conditioning; it pairs a behavior with a noxious stimulus so as to extinguish it. An example of this would be the use of disulfiram in patients who have alcohol dependence. Finally, progressive muscle relaxation is a relaxation technique in which patients gradually tense and relax various muscle groups to provide stress relief. *Answer: E*

23-3. A 45-year-old man with a history of major depression with psychosis, childhood abuse, and a genetic predisposition to depression is being treated with a combination of pharmacotherapy and psychotherapy. He has been gradually improving and is treated with an antidepressant and an atypical antipsychotic. Today he reports that he still occasionally experiences feelings of paranoia with concerns that people are trying to hurt him or at least are watching him. He occasionally hears his name called. There are no visual hallucinations and no history of self-harm or aggression. In talking further with the patient, the psychiatrist

learns of a conflict the patient had with a friend. The psychiatrist expresses interest in hearing more about this and helps the patient vent his frustration and sadness about the fight and his worries about the loss of the relationship. The psychiatrist advises the patient to talk further with his friend about their misunderstanding. This intervention is an example of:

A. Behavioral therapy
B. Cognitive psychotherapy
C. Couples therapy
D. Psychodynamic psychotherapy
E. Supportive psychotherapy

Supportive psychotherapy aims to help patients maintain or reestablish the best level of functioning, given the limitations of their illness, personality, native ability, and life circumstances. *Answer: E*

23-4. Two weeks later, the patient returns with no further auditory hallucinations, a better mood, good sleep, and increased energy. The psychiatrist notes ongoing mild paranoia now related to his work colleagues and instructs the patient to begin keeping a thought record describing the thoughts and feelings he experiences at work. He is told to rate the believability of the delusion that his colleagues are trying to get him in trouble with the boss. This intervention is an example of:

A. Behavioral therapy
B. Cognitive psychotherapy
C. Couples therapy
D. Psychodynamic psychotherapy
E. Supportive psychotherapy

Cognitive psychotherapy is based on the theoretic assumption that environmental events trigger cognitive processes and that these thoughts give an event personal meaning that leads to affective arousal. *Answer: B*

23-5. The following year, during a follow-up appointment with his psychiatrist, the patient begins to ask the psychiatrist about the possibility of further understanding the difficulty he has in keeping friendships and maintaining work colleagues. He has had a complete resolution of his psychotic symptoms, and his depression has been in full remission for 10 months. The psychiatrist wonders with the patient about his difficulty in trusting others and notes his history of abuse as a child. The patient has been in a stable marriage, has stable employment, and has had a good working relationship with his psychiatrist.

The type of psychotherapy that seems most indicated at this time is:

A. Behavioral therapy
B. Cognitive psychotherapy
C. Couples therapy
D. Psychodynamic psychotherapy
E. Supportive psychotherapy

The patient has been stable from a psychiatric perspective for some time. He has the ability to establish and maintain relationships despite his concerns about his ability to trust others. He has notable anxiety and dysphoria when he struggles to understand the motivations and actions of others as they relate to him. His early experience of unpredictable and often dangerous behavior (abuse) may have affected his ability to experience trust. Further exploration of the impact of these childhood experiences on his current presentation is warranted through psychodynamic psychotherapy.
Answer: D

References

Alexander F. The principle of corrective emotional experience. In: Alexander F, French TM, Bacon CL, et al., eds. *Psychoanalytic therapy: Principles and application*. New York: Ronald Press; 1946:66–70.

Andrasik F. What does the evidence show? Efficacy of behavioral treatments for recurrent headaches in adults. *Neurol Sci*. 2007;28(Suppl 2):S70–S77.

Bandelow B, Seidler-Brandler U, Becker A, et al. Meta-analysis of randomized controlled comparisons of psychopharmacological and psychological treatments for anxiety disorders. *World J Biol Psychiatry*. 2007;8(3):175–187.

Beck AT. *Cognitive theory and the emotional disorders*. New York: International Universities Press; 1976.

Beels CC. Family therapy. In: Talbott JA, Hales RE, Yudofsky SC, eds. *Textbook of psychiatry*. Washington, DC: American Psychiatric Press; 1988:929–930.

Bion WR. *Experiences in groups*. New York: Basic Books; 1961.

Bruch H. *Learning psychotherapy*. Cambridge: Harvard University Press; 1974.

Ciesla JA, Roberts JE. Rumination, negative cognition, and their interactive effects on depressed mood. *Emotion*. 2007;7(3):555–565.

Crits-Christoph P. The efficacy of brief-dynamic psychotherapy: A meta-analysis. *Am J Psychiatry*. 1992; 149:151–158.

Davanloo H. *Short-term dynamic psychotherapy*. New York: Jason Aronson Press; 1980.

Fiore J, Stoudemire A, Kriseman N. The family in human development and medical practice. In: Stoudemire A, ed. *Human behavior: An introduction for medical students*, 2nd ed. Philadelphia: JB Lippincott Co; 1994.

Gaarder K, Montgomery P. *Clinical biofeedback*. Baltimore: Williams & Wilkins; 1977.

Glick RA, Roose AP. Talking about medication. *J Am Psychoanal Assoc*. 2006;54(3):745–762.

Glynn SM, Cohen AN, Niv N. New challenges in family interventions in schizophrenia. *Expert Rev Neurother*. 2007;7(1):33–43.

Goldstein TR, Axelson DA, Birmaher B, et al. Dialectical behavior therapy for adolescents with bipolar disorder: A 1-year open trial. *J Am Acad Child Adolesc Psychiatry*. 2007;46(7):820–830.

Gossop M, Stewart D, Marsden J. Attendance at Narcotics Anonymous and Alcoholics Anonymous meetings, frequency of attendance, and substance use outcomes after residential treatment for drug dependence: A 5-year follow-up study. *Addiction*. 2008;103(1):119–125.

Hajek P, Stead LF. Aversive smoking for smoking cessation. *Cochrane Database Syst Rev*. 2004;(3): CD000546.

Heinrich H, Gevensleben H, Strehl U. Annotation: Neurofeedback—train your brain to train behaviour. *J Child Psychol Psychiatry*. 2007;48(1):3–16.

Kaplan HS. *The new sex therapy*. New York: Brunner/Mazel; 1974.

Karavidas MK, Tsai PS, Yucha C, et al. Thermal biofeedback for primary Raynaud's phenomenon: A review of the literature. *Appl Psychophysiol Biofeedback*. 2006;31(3):203–216.

Klerman GL, Weissman MM, Rounsaville BJ, et al. *Interpersonal Psychotherapy of Depression*. New York: Basic Books; 1984.

Lazar S. Epidemiology of mental illness in the United States: An overview of cost effectiveness of psychotherapy. *Psychoanal Inq*. 1998;(Suppl):4–16.

Lazarus A. *Behavior therapy and beyond*. New York: McGraw-Hill; 1971.

Lebovitz PS. Integrating psychoanalysis and psychopharmacology: A review of the literature of combined treatment for affective disorders. *J Am Acad Psychoanal Dyn Psychiatry*. 2004;32(4):585–596.

Leichsenring F. Are psychodynamic and psychoanalytic therapies effective? A review of empirical data. *Int J Psychoanal*. 2005;86(Pt 3):841–868.

Leichsenring F, Leibing E. Psychodynamic psychotherapy: A systematic review of techniques, indications and empirical evidence. *Psychol Psychother*. 2007;80(Pt 2):217–228.

Leichsenring F, Rabung S, Leibing E. The efficacy of short-term psychodynamic psychotherapy in specific psychiatric disorders: A meta-analysis. *Arch Gen Psychiatry*. 2004;61(12):1208–1216.

Linden W, Mosley JV. The efficacy of biofeedback for hypertension. *Appl Psychophysiol Biofeedback*. 2006;31(1):51–63.

Lynch TR, Trost WT, Salsman N, et al. Dialectical behavioral therapy for borderline personality disorder. *Annu Rev Clin Psychol*. 2007;3:181–205.

Luborsky L, Crits-Christoph P. *Understanding transference*. New York: Basic Books; 1990.

de Maat S, Dekker J, Schoevers R, et al. Short psychodynamic supportive psychotherapy, antidepressants, and their combination in the treatment of major depression: A mega-analysis based on three randomized clinical trials. *Depress Anxiety*. 2008;25(7):565–574.

Malan DH. *A study of brief psychotherapy*. New York: Plenum Press; 1975.

Mann J. *Time-limited psychotherapy*. Cambridge: Harvard University Press; 1973.

Mann K. Pharmacotherapy of alcohol dependence: A review of the clinical data. *CNS Drugs*. 2004;18(8):485–504.

Masters WH, Johnson VE. *Human sexual inadequacy*. Boston: Little, Brown and Company; 1970.

Nestoriuc Y, Martin A. Efficacy of biofeedback for migraine: A meta-analysis. *Pain*. 2007;128(1-2):111–127.

Pine F. Supportive psychotherapy: A psychoanalytic perspective. *Psychiatr Ann*. 1986;16:524–534.

Racker H. *Transference and countertransference*. New York: International Universities Press; 1968.

Reichmann FF. *Principles of intensive psychotherapy*. Chicago: University of Chicago Press; 1950.

Rockland LH. *Supportive therapy: A psychodynamic approach*. New York: Basic Books; 1989.

Rush AJ, Beck AT. Cognitive therapy. In: Frances A, Hales RE, eds. *American psychiatric press review of psychiatry*. Washington, DC: American Psychiatric Press; 1988:533–670.

Sandler J, Dare C, Holder A. *The patient and the analyst*. New York: International Universities Press; 1973.

Sifneos PE. *Short-term psychotherapy and emotional crisis*. Cambridge: Harvard University Press; 1972.

Trautmann E, Lackschewitz H, Kroner-Herwig B. *Cephalalgia*. 2006;26(12):1411–1426.

Turkington D, Sensky T, Scott J, et al. A randomized controlled trial of cognitive-behavior therapy for persistent symptoms in schizophrenia: A five-year follow-up. *Schizophr Res*. 2008;98(1-3):1–7.

Weissman MM. Recent non-medication trials of interpersonal psychotherapy for depression. *Int J Neuropsychopharmacol*. 2007;10(1):117–122.

Werman DS. *The practice of supportive psychotherapy*. New York: Brunner/Mazel; 1984.

Yalom I. Group psychotherapy. In: Frances A, Hales RE, eds. *American psychiatric press review of psychiatry*. Washington, DC: American Psychiatric Press; 1986:655–764.

Somatic Therapies

For many patients with psychiatric illness, medications and/or psychotherapy can be effective in reducing symptom load and improving overall function. However, a substantial minority of patients may receive inadequate benefit from these therapies. For example, up to 72% of patients with major depression may fail to achieve remission (i.e., complete resolution of symptoms), and >50% may not achieve an adequate antidepressant response (i.e., at least a 50% reduction in symptoms) following first-line therapy with a selective serotonin reuptake inhibitor (Trivedi et al., 2006). Importantly, subsequent therapeutic attempts are even less effective for patients who do not achieve remission with first-line treatment (Fava et al., 2006; Nierenberg et al., 2006; Rush et al., 2006; Trivedi et al., 2006), with only 6% to 14% of patients remitting after three prior treatment failures (McGrath et al., 2006). For those patients who have an acute response to treatment, relapse is unfortunately common in depression and many other psychiatric illnesses. Therefore, despite a number of available treatment strategies, many psychiatric patients remain significantly symptomatic.

When medications and psychotherapy fail to achieve a clinically sufficient response in psychiatric patients, more invasive somatic treatments may be considered. The nonpharmacologic somatic therapies currently in use or under investigation for the treatment of psychiatric illness include electroconvulsive therapy (ECT), vagus nerve stimulation (VNS), ablative neurosurgery, transcranial magnetic stimulation (TMS), magnetic seizure therapy (MST), and deep brain stimulation (DBS). ECT has a long-standing and well-established role in the treatment of mood disorders. VNS and TMS are approved by the U.S. Food and Drug Administration (FDA) for the treatment of medication-refractory depression. For the most treatment-refractory patients, focal ablative neurosurgical intervention is sometimes considered. MST and DBS are brain stimulation therapies currently under active investigation but not yet approved by the FDA for the treatment of any psychiatric illness.

At first glance, the risks associated with these interventions (especially ablative neurosurgery and DBS) may seem excessive. However, it is critical to recognize that untreated or undertreated psychiatric illness is often significantly disabling—no less so than treatment-resistant epilepsy, Parkinson disease, back pain, or a number of other conditions for which surgical and other invasive procedures are frequently considered.

In this chapter, these various somatic therapies will be reviewed in detail. After a brief history and description of each approach, the data supporting safety and efficacy will be reviewed. As appropriate, the role of each treatment in current clinical practice will be described, and the putative mechanism of action will be discussed. It is important to note that only ECT, VNS, and specific ablative procedures are currently used in clinical practice; TMS should become available for clinical use within the next several months. MST and DBS are currently only available in clinical trials.

ELECTROCONVULSIVE THERAPY

Background

ECT was developed in the mid-1930s when there were essentially no somatic treatments available for severely ill psychiatric patients (the clinical introduction of lithium—the first major psychotropic—occurred in 1949). In the 1950s, ECT was used to treat approximately one third of hospitalized psychiatric patients. In general, the use of ECT has decreased over the last several decades as more medications have become available to treat psychiatric illness (Eranti and McLoughlin, 2003). The introduction of anesthesia and the optimization of stimulation parameters have greatly improved the safety and tolerability of ECT, and it remains an important treatment option for patients with severe, treatment-refractory psychiatric illness.

Since its introduction, the basic approach to ECT has not changed: direct electrical current is delivered through scalp electrodes to cause a generalized seizure. Typical stimulation parameters include 0.5 to 8 seconds of stimulation given with a 0.3 to 2.0 millisecond pulse width at 20 to 130 Hz and a current of 500 to 800 milliamperes (mA). The induced seizure typically lasts 30 to 60 seconds, and recovery from the postictal state generally occurs within 15 to 45 minutes. With modern ECT, the patient is placed under general anesthesia (with sedation and paralysis) before treatment to prevent physical consequences from the seizure (i.e., the goal is to have no or very limited motor activity during the seizure).

Several different electrode placements have been evaluated and used clinically. The most common placements include (a) bitemporal (BT), with one electrode over each temporal lobe; (b) unilateral (typically, right unilateral [RUL]), with one electrode over the temporal lobe and one electrode over the parietal lobe of the same hemisphere; and (c) bifrontal (BF), with one electrode placed over the prefrontal cortex of each hemisphere (see Fig. 24-1).

Other electrode placements are less common but still used by some practitioners (such as asymmetric frontotemporal placement, with one electrode over the right temporal lobe and one electrode over the left prefrontal cortex). Each of these electrode placements is generally considered safe and effective, though some variability in acute efficacy and side effects may exist. Typically, ECT treatments are given two to three times per week, and most patients receive between 6 and 12 acute treatments.

Indications and Efficacy

Depression

The most common indication for ECT is major depression. ECT is generally considered one of the most effective acute treatments for a major depressive episode (MDE) with rates of antidepressant response (i.e., a reduction in depression severity of at least 50%) approaching 80% to 90% (Petrides et al., 2001; The UK ECT Review Group, 2003). The antidepressant efficacy of ECT has been confirmed in several controlled trials (Kho et al., 2003; Pagnin et al., 2004). Although treatment resistance (i.e., inadequate response to adequate antidepressant treatment with medications and psychotherapy) is not required for a referral to ECT, most patients who present for an ECT evaluation in fact are considered to have treatment-resistant depression (TRD). The efficacy of ECT may be somewhat lower in patients with TRD (Prudic et al., 1996). ECT appears to be effective in treating depression due to either major depressive disorder (unipolar depression) or bipolar disorder (bipolar depression), though far fewer patients with

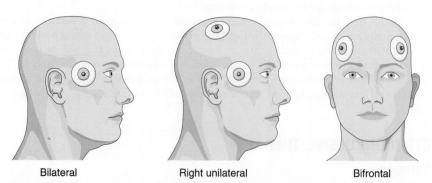

| Bilateral | Right unilateral | Bifrontal |

FIGURE 24-1. Commonly used electroconvulsive therapy (ECT) electrode placements (bitemporal, right unilateral, bifrontal). (Reprinted with permission from *New England Journal of Medicine*.)

bipolar depression have been included in ECT studies (Zornberg and Pope, 1993). Controlled studies suggest that high-dose RUL ECT is as efficacious as BT ECT and associated with fewer cognitive side effects (Sackeim et al., 2000; McCall et al., 2002; Tew et al., 2002).

Despite its demonstrated acute efficacy for treating depression, ECT is unfortunately associated with a high relapse rate following cessation of treatment, with approximately 50% of responders experiencing a return or worsening of depression within 6 months (Sackeim et al., 2001; Kellner et al., 2006). Optimized medication management following a successful course of ECT may decrease the relapse rate (Sackeim et al., 2001). Continuation ECT and maintenance ECT are two additional strategies for attempting to limit relapse following ECT. With continuation ECT, treatments are given at an increasing interval over time for 6 months following the acute course (e.g., on a schedule of once a week for four treatments, once every 10 days for four treatments, once every 2 weeks for four treatments). Maintenance ECT continues to provide treatments on a regular basis following a course of continuation ECT. The data supporting the efficacy of continuation ECT are limited: one large randomized, controlled study showed no difference between continuation ECT and medications in 6-month relapse rates (Kellner et al., 2006). The data supporting the efficacy of maintenance ECT are even more limited.

It is not completely clear which factors predict a good response to ECT. Clinical factors that appear to predict a better response to ECT include older age (O'Connor et al., 2001; Dombrovski et al., 2005) and psychotic and/or catatonic features (Petrides et al., 2001; Birkenhager et al., 2005). Clinical predictors of a poor response to ECT include chronic depression (Prudic et al., 1996; Dombrovski et al., 2005), treatment resistance (Devanand et al., 1991; Prudic et al., 1996), and personality disorder, especially borderline personality disorder (Feske et al., 2004). Patients with chronic and/or TRD may also be more likely to relapse following a successful course of ECT. Finally, ECT may be less effective in patients with comorbid disorders (such as severe anxiety disorders), substance abuse/dependence, and/or medical conditions.

Other Conditions

Beyond depression, a growing database supports the efficacy and safety of ECT for mania and catatonia (Fink, 2001). A more limited database supports at least transient efficacy for neuroleptic malignant syndrome (NMS), Parkinson disease (usually with only transient benefit), and Tourette

---

A CASE OF ECT FOR A PATIENT WITH TRD

Mrs. A is a 48-year-old woman with recurrent major depressive disorder. She has had two previous depressive episodes (at ages 22 and 35), each remitted with a combination of fluoxetine 20 to 40 mg per day and psychotherapy. Following her mother's death a year ago, Mrs. A developed a severe major depressive episode with depressed mood, profound anhedonia, insomnia, reduced appetite with a 20-lb weight loss (baseline weight was 145 lb), psychomotor agitation, impaired concentration, and increasing suicidal ideation (SI) with plan to overdose (but no current intent). Her Beck Depression Inventory (BDI) score is 36.

In this episode, she has unsuccessfully tried three different antidepressant medications (one selective serotonin reuptake inhibitor [SSRI], one serotonin-norepinephrine reuptake inhibitor [SNRI], and buproprion) at potentially therapeutic doses for at least 6 weeks each and several augmentation strategies. Her psychiatrist is very concerned about her lack of response and worsening SI; he refers her for an ECT evaluation.

After a careful psychiatric and medical evaluation, Mrs. A is found to be otherwise healthy, and a course of outpatient ECT is recommended. Right unilateral ECT given three times per week is initiated. After three treatments, she reports diminished SI and increased interest; her husband notes she is eating better and has gained 3 lb. She continues to have depressed mood and reports noticeable anterograde amnesia. Treatment frequency is reduced to twice per week. After eight treatments, she reports feeling "normal again." Her BDI is 9, and she denies adverse cognitive effects (her Mini-Mental Status Examination score is 30). ECT is discontinued.

syndrome (Fink, 2001; Fregni et al., 2005; Karadenizli et al., 2005). ECT does not appear to be particularly effective for chronic schizophrenia but may be beneficial for acute exacerbations (Tharyan and Adams, 2005).

Special Populations
Older adults

As discussed in the preceding text, older age is a good prognostic factor for response to ECT. However, the cognitive side effects of ECT may be more pronounced in older adults (Sackeim et al., 2007), with age-related comorbidities such as mild cognitive impairment, dementia, or cerebrovascular disease further increasing the risk (Flint and Gagnon, 2002). Therefore, ECT should be considered a viable treatment strategy for older adults with treatment-resistant mood disorders; however, careful attention should be paid to limiting cognitive side effects (e.g., by using unilateral lead placement) and carefully monitoring patients during the treatment course.

Pregnancy

In the past, ECT was considered an early treatment option for pregnant women with depression: the relative safety and efficacy of ECT were considered quite favorable compared to the potential adverse effects of available medications. As antidepressant medications with apparently better safety profiles have become available, the use of ECT in pregnancy is less common; however, it remains an important treatment option for women with treatment-resistant mood disorders, especially bipolar disorder (where typical mood stabilizers such as lithium and valproic acid have been associated with teratogenesis).

Children

The data on ECT in children and adolescents are very limited. Several case reports appear to support the safety and potential efficacy of ECT for severely depressed children who are nonresponsive to other available therapies (Ghaziuddin et al., 1996; Segal et al., 2004), though no prospective data are available. Patients younger than 18 years of age are rarely referred for ECT.

Risks and Side Effects

The most notable side effect of ECT is cognitive impairment. Nearly every patient has some degree of transient postictal confusion, which can be severe in some patients; rarely, ECT may be associated with postictal delirium. ECT is associated with minor and transient anterograde amnesia in almost all patients (e.g., patients may have difficulty remembering details of events between ECT treatments). Retrograde amnesia (especially for autobiographical information) can also occur. This is typically minor but may be severe in a minority of patients (Sackeim et al., 2007); however, long-term retrograde amnesia is rare. Older age and lower premorbid intellectual functioning are associated with greater risk of retrograde amnesia. Additionally, lead placement may predict cognitive disturbance, with BT ECT associated with greater cognitive impairment than RUL or BF ECT (Sackeim et al., 2000; Bakewell et al., 2004).

In addition to cognitive impairment, ECT may be associated with other minor and some potentially major complications. Common minor side effects include headache, nausea, and muscle aches—if present, these can usually be managed with pre- or posttreatment interventions (such as ketorolac for headache or ondasentron for nausea). Severe and clinically significant postictal confusion may be minimized by giving a short-acting benzodiazepine (such as midazolam) immediately after the treatment or an injectable antipsychotic (such as intramuscular olanzapine or ziprasidone) before the treatment. More serious complications of ECT include those associated with increased cardiac demand and intracranial pressure: arrhythmias, myocardial infarction, and stroke. Patients with known intracranial lesions (such as a brain tumor) are at increased risk of herniation due to intracranial pressure associated with ECT. Careful screening and perioperative management can significantly reduce the risk of these events. Patients with compromised pulmonary function may have difficulty tolerating and recovering from the general anesthesia used during treatments. Patients with pseudocholinesterase deficiency may have a prolonged recovery from succinylcholine (the agent used most often for paralysis); for patients with significant pseudocholinesterase deficiency, a different paralytic (such as rocuronium) might be used. Contrary to perception among the lay public, ECT is not associated with brain damage.

Despite potential side effects, it is critical to recognize that the vast majority of patients tolerate ECT very well. In a study assessing patients' views on the benefits of and possible memory loss from ECT, >80% of patients were satisfied and would be willing to have ECT again if recommended (Rose et al., 2003). Additionally, untreated depression itself is a disabling and potentially lethal illness; therefore, the risks of not treating a depressed patient (including risk of death) may be greater than the risks associated with ECT (Avery and Winokur, 1976; Avery and Winokur, 1978; Wulsin et al., 1999; Cuijpers and Smit, 2002).

Clinical Use

Currently, ECT is an important treatment option to consider for depressed patients who have not responded to other conventional therapies. Beyond depression, patients with severe, treatment-resistant mania or catatonia may be appropriate for ECT. ECT may also be an option for patients with other treatment-refractory psychiatric illnesses, but the risks and potential benefits must be carefully considered, given the limited database.

If a patient is deemed appropriate for ECT, a careful workup must be performed to rule out other treatable causes of depression and/or treatment resistance and assess the safety of ECT in a particular patient. Evaluation should include a careful psychiatric examination, physical examination (including a detailed neurologic examination), complete medical and surgical history, and a review of current mental and physical symptoms. Cognitive status should be carefully evaluated before a course of ECT and before each treatment. Laboratory workup should include a complete blood count, electrolytes, and renal function testing in all patients; thyroid function should also be checked (if not tested within the past 6 to 12 months); other laboratory workups may be needed for specific patients (e.g., B_{12} level for an older patient with new-onset depression and cognitive impairment). For patients with no history of cardiac disease, an electrocardiogram (ECG) is usually sufficient to rule out cardiac abnormalities that may increase the risk of ECT. Similarly, for patients with no history of neurologic disease (especially stroke, seizure disorder, traumatic brain injury, multiple sclerosis, or neoplasm), a computed tomography scan or magnetic resonance imaging of the head without contrast is usually sufficient to rule out major central nervous system (CNS) abnormalities that may increase the risk of ECT.

In general, patients should remain on psychotropic medications during a course of ECT. Exceptions may include lithium (which may increase the cognitive impairment associated with ECT) and benzodiazepines/anticonvulsants (which may limit the ability to achieve a therapeutic seizure, though flumazenil may be given to a patient on benzodiazepines to temporarily reverse the anticonvulsant effects of these agents). The majority of patients presenting for ECT have shown an incomplete response to current medications. Therefore, a careful evaluation should be performed to identify potential medication strategies that may increase maintenance of response following ECT treatment. Although the data supporting continuation and maintenance ECT are limited, a subset of patients may benefit from these approaches; therefore, for a patient with a good response to ECT but rapid relapse (despite optimal medication and psychotherapeutic management), continuation and maintenance ECT should be considered.

Mechanism of Action

Despite its clear efficacy for depression and other psychiatric diseases, the mechanism of action of ECT remains obscure. Data from human and animal studies have shown that ECT has effects on monoaminergic systems (including serotonin, norepinephrine, and dopamine), reduces corticotropin releasing factor (CRF) hypersecretion (which has been associated with depression), and modulates a number of other neurotrophic factors potentially involved in the pathophysiology of depression (Nemeroff et al., 1991; Wahlund and von Rosen, 2003). Similar to other antidepressant treatments, ECT increases hippocampal neurogenesis (Perera et al., 2007). It may be that ECT acts through mechanisms related to its anticonvulsant activity. ECT is clearly anticonvulsant (with an almost ubiquitous increase in the seizure threshold over the course of treatment), and certain anticonvulsant medications have established beneficial effects for mood disorders. The anticonvulsant properties of ECT are likely mediated through modulation of γ-aminobutyric acid (GABA) neurotransmission.

VAGUS NERVE STIMULATION
Background

VNS is currently approved by the FDA for adjunctive treatment of medication-refractory epilepsy and medication-resistant depression. To achieve VNS, surgery is performed to attach a stimulating electrode to the patient's left vagus nerve (cranial nerve X), which is then connected to a programmable pulse generator implanted subcutaneously in the patient's chest (see Fig. 24-2).

The stimulator can then be programmed to deliver electrical pulses to the vagus nerve at various frequencies and currents. The best-studied stimulation parameters are 0.25 mA, 20 to 30 Hz, 250 to 500 μs pulse width, and an on/off cycle of 30 seconds every 3 to 5 minutes. Other stimulation parameter combinations are possible; however, the relative safety and efficacy of different parameter combinations have not been studied in detail.

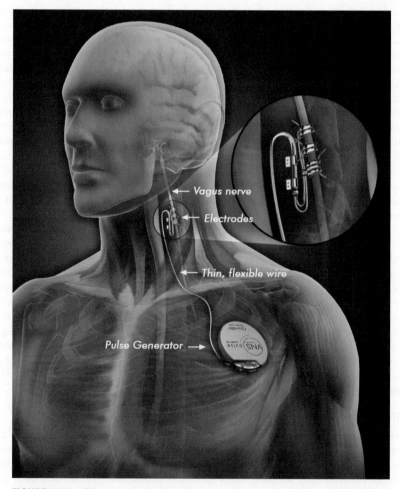

FIGURE 24-2. Diagram of an implanted vagus nerve stimulation (VNS) system. A stimulating lead is attached to the left vagus nerve (inset) and connected to a programmable pulse generator/battery pack that is implanted in the subcutaneous tissue of the patient's chest wall. (Courtesy of Cyberonics, Inc.)

Indications and Efficacy

VNS was originally tested as a treatment for epilepsy that had not fully responded to anticonvulsant medications (Ben-Menachem, 2002). Two small studies in epilepsy patients suggested that VNS was associated with mood improvements in some patients (Elger et al., 2000; Harden, 2002). When evaluated in an open-label study in medication-refractory depressed patients, VNS was associated with potentially clinically meaningful antidepressant effects at 3 months (Sackeim et al., 2001), which were more pronounced at 1 year (Marangell et al., 2002).

On the basis of these data, VNS was tested in a large placebo-controlled study of patients with TRD. In this study, all patients received VNS surgery, but the device was turned on in only half of the participants for the first 3 months; after the first 3 months, the device was turned on in all participants and other changes in treatment were allowed, including changing or adding medications, adding psychotherapy, or referring for ECT. The acute 3-month study did not find a statistically significant antidepressant benefit for VNS (Rush et al., 2005). After 1 year of open treatment with VNS combined with treatment-as-usual (i.e., standard treatment, including medications, psychotherapy, and ECT), approximately 27% of patients with TRD showed an antidepressant response, with approximately 16% of patients in remission (i.e., absence of depressive symptoms) (Rush et al., 2005). These antidepressant effects were shown to be greater than the 13% response and 7% remission rates in a cohort of patients with TRD receiving treatment-as-usual alone (without ever having had VNS surgery)—however, the groups were not randomized, and no placebo control was included in this comparison. It appears that approximately 50% to 75% of patients who respond to VNS by 3 or 12 months maintain this improvement over the ensuing 1 to 2 years (Nahas et al., 2005; Sackeim et al., 2007), compared to a much lower percentage of patients (~38%) maintaining response with treatment-as-usual alone (Dunner et al., 2006).

Risks and Side Effects

VNS surgery is a relatively minor procedure. Once a VNS system has been implanted, the battery in the pulse generator may need to be replaced every few years. The most common side effect of surgery is incisional pain; other surgical complications (such as infection and autonomic effects) are rare. The most common side effects of chronic VNS include voice changes, hoarseness, and coughing typically occurring during the 30-second "on" period of stimulation. Clinical studies have shown VNS to be well tolerated in 80% to 90% of patients.

Clinical Use

The FDA conditionally approved VNS for the adjunctive treatment of TRD in 2005. However, based on a separate review of the evidence, the Centers for Medicare and Medicaid Services (CMS) determined in 2007 that VNS was not "a reasonable and necessary" treatment for TRD; therefore, Medicare and Medicaid claims to cover VNS for TRD would not be paid. Several other third-party payors have also refused to reimburse for VNS for TRD. These decisions have limited the availability of VNS for patients with TRD, and few patients with TRD are currently referred for VNS surgery.

Mechanism of Action

The mechanism of action of VNS is not fully known. The central afferent projections of the vagus nerve, through the nucleus tractus solitarius, include brain regions previously implicated in mood regulation, and functional brain imaging studies have confirmed that VNS alters activity of many of these regions (Chae et al., 2003). VNS may affect GABA function (Ben-Menachem et al., 1995; Marrosu et al., 2003), possibly explaining its ability to reduce seizure frequency. As with ECT, antidepressant effects of VNS may be related to its anticonvulsant properties. VNS also has effects on dopamine (Carpenter et al., 2004), serotonin (Dorr and Debonnel, 2006), and norepinephrine (Lechner et al., 1997; Krahl et al., 1998; Hassert et al., 2004; Groves et al., 2005) systems. Neuroimaging studies (primarily using positron emission tomography) have shown that VNS is associated with activity changes in brain regions known to be involved in mood regulation and depression (Chae et al., 2003; Zobel et al., 2005; Conway et al., 2006).

ABLATIVE NEUROSURGERY

Background

By the late 19th century, animal experiments and observations of humans after brain injury suggested that the frontal lobes of the brain were involved in emotion and behavior. On the basis of this, surgeons in the late 19th and early 20th centuries attempted various frontal lobe surgeries to treat patients with severe and disabling mental illness. It is important to recognize that at this time, there were essentially no useful treatments for patients with severe psychiatric disease, many of whom exhibited dangerous behaviors and required constant restraint for their own safety and the safety of others.

In 1936, Egas Moniz, a Portuguese neurologist, expanded on early efforts to surgically treat psychiatric patients. With the help of neurosurgeon Almeida Lima, he developed prefrontal leucotomy, the goal of which was to sever the white matter connections between the ventral prefrontal cortex and the thalamus. He reported that 14 of 20 patients exhibited significant improvement following the procedure (Moniz, 1937). Moniz won the Nobel Prize in Medicine and Physiology in 1949.

In the 1940s and 1950s, neurologist Walter Freeman and neurosurgeon James Watts helped popularize prefrontal leucotomy (also called *prefrontal lobotomy*) in the United States. Between the 1950s and 1970s, prefrontal lobotomy was commonly recommended for and performed in treatment-resistant psychiatric patients, and modifications of the procedure that attempted to preserve the clinical benefit and limit side effects were reported. However, because of increasing criticism of the widespread and often indiscriminate use of these procedures in psychiatric patients, and the advent of new classes of medications that could be used to treat severe psychiatric illness (such as chlorpromazine in 1954), neurosurgery for mental illness declined over the last three to four decades of the 20th century.

Despite this decline, neurosurgery continues to be offered in certain specialty centers for those patients who are the most severely ill and most resistant to available treatments (Cosgrove, 2000). The procedures most commonly performed include anterior cingulotomy (a lesion is made in the dorsal anterior cingulate), anterior capsulotomy (a lesion is made in the ventral portion of the anterior limb of the internal capsule), subcaudate tractotomy (a lesion is made in the white tracts ventral to the caudate nucleus), and limbic leucotomy (which combines anterior cingulotomy with subcaudate tractotomy) (see Fig. 24-3).

Indications and Efficacy

The primary indications for neurosurgical procedures in psychiatry are treatment-resistant mood disorders (including depression and bipolar disorder) and anxiety disorders, especially obsessive-compulsive disorder (OCD). Early reports suggested an efficacy up to 70% in patients receiving

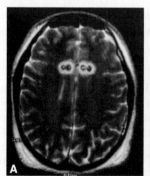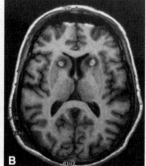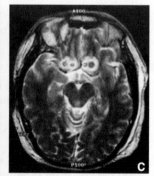

FIGURE 24-3. Postoperative magnetic resonance imaging (MRI) of three ablative neurosurgical procedures currently available: **A:** anterior cingulotomy; **B:** anterior capsulotomy; **C:** subcaudate tractotomy. A limbic leucotomy is achieved by combining an anterior cingulotomy **(A)** with a subcaudate tractotomy **(C)**. (Courtesy of G. Rees Cosgrove, MD, Massachusetts General Hospital, Boston.)

A CASE OF ABLATIVE NEUROSURGERY TO TREAT OCD

Mr. B is a 27-year-old man with a history of obsessive-compulsive disorder (OCD) with predominant cleanliness, order, and symmetry obsessions/compulsions. He was diagnosed at age 15 after being consistently late for school due to complex morning rituals (e.g., his shower would take at least 45 minutes, and he would need to dress and redress at least seven times). For several years, he had reasonable symptom control with fluvoxamine 300 to 400 mg per day but maintained only limited part-time employment as a stocker at a local convenience store. Over the last 5 years, his symptoms have increased in severity and complexity such that he is now homebound and currently weighs 120 lb (height is 5 ft 8 in.). He has tried multiple medications and augmentation strategies, including every SSRI, several atypical antipsychotics, pimozide, buspirone, anticonvulsants, and benzodiazepines. He has been unable to participate in minimal cognitive behavioral therapy. His Yale-Brown Obsessive Compulsive Scale (Y-BOCS) score is 36.

Because of the chronicity and severity of his illness, Mr. B is referred for ablative neurosurgery. After a careful psychiatric, neuropsychological, and medical examination, he is deemed an appropriate candidate. Bilateral anterior capsulotomy is performed without adverse effects. By 6 months after surgery, he notes a significant decrease in symptom severity. His Y-BOCS score is 22 (39% decrease from baseline). He is not yet able to work but can now leave his house to complete various errands. He rates himself as "much improved."

prefrontal leucotomy. Open-label studies of the surgical procedures performed currently show significant improvement in 35% to 65% of patients; placebo-controlled trials have not been reported for any of the currently used procedures.

Risks and Side Effects

Potential adverse events of ablative surgery for psychiatric conditions include confusion, seizures, apathy, behavioral disinhibition, cognitive dysfunction, personality change, and stroke (due to intracranial hemorrhage) (Greenberg et al., 2003). Prefrontal leucotomy was commonly associated with significant adverse events, likely due to the often large extent of the lesion. Adverse events appear less frequent with the procedures currently available, though accurate rates are difficult to determine due to inadequate and incomplete reporting. Because ablation is the goal of these procedures, adverse effects are generally irreversible if they occur.

Clinical Use

Ablative neurosurgery for psychiatric illness is available at several centers throughout the United States and other countries. Because these procedures use devices and techniques already clinically available, FDA approval is not specifically required. However, most insurance companies will not reimburse for these procedures such that practical availability is limited.

Mechanism of Action

Ablative neurosurgical procedures are thought to work by altering function within the neural networks involved in the regulation of mood, thought, and behavior. Generally, this is achieved by disrupting the white matter tracts connecting brain regions in these networks.

TRANSCRANIAL MAGNETIC STIMULATION AND MAGNETIC SEIZURE THERAPY

Background

TMS uses an electromagnetic coil placed on the scalp to generate a rapidly changing magnetic field that then induces an electrical current in the cerebral cortex (see Fig. 24-4). This current can focally depolarize cortical neurons; for example, a TMS pulse delivered over a focal area of the motor cortex can cause a contraction in the corresponding muscle group. Because magnetic fields

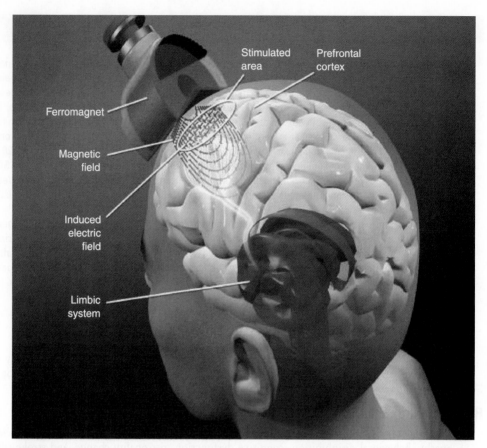

FIGURE 24-4. Schematic of how transcranial magnetic stimulation results in cortical stimulation. A ferromagnetic coil is placed against the scalp, and a rapidly changing magnetic field is generated. This magnetic field passes unimpeded through the skin and skull to reach the cortex. This rapidly changing magnetic field induces an associated electrical field that can depolarize cortical neurons. Although stimulation is limited to cortical structures, "downstream" effects in other brain regions (such as limbic structures) may be involved in behavioral effects. (Courtesy of Neuronetics, Inc.)

do not experience any resistance from the skin, skull, or membranes covering the brain, a very focal electrical current can be delivered safely and relatively painlessly, with the subject awake and without anesthesia.

Single-pulse TMS (where a discrete electrical pulse is generated in a given brain area) is an established research tool in humans (Anand and Hotson, 2002), though it is not approved for clinical use for any condition. Repetitive TMS (rTMS) is achieved by delivering multiple TMS pulses over a short period of time. rTMS has physiological effects that are quite distinct from single-pulse TMS. rTMS is currently approved by the FDA for the treatment of depression that has not responded to one or more antidepressant medications. It is also available in a number of FDA-approved research protocols for other conditions.

As with VNS, rTMS parameters can vary widely. The major variability between rTMS stimulation parameters relates to differences in frequency, intensity, and location of the stimulation. Frequency can vary from 1 Hz or less (referred to as low-frequency or slow rTMS) to 5 Hz or more (referred to as high-frequency or fast rTMS). rTMS delivered at different frequencies can have widely different biological effects; for example, high-frequency rTMS over the motor cortex has been shown to increase cortical excitability, while low-frequency rTMS has been shown to decrease motor cortical excitability (Pascual-Leone et al., 1994; Chen et al.,

1997). Treatment intensity is typically defined by reference to each patient's motor threshold (MT), the level of stimulation required to generate a motor response in one of the small hand muscles in approximately 50% of single-pulse trials. Because the intensity of the magnetic field decreases significantly with distance from its source, treatment location is generally limited to 2 to 3 cm below the coil. At this distance, which allows stimulation of most surface cortical sites, the diameter of stimulation is approximately 2 to 3 cm. During an rTMS treatment session, one to several bursts of pulses are delivered. rTMS can be provided daily for a specified number of treatment sessions.

Indications and Efficacy

rTMS has been a subject of clinical investigation for approximately 15 years, with most studies focusing on the treatment of depression. The most common parameters tested in depression are high-frequency rTMS delivered over the left dorsolateral prefrontal cortex (DLPFC) at 80% to 120% of the subject's MT. A smaller number of studies have explored the use of low-frequency rTMS delivered over the right DLPFC.

Meta-analyses of the several open and controlled studies of rTMS for depression have concluded that high-frequency rTMS applied to the left DLPFC for at least 10 sessions has statistically significant antidepressant effects (Holtzheimer et al., 2001; Burt et al., 2002; Kozel and George, 2002; Martin et al., 2002). More treatment sessions may be associated with a greater antidepressant effect (Gershon et al., 2003; Avery et al., 2006). Response rates across all rTMS studies in depression have generally been quite small (often lower than 20%) and of questionable clinical significance (Martin et al., 2002; Schlaepfer et al., 2003), though response rates are often much greater than those seen with sham rTMS. A large industry-sponsored, multisite trial recently revealed that high-frequency left DLPFC rTMS was more effective than sham rTMS in treating depression, with an 18% response rate after 4 weeks of treatment (versus a 11% response rate with sham) (O'Reardon et al., 2007). A limited but growing database supports statistically significant antidepressant effects for low-frequency rTMS applied to the right DLPFC (Klein et al., 1999; Fitzgerald et al., 2003; Rossini et al., 2005; Januel et al., 2006).

Beyond depression, rTMS may have efficacy in treating treatment-resistant auditory hallucinations in patients with chronic schizophrenia (Hoffman et al., 2000), pain (Avery et al., 2007; Passard et al., 2007), and tinnitus (Rossi et al., 2007). rTMS has not shown consistent efficacy in treating mania, OCD, or post-traumatic stress disorder.

Risks and Side Effects

rTMS appears to be generally safe and well tolerated (Martin et al., 2003; O'Reardon et al., 2007) and is associated with no negative cognitive side effects (Loo et al., 2001; Martis et al., 2003; O'Reardon et al., 2007). Common side effects with rTMS include pain with stimulation and headache. A generalized seizure may be induced with rTMS (Wassermann, 1998), though this is more common with high-frequency rTMS used beyond established safety parameters (Wassermann, 1998).

Clinical Use

The FDA recently approved an rTMS device for the treatment of depression not responding to one or more antidepressant medications. It is expected that rTMS will become more clinically available over the next several months.

Mechanism of Action

The mechanism of action for rTMS is not completely known. The rationale for rTMS for depression was initially based on imaging studies showing consistent differences in regional blood flow and metabolism in the left DLPFC between depressed patients and controls (George et al., 1995). It was hypothesized that rTMS might help normalize activity in this brain region in patients with depression. Subsequent studies have expanded on this hypothesis by suggesting that rTMS may alter activity throughout a mood regulation network (Speer et al., 2000), perhaps by modulating functional connectivity. rTMS has been shown to have antidepressant-like effects in various animal models (Muller et al., 2000; Post and Keck, 2001). rTMS applied to frontal cortical regions results in dopamine release in subcortical structures, which may be related to its therapeutic effects (Strafella et al., 2001; Keck et al., 2002; Zangen and Hyodo, 2002; Strafella et al., 2003; Kanno et al., 2004; Ohnishi et al., 2004). Other neurotransmitter systems may also be affected (Ben-Shachar et al., 1999).

Magnetic Seizure Therapy

MST uses an rTMS system to induce a generalized seizure. This is similar to ECT in that a generalized seizure is induced, but differs by using a much more focal initial stimulation. Theoretically, such focused stimulation should result in antidepressant efficacy with fewer cognitive side effects. Preliminary data support this by showing that MST (compared with ECT) has antidepressant effects with fewer cognitive side effects (Kosel et al., 2003; Lisanby et al., 2003; White et al., 2006). Although the antidepressant efficacy of MST may be less robust than that of ECT (White et al., 2006), the better cognitive side effect profile may support MST as a potential treatment option for depressed patients that may not otherwise tolerate ECT. Currently, MST is not available for clinical use.

DEEP BRAIN STIMULATION

Background

DBS allows for a specific brain region to be focally stimulated through implanted electrodes. DBS allows for direct electrical stimulation of deep cortical and/or subcortical brain regions that cannot otherwise be focally stimulated with other approaches (such as TMS or VNS). Additionally, DBS is associated with little to no tissue damage such that it is essentially reversible (i.e., the system can be removed if not effective), unlike ablative neurosurgical approaches.

Implanted DBS electrodes are connected through subcutaneous connecting wires to a pulse generator implanted in the chest wall (see Fig. 24-5). Typical stimulation parameters are 60 to

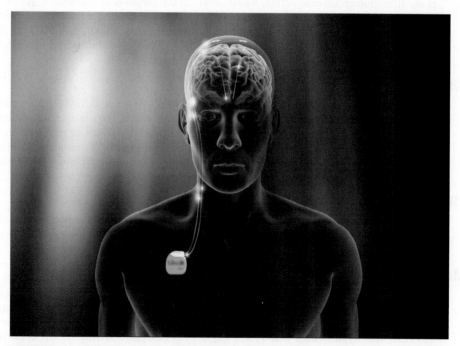

FIGURE 24-5. Depiction of an implanted DBS system. A stimulating electrode is implanted directly into the brain and connected via subcutaneous wires to a pulse generator implanted in the chest wall. (Courtesy of Advanced Neuromodulation Systems/St. Jude Medical, Inc.)

130 Hz, 60 to 90 μs pulse width, and 3 to 6 mV (corresponding to 3 to 6 mA in most patients). DBS (of various subcortical regions) is an established treatment for patients with treatment-refractory Parkinson disease (Deuschl et al., 2003), essential tremor (Rehncrona et al., 2003), and dystonia (Halbig et al., 2005). The ability of DBS to focally modulate activity in neural networks makes it an attractive treatment option for patients with treatment-refractory psychiatric illnesses, which are likely associated with aberrant function of neural networks involved in regulation of mood, thought and behavior.

Indications and Efficacy

The first psychiatric condition to become a focus for DBS research was OCD. This was largely based on the apparent efficacy of ablative neurosurgical approaches in this disorder. Available open-label data suggest that DBS of the anterior limb of the anterior internal capsule (i.e., the target for capsulotomy) may be therapeutic for patients with severe, treatment-resistant OCD (Nuttin et al., 2003; Greenberg, 2004; Greenberg et al., 2006).

Depression has been clearly associated with dysfunction within a neural network involved in mood regulation (Mayberg, 2003). On the basis of converging neuroimaging and neuropathological data, the subgenual cingulate white matter was proposed as a potential target for DBS in patients with severe TRD, and a small open study showed that subgenual cingulate white matter DBS was associated with an antidepressant response in four of six patients with severe TRD (Mayberg et al., 2005). Antidepressant effects have also been reported with DBS of the anterior limb of the internal capsule/ventral striatum (Malone et al., 2009). A related DBS target under investigation is the nucleus accumbens (Schlaepfer and Lieb, 2005).

Risks and Side Effects

Major risks of DBS surgery include hemorrhagic stroke (during implantation of the electrode), infection, and complications associated with anesthesia. In patients with Parkinson disease, the risk of major complications associated with DBS surgery is approximately 10%. Adverse effects of chronic DBS are related to the site of stimulation. To date, the procedure and long-term stimulation appear to be well tolerated in psychiatric patients (Mayberg et al., 2005; Greenberg et al., 2006).

Clinical Use

DBS is not currently available for clinical use in psychiatric patients. It is available in a number of ongoing research studies focused on OCD and depression.

Mechanism of Action

As with other brain stimulation approaches to treating psychiatric disease, the mechanisms of action of DBS are not known. By modulating local neuronal activity, DBS appears to alter neural network function (McIntyre et al., 2004). DBS of the subgenual cingulate white matter for TRD was associated with changes in blood flow in brain regions involved in depression (Mayberg et al., 2005). It remains to be tested whether these changes resulted from *deactivation* of a critical node (e.g., the subgenual cingulate) or *activation* of compensatory neural pathways.

SUMMARY

Treatment-refractory psychiatric illness is unfortunately common, and patients with such illness may benefit from nonpharmacological somatic treatments. ECT is an established treatment for treatment-refractory depression and may have efficacy for a number of other conditions. VNS is approved for the treatment of medication-resistant depression, but third-party funding issues currently limit its availability. Ablative neurosurgical procedures may be helpful for patients with severe treatment-refractory mood or anxiety disorders. TMS, MST, and DBS are under active investigation for the treatment of severe treatment-refractory psychiatric illness (primarily depression and OCD). The mechanisms of action of these various treatments remain obscure, but it is likely that all work through modulation of dysfunctional neural networks involved in the regulation of mood, thought, and behavior.

Clinical Pearls

- A substantial minority of patients with psychiatric illness do not respond to currently available treatments and few evidence-based treatments are available for them.
- For patients with treatment-resistant psychiatric illness, more invasive somatic treatments may be appropriate, which may carry risks greater than those associated with medications and psychotherapy, but these are justified by the distress and disability associated with treatment-resistant psychiatric illness.
- ECT has been established as a safe and effective *acute* treatment for treatment-resistant depression and may have efficacy in several other psychiatric illnesses.
- Relapse after ECT is common, and the efficacy of continuation or maintenance ECT has not been established for any psychiatric illness.
- VNS is FDA-approved for the long-term adjunctive treatment of medication-refractory depression, though the magnitude of response is limited, and maintenance of response over time is promising but uncertain.
- Ablative neurosurgery is occasionally recommended for patients with severe, intractable psychiatric illness (usually OCD or major depression), but efficacy is limited, and no controlled data are available.
- TMS is well tolerated and may have antidepressant efficacy; response rates are generally small in patients with treatment-resistant depression. TMS is FDA approved for the treatment of medication-refractory depression.
- MST may offer a safer alternative to ECT, although data are very limited at this time. MST is not FDA approved for treatment of any psychiatric illness.
- DBS may be safe and efficacious for severe, medication-refractory OCD, although no controlled data are available. It is currently under investigation as a treatment for treatment-resistant depression but not FDA approved for treatment of any psychiatric illness.
- The mechanism of action of brain stimulation therapies in psychiatric illness is largely unknown. However, it is presumed that these treatments act through modulation of activity in neural networks involved in the regulation of mood, cognition, and behavior.

Self-Assessment Questions and Answers

24-1. Which of the following is an indication for electroconvulsive therapy (ECT)?

A. Acute, treatment-resistant major depression
B. Borderline personality disorder
C. Chronic, disabling obsessive-compulsive disorder
D. Schizophrenia, chronic paranoid type

The most common indication for ECT is major depression. *Answer: A*

24-2. Which of the following is a *rare* side effect of ECT?

A. Anterograde amnesia
B. Long-term retrograde amnesia
C. Transient postictal confusion
D. Headache

The most notable side effect of ECT is cognitive impairment, and nearly every patient has some degree of transient postictal confusion. ECT is also associated with minor and transient anterograde amnesia in almost all patients, but long-term retrograde amnesia is rare. *Answer: B*

24-3. Which of the following is an approved indication for vagus nerve stimulation (VNS)?

A. Medication-refractory borderline personality disorder
B. Medication-refractory depression
C. Medication-refractory mania
D. Medication-refractory obsessive-compulsive disorder

VNS is currently approved by the FDA for adjunctive treatment of medication-refractory epilepsy and medication-resistant depression. *Answer: B*

24-4. Which of the following disorders is *most* likely to improve following ablative neurosurgery?

A. Anorexia nervosa
B. Dysthymia
C. obsessive-compulsive disorder
D. Post-traumatic stress disorder

Treatment-resistant mood disorders (including depression and bipolar disorder) and anxiety disorders, especially obsessive-compulsive disorder (OCD), are primary indications for neurosurgical procedures in psychiatry, with early reports suggesting an efficacy up to 70% in patients receiving prefrontal leucotomy. *Answer: C*

24-5. Which of the following is NOT a U.S. Food and Drug Administration (FDA)–approved treatment for depression?

A. Electroconvulsive therapy

B. Deep brain stimulation of the subgenual cingulate gyrus

C. Vagus nerve stimulation

D. Transcranial magnetic stimulation

Electroconvulsive therapy (ECT) is an established treatment for treatment-refractory depression. Vagus nerve stimulation (VNS) and transcranial magnetic stimulation (TMS) are approved by the FDA for the treatment of medication-refractory depression. Deep brain stimulation (DBS) is currently under active investigation for the treatment of depression, but it is not yet approved by the FDA for the treatment of any psychiatric illness. *Answer: B*

References

Anand S, Hotson J. Transcranial magnetic stimulation: Neurophysiological applications and safety. *Brain Cogn.* 2002;50(3):366–386.

Avery D, Winokur G. Mortality in depressed patients treated with electroconvulsive therapy and antidepressants. *Arch Gen Psychiatry.* 1976;33(9):1029–1037.

Avery D, Winokur G. Suicide, attempted suicide, and relapse rates in depression. *Arch Gen Psychiatry.* 1978;35(6):749–753.

Avery DH, PE Holtzheimer PE III, Fawaz W, et al. A controlled study of repetitive transcranial magnetic stimulation in medication-resistant major depression. *Biol Psychiatry* 2006;59(2):187–194.

Avery, DH, PE Holtzheimer PE III, Fawaz W, et al. Transcranial magnetic stimulation reduces pain in patients with major depression: A sham-controlled study. *J Nerv Ment Dis.* 2007;195(5): 378–381.

Bakewell CJ, Russo J, Tanner C, et al. Comparison of clinical efficacy and side effects for bitemporal and bifrontal electrode placement in electroconvulsive therapy. *J ECT.* 2004;20(3):145–153.

Ben-Menachem E. Vagus-nerve stimulation for the treatment of epilepsy. *Lancet Neurol.* 2002;1(8): 477–482.

Ben-Menachem E, Hamberger A, Hedner T, et al. Effects of vagus nerve stimulation on amino acids and other metabolites in the CSF of patients with partial seizures. *Epilepsy Res.* 1995;20(3):221–227.

Ben-Shachar D, Gazawi H, Riboyad-Levin J, et al. Chronic repetitive transcranial magnetic stimulation alters beta-adrenergic and 5-HT2 receptor characteristics in rat brain. *Brain Res.* 1999;816(1):78–83.

Birkenhager TK, van den Broek WW, Mulder PG, et al. One-year outcome of psychotic depression after successful electroconvulsive therapy. *J ECT.* 2005;21(4):221–226.

Burt T, Lisanby SH, Sackeim HA. Neuropsychiatric applications of transcranial magnetic stimulation: A meta-analysis. *Int J Neuropsychopharmacol.* 2002;5(1):73–103.

Carpenter LL, Moreno FA, Kling MA, et al. Effect of vagus nerve stimulation on cerebrospinal fluid monoamine metabolites, norepinephrine, and gamma-aminobutyric acid concentrations in depressed patients. *Biol Psychiatry.* 2004;56(6):418–426.

Chae JH, Nahas Z, Lomarev M, et al. A review of functional neuroimaging studies of vagus nerve stimulation (VNS). *J Psychiatr Res.* 2003;37(6):443–455.

Chen R, Classen J, Gerloff C, et al. Depression of motor cortex excitability by low-frequency transcranial magnetic stimulation. *Neurology.* 1997;48(5):1398–1403.

Conway CR, Sheline YI, Chibnall JT, et al. Cerebral blood flow changes during vagus nerve stimulation for depression. *Psychiatry Res.* 2006;146(2):179–184.

Cosgrove GR. Surgery for psychiatric disorders. *CNS Spectr.* 2000;5(10):43–52.

Cuijpers P, Smit F. Excess mortality in depression: A meta-analysis of community studies. *J Affect Disord.* 2002;72(3):227–236.

Deuschl G, Wenzelburger R, Kopper F, et al. Deep brain stimulation of the subthalamic nucleus for Parkinson's disease: A therapy approaching evidence-based standards. *J Neurol.* 2003;250(Suppl 1): I43–I46.

Devanand DP, Sackeim HA, Prudic J. Electroconvulsive therapy in the treatment-resistant patient. *Psychiatr Clin North Am.* 1991;14(4):905–923.

Dombrovski AY, Mulsant BH, Haskett RF, et al. Predictors of remission after electroconvulsive therapy in unipolar major depression. *J Clin Psychiatry.* 2005;66(8):1043–1049.

Dorr AE, Debonnel G. Effect of vagus nerve stimulation on serotonergic and noradrenergic transmission. *J Pharmacol Exp Ther*. 2006;318(2):890–898.

Dunner DL, Rush AJ, Russell JM, et al. Prospective, long-term, multicenter study of the naturalistic outcomes of patients with treatment-resistant depression. *J Clin Psychiatry*. 2006;67(5):688–695.

Elger G, Hoppe C, Falkai P, et al. Vagus nerve stimulation is associated with mood improvements in epilepsy patients. *Epilepsy Res*. 2000;42(2-3):203–210.

Eranti SV, McLoughlin DM. Changing use of ECT. *Br J Psychiatry*. 2003;183:173.

Fava M, Rush AJ, Wisniewski SR, et al. A comparison of mirtazapine and nortriptyline following two consecutive failed medication treatments for depressed outpatients: A STAR*D report. *Am J Psychiatry*. 2006;163(7):1161–1172.

Feske U, Mulsant BH, Pilkonis PA, et al. Clinical outcome of ECT in patients with major depression and comorbid borderline personality disorder. *Am J Psychiatry*. 2004;161(11):2073–2080.

Fink M. Convulsive therapy: A review of the first 55 years. *J Affect Disord*. 2001;63(1-3):1–15.

Fitzgerald PB, Brown TL, Marston NA, et al. Transcranial magnetic stimulation in the treatment of depression: A double-blind, placebo-controlled trial. *Arch Gen Psychiatry*. 2003;60(10):1002–1008.

Flint AJ, Gagnon N. Effective use of electroconvulsive therapy in late-life depression. *Can J Psychiatry*. 2002;47(8):734–741.

Fregni F, Simon DK, Wu A, et al. Non-invasive brain stimulation for Parkinson's disease: A systematic review and meta-analysis of the literature. *J Neurol Neurosurg Psychiatry*. 2005;76(12):1614–1623.

George MS, Wassermann EM, Williams WA, et al. Daily repetitive transcranial magnetic stimulation (rTMS) improves mood in depression. *Neuroreport*. 1995;6(14):1853–1856.

Gershon AA, Dannon PN, Grunhaus L, et al. Transcranial magnetic stimulation in the treatment of depression. *Am J Psychiatry*. 2003;160(5):835–845.

Ghaziuddin N, King CA, Naylor MW, et al. Electroconvulsive treatment in adolescents with pharmacotherapy-refractory depression. *J Child Adolesc Psychopharmacol*. 1996;6(4):259–271.

Greenberg B. Deep brain stimulation: Clinical findings in OCD and depression. *59th Annual Meeting of the Society of Biological Psychiatry*. New York, 2004.

Greenberg BD, Malone DA, Friehs GM, et al. Three-year outcomes in deep brain stimulation for highly resistant obsessive-compulsive disorder. *Neuropsychopharmacology*. 2006;31(11):2384–2393.

Greenberg BD, Price LH, Rauch SL, et al. Neurosurgery for intractable obsessive-compulsive disorder and depression: Critical issues. *Neurosurg Clin N Am*. 2003;14(2):199–212.

Groves DA, Bowman EM, Brown VJ. Recordings from the rat locus coeruleus during acute vagal nerve stimulation in the anaesthetised rat. *Neurosci Lett*. 2005;379(3):174–179.

Halbig TD, Gruber D, Kopp UA, et al. Pallidal stimulation in dystonia: Effects on cognition, mood, and quality of life. *J Neurol Neurosurg Psychiatry*. 2005;76(12):1713–1716.

Harden CL. The co-morbidity of depression and epilepsy: Epidemiology, etiology, and treatment. *Neurology*. 2002;59(6 Suppl 4):S48–S55.

Hassert DL, Miyashita T, Williams CL. The effects of peripheral vagal nerve stimulation at a memory-modulating intensity on norepinephrine output in the basolateral amygdala. *Behav Neurosci*. 2004;118(1):79–88.

Hoffman RE, Boutros NN, Hu S, et al. Transcranial magnetic stimulation and auditory hallucinations in schizophrenia. *Lancet*. 2000;355(9209):1073–1075.

Holtzheimer PE III, Russo J, Avery DH. A meta-analysis of repetitive transcranial magnetic stimulation in the treatment of depression. *Psychopharmacol Bull*. 2001;35(4):149–169.

Januel D, Dumortier G, Verdon CM, et al. A double-blind sham controlled study of right prefrontal repetitive transcranial magnetic stimulation (rTMS): Therapeutic and cognitive effect in medication free unipolar depression during 4 weeks. *Prog Neuropsychopharmacol Biol Psychiatry*. 2006;30(1):126–130.

Kanno M, Matsumoto M, Togashi H, et al. Effects of acute repetitive transcranial magnetic stimulation on dopamine release in the rat dorsolateral striatum. *J Neurol Sci*. 2004;217(1):73–81.

Karadenizli D, Dilbaz N, Bayam G. Gilles de la Tourette syndrome: Response to electroconvulsive therapy. *J Ect*. 2005;21(4):246–248.

Keck ME, Welt T, Muller MB, et al. Repetitive transcranial magnetic stimulation increases the release of dopamine in the mesolimbic and mesostriatal system. *Neuropharmacology*. 2002;43(1):101–109.

Kellner CH, Knapp RG, Petrides G, et al. Continuation electroconvulsive therapy versus pharmacotherapy for relapse prevention in major depression: A multisite study from the Consortium for Research in Electroconvulsive Therapy (CORE). *Arch Gen Psychiatry*. 2006;63(12):1337–1344.

Kho KH, van Vreeswijk MF, Simpson S, et al. A meta-analysis of electroconvulsive therapy efficacy in depression. *J ECT*. 2003;19(3):139–147.

Klein E, Kreinin I, Chistyakov A, et al. Therapeutic efficacy of right prefrontal slow repetitive transcranial magnetic stimulation in major depression: A double-blind controlled study. *Arch Gen Psychiatry*. 1999;56(4):315–320.

Kosel M, Frick C, Lisanby SH, et al. Magnetic seizure therapy improves mood in refractory major depression. *Neuropsychopharmacology*. 2003;28(11):2045–2048.

Kozel FA, George MS. Meta-analysis of left prefrontal repetitive transcranial magnetic stimulation (rTMS) to treat depression. *J Psychiatr Pract*. 2002;8(5):270–275.

Krahl SE, Clark KB, Smith DC, et al. Locus coeruleus lesions suppress the seizure-attenuating effects of vagus nerve stimulation. *Epilepsia*. 1998;39(7):709–714.

Lechner SM, Curtis AL, Brons R, et al. Locus coeruleus activation by colon distention: Role of corticotropin-releasing factor and excitatory amino acids. *Brain Res*. 1997;756(1-2):114–124.

Lisanby SH, Luber B, Schlaepfer TE, et al. Safety and feasibility of magnetic seizure therapy (MST) in major depression: Randomized within-subject comparison with electroconvulsive therapy. *Neuropsychopharmacology*. 2003;28(10):1852–1865.

Loo C, Sachdev P, Elsayed H, et al. Effects of a 2- to 4-week course of repetitive transcranial magnetic stimulation (rTMS) on neuropsychologic functioning, electroencephalogram, and auditory threshold in depressed patients. *Biol Psychiatry*. 2001;49(7):615–623.

Malone DA, Dougherty DD, Rezai AR, et al. Deep brain stimulation of the ventral capsule/ventral striatum for treatment-resistant depression. *Biol Psychiatry*. 2009;65(4):267–275.

Marangell LB, Rush AJ, George MS, et al. Vagus nerve stimulation (VNS) for major depressive episodes: One year outcomes. *Biol Psychiatry*. 2002;51(4):280–287.

Marrosu F, Serra A, Maleci A, et al. Correlation between GABA(A) receptor density and vagus nerve stimulation in individuals with drug-resistant partial epilepsy. *Epilepsy Res*. 2003;55(1-2):59–70.

Martin, JL, MJ Barbanoj, Schlaepfer TE, et al. Transcranial magnetic stimulation for treating depression *Cochrane Database Syst Rev*. 2002;(2):CD003493.

Martin JL, Barbanoj MJ, Schlaepfer TE, et al. Repetitive transcranial magnetic stimulation for the treatment of depression: Systematic review and meta-analysis. *Br J Psychiatry*. 2003;182:480–491.

Martis B, Alam D, Dowd SM, et al. Neurocognitive effects of repetitive transcranial magnetic stimulation in severe major depression. *Clin Neurophysiol*. 2003;114(6):1125–1132.

Mayberg HS. Modulating dysfunctional limbic-cortical circuits in depression: Towards development of brain-based algorithms for diagnosis and optimised treatment. *Br Med Bull*. 2003;65:193–207.

Mayberg HS, Lozano AM, Voon V, et al. Deep brain stimulation for treatment-resistant depression. *Neuron*. 2005;45(5):651–660.

McCall WV, Dunn A, Rosenquist PB, et al. Markedly suprathreshold right unilateral ECT versus minimally suprathreshold bilateral ECT: Antidepressant and memory effects. *J ECT*. 2002;18(3):126–129.

McGrath PJ, Stewart JW, Fava M, et al. Tranylcypromine versus venlafaxine plus mirtazapine following three failed antidepressant medication trials for depression: A STAR*D Report. *Am J Psychiatry*. 2006; 163(9):1531–1541.

McIntyre CC, Savasta M, Goffc LK, et al. Uncovering the mechanism(s) of action of deep brain stimulation: Activation, inhibition, or both. *Clin Neurophysiol*. 2004;115(6):1239–1248.

Moniz E. Prefrontal leucotomy in the treatment of mental disorders. *Am J Psychiatry*. 1937;93:1379–1385.

Muller MB, Toschi N, Kresse AE, et al. Long-term repetitive transcranial magnetic stimulation increases the expression of brain-derived neurotrophic factor and cholecystokinin mRNA, but not neuropeptide tyrosine mRNA in specific areas of rat brain. *Neuropsychopharmacology*. 2000;23(2):205–215.

Nahas Z, Marangell LB, Husain MM. Two-year outcome of vagus nerve stimulation (VNS) for treatment of major depressive episodes. *J Clin Psychiatry*. 2005;66(9):1097–1104.

Nemeroff CB, Bissette G, Akil H, et al. Neuropeptide concentrations in the cerebrospinal fluid of depressed patients treated with electroconvulsive therapy. Corticotrophin-releasing factor, beta-endorphin and somatostatin. *Br J Psychiatry*. 1991;158:59–63.

Nierenberg AA, Fava M, Trivedi MH, et al. A comparison of lithium and T3 augmentation following two failed medication treatments for depression: A STAR*D Report. *Am J Psychiatry*. 2006;163(9): 1519–1530.

Nuttin BJ, Gabriels LA, Cosyns PR, et al. Electrical stimulation of the anterior limbs of the internal capsules in patients with severe obsessive-compulsive disorder: Anecdotal reports. *Neurosurg Clin N Am*. 2003;14(2):267–274.

O'Connor MK, Knapp R, Husain M, et al. The influence of age on the response of major depression to electroconvulsive therapy: A C.O.R.E. Report. *Am J Geriatr Psychiatry*. 2001;9(4):382–390.

O'Reardon JP, Solvason HB, Janicak PG, et al. Efficacy and safety of transcranial magnetic stimulation in the acute treatment of major depression: A multisite randomized controlled trial. *Biol Psychiatry*. 2007;62:1208–1216.

Ohnishi T, Hayashi T, Okabe S, et al. Endogenous dopamine release induced by repetitive transcranial magnetic stimulation over the primary motor cortex: An [11C] raclopride positron emission tomography study in anesthetized macaque monkeys. *Biol Psychiatry*. 2004;55(5):484–489.

Pagnin D, de Queiroz V, Pini S, et al. Efficacy of ECT in depression: A meta-analytic review. *J ECT*. 2004; 20(1):13–20.

Pascual-Leone A, Valls-Sole J, Wassermann EM, et al. Responses to rapid-rate transcranial magnetic stimulation of the human motor cortex. *Brain*. 1994;117(Pt 4):847–858.

Passard A, Attal N, Benadhira R, et al. Effects of unilateral repetitive transcranial magnetic stimulation of the motor cortex on chronic widespread pain in fibromyalgia. *Brain*. 2007;130(Pt 10):2661–2670.

Perera TD, Coplan JD, Lisanby SH, et al. Antidepressant-induced neurogenesis in the hippocampus of adult nonhuman primates. *J Neurosci*. 2007;27(18):4894–4901.

Petrides G, Fink M, Husain MM, et al. ECT remission rates in psychotic versus nonpsychotic depressed patients: A report from CORE. *J ECT*. 2001;17(4):244–253.

Post A, Keck ME. Transcranial magnetic stimulation as a therapeutic tool in psychiatry: What do we know about the neurobiological mechanisms? *J Psychiatr Res*. 2001;35(4):193–215.

Prudic J, Haskett RF, Mulsant B, et al. Resistance to antidepressant medications and short-term clinical response to ECT. *Am J Psychiatry*. 1996;153(8):985–992.

Rehncrona S, Johnels B, Widner H, et al. Long-term efficacy of thalamic deep brain stimulation for tremor: Double-blind assessments. *Mov Disord*. 2003;18(2):163–170.

Rose D, Fleischmann P, Wykes T, et al. Patients' perspectives on electroconvulsive therapy: Systematic review. *Br Med J*. 2003;326(7403):1363.

Rossi S, De Capua A, Ulivelli M, et al. Effects of repetitive transcranial magnetic stimulation on chronic tinnitus: A randomised, crossover, double blind, placebo controlled study. *J Neurol Neurosurg Psychiatry*. 2007;78(8):857–863.

Rossini D, Lucca A, Zanardi R, et al. Transcranial magnetic stimulation in treatment-resistant depressed patients: A double-blind, placebo-controlled trial. *Psychiatry Res*. 2005;137(1-2):1–10.

Rush AJ, Marangell LB, Sackeim HA, et al. Vagus nerve stimulation for treatment-resistant depression: A randomized, controlled acute phase trial. *Biol Psychiatry*. 2005;58(5):347–354.

Rush AJ, Sackeim HA, Marangell LB, et al. Effects of 12 months of vagus nerve stimulation in treatment-resistant depression: A naturalistic study. *Biol Psychiatry*. 2005;58(5):355–363.

Rush AJ, Trivedi MH, Wisniewski SR, et al. Bupropion-SR, sertraline, or venlafaxine-XR after failure of SSRIs for depression. *N Engl J Med*. 2006;354(12):1231–1242.

Sackeim HA, Brannan SK, John RA, et al. Durability of antidepressant response to vagus nerve stimulation (VNSTM). *Int J Neuropsychopharmacol*. 2007;1–10.

Sackeim HA, Haskett RF, Mulsant BH, et al. Continuation pharmacotherapy in the prevention of relapse following electroconvulsive therapy: A randomized controlled trial. *JAMA*. 2001;285(10):1299–1307.

Sackeim HA, Prudic J, Devanand DP, et al. A prospective, randomized, double-blind comparison of bilateral and right unilateral electroconvulsive therapy at different stimulus intensities. *Arch Gen Psychiatry*. 2000;57(5):425–434.

Sackeim HA, Prudic J, Fuller R, et al. The cognitive effects of electroconvulsive therapy in community settings. *Neuropsychopharmacology*. 2007;32(1):244–254.

Sackeim HA, Rush AJ, George MS, et al. Vagus nerve stimulation (VNS) for treatment-resistant depression: Efficacy, side effects, and predictors of outcome. *Neuropsychopharmacology*. 2001;25(5):713–728.

Schlaepfer TE, Kosel M, Nemeroff CB. Efficacy of repetitive transcranial magnetic stimulation (rTMS) in the treatment of affective disorders. *Neuropsychopharmacology*. 2003;28(2):201–205.

Schlaepfer TE, Lieb K. Deep brain stimulation for treatment of refractory depression. *Lancet*. 2005; 366(9495):1420–1422.

Segal J, Szabo CP, du Toit J, et al. Child and adolescent electroconvulsive therapy: A case report. *World J Biol Psychiatry*. 2004;5(4):221–229.

Speer AM, Kimbrell TA, Wassermann EM, et al. Opposite effects of high and low frequency rTMS on regional brain activity in depressed patients. *Biol Psychiatry*. 2000;48(12):1133–1141.

Strafella AP, Paus T, Barrett J, et al. Repetitive transcranial magnetic stimulation of the human prefrontal cortex induces dopamine release in the caudate nucleus. *J Neurosci*. 2001;21(15):RC157.

Strafella AP, Paus T, Fraraccio M, et al. Striatal dopamine release induced by repetitive transcranial magnetic stimulation of the human motor cortex. *Brain*. 2003;22:22.

Tew JD Jr, Mulsant BH, Haskett RF, et al. A randomized comparison of high-charge right unilateral electroconvulsive therapy and bilateral electroconvulsive therapy in older depressed patients who failed to respond to 5 to 8 moderate-charge right unilateral treatments. *J Clin Psychiatry*. 2002;63(12):1102–1105.

Tharyan, P, Adams CE. Electroconvulsive therapy for schizophrenia. *Cochrane Database Syst Rev*. 2005;2: CD000076.

The UK ECT Review Group. Efficacy and safety of electroconvulsive therapy in depressive disorders: A systematic review and meta-analysis. *Lancet*. 2003;361:799–808.

Trivedi MH, Fava M, Wisniewski SR, et al. Medication augmentation after the failure of SSRIs for depression. *N Engl J Med*. 2006;354(12):1243–1252.

Trivedi MH, Rush AJ, Wisniewski SR, et al. Evaluation of outcomes with citalopram for depression using measurement-based care in STAR*D: Implications for clinical practice. *Am J Psychiatry*. 2006; 163(1):28–40.

Wahlund B, von Rosen D. ECT of major depressed patients in relation to biological and clinical variables: A brief overview. *Neuropsychopharmacology*. 2003;28(Suppl 1):S21–S26.

Wassermann EM. Risk and safety of repetitive transcranial magnetic stimulation: Report and suggested guidelines from the International Workshop on the Safety of Repetitive Transcranial Magnetic Stimulation, June 5–7, 1996. *Electroencephalogr Clin Neurophysiol*. 1998;108(1):1–16.

White PF, Amos Q, Zhang Y, et al. Anesthetic considerations for magnetic seizure therapy: A novel therapy for severe depression. *Anesth Analg*. 2006;103(1):76–80, table of contents.

Wulsin LR, Vaillant GE, Wells VE, et al. A systematic review of the mortality of depression. *Psychosom Med*. 1999;61(1):6–17.

Zangen A, Hyodo K. Transcranial magnetic stimulation induces increases in extracellular levels of dopamine and glutamate in the nucleus accumbens. *Neuroreport*. 2002;13(18):2401–2405.

Zobel A, Joe A, Freymann N, et al. Changes in regional cerebral blood flow by therapeutic vagus nerve stimulation in depression: An exploratory approach. *Psychiatry Res*. 2005;139(3):165–179.

Zornberg GL, Pope HG Jr. Treatment of depression in bipolar disorder: New directions in research. *J Clin Psychopharmacol*. 1993;13(6):397–408.

Therapeutic Response to Chronic Pain

Community studies suggest that the lifetime prevalence of chronic pain is 15% to 25%. In the elderly, that number increases to 50%. Yet, although common, pain remains a private experience, difficult to define and harder to quantify. In describing pain, the Institute of Medicine wrote, "The experience of pain is more than a simple sensory process. It is a complex perception involving higher levels of the central nervous system, emotional status, and higher order mental processes" (Osterweis et al., 1987).

Pain serves an important signaling function and often leads to recognition of some underlying disease that can be remedied. However, pain remains hard to describe and quantify. Of more concern is that it is often inadequately treated.

This chapter will concentrate on the management of chronic pain. However, proper treatment of pain requires a proper understanding of pain; therefore, this chapter will begin with a brief discussion of the assessment of pain.

ASSESSMENT OF PAIN

Currently there is no universal "gold standard" for pain assessment, and such an assessment is necessarily subjective and must recognize the many dimensions of the pain experience.

The Immediate Pain Experience

When a patient complains of "pain," the physician must first attempt to understand what the patient means by quantifying and qualifying the nature of the patient's experience.

Intensity

Clinicians can use various approaches to quantify the intensity of pain, including verbal, numerical, and visual scales. Typically, the patient is asked to assign a numerical value to the pain intensity, from 1 to 10 (1 = no pain, 10 = the most pain imaginable). Such an approach is rapid, simple, and easily comprehended and can be used to track changes over time. However, such scales are ordinal, the distance between intervals is not always consistent, and the patient may be affected by recall bias. Still, this method is very practical at the bedside.

Another approach is to employ visual analog scales, in which the clinician asks the patient to indicate the intensity of the pain with a mark on a line. The line is usually 10 cm to 15 cm long and has no anchors on it except at the ends ("no pain" on one end and "the most intense pain imaginable" on the other). This method may have the advantage of reflecting changes in pain intensity. The major drawbacks are the need for prepared materials and the time spent scoring the instrument.

The Affective Response to Pain

Individuals can usually distinguish between the intensity of pain and their feelings associated with the pain. An affective response can involve many dimensions, but most typically involve the degree of unpleasantness. Compared with pain intensity the affective response is more influenced by the context of the pain and can be assessed using the same methods as for pain intensity, including verbal, numerical, or visual analog scales.

Location

Pain location is usually assessed graphically. Patients are shown figures of a human body on which they draw the locations of their pain. Different symbols can represent different qualities of pain (for example "oo" for "pins and needles," "xx" for "burning").

Pain Scales and Instruments

A number of pain scales and instruments have been devised to measure other aspects of pain, such as the behavioral aspects of pain or the impact of pain on a patient's life. These tend to be larger, multidimensional scales. For example, the American Pain Society's Patient Outcome Questionnaire (Dihle et al., 2006) looks not only at pain severity but also the patient's reports of quality of life and satisfaction with treatment, and the McGill Pain Questionnaire (Melzack, 2005) is a comprehensive scale combining multiple domains, including affective and temporal quality, intensity, and location.

A number of tools can assess pain in special populations. For example, with children clinicians often use pictograms, such as the FACES scale (Wong and Baker, 1988), which, as implied, shows a series of increasingly distressed faces. Similarly, scales designed for the elderly may rely on nonverbal cues of pain behaviors.

Physical Functioning

In evaluating physical function, clinicians must distinguish among concepts of impairment, functional limitation, and disability.

Impairment refers to any objective abnormality or loss. These can be anatomic (e.g., loss of limb, physical deformity), physiologic (e.g., decreased cardiac output, muscle weakness), or psychological (e.g., changes in cognition). They can usually be objectively measured.

Functional limitations are any restrictions in an individual's normal functioning. They are the practical result of impairment. In evaluating for functional limitations, an attempt is made to measure physical functioning in specific activities judged necessary for daily living. There is no agreement on exactly what these activities are. Most evaluations include measurements of the range of motion at major joints, strength testing in major muscle groups, and endurance for specific tasks.

Disability refers to the inability to do one's usual activities or duties as the result of impairment. It is task specific, and again, there is no gold standard of assessment. Different organizations that evaluate and compensate disability will require that specific factors be assessed. For example, social security relies primarily on objective measures of impairment over subjective symptoms such as pain.

Psychological Factors

No pain should ever be viewed as either physical or psychological. Psychological evaluation is important for every patient with pain and may be the most reliable predictor of functional outcome.

In performing a psychological assessment in a patient with pain, the goal is to find factors that *influence* pain, rather than *cause* it. It is often helpful to make this goal clear to the patient, who may be skeptical of psychological questions. Most patients will be defensive at the implication that the pain they experience is "just in their heads." They are usually quite willing, however, to consider how stresses in their lives influence their pain.

A proper assessment should include both the patient and other significant persons. The clinician should try to identify events that exacerbate pain and how the patient copes with this pain. In addition, the clinician should review a patient's usual daily activities and appraise how these activities have changed because of the pain. Possible sources of reinforcement of the pain, whether financial, sympathetic, or avoidance, should be tactfully explored. The patient should be asked about past events that may resonate with the current situation. For example, a large survey found that chronic pain in women was significantly associated with a childhood history of sexual abuse (Walsh et al., 2007). A family history of similar pain problems should be recorded. Any psychiatric illnesses may affect pain, and the doctor should ask about these. Finally, the clinician should try to understand the patient's beliefs about the pain, including beliefs about etiology, such as issues of retribution or blame.

PAIN DISORDER ASSOCIATED WITH PSYCHOLOGICAL FACTORS

A 43-year-old woman presents to an emergency department saying, "If someone cannot help my pain, I am going to kill myself." She reports several types of pain, including chronic headaches, sharp pains in her lower back, and "fibromyalgia" pain in her joints. Physical therapy and multiple medication regimens, including opioids, have not helped significantly. She says that, despite a childhood history of sexual abuse, she was a highly successful physician until age 30. At that time, she discovered her husband was having an affair, which resulted in a painful divorce. Shortly after, she had a minor car accident, and despite multiple medical workups showing no explanatory pathology, she began complaining of pain, which has only worsened with time. She has not been able to return to work and currently supports herself through disability. On reflection, she admits that her pain seems to worsen under stress but says, "I am stressed most of the time." In addition to her pain, she notes feeling depressed and constantly tired. She admits, "I know everyone thinks this pain is just in my head, but if it is, show me how to stop it, because it is ruining my life."

Pain Behavior

Patients can exhibit predictable behaviors associated with their pain. They are reinforced over time—that is, they are learned behaviors. Most important, they represent potential targets for behavioral intervention.

Assessment of pain behavior is done through observation of verbal and nonverbal behaviors, because patients may not be aware of their behavior. Examples of verbal behaviors include complaining of pain or using other vocalizations (e.g., moaning). Nonverbal behavior can be general, involving movement (e.g., pacing) or position, or can be more specific (e.g., guarding a painful joint).

Physical Correlates of Pain

The relationship between organic pathology, physiological functioning, and pain report is poorly understood. Any correlations between these objective and subjective factors are weak and difficult to predict. Most physiological measures remain only research tools, but some have clinical value. Examples include the use of electromyography in evaluating temporomandibular joint syndrome. In each case, physiological measures serve as adjuncts, not substitutes, for the subjective evaluation.

CATEGORIZING PAIN

Pain is usually categorized by its course and differentiated by whether it is acute or chronic. Acute pain is not only brief but also usually associated with clear injury or disease, such as postsurgical pain, in which the pain is reasonably well correlated to the degree of injury and healing. A better term might be *nociceptive pain*.

Chronic pain is more complicated. Although it is often initially associated with an injury, this association is less clear over time. Therefore, it may persist well beyond the usual length of an injury and seem to be "self perpetuating." Some types of chronic pain wax and wane (e.g., fibromyalgia), whereas others are likely to progress in concert with a disease process (e.g., cancer pain).

Chronic pain is usually categorized by its presumed etiology. An example is neuropathic pain, in which the pathology is thought to reside not merely in nociception but also in the transmission of the signal to the brain and in the subsequent processing within the brain. A classic example is phantom limb pain. Other examples include postherpetic neuralgia, trigeminal neuralgia, diabetic neuropathies, myelopathic and radiculopathic pain, and central pain. Assumptions are made about the etiology of chronic pain based on the clinical description; for example, neurologic pains are often described as having a "burning" or "electrical" quality, as opposed to the sharp, stabbing quality of an acute pain.

Many types of chronic pain have an unclear or mixed etiology. Examples include chronic recurrent headaches, vasculopathic pain, and complex regional pain. Complex regional pain (also historically called *reflex sympathetic dystrophy*) is a particularly confusing type of pain, with both nociceptive and neuropathic elements, which is associated with abnormal activity of the sympathetic nervous system.

Pain from a Psychiatric Perspective

In the *Diagnostic and Statistical Manual of Mental Disorders,* Third Edition (DSM-III) (American Psychiatric Association, 1980), psychogenic pain disorder had to be either incompatible with organic disease, or "grossly in excess" of what one would expect from the physical findings. It also stipulated that psychological factors were judged to be "etiologically related" to pain development. Obviously, this was difficult to use because most patients with chronic pain have some organic pathology, and it seems judgmental to say what pain is "in excess" of the pathology. DSM-III-R (American Psychiatric Association, 1987), therefore, dropped this last criterion and renamed the disorder somatoform pain disorder.

DSM-IV (American Psychiatric Association, 1994) simplified the name to pain disorder and suggested three main criteria: that pain is the predominant focus of clinical attention, it causes substantial distress or impairment, and psychological factors are judged to have a role in its onset or expression. The disorder is further subdivided based on whether it is associated with just psychological or both psychological and medical factors and whether it is acute or chronic.

This further revision continues to present problems for the clinician treating patients with chronic pain, because one must decide the relative importance of psychological factors. It can be argued that psychological factors are always important in the expression of pain, and it is likely that any patient with any type of chronic pain would meet the criteria of this disorder (Boland, 2002), thereby making its status as a psychiatric disorder questionable.

TREATMENT OF PAIN

Alleviating pain is one of the clinician's most fundamental roles. At times, this can be complex and frustrating. Often, however, through understanding some fundamental principles of pain management, even the inexperienced clinician gives some relief to the suffering patient.

Ethical and Legal Perspectives on a Patient's Right to Pain Management

Historically, the undertreatment of pain was an all-too-frequent reality. Well into the modern medical era there remained many barriers to adequate pain management, including cultural attitudes about pain as an inevitable part of the human condition, fear of analgesic misuse or disciplinary action against those who prescribe such analgesics, and inadequate medical training in pain management. These problems continue into the present; however, there has been a gradual shift in attitudes about a patient's right to adequate treatment, which has evolved from being viewed as good medical practice to a fundamental human right.

This right has gained legal grounding. The Supreme Court has supported the contention, in two cases related to palliative care, that patients have a constitutional right to adequate symptomatic relief.

The right to pain relief is gaining statutory support as well. Several states, including California and New York, require continuing education in pain management. Some state medical boards have protocols for the investigation of physicians who inadequately treat pain and have disciplined such physicians. Successful civil cases have been brought against health care workers for inadequate pain treatment. Additionally, health care providers who did not provide adequate pain relief to elderly patients have been criminally prosecuted for elder abuse (Brennan et al., 2007).

PHARMACOLOGIC TREATMENT FOR PAIN

Most patients who seek medical attention for pain will eventually receive medication. As with all medications, it is important to follow a clear rationale. The physician and patient must have mutually understood goals and a plan of what to do when relief is not adequate.

All regimens should be individualized; however, in general, it is usually best to begin with the least potent medication, the simplest dosing regimen, and the least invasive route of administration and to work up from there.

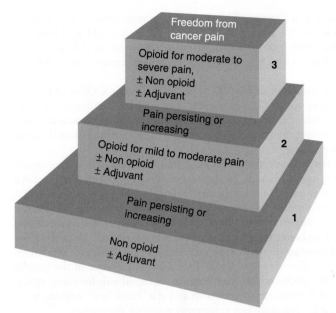

FIGURE 25-1. The World Health Organization (WHO) Pain Ladder. (Reproduced with permission from WHO. *Cancer pain relief*, 2nd ed. Geneva: World Health Organization; 1996.)

The World Health Organization (WHO) has suggested a rational titration of pain medication, called the *WHO Pain Ladder* (see Fig. 25-1). This stepwise approach was devised for the treatment of cancer pain but is applicable to many pain situations.

The first step in the approach is the use of nonsteroidal anti-inflammatory drugs (NSAIDs) for mild to moderate pain. Adjuvant drugs may also be used at any step. When pain persists, a low-potency opioid should be added to this regimen. The NSAID should be maintained because it may provide additive analgesia. Pain that persists despite this regimen should be treated with opioids that are more potent. For pain that is moderate to severe at the outset, opioids should be the first choice.

This approach emphasizes the importance of simplicity—both in drug choice and in dose scheduling. Single agents are more easily titrated and their side effects are more predictable. Adjuvant medications should be added only when indicated.

Simple dosing that incorporates knowledge of a drug's pharmacokinetics is equally important. Ordering a short-acting agent such as morphine to be given every 4 to 6 hours betrays an overestimation of the drug's likely length of effect. Similarly, medications for persistent pain should be scheduled with dosing "around the clock" to ensure a constant effective blood level.

"As needed" or p.r.n. (*pro re nata,* literally, "for the thing born," loosely meaning "as the situation arises") medication can be added to the regimen but should not be used alone, because it can result in erratic blood levels, and treatment with this approach is usually "too little, too late."

Nonsteroidal Anti-Inflammatory Drugs

All NSAIDs inhibit cyclooxygenase (COX). COX is an enzyme responsible for the synthesis of prostaglandins. Prostaglandins are metabolized from arachidonic acid—this process occurs at sites of tissue damage and seems to help sensitize nociceptors to painful stimuli. COX has three known isoenzymes; two are of clinical importance here: those prostaglandins involved in the maintenance and protection of the gastrointestinal tract (COX-1) and those involved in the inflammatory response to pain (COX-2). Most NSAIDs inhibit both COX-1 and COX-2.

NSAIDs are helpful for treating many types of pain, ranging from minor aches and sprains to bony metastases. There is no clear relationship between serum levels of NSAIDs and analgesia. NSAIDs may be used alone or in conjunction with other analgesics employing different mechanisms of action, such as opioids.

The most common side effect is gastric irritation. The decrease in prostaglandin caused by NSAIDs reduces gastric mucus and increases gastric acidity. Other side effects include salt and fluid retention, platelet inhibition, and tinnitus. The drugs are excreted renally, and patients with renal insufficiency may be at risk for toxicity. NSAIDs may decrease renal blood flow and may cause renal failure. The latter effect is of most concern in patients who are elderly, volume depleted, or taking nephrotoxic drugs or who have preexisting renal impairment, heart failure, or hepatic dysfunction.

Acetaminophen, strictly speaking, is not an NSAID; it has little effect on COX-1 or COX-2 and is not a potent anti-inflammatory agent. The mechanism of action of acetaminophen is still a subject of debate. However, it has similar analgesic potency to that of the NSAIDs and is included here for simplicity. It has few gastrointestinal side effects; however, it carries the additional hazard of possible liver damage from an overdose.

The introduction of agents that were selective for COX-2, including celecoxib and rofecoxib, was thought to be a major advance in NSAIDs in that they could be specific for the anti-inflammatory effect while minimizing gastrointestinal side effects. Early reports suggested that the drugs had improved side effect profiles, but later data suggested that with chronic use the gastrointestinal benefits are not as apparent. In addition, the rates of other NSAID-related side effects, such as renal failure, were no better than with other NSAIDs. Celecoxib has a structure similar to that of sulfa and could cause an allergy in some patients who are allergic to sulfa drugs. However, of most concern was the discovery that COX-2 inhibitors lack some of the platelet inhibiting properties of nonspecific NSAIDs and may have an increased risk for heart attack, thrombosis, and stroke. Because of these concerns, celecoxib added a "black box" warning to its prescription information, and in 2004 rofecoxib was voluntarily taken off the market.

Opioid Analgesia

Opioids remain the "gold standard" of pharmacologic treatment for the patient with pain.

Narcotics act by mimicking the effect of endogenous opioids, the most potent being β-endorphin. All opioids, endogenous and exogenous, bind to specific opioid receptors in the brain and peripheral nervous system. Most of the opioids bind to μ receptors. The potency of opioids is related to their affinity for this receptor.

There are two classes of μ receptor, $\mu 1$ and $\mu 2$. The first is involved in analgesia, and the second is responsible for respiratory depression. No opioid can bind $\mu 1$ alone. Of the other receptors, the most important are δ and κ, which are important in spinal analgesia. Of note is that use of Greek letters may soon be obsolete: the International Union of Pharmacology has reclassified these receptors as OP1 (δ), OP2 (κ), and OP3 (μ).

Opioids are the most effective agents available for treating acute pain. They are used in a variety of other types of pain, including cancer pain and such noncancer chronic pain as neuropathic pain. The drugs within the class are very similar, and most differences are pharmacokinetic rather than pharmacodynamic. That is, all opioids can be made equipotent by adjusting their dose or route of administration.

Perhaps most central to the use of opioids is the idea of minimum effective concentration (MEC). The MEC is a hypothetical plasma concentration below which a drug is ineffective. The MEC for an opioid—that is, the plasma level at which analgesia is effective—can vary greatly among different individuals. Therefore, when choosing an opioid dose for a patient, the only way to find the effective dose is through empirical titration. Recommended doses and comparative potencies found in various references can only be considered rough guidelines.

Side Effects

The most problematic side effect of opioids is respiratory depression. This is due to a reduction in brainstem responsiveness to PCO_2 and to the depression of the pontine and medullary centers involved in the regulation of breathing. Respiratory depression can be reversed by naloxone; however, the drug requires careful monitoring because it has a short half-life.

The most common opioid side effects are nausea and sedation. Opioids can also cause alterations in mood and alertness. They decrease gastrointestinal peristalsis and increase sphincter tone, causing constipation. This effect on sphincter tone can also increase biliary pressure and urinary retention. Although rare, opioids can depress cardiac function and cause bradycardia.

The incidence and severity of side effects seen with different opioids are probably similar at equianalgesic doses (meperidine may be an exception and is discussed separately). Switching opioids is unlikely to improve side effects, and the clinician should be familiar with the symptomatic treatment of these side effects. An example is the prophylactic use of laxatives for chronic opioid use.

Meperidine

Meperidine has a very short duration of action, making it inappropriate for all but brief courses of treatment. It is lower in potency than similar opioids and often underdosed in patients. Its metabolite, normeperidine, can be toxic and cause central nervous system irritation, including dysphoria, delirium, and even seizures. The medication is strongly anticholinergic. Moreover, the belief that meperidine causes less sphincter spasm than other opioids was disproved a decade ago (Sherman and Lehman, 1994). For these reasons, meperidine is best avoided.

Tolerance, Physical Dependence, and Addiction

The greatest barrier to long-term opiate use is the fear of causing addiction. In understanding this, it is important to distinguish among tolerance, physical dependence, and withdrawal. Tolerance is the decline in potency of an opioid experienced with continued use, so that higher doses are needed to achieve the same effect. Physical dependence refers to the development of withdrawal symptoms once a drug is stopped. Typical symptoms of opioid withdrawal include yawning, diaphoresis, lacrimation, coryza, and tachycardia, followed by abdominal cramps, nausea, and vomiting.

Tolerance and dependence are physiological phenomena and not the same as addiction. Addiction is a compulsion to use a drug, usually for its psychic, rather than therapeutic, effects. This is a behavioral problem, with psychological as well as physical dependence. Although DSM-IV-TR (American Psychiatric Association, 2000) does not use the term *addiction*, the diagnosis of substance dependence within DSM-IV-TR corresponds more to an addiction than physical dependence. One can have tolerance or dependence without addiction, and the reverse is true as well.

Clearly, individuals with histories of opiate addiction are at risk of continued addictive use if they are prescribed opioids. The question remains, however, whether patients without such a history are at risk to become addicted to opioids. In clinical investigations of the question, it appears that iatrogenic addiction is a rare event. In a large review of >11,000 Medicare inpatients who received narcotics, only four cases of iatrogenic narcotic addiction were documented (Porter and Jick, 1980); however, this was a retrospective review, including patients with various types of pain. In patients using opioids for chronic pain, various ranges have been reported for the incidence of addiction, from a low of 3% to a high of 19% (Weaver and Schnoll, 2007). Taken as a whole, these ranges are roughly similar to the rates of addiction reported in the general population, and opioids do not appear to increase the baseline risk of addiction.

Route of Administration

Drugs administered into the gastrointestinal tract go through the portal circulation to the liver. In the liver, opioids are extensively metabolized ("first-pass" metabolism) to inactive products. Therefore, most of the oral dose never reaches the target receptor. The amount of active medication that is available after first-pass metabolism varies greatly among agents. Generally, the oral to parenteral potency ratio for morphine is 1:6 for acute use and 1:2-3 for chronic use.

Several compounds have sustained-release preparations, including morphine and oxycodone. It remains a challenge to develop oral agents that can maintain a stable blood level over time. Factors such as eating and physical activity may also alter a sustained-release drug's kinetics.

Many methods of administration can circumvent the gastrointestinal tract. Some, such as sublingual, rectal, and transnasal administration, are potentially helpful but rarely used in the United States. Intramuscular (IM) administration is common; however, the pharmacokinetics of IM injections are unpredictable and the method can be painful. Therefore, IM administration should be avoided when another method is available. Subcutaneous administration is also common, but the pharmacokinetics are not well understood. This route of administration is becoming more compelling with the development of portable pumps that can deliver continuous infusions. The delivery of opioids in a transdermal patch offers another method of continuous analgesia. Fentanyl is available in this formulation. Its peak serum concentration remains relatively constant for 3 days. Transdermal fentanyl is a popular choice for ambulatory chronic pain patients.

Intravenous (IV) administration remains the most rapid and effective means of delivering opioids to the systemic circulation. Generally reserved for acute pain treatment, it is occasionally given in long-term institutional or home care settings, in scheduled boluses or continuous infusion. Proper use of this method requires understanding the pharmacokinetics of a drug, to ensure that the drug is given frequently enough to keep the blood level above the MEC.

The direct administration of opioids to receptor sites is possible through intrathecal, epidural, and intracerebroventricular administration. Enthusiasm for this technique is tempered by the occurrence of severe delayed-onset respiratory depression, which occurs in perhaps 1 of 1,000 patients receiving epidural morphine.

Patient Contracts

The Federation of State Medical Boards of the United States (2004) has suggested that in cases where patients are prescribed long-term opioids, there be a written contract between the doctor and patient. Components of this contract should include outlining such provisions as drug testing, set amounts of medications and refills, and situations under which medications may be discontinued.

Adjunctive Medications

Opioids and NSAIDs are the most important pharmacologic options in pain management. However, opioids or NSAIDs remain inadequate, intolerable, or inappropriate for some patients.

Antidepressants

Antidepressants are the most commonly used adjunctive agents. They have become common in the treatment of certain types of pain.

Various explanatory mechanisms for their analgesic effect have been suggested. Monoamine neurotransmitters, such as norepinephrine and serotonin, may influence the transmission of pain. This influence is thought to be a central phenomenon. However, sympathetic neurons are located near nociceptors and may play a role in peripheral pain modulation.

Most data suggest that antidepressants have independent analgesic effects. In addition, many studies suggest that effective analgesic doses for antidepressants are much less than those used for depression.

Antidepressants are most frequently used for neuropathies, such as those caused by diabetes mellitus. They have also been shown useful for treating migraine headaches. Beyond that, there are isolated accounts of their use in almost every pain imaginable.

It appears that the best antidepressants for pain treatment are those that act on both norepinephrine and serotonin, such as many of the tricyclic antidepressants, venlafaxine, and duloxetine. In one comparison of several antidepressants in patients with diabetic neuropathies (Max et al., 1992), the tricyclic antidepressants amitriptyline and desipramine were superior to both fluoxetine and placebo.

More recently, investigators have looked at duloxetine, a serotonin-norepinephrine reuptake inhibitor (SNRI). Duloxetine has the potential benefit of being both a serotononergic and noradrenergic agonist without having the side effect profile of tricyclic antidepressants. It has been successfully used for a number of chronic pain disorders, including diabetic peripheral neuropathic pain and fibromyalgia pain (Perahia et al., 2006).

Anticonvulsants

Anticonvulsants are also used for neuropathic pain. Several are approved by the Food and Drug Administration for pain management, including carbamazepine for trigeminal neuralgia and gabapentin for postherpetic neuralgia. There is good evidence to support the use of carbamazepine, gabapentin, and pregabalin for diabetic neuropathy as well and preliminary evidence for lamotrigine (Vinik, 2005). Valproic acid and topiramate have not been as successful, and phenytoin may cause a peripheral neuropathy.

Anticonvulsants may act by suppressing neuronal firing in the area of damaged neurons. Usually, dosing is started slowly and gradually increased to minimize side effects, which commonly include dizziness, ataxia, drowsiness, blurred vision, and gastrointestinal irritation. Specific organ toxicities can present a problem: carbamazepine can cause bone marrow suppression, sodium valproate can cause liver toxicity, and both drugs require blood monitoring.

Local Analgesics

Lidocaine and 2-chlorprocaine are used for peripheral neuropathies and generally given intravenously. There is some suggestion that patients who describe their neuropathic pain as constant are more likely to benefit from these agents, whereas those with episodic pain benefit more from anticonvulsants.

Another locally acting agent is capsaicin, an alkaloid irritant derived from chili peppers. Its analgesic effect appears to relate to desensitization of the transient receptor potential vanilloid subfamily, member 1 (TRPV1) nociceptor (Knotkova et al., 2008). Capsaicin has been shown to be effective for a number of syndromes, including diabetic neuropathy, osteoarthritis, postherpetic neuralgia, and psoriasis. It is available as a cream that is applied topically to painful areas; however, this cream may have erratic skin absorption, and more potent patches as well as injectable forms of the substance are being developed.

Antihistamines

Antihistamines are probably weakly analgesic. Antihistamines such as hydroxyzine are sometimes used to potentiate the effects of opioids; however, they are more likely to add to opioid side effects, particularly sedation and confusion.

Antipsychotics

Although rarely used as single agents, antipsychotics are thought to potentiate the action of opioids. Most of the support for this is anecdotal. Antipsychotics may be useful for opioid-induced side effects, such as nausea and confusion.

Benzodiazepines

Benzodiazepines do not appear to have any analgesic properties; however, they may modify the affective experience of pain. They also act as muscle relaxants, which can be useful in musculoskeletal pain.

Stimulants

Stimulants include the amphetamines, caffeine, and cocaine. All act as sympathomimetics and can potentiate the action of opiates. It is not clear whether this effect is long term or short term. Amphetamines have been combined with opiates, and caffeine has been used to potentiate NSAIDs. An advantage of stimulants is that they often act quickly, and their efficacy can often be judged after only a few days.

Cannabinoids

A number of states have passed legislation removing state-level penalties for medically justified marijuana use. Chronic pain and arthritis are among the recognized indications for marijuana use in many of these states. Cannabinoids appear to have a moderate analgesic effect mediated by nonopioid receptors, and they have been shown to be effective in several types of chronic pain, including cancer and neuropathic pain. Some studies suggest that they can be effective for patients who are refractory to other analgesics (Ashton and Milligan, 2008). In the past, the negative side effect profile of these drugs has been emphasized; in reality, they are unlikely to be any more harmful than other available analgesics. Side effects include sedation, hypotension, and bradycardia, but the psychoactive effects limit the dose. An orally available cannabinoid (the synthetic cannabinoid dronabinol) is less potent and likely less effective for pain relief. The development of cannabinoid-like medications with improved therapeutic profiles would likely be of great benefit to chronic pain sufferers.

PROCEDURAL TREATMENTS

Nonsurgical Procedures

Cutaneous Stimulation

Cutaneous stimulation involves the application of heat, cold, or mechanical pressure to a superficial area. Heat may decrease pain through vasodilatation and reduction of joint stiffness.

Cold causes vasoconstriction and local hyperesthesia, which reduces inflammation in an affected area. Mechanical pressure is typified by massage, which can relax muscular aches.

Electrical Stimulation

The rationale for electrical stimulation to modulate pain is based on the gate theory of pain. Here, an electrical charge excites large peripheral fibers, and other nociceptive information is blocked in the process. Transcutaneous electrical nerve stimulation (TENS) uses low-intensity stimulation of muscle and skin in a particular segmental distribution. Dorsal column stimulation uses a high-frequency current over the dorsal spinal cord and has been useful in deafferentation pain syndromes.

Acupuncture

Theoretically, acupuncture analgesia is similar to electrical stimulation, except that manual stimulation is used. The stimulation is produced through rotation of small needles at certain body sites. The resulting sensation (*teh chi*) confers not only local analgesia but also a more generalized phenomenon. This generalized effect may result from stimulation of chemical modulators, although the actual mechanism of action remains poorly understood. Most studies investigating acupuncture suffer from methodological difficulties; however, there is strong evidence for the efficacy of acupuncture for dental pain and preliminary data for lower back pain, headache, and fibromyalgia (Sierpina and Frenkel, 2005).

Exercise

In cases of acute pain, immobilization is often needed. Prolonged immobilization, however, can cause joint contractures, muscle atrophy, and cardiovascular deconditioning and should be avoided whenever possible. Appropriate exercises depend on the specific injury or pathology and can range from passive motion and positional change to weight-bearing exercises and aerobic conditioning.

Surgical Treatment

Neural Blockade

Typically, nerve transmission to an area is blocked through injection of an agent. The injection sites can be around the peripheral nerves and somatic plexuses and at the dorsal roots. Short-acting agents (e.g., lidocaine) can be used for acute pain, whereas more permanent blockade (e.g., alcohol) is used for chronic pain. In the latter case, diagnostic blocks are done first, in which short-acting agents can help localize the pain pathway.

Surgical lesions can also be used to block a pain pathway permanently. Side effects of this treatment mainly result from the fact that it is not possible to isolate the pain fibers completely. Therefore, other motor and sensory information may be lost as well.

The efficacy of these treatments is unpredictable, and neuronal block is often unreliable in chronic pain situations. When weighing the above side effects against a questionable benefit, permanent neuronal block is not usually appropriate in chronic pain situations. It is also not appropriate for non-nociceptive pain, such as neuropathic pain. Neurodestructive techniques sometimes worsen neuropathic pain. Such techniques may be appropriate in cases where the life expectancy is short. Even then, it should only be considered when other approaches to pain management have been exhausted.

Prolotherapy

Prolotherapy is the injection of small amounts of irritants that cause local inflammatory responses and are thought to cause hypertrophy and strengthening of ligaments and tendons, ultimately relieving pain in the process. They have been used both in chronic musculoskeletal and arthritic pain, particularly with sports-related injuries. Most of the support for this treatment is from case reports and open trials, and the few randomized controlled trials performed have had conflicting results (Rabago et al., 2005).

PSYCHOLOGICAL TREATMENTS

Psychoeducation

Properly educating a patient about pain treatment can help make the patient an active participant in the pain management. Education can lessen potential misunderstandings. For example, patients may fear that they may become addicted to pain medication. Similarly, patients often believe that they should avoid pain medication until they can no longer bear their pain. Proper education can allay their fears about addiction and help them understand that their pain is better treated early than when it reaches peak intensity.

Hypnosis

It has been known for more than a century that hypnosis can help treat pain, but hypnosis remains an underused option for pain management. Hypnosis works through a combination of effects, including relaxation, distraction, and perceptual alteration. Most intriguing is the ability of hypnosis to alter perceptions. Most individuals can learn to alter their sensations somewhat, and this ability improves with practice. A patient will typically receive the suggestion that the pain is another sensation, such as the sense of warmth. An advantage of hypnosis is that, with training, patients can learn to hypnotize themselves.

Behavioral Treatment of Pain

Behavioral treatment of pain is derived from learning theory, in which most behavior is assumed to be learned through reinforcement. For pain treatment, the focus is on pain-related behaviors. The goal of treatment is to decrease the factors that are reinforcing such behaviors. A simple example is on hospital wards, where staff members pay more attention to patients with problems, thereby reinforcing the behavior.

Relaxation Training

Relaxation training, a simple behavioral technique, involves teaching patients to relax each of their muscle groups systematically. This can be useful in a variety of pain conditions, particularly where tension may play a role (e.g., tension headaches). Usually patients are also taught to imagine a pleasant scene. With practice, the patient can perform this technique without assistance.

Biofeedback

In biofeedback, imperceptible physiological responses are amplified and made accessible. Once made aware of these responses, an individual can attempt to modify them. For example, a patient with tension headaches might hear an audible electromyogram, representing the frequency of muscle contractions in selected muscle groups, and then learn to reduce such contractions.

Cognitive Behavioral Therapy

In cognitive behavioral therapy, the focus is on both pain behavior and the conscious thoughts that influence such behavior. The therapist thoroughly explores all aspects of the pain experience: thoughts and feelings preceding, accompanying, and following the experience. The goal is not so much to eliminate pain as it is to lessen the disability associated with the pain. Given the complexity of the pain experience and biopsychosocial interactions, it is not unusual for patients to perceive some lessening in pain intensity as well.

Many studies have documented the efficacy of cognitive behavioral therapy for pain. Although they differ widely in methodology, patient selection, and outcome measures, certain themes seem to emerge from these studies. The treatment can have an effect on both the perception of pain and on functional outcome. Individual response varies widely. Negative predictors of outcome include high levels of distress, whereas positive predictors include comparatively low negative emotional responses to pain, low perceptions of disability, and higher motivation and orientation toward self-management strategies (McCracken and Turk, 2002).

MULTIDISCIPLINARY PAIN REHABILITATION

Perhaps the best treatment for chronic pain is given by a multidisciplinary group, as opposed to the traditional medical system, in which different consultants act in relative isolation from each other and the primary medical doctor. A multidisciplinary rehabilitation program employs professionals from various disciplines working in tandem. The goals of treatment are usually multiple as well, simultaneously including decreasing pain intensity and use of medication and medical services and increasing activity level. Such a program is expensive, although it may be cost effective when compared with traditional medical/surgical interventions and diagnostic procedures.

SOME SPECIFIC PAIN SITUATIONS

Pain, Mood, and Anxiety

The relationship between pain and depression is complicated, and each can affect the other. In experimental conditions, participants who are depressed have a lower threshold for pain. In clinical situations, approximately half of patients with depression report having physical pain (Katona et al., 2005). Reciprocally, many—perhaps most—patients with chronic pain have depression.

Pain and anxiety are also closely linked and correlate highly in both clinical and experimental settings. The question ultimately arises about whether this represents a mislabeling phenomenon, in which an individual cannot distinguish pain from anxiety. Some studies suggest a classical conditioning model in which pain becomes paired with anxiety. Anxiety can worsen pain, both through psychological mechanisms (e.g., worsening the context of the pain) and physical mechanisms (e.g., through increased muscle tension).

The clinician often confronts a situation involving the "chicken or the egg" dilemma in which it can be difficult to sort out whether the pain is the cause of the anxiety or depression or *vice versa*. It is usually not productive to try to sort this out. Instead, the clinician should identify signs and symptoms of significant anxiety or depression and explain to the patient (and staff) that psychological distress and pain often coexist in a feedback loop in which they reinforce each other. The clinical strategy is to intervene in both areas: treat the physical basis for the pain as aggressively as possible and simultaneously address the anxiety or depression.

Pain in Children

Pain syndromes have long been recognized in children, but little attempt has been made to study pain in children. Nonspecific limb and muscle aches—"growing pains"—are common and usually do not reach medical attention. The most common pain complaint in children is probably that of headaches. Also common is recurrent abdominal pain (RAP), defined as three or more episodes of pain that is severe enough to affect activities and that occurs for longer than 3 months. The vast majority of these cases have no identifiable pathology and are caused by problems with normal physiological functioning (e.g., stool retention). They often relate to stressful life events, such as family pathology. With or without clear family pathology, treatment of childhood pain syndromes involves a psychosocial approach that must include the family.

Nonmalignant Chronic Pain

Nonmalignant chronic pain may affect more than 50 million people in the United States and cost billions of dollars in lost productivity. In many cases, the cause of the pain is unclear, or the pathology, if identified, seems inadequate to explain the level of disability caused by the pain. Clinicians often expect direct associations between physical pathology and reports of pain. Unfortunately, pain is not that simple. Often a clear pathology causing pain cannot be demonstrated. Some of this may represent limitations in technology. Even when pathology is proved, it often correlates poorly with pain reports: for example, lower back pain seems to correlate poorly with the degree of degenerative disc disease.

Should clinicians use opioids to treat chronic pain? Opinions range from complaints that opioids are underused to statements that they are completely inappropriate. Some of this controversy may be due to patient populations: clinicians in specialty pain clinics are often more critical of opioid use than those in cancer pain centers. There is little doubt now that in the treatment of cancer pain, opioids have an important role; therefore, much of the controversy now revolves around chronic, noncancerous pain.

Beyond moral or ethical issues, the clinician first should consider whether opioids are efficacious for chronic, noncancerous pain. Unfortunately, to date, there are limited data to guide this decision. In general, the data are strongest for the treatment of chronic pain of nociceptive origin, as in osteoarthritis and other musculoskeletal conditions (Nicholson and Passik, 2007). However, even in these cases, the data are mixed: In a meta-analysis of studies examining the treatment of chronic lower back pain (Martell et al., 2007), it was found that opioids were only helpful for short-term treatment; the data for long-term treatment were too inconsistent to support any statement of efficacy. The long-term use of opioids for chronic arthritis sufferers remains controversial as well, although existing data, including several studies with good methodology, suggest that opioid treatment consistently provides effective pain relief with only minimal side effects and a low abuse potential (Bloodworth, 2005).

The data are more mixed for neurologic and other non-nociceptive sources of pain. One study (Rowbotham et al., 2003) compared the use of low- and high-dose levorphanol in the treatment of neuropathic pain. It not only found that the higher-dosed patient had greater improvement in pain relief but also had more side effects and no improvement in other outcome measures (quality of life, psychological and cognitive functioning). Furlan et al. (2006), in a meta-analysis of 41 randomized studies involving >6,000 patients with various types of chronic, noncancerous pain, found that opioids were preferable to placebo in improving both pain and function for these patients. When compared with other medications, high-potency opioids provided better pain relief than nonsteroidal analgesics and antidepressants; however, patients treated with the latter two medications appeared to have better functional outcome. This last finding was based mostly on a single study that compared dextropropoxyphene, a weak opioid, with diclofenac.

It seems safe to say that the further the patient is from nociceptive pain, the more controversial treatment with opioids becomes. At the same time, most types of pain have at least some evidence for the use of opioids. In neuropathic pain, the strategy is generally to first use nonopioid medications for prophylaxis, reserving opioids for crisis management or poor response to other treatments (Harden, 2005).

Many of the studies cited above report high dropout rates, suggesting that patients find the drugs inadequately effective or the side effects too unpleasant to justify continuing in the studies.

Pain Treatment in the Patient Addicted to Opioids

In situations involving acute pain treatment in the patient with narcotic addiction, it is often helpful to keep the management of the addiction separate from the management of the pain. For example, the patient's underlying narcotic addiction can be managed with methadone. Most street addicts can be adequately managed on an oral dose of methadone between 20 and 40 mg

PAIN DISORDER ASSOCIATED WITH A GENERAL MEDICAL CONDITION

A 54-year-old man began having back pain while lifting a heavy box at work. Several reparative surgeries did not help his pain, and he refused further surgical intervention. His primary care doctor prescribed p.r.n. hydrocodone with acetaminophen, not to exceed three tablets per day, but became alarmed when the patient exceeded his dose and sent him for psychiatric evaluation of a presumed addiction. The patient told the psychiatrist he did indeed use extra medication because the prescribed dose wore off too quickly. He admitted to frustration over his continued pain and anger at his doctor but denied other psychiatric symptoms. A regimen of controlled release oxycodone was begun. After 1 week, the patient reported partial improvement. A dose increase gave greater relief, but the patient complained of feeling "drugged," and the dose was lowered. He reported satisfactory improvement, saying, "The pain is still there, but at least I can play with my kids." Soon after, he returned to work on the stipulation that he not be required to do heavy lifting.

per day (or an IM dose between 10 and 20 mg per day). With methadone used for maintenance of the underlying addiction, the pain can then be treated as a separate issue, using a different narcotic at doses 50% greater than normal.

More controversial is the use of long-term opioid pain management in patients with concurrent addiction. Although many physicians may be understandably apprehensive about treating such patients, it does not follow that such apprehension can be the only factor in deciding the appropriate treatment for a patient. As already discussed in this chapter, pain relief has moved from being thought of as good clinical practice to a fundamental human right, and it seems antithetical to principles of humanistic medicine to deny patients this right if they have an addiction.

In treating patients with concomitant chronic pain and addiction, certain caveats must apply. The patient should concurrently be in treatment for the addiction as a way to maintain abstinence, and such treatment is likely to include regular attendance at a support group such as Narcotics or Alcoholics Anonymous. Furthermore, a system of monitoring should be in place to identify early signs of relapse, with the specifics specified in a written contract of treatment (Weaver and Schnoll, 2007).

Every effort should be made to obtain proper addiction treatment for patients currently using illicit substances or for those who have a relapse. However, treatment of pain with controlled substances cannot continue in patients who refuse or fail addiction treatments. The reason for this refusal to prescribe opioids is not that the patient no longer "deserves" the treatment but that the treatment is almost sure to fail in a patient who is actively abusing substances, and the risks of supporting the addiction outweigh any potential gain in pain relief.

Pain Management in the Palliative Care Setting

Palliative care is a specialized medical treatment that focuses on *palliating*, or alleviating, symptoms (Morrison and Meier, 2004). As such, the goal is comfort more than cure. It is usually intended for those at imminent risk of dying but may also be appropriate for those with advanced chronic disease. Although frequently associated with hospice, the two are distinct concepts: hospice refers to the care of dying patients, as well as the site at which that care takes place. Palliative care, with its emphasis on providing comfort, is an important part of hospice care.

Pain management is central to palliative care. The principles of pain management emphasized by palliative care specialists are similar to those discussed elsewhere in the chapter: proper assessment of pain, proper use of nonpharmacologic techniques, appropriate use of pharmacologic analgesia, and anticipating and minimizing the side effects of analgesia.

Although the principles are the same, the practice is often different. In the palliative care setting, treatment decisions require greater speed, the management of side effects is more difficult, and the need to give proper relief of symptoms is more urgent. As such, treatment is a group effort, and a multidisciplinary approach, as discussed earlier, is even more important.

The Role of the Psychiatrist in Pain Management

Usually, psychiatrists are called in around conceptual crises in which the patient is seen as a "problem." The patient may be perceived as drug seeking, or the clinicians may have decided that the pain is "just in the patient's head." Even in the face of clear physical pathology, clinicians are often inclined to interpret complex pain as being "out of proportion for the pathology."

In addressing a pain problem, the psychiatrist should always try to decide whether the pain has been adequately assessed and categorized. Psychiatric consultation is commonly requested for a patient whose pain problem has exhausted other providers. Such situations are common with patients who have low back pain and are admitted for a myelogram that is read as questionable or negative or with patients who have chronic abdominal pain, multiple surgeries, and "million-dollar" workups. Medical patients and providers are used to thinking of pain in terms of an acute paradigm (i.e., "What can be done now?") and often overlook the broader picture, that what they are seeing is better conceptualized as a chronic pain syndrome. Instead of more diagnostic testing or battles over drugs or doses, a shift in management philosophy is required. Although the ability to view a patient from a holistic perspective is not limited to psychiatry, the psychiatrist has special expertise in this area. In that sense, the psychiatrist's role is not merely to recognize the psychiatric aspects of pain but to help offer a broader perspective of the patient with chronic pain.

CONCLUSION

Pain is complex, transmitted by multiple pathways, many of which are bidirectional, and modulated at various levels of the brain. It should be no surprise that pain is different from other senses and that its evaluation and management are difficult. This should not invite nihilism. There have been great strides in the evaluation and management of pain. In many cases, patients can be freed of their pain altogether, and in most cases, at least some relief is possible. This is important, because relief from suffering is a fundamental role of physicians, and appropriate pain relief is a right of patients.

Nevertheless, challenges remain, such as treating non-nociceptive pain and determining when opioid medications are appropriate. Opioids remain the most powerful analgesic in the physician's armamentarium, but some types of pain do not respond well to them, they have significant side effects, and addiction remains a concern for most physicians. Choosing the appropriate treatment for patients at high risk for addiction is one of the more controversial areas in clinical medicine. Some guidelines for approaching such patients are given in this chapter, but the decision to use opioids requires comparing risks against benefits. As Turk (1996) suggests, we must ask ourselves, "How much suffering are we willing to accept to prevent what amount of abuse and negative side effects?"

Clinical Pearls

- Pain is subjective. A lack of objective findings is not by itself a reason not to treat a patient's complaint of pain.
- Adequate relief of pain is a fundamental human right.
- A comprehensive assessment is necessary. Consider not only intensity but also other dimensions of the pain experience, such as the course of the pain, affective response to pain, psychological factors, and beliefs about the pain.
- True "psychogenic" pain is probably very rare and should never be assumed without overwhelming supportive evidence.
- When approaching long-term pharmacologic treatment, use the WHO Pain Ladder as a guideline, beginning with lower potency agents and increasing as needed for adequate pain relief.
- When analgesics prove inadequate, consider adjunctive treatment, including antidepressants and anticonvulsants.
- For neuropathic and other non-nociceptive pain, consider adjunctive medication earlier in the treatment, possibly as first-line treatment.
- Anticipate the side effects of opioids. Constipation is usually present in patients who use them, and an appropriate bowel regimen should be part of the treatment.
- Fixed-dose regimens are preferable to as-needed regimens.
- Avoid partial agonists, agonist-antagonists, and meperidine.

Self-Assessment Questions and Answers

25-1. Mr. Smith is a 32-year-old man with a history of chronic pain for 2 years after a fall from a ladder. For this pain, he has taken consistently for the last 2 years the prescribed opioid oxycodone controlled release 20 mg twice a day. He was content with this dose but then noticed that the pain seemed much worse and that the oxycodone was not working as well. He began taking an extra dose each day, which seemed to help his pain more. However, he ran out of his oxycodone early, and when he called his doctor to explain, the doctor refused to refill the prescription.

He presents to the emergency room after awaking in the night, shivering and feeling anxious and sick to his stomach. On examination, he is noted to have gooseflesh and dilated pupils. He is sweating and appears very uncomfortable. He says that he regrets taking the extra medication, but "my pain was getting intolerable." He denies ever feeling high on his medication or taking the medication for any reason besides pain: "I just need to be able to function, or I will lose my job." He says that he and his doctor had never discussed the procedures for altering his dose, nor the ramifications should he fail his regimen.

Mr. Smith's need to take additional oxycodone is an example of which of the following?

A. Abuse
B. Craving
C. Dependence
D. Tolerance
E. Withdrawal

Physical dependence and tolerance are common results of long-term opioid use. Addiction is not and requires evidence of craving and inappropriate use (i.e., for psychogenic rather than therapeutic effects). The only sign of inappropriate use is that Mr. Smith used more medication than that prescribed, causing him to run out early. Although of concern, this alone is not sufficient to make a diagnosis of addiction, particularly when a more likely explanation is that the patient has become too tolerant of the current dose, after 2 years of continuous use.

It may be appropriate at this point to increase the patient's dose. However, for the future, the physician should create an explicit written contract with the patient to make clear both acceptable and unacceptable behaviors and the appropriate actions the patient can take should his pain worsen. *Answer: D*

25-2. Ms. Jones, a 68-year-old woman with a history of diabetes, has begun to notice pain in her lower extremities. She describes severe burning sensations in both soles of her feet, which worsen at night and disturb her sleep. On physical examination, her skin on both feet is hypersensitive to touch and pressure. Which of the following medications is best indicated for her complaint?

A. Citalopram
B. Gabapentin
C. Lorazepam
D. Meperidine
E. Phenytoin

Ms. Jones most likely has symptoms of painful diabetic neuropathy. Among the choices, gabapentin has the best evidence for use in diabetic neuropathy. It should be noted that citalopram and lorazepam have little support for an analgesic effect, phenytoin can worsen neuropathies, and meperidine is not recommended for chronic pain. *Answer: B*

25-3. Among the antidepressants, which of the following has the best evidence to support its use as an analgesic?

A. Amitriptyline
B. Bupropion
C. Fluoxetine
D. Mirtazapine
E. Venlafaxine

Among the antidepressants, those that act on norepinephrine and serotonin appear to be the most efficacious for pain. Amitriptyline and venlafaxine both act to inhibit norepinephrine and serotonin reuptake; of the two, amitriptyline has much more evidence of an analgesic effect. *Answer: A*

25-4. Which of the following scales would be most appropriate to use when assessing pain in a 5-year-old child?

A. Descriptor Differential Scale
B. FACES scale
C. 100 mm line
D. Pain perception profile
E. Unmet analgesic needs scale

Nonverbal scales such as the FACES scale, which shows pictures of increasingly distressed faces, are preferred in assessing pain in children. *Answer: B*

25-5. A 56-year-old man sustains a back injury after falling from a ladder. He undergoes a laminectomy but continues to have back pain following the surgery. He describes the pain as sharp, stabbing, and localized to his lower back. He takes ibuprofen 800 mg four times a day, which gives only partial relief of his symptoms. He expresses frustration and some depression over being unable to return to work. Which of the following treatments would most likely give the patient improved pain relief?

A. Hydrocodone
B. Hydroxyzine
C. Prolotherapy
D. Topiramate
E. Transcutaneous electrical nerve stimulation

Although originally developed for cancer pain, the WHO Pain Ladder provides a useful guideline in treating chronic pain of other causes. In this case, the patient has pain following a back injury. It is common for surgical intervention to restore function but not relieve pain. For such pain, presumably of nociceptive origin, opioid medication is most likely to provide relief. Of the other choices, transcutaneous electrical nerve stimulation (TENS) is a possible nonsurgical option. Prolotherapy has primarily anecdotal evidence. Topiramate may have a role in neuropathic pain, and hydroxyzine has at best weak analgesic properties. *Answer: A*

References

American Psychiatric Association. Task Force on Nomenclature and Statistics. *Diagnostic and statistical manual of mental disorders*. Washington, DC: American Psychiatric Association; 1980.

American Psychiatric Association. Work Group to Revise DSM-III. *Diagnostic and statistical manual of mental disorders: DSM-III-R*. Washington, DC: American Psychiatric Association; 1987.

American Psychiatric Association. Task Force on DSM-IV. *Diagnostic and statistical manual of mental disorders: DSM-IV*. Washington, DC: American Psychiatric Association; 1994.

American Psychiatric Association. *Diagnostic and statistical manual of mental disorders*, 4th ed, text revision. Washington, DC: American Psychiatric Association; 2000.

Ashton JC, Milligan ED. Cannabinoids for the treatment of neuropathic pain: Clinical evidence. *Curr Opin Investig Drugs*. 2008;9:65–75.

Bloodworth D. Issues in opioid management. *Am J Phys Med Rehabil*. 2005;84:S42–S55.

Boland RJ. How could the validity of the DSM-IV pain disorder be improved in reference to the concept that it is supposed to identify? *Curr Pain Headache Rep*. 2002;6:23–29.

Brennan F, Carr DB, Cousins M. Pain management: A fundamental human right. *Anesth Analg*. 2007; 105:205–221.

Dihle A, Helseth S, Kongsgaard UE, et al. Using the American Pain Society's patient outcome questionnaire to evaluate the quality of postoperative pain management in a sample of Norwegian patients. *J Pain*. 2006;7:272–280.

Federation of State Medical Boards of the United States. *Model policy for the use of controlled substances for the treatment of pain*. Dallas, TX: Federation of State Medical Boards of the United States; 2004.

Furlan AD, Sandoval JA, Mailis-Gagnon A, et al. Opioids for chronic noncancer pain: A meta-analysis of effectiveness and side effects. *CMAJ*. 2006;174:1589–1594.

Harden RN. Pharmacotherapy of complex regional pain syndrome. *Am J Phys Med Rehabil*. 2005; 84:S17–S28.

Katona C, Peveler R, Dowrick C, et al. Pain symptoms in depression: Definition and clinical significance. *Clin Med*. 2005;5:390–395.

Knotkova H, Pappagallo M, Szallasi A. Capsaicin (TRPV1 Agonist) therapy for pain relief: Farewell or revival? *Clin J Pain*. 2008;24:142–154.

Martell BA, O'Connor PG, Kerns RD, et al. Systematic review: Opioid treatment for chronic back pain: Prevalence, efficacy, and association with addiction. *Ann Intern Med*. 2007;146:116–127.

Max MB, Lynch SA, Muir J, et al. Effects of desipramine, amitriptyline, and fluoxetine on pain in diabetic neuropathy. *N Engl J Med*. 1992;326:1250–1256.

McCracken LM, Turk DC. Behavioral and cognitive-behavioral treatment for chronic pain: Outcome, predictors of outcome, and treatment process. *Spine*. 2002;27:2564–2573.

Melzack R. The McGill pain questionnaire: From description to measurement. *Anesthesiology*. 2005; 103:199–202.

Morrison RS, Meier DE. Clinical practice. Palliative care. *N Engl J Med*. 2004;350:2582–2590.

Nicholson B, Passik SD. Management of chronic noncancer pain in the primary care setting. *South Med J*. 2007;100:1028–1036.

Osterweis M, Kleinman A, Mechanic D. *Pain and disability: Clinical, behavioral, and public policy perspectives*. Washington, DC: National Academy Press; 1987.

Perahia DG, Pritchett YL, Desaiah D, et al. Efficacy of duloxetine in painful symptoms: An analgesic or antidepressant effect? *Int Clin Psychopharmacol*. 2006;21:311–317.

Porter J, Jick H. Addiction rare in patients treated with narcotics. *N Engl J Med*. 1980;302:123.

Rabago D, Best TM, Beamsley M, et al. A systematic review of prolotherapy for chronic musculoskeletal pain. *Clin J Sport Med*. 2005;15:376–380.

Rowbotham MC, Twilling L, Davies PS, et al. Oral opioid therapy for chronic peripheral and central neuropathic pain. *N Engl J Med*. 2003;348:1223–1232.

Sherman S, Lehman GA. Opioids and the sphincter of Oddi. *Gastrointest Endosc*. 1994;40:105–106.

Sierpina VS, Frenkel MA. Acupuncture: A clinical review. *South Med J*. 2005;98:330–337.

Turk DC. Clinicians' attitudes about prolonged use of opioids and the issue of patient heterogeneity. *J Pain Symptom Manage*. 1996;11:218–230.

Vinik A. Clinical Review: Use of antiepileptic drugs in the treatment of chronic painful diabetic neuropathy. *J Clin Endocrinol Metab.* 2005;90:4936–4945.

Walsh CA, Jamieson E, Macmillan H, et al. Child abuse and chronic pain in a community survey of women. *J Interpers Violence.* 2007;22:1536–1554.

Weaver M, Schnoll S. Addiction issues in prescribing opioids for chronic nonmalignant pain. *J Addict Dis.* 2007;1:2–10.

Wong DL, Baker CM. Pain in children: Comparison of assessment scales. *Pediatr Nurs.* 1988;14:9–17.

CHAPTER 26

Brian D. Smith and Madhvi Phadtare Richards

Therapeutic Response to Psychiatric Emergencies

Psychiatric emergencies are changes in mood, behavior, or thought that acutely threaten someone's life or health. They may arise in the context of a psychiatric or medical illness, drug intoxication or withdrawal, or an adverse drug reaction (Roy and Fauman, 2004). They are not only seen in the psychiatric emergency room (ER) but also very commonly in the general emergency department, where ideally a psychiatrist should be consulted.

EPIDEMIOLOGY

Men and women are seen equally in the psychiatric ER and single persons more than married. Approximately 20% of these patients are suicidal and about 10% are violent. Patients also frequently present with anxiety or psychosis. The diagnostic groups often seen are mood disorders, schizophrenia, panic disorders, and alcohol dependence. Approximately 40% of such patients require hospitalization (Sadock and Sadock, 2003).

THE EVALUATION PROCESS

In a psychiatric emergency, the goals of the evaluation are to identify a tentative diagnosis, provide emergency treatment, and arrange for appropriate disposition (Piechniczek-Buczek, 2006). (See Chapter 4 for more on the differential diagnosis of mental illness.) It is very important to consider the various possible organic etiologies for the presenting symptoms, particularly among the geriatric population. There should be greater concern for an underlying medical condition with acute onset of psychiatric symptoms in patients older than 45 years, known medical illness, perceptual disturbances other than auditory hallucinations, neurologic symptoms, and cognitive impairment (Meyers and Stein, 2000). Acute onset is often indicative of delirium, especially with fluctuating sensorium, including impaired alertness, thinking, memory, perception, concentration, attention, and disorientation. Delirium is usually a reversible disturbance of cerebral functioning caused by a toxic, neurologic, or metabolic insult (Dubin, 1998). (See Chapter 8 for additional information regarding delirium and other disorders associated with cognitive impairment.)

Organic etiologies include not only medical disorders but also various medication-related adverse effects or substance intoxication or withdrawal. (See Chapter 9 for additional information regarding substance-related disorders). Neuroleptic malignant syndrome (NMS) is a rare, but sometimes fatal, psychiatric emergency most often caused by exposure to neuroleptic drugs. The patient often presents with the clinical triad of alteration in mental status, autonomic instability, and rigidity. Treatment involves stopping the offending agent, supportive therapies such as rehydration and restoring electrolyte balance, and sometimes pharmacotherapy (most often dopamine agonists) or electroconvulsive therapy (Kipps et al., 2005). (See Chapter 22 for more on psychopharmacological therapies, including NMS.)

Once organic etiologies have been ruled out, the clinician can proceed with treatment options for the psychiatric disorder as the primary diagnosis, typically referred to as *medical clearance*, which includes a thorough history, physical examination, laboratory evaluation, and other ancillary testing at times (Williams and Shepherd, 2000). (See Chapter 5 for additional information on neuroimaging and laboratory evaluation.)

In this chapter, the most common presentations of psychiatric emergencies, namely, aggression/agitation and suicide risk, will be reviewed in greater depth. The most frequent presentation to a psychiatric emergency setting is agitation followed by suicidal or assaultive threats or behavior.

AGGRESSION/AGITATION

Aggression has been defined as "forceful, goal-directed action that may be verbal or physical; the motor counterpart of the affect of rage, anger, or hostility" (Sadock and Sadock, 2004, p. 282). Most studies tend to use *aggression* and *violence* as synonyms.

Agitation is defined as an excessive motor or verbal activity and exemplified by hyperactivity, assaultiveness, verbal abuse, threatening gestures, physical destructiveness, vocal outbursts, and excessive verbalization of distress (Piechniczek-Buczek, 2006).

Agitation and/or aggression can be seen in patients with traumatic brain injuries, cerebral infections, metabolic diseases, drug intoxication (especially from phencyclidine [PCP], cocaine, amphetamines, and alcohol), drug withdrawal (especially from cocaine, opioids, and alcohol), side effects of medication (such as steroids), personality disorders, developmental disabilities, dementia, delirium, bipolar affective disorders, and schizophrenia (most often with acute psychosis) (Rocca et al., 2006).

Demographics

Violent patients are definitely not a homogeneous group. In general, though, "the best predictors of potential violent behavior are excessive alcohol intake, a history of violent acts with arrests or criminal activity, and a history of childhood abuse" (Sadock and Sadock, 2004, p. 904). While assessing for risk of violence among psychiatric patients, the clinician should consider some additional factors as shown in Table 26-1 (Rocca et al., 2006).

Neurobiology

Various neurotransmitters have been considered to explain the origin of aggression and impulsivity, including serotonin, norepinephrine, dopamine, and γ-aminobutyric acid (GABA). Aggression and impulsivity may result from a failure of the balance between dopamine and serotonin. Dopamine plays a strong role in activation and initiation of behavior, and serotonin plays a role in inhibitory control. In addition, impulsivity may be caused by changes in noradrenergic activity associated with stress and overstimulation. The balance between excitatory (glutamate) and inhibitory (GABA) amino acid function has an important role in the level of arousal as well (Davidson et al., 2000; Krakowski, 2003; Lesch and Merschdorf, 2000; Rocca et al., 2006; Swann, 2003; Yildiz et al., 2003).

Evaluation

The evaluation of an agitated/aggressive patient can be quite difficult and should be performed with caution. Here are some considerations.

TABLE 26-1	Risk Factors for Violence
Demographics	Male, age between 15 and 25 years, lower socioeconomic status, uneducated, unemployed, lack of social support system
Past history	History of childhood abuse (physical, sexual), childhood exposure to violence, history of substance abuse, head injury, history of being violent in the past
Diagnostic groups	Organic brain disorder, personality disorder, psychosis, substance abuse (intoxication/withdrawal)
Clinical features	Command auditory hallucinations, paranoid delusions, poor impulse control, nonadherence with treatment, low IQ, low frustration tolerance, low self-esteem, irritability

IQ, intelligence quotient.

Setting

One must consider the optimal setting that would best serve both the clinician and the patient from the standpoint of safety and preventing any further escalation, such as a big and quiet room that is easily accessible by other staff if needed. Security staff should be on hand. Ideally the room would have an emergency call button; alternatively, the clinician may carry a personal alarm. The clinician must sit between the patient and the door to ensure easy exit from the room if needed. ER staff and physicians should be trained in safe interventions with agitated patients.

Approach

Maintaining a very calm and neutral approach toward the violent patient is essential. Talking down the patient may de-escalate the situation and eliminate the need for any forceful form of intervention. A clinician must never interview an armed patient. Many emergency departments scan patients for weapons. Explaining to the patient that he or she is in a safe setting that does not require weapons for protection may also be helpful. Additional pointers on how to approach a potentially violent patient are summarized in Table 26-2 (Rocca et al., 2006).

Signs of Imminent Danger

Typically, violent behavior follows a preliminary period in which early signs may predict imminent danger, such as tense posture, clenched fist or jaw, answering questions with an increase in irritable tone, yelling, cursing, and open hostility toward the clinician. If the patient appears about to lose control, it may be beneficial to acknowledge this and explain what intervention will be done to ensure everyone's safety (Rocca et al., 2006). If the patient were to make threats toward a third party, the clinician has the duty to protect and/or warn the third party. (The Tarasoff rule and other psychiatric legal issues are discussed in greater depth in Chapter 2.)

Scales Used for Evaluating Agitation

Several scales have been used to help assess agitation or violence in a patient and most have been validated for use in patients with a psychiatric illness. Scales such as the Behavioral Activity Rating

TABLE 26-2 How to Approach the Potentially Violent Patient
Remain calm and nonjudgmental
Be empathic and validate the patient
Explicitly recognize the patient's emotional state, e.g., "You seem frustrated." "What is angering you?"
Introduce yourself and explain what you are going to do
Keep a distance and do not hover over the patient (agitated patients tend to need more room)
Avoid sustained eye contact
Offer something to eat or drink (preferably not hot beverages)
Never turn your back to the patient
If others are causing an escalation in the patient's agitation, have them leave the room
Help the patient understand what is happening and reassure the patient about diagnostic and therapeutic procedures
Encourage the verbal expression of feelings, which may release tension
Allow the patient to make his or her own decisions, within reason
At times, taking the patient's blood pressure or a physical examination may be calming
Discourage the patient from acting out by making it clear that he or she will be held responsible for his or her actions
Communicate your decision clearly and simply

A CASE OF AGITATION

A 25-year-old man with a history of auditory hallucinations, sometimes command in nature, and paranoid delusions as part of schizophrenia was seen standing outside of his house screaming that the neighbor was the devil. He had ingested four to five beers earlier in the day and had not taken his antipsychotic medication for the last week. He believes that his doctor is trying to poison and control him with the medication. The neighbor called the police, who in turn transported the patient in handcuffs to the emergency department. While there, the patient was agitated and pacing, mumbling to himself and looking at everyone with suspicion. When a nurse approached, he threatened to hurt her. The physician on duty ordered that he be given 2 mg of risperidone and 2 mg of lorazepam orally. At first he refused to take the medications, but after the physician explained the benefits of taking the medications orally versus intramuscularly, he finally agreed. Within 45 minutes, he was more calm and willing to be admitted to the inpatient psychiatric facility.

Scale (BARS), Overt Agitation Severity Scale (OASS), and Positive and Negative Syndrome Scale, Excited Component (PANSS-EC) are not diagnostic but can aid the evaluation (Battaglia et al., 2007).

The Management Process

With aggressive/agitated patients, always consider the least restrictive mode of intervention appropriate for the situation. The first step to contain agitation and aggression is the talk down process, which typically begins during the clinical interview and the evaluation (as mentioned earlier). If less restrictive interventions are not effective in stopping an aggressive patient, the clinician needs to consider a more restrictive line of management.

Show of Force

Having security or other staff back up clinicians as a show of force can help patients realize that they will be held responsible for their actions. Clinicians should make it clear to patients that the extra staff is there to help contain their aggression and protect others. The presence of added security also helps give the clinician the confidence to make the necessary management decisions (Rocca et al., 2006).

Pharmacologic Interventions

If nonpharmacologic methods fail to de-escalate an aggressive patient, the next treatment includes rapid tranquilization (RT), chemical measures for confining a patient's bodily movements, thereby preventing injury to self or others and reducing agitation (De Fruyt and Demyttenaere, 2004; Sailas and Fenton, 2000).

Medications used in rapid tranquilization include antipsychotics (typical and atypical) and benzodiazepines. The goal is behavioral control, not sedation. The patient should be calm enough that aggression toward others is averted and the evaluation can be successfully completed. In addition to targeting behavioral control, the clinician could attempt to target the underlying illness as well, depending on the medication chosen (e.g., using an antipsychotic in an aggressive patient with a history of psychosis or using a benzodiazepine in an aggressive patient with drug withdrawal). Oral administration (tablet or liquid) of the medication should be offered first. If it is clear that the patient is unwilling to take the medication this way, involuntary administration intramuscularly or intravenously may be necessary. The clinician may be able to maintain some degree of an alliance with the patient by allowing him or her to take the medication voluntarily. The only clear advantage of intramuscular and intravenous medications is that they can be given involuntarily.

The effectiveness of antipsychotics and benzodiazepines alone and in combination has been confirmed with numerous studies. The most common combination includes haloperidol and lorazepam (De Fruyt and Demyttenaere, 2004; Sailas and Fenton, 2000). However, with the arrival and now established effectiveness of atypical antipsychotics, the combination of an atypical antipsychotic and a benzodiazepine is becoming more commonplace. The subsequent text describes some medications commonly utilized to target agitation and/or aggression.

Typical antipsychotics

High potency antipsychotics, such as haloperidol, used to be the most commonly used medications for treatment of aggression, especially in psychosis. These agents were preferred due to their efficacy, ease of use, and titration and their availability in the form of tablet, liquid, and intramuscular injections. However, with better tolerated alternative pharmacologic interventions, their use has become more limited due to a number of side effects, including extrapyramidal symptoms (tremor, akathisia, dystonia), hypotension, lowering of seizure threshold, and anticholinergic effects. In adults, 5 to 10 mg of haloperidol can be given orally or intramuscularly and repeated in 20- to 30-minute intervals until the patient is calm. With haloperidol there is some risk of QT prolongation, which may lead to sudden cardiac death. Droperidol had also become a standard form of emergency treatment for the aggressive patient. It resulted in more rapid control of the agitated patient than haloperidol. However, following several reports of death associated with QT prolongation and *torsade de pointes*, the U.S. Food and Drug Administration (FDA) mandated a black box warning (Rocca et al., 2006).

Atypical antipsychotics

Atypical antipsychotics, also known as *second generation antipsychotics*, have become progressively more common in the ER. They have a broader spectrum of action and lower rates of acute side effects, particularly lower risk of dystonic reactions. Given that these medications are much better tolerated by the patient, they are becoming the mainstay of treatment for aggression/agitation in the ER and are often given in combination with a benzodiazepine, such as lorazepam. Table 26-3 summarizes commonly used atypical antipsychotics.

Benzodiazepines

Benzodiazepines are often used as monotherapy or in combination with antipsychotics while treating aggression/agitation. Their side effect profile is relatively benign. Some of the short-term disadvantages include sedation, respiratory depression, and memory impairment. These medications tend to be the preferred choice when there are no data to support a provisional diagnosis, for agitation suspected from post-traumatic stress disorder, for agitation presumed to be secondary to a general medical condition, and most substance intoxication or withdrawal. They are given in combination with an antipsychotic in psychotic depression, schizophrenia, and mania. The most commonly used benzodiazepines in the ER are lorazepam (1 to 2 mg oral,

TABLE 26-3 Commonly Used Atypical Antipsychotics for Agitation and/or Aggression

Atypical Antipsychotic	Form	Typical mg per Dosage in the ER	Caution
Risperidone	Tablet/liquid/oral disintegrating/IM	1–2 mg (maximum of 8 mg/day)	Dystonic reaction
Olanzapine	Tablet/oral disintegrating/IM	5–10 mg (maximum of 30 mg/day)	When given in combination with lorazepam, there can be cardiorespiratory suppression
Ziprasidone	Oral/IM	20 mg PO/10–20 mg IM (maximum of 40 mg/day)	QTc interval prolongation
Aripiprazole	Tablet/liquid/oral disintegrating/IM	10–15 mg PO/9.75 mg IM (maximum of 30 mg/day)	Nausea, akathisia
Quetiapine	Oral	25–50 mg	Sedation

Lower doses should be considered in the elderly and the medically frail.

sublingual or IM/IV) and diazepam (5 to 10 mg oral or IM/IV) (Rocca et al., 2006). However, lorazepam and diazepam are both absorbed relatively slowly if given intramuscularly, and other routes or medications may be more appropriate for acutely agitated patients.

Physical Restraint and Seclusion

If less restrictive interventions are not effective in managing an aggressive patient, it may become necessary to use the most restrictive approach as a final response: physical restraint and/or seclusion. These have been defined by the Joint Commission on Accreditation of Healthcare Organizations (JCAHO) as follows:

> Restraint: Direct application of physical force to a patient, with or without the patient's permission, to restrict his or her freedom of movement. The physical force may be human, mechanical devices, or a combination thereof (Rocca et al., 2006, p. 591).
>
> Seclusion: involuntary confinement of a person alone in a locked room. The behavioral health care reasons for the use of restraint and seclusion are primarily to protect the patient against injury to self or others because of an emotional or behavior disorder (Rocca et al., 2006, p. 591).

In 2006 JCAHO attributed 153 deaths to seclusion and restraint in the United States, mostly due to asphyxiation (D'Orio, 2007). JCAHO and the Centers for Medicare and Medicaid Services (CMS) both mandated standards for seclusion and restraint as tools to reduce risk. The use of restraints must be performed by well-trained and experienced staff to avoid harming the staff and/or patient, including physical and psychological trauma or even death. Before attempting to restrain a patient, the patient must be told what is about to take place and given another chance to comply voluntarily (Currier and Allen, 2000). During the entire process of seclusion and restraint, every effort must be made to ensure the respect of the patient's rights, dignity, and privacy.

Table 26-4 describes the proper use of restraints, and Table 26-5 shows the advantages and disadvantages of RT versus physical restraint.

SUICIDE

Suicide risk assessment is a vital component of psychiatric emergency care. Suicide is a fatal, self-inflicted, destructive act with explicit or inferred intent to die. A suicide attempt occurs

TABLE 26-4 Proper Use of Restraints
A licensed independent practitioner may give the order for restraint
Inform the patient that he or she is about to be placed in restraints
Explain the reason for restraints to the patient
A minimum of four individuals are required to restrain the patient
Leather restraints are considered to be the safest form
Reassure the patient during the process
Patients are typically restrained with legs spread, one arm to one side and the other arm over the patient's head
Ensure that the patient's arm that is restrained to the side is positioned such that an intravenous line may be placed if needed
The patient's head is typically raised during the process of restraints
A physician must examine the patient within an hour of placement of restraints
The nursing staff must examine the patient every 15 minutes
In adults, an order for restraints is limited to 4 hours
Once the patient is calm, the first two restraints must be removed one at a time within 5 minutes of each other; the last two restraints are removed at the same time
A thorough documentation is necessary regarding reason for restraint, course of treatment, and the patient's response

TABLE 26-5	Rapid Tranquilization Versus Physical Restraint	
Rapid Tranquilization	**Physical Restraint**
Less restrictive	Much more restrictive
Less physically, and possibly emotionally, traumatic	Trauma/death may occur
Patients tend to prefer medication	Used as last resort
Side effects may occur	No medication side effects
May alter mental status, thereby making further evaluation difficult	This intervention may be discontinued without lingering side effects

when the act is nonfatal, and suicidal ideation involves thoughts of harming or killing oneself (Goldsmith et al., 2002; Mann and Currier, 2007; Roy and Fauman, 2004). Parasuicide involves acts of self-harm with nonlethal intent, such as superficial cutting or ingestion (American Academy of Child and Adolescent Psychiatry, 2001).

Epidemiology

Suicide is a major preventable public health problem. In 2004, it was the 11th leading cause of death in the United States, accounting for 32,439 deaths, and third for the 15- to 24-year-old age group. The overall rate was approximately 11 suicide deaths per 100,000 people (National Institute of Mental Health, 2007).

It is estimated that there are 25 suicide attempts for every death by suicide across all age groups (Mann and Currier, 2007). Rates are highest in the spring and, against popular myth, lower in the winter (Centers for Disease Control, 2007). It is estimated that 13.5% of the U.S. population will have suicidal ideation at some point in their lives, but <1% will kill themselves (Welton, 2007).

Suicide accounts for the largest number of malpractice suits against psychiatrists, even though it is well established that individual cases of suicide cannot be predicted (Rives, 1999; Simon and Shuman, 2006; Welton, 2007). Suicide is relatively rare, with a multitude of contributory factors, and trying to predict who is at risk of attempt or completion is daunting (Baldessarini et al., 1988; Mann and Currier, 2007). No suicide risk assessment model has been empirically tested for reliability and validity (Simon and Shuman, 2006). However, it is expected as the standard of care that an adequate suicide risk assessment be performed and documented and interventions enacted in accordance with the assessment.

Risk Factors

Suicide risk factors may be significant statistically and of limited help in planning interventions, but they are not specific to suicide completion when used for individual patients and lead to many false positives (Welton, 2007; Cooper et al., 2006). Suicide is a multidetermined act with psychiatric, social, psychological, biological, genetic, and physical risk factors. The stress-diathesis model can assist in explaining the interactions among these risk and protective factors. A set of enduring conditions or traits predisposes an individual to suicidal behavior when the individual encounters a stressor (Gould et al., 2003; Mann et al., 1999).

Risk factors may be divided into historical (i.e., static) and changeable (i.e., dynamic) personal variables. The clinician must carefully weigh both static and dynamic risks during the suicide assessment.

Static Risk Factors

Past attempts may be the best indicator of increased risk of suicide. When coupled with current suicidal ideation, past attempts are an even better predictor of imminent risk (Mann and Currier, 2007). One of every 100 survivors of suicide attempts will die by suicide within 1 year of the index attempt, a suicide risk approximately 100 times that of the general population. Approximately 10% of people who make a suicide attempt will eventually die by suicide (Hawton, 1992; Porter and Kaplan, 2005). The American Association of Suicidology Working Group also considers talking or writing about death, dying, or suicide a warning sign of the highest concern

(Rudd et al., 2006). Presenting with self-harm also increases the risk of suicide (Cooper et al., 2006). Of depressed patients who commit suicide, 40% have a history of previous attempts, and the risk of a second attempt is highest within 3 months of the first. However, for 60% to 80% of suicide victims, the first attempt is lethal (Rives, 1999). Other risk factors include histories of violent behavior and previous psychiatric hospitalization, especially the postdischarge period (Mann and Currier, 2007; Roy and Fauman, 2004).

Gender is another static risk factor. Men commit suicide more than four times as often as women. However, women attempt suicide three to four times as often as men. The highest rate of suicide attempts occurs in females aged 15 to 19 years (Centers for Disease Control, 2007; Mann and Currier, 2007). Men tend to choose more lethal means, such as firearms, with greater frequency than women, who are more likely to use such means as drug overdoses.

Ethnicity influences risk, with white males having the highest risk followed by American Indian and Native Alaskan men (Centers for Disease Control, 2007). Suicide rates among whites are approximately twice that of nonwhites. The suicide rate is also elevated for inner-city youth, along with immigrants.

Rates tend to increase with age. There is a significant increase in risk from childhood to adolescence/early adulthood (0.6 to 9.7 per 100,000 per year). Being older than age 45 and male are high-risk characteristics. Elderly white males aged 85 and older have the highest risk, at 16.9 per 100,000 per year (Welton, 2007), although psychiatric patients who commit suicide tend to be relatively young (Roy and Fauman, 2004).

Family history of suicide increases risk to roughly two to six times that of the general population (Cheng et al., 2000; Gould et al., 2003; Schulsinger et al., 1979). As an example, Margaux Hemingway's suicide was the fifth among four generations of the Ernest Hemingway family (Roy and Fauman, 2004). Research scientists are currently looking at candidate genes that may be associated with risk, including tryptophan hydroxylase, the serotonin transporter gene, and the serotonin receptor gene (Gould et al., 2003). Parental psychopathology, particularly depression and substance abuse, also increases the risk of suicide in offspring (Brent et al., 1994). Exposure to real or fictional accounts of suicide may also increase risk through contagion (the increased probability of an individual engaging in a behavior when exposed to others engaging in that same behavior) (American Academy of Child and Adolescent Psychiatry, 2001).

Life situation and stressful life events have a significant association with completed suicides. Most of these psychosocial stressors have to do with themes of loss: separation/divorce, job loss, legal troubles, bereavement (especially suicide-bereaved when identifying with the victim), financial pressures, recent migration (Cheng et al., 2000). Single persons have a suicide rate twice that of married persons. Divorced, separated, or widowed individuals have a rate four to five times higher than that of married persons. Unemployment constitutes a risk factor for suicide; however, higher social status also correlates with a greater risk of suicide, especially with a fall in social status. Lack of social support, including the warning sign of withdrawing from friends, is also of concern (Welton, 2007).

Additional static suicide risk factors include recent hospital discharge, a history of violent behavior, diverse sexual orientation (with a two- to six-fold increased risk of nonlethal suicidal behavior for homosexual and bisexual youths), and being a victim of abuse (Gould et al., 2003; Molnar et al., 2001).

Physicians are also at increased risk for suicide. Women physicians have a higher risk of suicide than other women (Roy and Fauman, 2004). Among the medical specialties, psychiatrists may have the greatest risk.

Dynamic Risk Factors

Psychopathology is found in >90% of completed suicides, and approximately half of completers had two or more axis I diagnoses and at least one diagnosis on axis III (Roy and Fauman, 2004). However, most patients who are at risk of suicide are unlikely to meet with mental health professionals and may present instead in the emergency department due to the stigma attached to mental health and substance abuse disorders or suicidal thoughts (Baldessarini et al., 2006; Centers for Disease Control, 2007).

Mood disorders have the highest risk of suicide of any other psychiatric or medical disorder, especially early in the course of bipolar disorder in the depressive or mixed states and recurrent unipolar depression severe enough to require hospitalization (Baldessarini et al., 2006). Mood disorders account for 45% of suicides, and approximately 10% of individuals with major depression commit suicide, compared to approximately 20% of bipolar individuals (Mann and Currier, 2007; Welton, 2007).

People with schizophrenia also have a high risk of suicide; 10% eventually commit suicide, with the greatest risk occurring during the first few years of the illness (Welton, 2007). Command hallucinations instructing the patient to commit suicide are particularly worrisome, with many individuals obeying command hallucinations to harm themselves. Eating disorders, particularly anorexia, increase suicide risk. Personality disorders (borderline and antisocial in particular, along with narcissistic injury) and sudden changes in personality are also risk factors. Axis II diagnoses are found in approximately one third of suicide completers.

Particular psychiatric presenting symptoms heighten the concern for suicide. Anxiety and/or agitation, especially panic attacks when comorbid with depression, are risk factors. Changes in sleeping patterns are worrisome (Rudd et al., 2006), and hopelessness has also been associated with all forms of suicidality (Beck et al., 1990).

Substance abuse is a significant contributor to completed suicide, with >20% of victims intoxicated at the time of death and half of suicide attempts involving intoxication. Alcohol-dependent persons account for 23% of suicides, with up to 15% of individuals with alcoholism committing suicide, a rate that is 50 times higher than that of the general population (Porter and Kaplan, 2005). Heroin addicts have 20 times the risk of the general population. Availability of lethal amounts of drugs, intravenous use, associated antisocial personality disorder, chaotic lifestyle, and impulsivity further heighten the suicide risk in substance abusers (Roy and Fauman, 2004). Substance use disorders are more often seen in suicide completers younger than age 30, whereas mood disorders are more often seen in completers older than age 30.

Physical illness, especially of a severe and chronic nature, also increases suicide risk and is often found in suicide completers older than age 30. The risk is especially marked with loss of mobility, disfigurement, and chronic intractable pain. Some conditions in particular carry significantly increased risk, including acquired immunodeficiency syndrome (AIDS), cancer, epilepsy, spinal cord injuries, head trauma, and Huntington chorea, for which a psychiatric evaluation is often required before a patient may undergo genetic testing (Stern et al., 1997).

Access to firearms is a significant risk factor—55% of suicides are committed with a firearm, making gunshot wounds the leading cause of completed suicide in both men and women (Centers for Disease Control, 2007; Gould et al., 2003; Rives, 1999). See Table 26-6 for a summary of static and dynamic risk factors for suicide.

TABLE 26-6 Static and Dynamic Risk Factors for Suicide	
Static Risk Factors	**Dynamic Risk Factors**
Past suicide attempt	Access to firearms
Past violent behavior	Psychopathology (mood disorders, acute anxiety,
Previous psychiatric hospitalizations (especially with	schizophrenia, eating disorders, substance abuse)
recent discharge)	Personality disorders (especially borderline)
Male gender	Physical illness (chronic pain, loss of mobility, dis-
White or American Indian	figurement, etc.)
Age 85 and older	
Family history of suicide	
Family history of depression, substance abuse	
Recent loss (separation, divorce, legal issues, bereave-	
ment, financial trouble, etc.)	
Single person	
Unemployment	
Lack of social support	
Victim of abuse	

Protective Factors

Family and community support, religions that discourage suicide (e.g., rates are lower among Jews and Catholics), skills in problem solving, effective clinical mental health care, and ongoing relationships with mental health and medical providers may prove protective against suicide (Centers for Disease Control, 2007).

The possibility of malingering should also be considered. Malingering is when the patient fabricates suicidality for primary gain. Patients who threaten suicide or exaggerate suicidal symptoms to gain hospital admission are more likely to be substance dependent, antisocial, homeless, unmarried, or in legal difficulty. Subsequent suicides are uncommon (Lambert and Bonner, 1996). Motives for feigning psychiatric disorders or conditions include the desire for food and shelter, financial gains, and avoidance of jail, work, or family.

Biological Factors

Evidence supports a link between central serotonin hypofunction/dysregulation and suicidality. Findings consistent with this link include low concentrations of metabolite 5-hydroxy-indoleacetic acid (5-HIAA) in lumbar cerebrospinal fluid (CSF), and reductions in the number and binding capacity of serotonin 1A receptors and serotonin transporter receptors in the brain (Gould et al., 2003). Deficits in serotonin function have been linked to traits of impulsivity and aggression, which have been correlated with increased likelihood of past suicide attempts and future completed suicides (Coryell, 2006). Approximately two thirds of suicide attempts are impulsive, and most adolescent suicides appear to be impulsive, often preceded by a stressful event (American Academy of Child and Adolescent Psychiatry, 2001; Mann and Currier, 2007). Acting recklessly and engaging in risky behaviors are also warning signs for suicide (Rudd et al., 2006). Head injury increases the risk for suicide, and individuals with head injuries often act impulsively and aggressively and have emotional instability (Oquendo et al., 2006).

In addition to serotonin abnormalities, the hypothalamic-pituitary-adrenal (HPA) axis has been implicated in suicide risk. The HPA axis is an integral part of the stress response and may be affected by early life adversity (Mann and Currier, 2007). HPA axis hyperactivity has been identified as a risk factor for suicide in depressive disorder (Coryell, 2006).

Assessment

Assessment of suicide potential involves a complete psychiatric history, thorough examination of mental state, and direct inquiry about suicidal thoughts, behaviors/attempts, intents, and plans. The American Psychiatric Association (2004) describes this approach in detail. Part of conducting a thorough psychiatric evaluation includes identifying psychiatric signs and symptoms that may influence suicide risk in particular. Past suicidal behavior, past psychiatric and medical history, family history of suicide, mental illness, and dysfunction are assessed, psychosocial stressors are considered, and the strengths and vulnerabilities of the individual patient are appreciated. Three other steps are described: asking very specific questions about suicidality, estimating level of suicide risk, and using modifiable risk and protective factors as the basis for treatment planning (Jacobs and Brewer, 2006). Sometimes a distinction is made between a risk factor, as noted earlier, and a warning sign. A warning sign has been defined as, "the earliest detectable sign that indicates heightened risk for suicide in the near-term" (Rudd et al., 2006, p. 258).

Approaching the Patient During a Suicide Risk Assessment

In a suicide risk assessment, the clinician approaches the patient in an empathic, objective, nonjudgmental, and concerned manner and spends the necessary time to listen to the patient. The clinician can ask directly about suicidality; asking does not increase risk. It is important to repeat suicide assessments over time, because of the waxing and waning nature of suicidality (American Psychiatric Association, 2004). Patient self-report is most often reliable (Posner et al., 2007). However, if the clinician's assessment relies solely on the patient's denial of suicidal ideation, intent, or plan, the assessment is insufficient (Simon and Shuman, 2006). Additional clarifying questions are of the utmost importance, especially to take an inventory of risk and protective factors for suicide. What prevented the patient from acting on his or her thoughts? Under what conditions would the patient consider suicide?

The clinician assesses any suicide attempts and inquires about possible precipitating events. Low lethality acts should not be discounted. Intent and lethality may not actually be directly associated; the patient's belief about the lethality is most important (Posner et al., 2007). The clinician will benefit from examining the chance of discovery and possibility of rescue in relation to a suicide attempt. Planning is concerning, including giving away personal property, making a will, and lacking plans for the future. The clinician can ask how the patient feels about still being alive and the potential to harm others. The suicide risk assessment also includes identifying risk factors as detailed earlier, intervening when appropriate in regard to dynamic risk factors, and identifying protective factors that may decrease suicide risk, such as pregnancy, religiosity, and positive social support (American Psychiatric Association, 2004).

The clinician should address the patient's immediate environment, making sure it is free of hazards (sharps, belts, etc.) and removing any potentially hazardous items. Searching or scanning (possibly with metal detectors) the patient for weapons and inquiring about the presence of a firearm or other weapons in the home or workplace are important. The interview should ideally be performed in a quiet setting with the lowest stimulation possible.

Throughout this process the patient must constantly be observed and/or supervised, with a one-to-one sitter or continuous closed-circuit television monitoring (American Psychiatric Association, 2004). The patient must be detained until a proper suicide risk assessment has been completed.

Mental Status Examination

Clinicians may consider performing a formal Mini-Mental State Examination (MMSE) if they are concerned about a cognitive disturbance and a drug or alcohol screen, which may also check for possible ingestions. Intoxicated patients should be reassessed at a later time. Most states allow for a 24-hour period of involuntary detention to protect patients from themselves (Rives, 1999).

No standardized suicide risk prediction scale identifies which patients will commit suicide (Busch et al., 1993). Suicide assessment scales have very low predictive values and do not provide reliable estimates of suicide risk. They may help open communication with a patient about this subject matter, though, and provide a thorough line of questioning about suicide (American Psychiatric Association, 2004; United States Preventive Services Task Force, 2004). Suicide scale questionnaires may complement a thorough assessment, but should never take the place of or substitute for any aspect of assessment (American Academy of Child and Adolescent Psychiatry, 2001).

Even though patients are often reliable historians, obtaining information from collateral informants is vital (e.g., family, friends, other treatment providers, bystanders, police, emergency medical service [EMS]). In an emergency a clinician may break confidentiality as relates to acting in the patient's best interest, and there is implied consent for treatment to prevent harm (Simon and Shuman, 2006). The safety of the patient and others takes precedence over confidentiality (American Psychiatric Association, 2004).

A CASE OF A SUICIDE ATTEMPT

A 15-year-old girl presents to the emergency department after ingesting an unknown number of 500 mg acetaminophen capsules. She was reportedly arguing with her mother and stepfather and then shut herself in her room. An hour later, her parents discovered her there unconscious, with the empty pill bottle next to her. She currently describes the overdose as "stupid" and "impulsive" and denies active suicidal intent. She has a history of alcohol and marijuana abuse and self-injury through cutting with a razor blade. She describes the self-injury as "calming." She does not have a history of prior possible suicide attempts. Her primary care physician had prescribed fluoxetine for depression, but she admits treatment nonadherence. After acute medical interventions in the ER, she was admitted to the intensive care unit for ongoing treatment and monitoring of her liver functioning, and a psychiatric consultation was ordered. Her parents are advised to secure both over-the-counter and prescription medications at home, along with anything else that could be used for self-harm, such as knives or firearms. After she is medically cleared, the consulting psychiatrist agrees that an inpatient psychiatry admission is not mandatory and helps arrange for follow-up with her outpatient psychiatrist for 2 days after discharge and also arranges for her to see a therapist for both individual and family counseling.

Interventions

The interview itself, especially if approached in the right way, can be a positive intervention for suicide. Following an assessment of the static and dynamic risk factors and protective factors, interventions should be targeted toward minimizing risk and maximizing protective elements as part of patient treatment and safety management (Simon and Shuman, 2006). There should be an engaging of supports for the patient and possible sharing of information with the family and outpatient provider.

Medications may target insomnia, anxiety, and agitation. Benzodiazepines may be used for all of these symptoms, with consideration of nonbenzodiazepine receptor agonists for insomnia. Medications with evidence for decreasing suicidal risk in the short term include clozapine and lithium. Lithium appears to significantly reduce suicide risk for bipolar patients or patients with recurrent major depression beyond its mood stabilizing effects, as clozapine appears to reduce risk for schizophrenics beyond its antipsychotic effects (Baldessarini et al., 2006). It is possible that selective serotonin reuptake inhibitors (SSRIs) may reduce long-term suicide risk (Gould et al., 2003; Mann and Currier, 2007). However, there may be consideration of stopping an SSRI if started within a week or two of presentation if it is felt that it may be poorly tolerated or otherwise increasing the risk for nonfatal or fatal suicidal behavior (Mann and Currier, 2007).

Electroconvulsive therapy (ECT) is also an option, and psychotherapy has been shown to reduce suicidal ideation and behavior in some clinical trials, including problem-solving and interpersonal therapies in general therapy and dialectical behavior therapy (DBT) and psychoanalytically oriented partial hospitalization for people with borderline personality disorder (Mann et al., 2005). DBT is a form of psychotherapy shown in randomized controlled trials to reduce suicidality in adults with borderline personality disorder (Linehan et al., 2006).

Suicide prevention contracts, in which patients sign a document agreeing to not kill themselves, are not recommended in many situations, including emergency settings, and may falsely lower clinical vigilance without altering patients' suicidal state (American Psychiatric Association, 2004). Lewis (2007) states, "The existing research does not support the use of such (no-harm) contracts as a method for preventing suicide, nor for protecting clinicians from malpractice litigation in the event of a client suicide" (p. 50). However, an unwillingness to commit to safety mandates a reassessment of therapeutic alliance and level of suicide risk. No-suicide contracts also may be viewed as utilizing the potential power of the relationship or at the very least honoring of a social contract (American Psychiatric Association, 2004; Lewis, 2007).

Interventions should involve treating the patient in the setting that is least restrictive while erring on the side of safety. Hospitalization (voluntary versus involuntary) must be considered versus outpatient management. Hospitalization has switched from a treatment to dangerousness model. Clinicians should be prepared to hospitalize patients who attempt suicide, especially with highly lethal methods; who have a persistent wish to die; or who have a clearly abnormal mental state, even without randomized controlled trials to determine whether hospitalizing high-risk suicide attempters saves lives. Mental status features of concern include an inability to form a therapeutic alliance, lack of truthfulness, inability to discuss or regulate emotion or behavior, and psychotic thinking (American Academy of Child and Adolescent Psychiatry, 2001). Additional indications for hospitalization include the absence of a strong social support system, including living alone; a history of impulsive behavior; and suicidal intent with plan of action and means (Roy and Fauman, 2004). An involuntary hospitalization involves the clinician filling out a formal document explicitly stating the patient's need for hospitalization in terms of danger toward self or others, inability to care for self, and inability to understand need for treatment. Safe transport to the hospital setting is needed; the clinician should not rely on family or friends to provide transportation, especially for involuntary hospitalizations. Most often the police or an ambulance is required.

Partial hospitalization may be a less restrictive option that still offers multidisciplinary treatments and skilled observation and support (American Academy of Child and Adolescent Psychiatry, 2001). Partial hospitalization may be preferable for patients with borderline personality disorder and chronic suicidality or other individuals with a number of risk factors but no clear imminent dangerousness (Paris, 2002).

Throughout this process the clinician provides education to the patient and family and demonstrates the empathic approach described earlier to promote adherence to the treatment plan. Coordinating care and collaborating with other clinicians, including outside providers and current team members, are important.

If it is determined that the patient is not under imminent risk of suicide, outpatient interventions may be appropriate. These commonly involve increased vigilance, including restricting access to potential weapons, more frequent visits and/or telephone contact with providers, and possible assistance of family members or other close persons as part of engaging existing support systems (Mann and Currier, 2007). Access to potential weapons is restricted by having them removed from the patient's environment or secured (especially firearms, along with sharps and large supplies of medications, including consideration of dispensing prescriptions in weekly amounts).

A follow-up appointment can be made for the next day, whether as a home visit by a mobile outreach unit or an increased frequency of therapy visits, or the patient may be referred to DBT.

Another common strategy is the development of a crisis plan, a detailed list of steps for the patient to follow when he or she is suicidal (Joiner et al., 1999). Crisis plans include identifying potential precipitants for suicidal thinking, problem-solving ways to avoid or minimize the precipitants, preventing recurrence of suicidal thinking, and coping with suicidal thoughts when they recur (American Academy of Child and Adolescent Psychiatry, 2001). Part of the crisis plan may involve agreeing to call the provider (or other agreed-upon supports) when the patient is uncertain about his or her ability to control suicidal impulses (Welton, 2007).

Clinicians (or suitable coverage) should be available to the patient 24 hours a day. It may be preferable for the patient to not be alone. Any family members or friends asked to watch the patient in lieu of hospitalization should be informed of the potential risk for suicide (Welton, 2007).

Documentation

Documenting the evaluation of a suicidal patient reflects the thoughtfulness that goes into a thorough suicide risk assessment (Ballas, 2007). The report should clearly communicate how clinical judgment of the pertinent positive and negative risk factors led to the final assessment and plan. Medicolegally, if something is not clearly documented in the record, it is as if it did not happen.

SUMMARY

Patients frequently present to general emergency departments with psychiatric emergencies, most commonly agitation and suicidality. The process of evaluation and intervention for such patients should be performed carefully and systematically. Having the patient "medically cleared" by excluding organic etiologies, substance intoxication or withdrawal, and medication side effects is an important first step. Knowing the various risk factors for suicidality and violence toward others is key to formulating a treatment plan. Appropriate caregiver responses to psychiatric emergencies may result in the avoidance of harm to patients or others both inside and outside emergency settings.

Clinical Pearls

- Psychiatric emergencies, which often include agitation, aggression, or suicidality, commonly present to the general emergency department.
- In addition to consideration of psychiatric disorders, possible organic etiologies for the presenting signs or symptoms, such as medical disorders, drugs of abuse, or adverse effects of prescription medications, must be ruled out in a process known as *medical clearance*.
- Agitation and aggressive behavior have been linked to abnormalities in dopaminergic, serotonergic, noradrenergic, and glutaminergic-GABAergic systems. Evidence links serotonin and/or HPA axis dysregulation and suicide risk.
- Depending on the risk assessment and provisional diagnosis, monotherapy with either an antipsychotic or a benzodiazepine may be sufficient to reduce agitation/aggression. Combined

continued

use of an antipsychotic and benzodiazepine may produce an antiagitation effect that is superior to either one alone.

- Atypical antipsychotics provide a much safer acute side effect profile than the typical antipsychotics and are now used more for treatment of nonspecific agitation and/or aggression.
- Even though it is well established that individual cases of suicide cannot be predicted, it is expected as the standard of care that an adequate suicide risk assessment be performed and documented and then appropriate interventions enacted.
- Past suicide attempts may be the best indicator of increased risk of suicide, particularly when coupled with current suicidal ideation, and one of the best predictors of violence is a history of past violence.
- Men commit suicide more than four times as often as women, even though women attempt suicide three to four times as often as men. Men tend to choose more lethal means, such as firearms.
- Psychopathology is found in >90% of completed suicides, especially mood disorders, and substance abuse is often a contributing factor.
- While erring on the side of safety, ideally psychiatric interventions should involve the least restrictive or invasive options, such as oral medication as opposed to intramuscular or intravenous, calming approaches or rapid tranquilization as opposed to physical restraint, and outpatient management or partial hospitalization versus psychiatric hospitalization.

Self-Assessment Questions and Answers

26-1. A patient presents to the emergency department with irritability and threatening physical harm to others. Which of the following additional factors constitutes the greatest risk for violent behavior?

A. The patient is a 10-year-old boy recently suspended from school.

B. The patient is a 75-year-old man whose wife recently died from cancer.

C. The patient is a 24-year-old man who recently lost his job and has a history of alcohol abuse.

D. The patient is a 45-year-old woman with anxiety.

Risk increases if the patient is a young male. Unemployment and substance abuse or dependence further increase the risk. *Answer: C*

26-2. A patient presents to the ER with aggression and agitation. Which would be the first most appropriate step in the care of this patient?

A. Approach the patient in an empathic manner and try to talk him down.

B. Order IM haloperidol 5 mg.

C. Order oral lorazepam 2 mg.

D. Send the patient to a seclusion room and prepare for restraint.

The preferred means of treatment is always the least restrictive intervention, including the talk-down process. *Answer: A*

26-3. A 30-year-old woman presents to the ER with superficial cuts on her arm. She recently found out that her boyfriend of 2 months wants to end their relationship. When the physician approaches, she appears very anxious and agitated and becomes quite frantic. Which of the following would be an appropriate option given her symptoms?

A. 2 mg oral lorazepam

B. 2 mg IM risperidone

C. 5 mg oral haloperidol

D. 5 mg IM haloperidol

Given the symptoms of anxiety and no data to support any other provisional diagnosis, a benzodiazepine would be preferred in this case. *Answer: A*

26-4. A patient presents to the emergency department and endorses suicidal ideation. Which additional factors constitute the greatest additional risk for suicide?

A. The patient is a 12-year-old white girl with a history of deliberate self-injury.

B. The patient is a 35-year-old African American woman with generalized anxiety disorder.

C. The patient is a 35-year-old Asian male with insomnia and cannabis dependence.

D. The patient is an 85-year-old recently widowed white man with untreated depression.

Risk increases with advancing age. White ethnicity, male gender, depression, and recent significant life stress constitute additional risk factors.
Answer: D

26-5. Which outpatient intervention following a suicide risk assessment is most likely to be counterproductive?

A. Ask the patient to call when uncertain about ability to control suicidal impulses.

B. Limit access to firearms.

C. Make an appointment to follow up the next day.

D. Recommend that the patient spend time alone to limit environmental stress.

Being unsupervised and in the absence of social supports may constitute a risk factor for suicide. Access to firearms should be limited. An appropriate crisis plan may involve coping skills and an agreement to contact a provider when uncertain as to ability to resist suicidal thoughts. Targeting insomnia with medication may be an appropriate intervention, and setting up follow-up is essential.
Answer: D

References

American Academy of Child and Adolescent Psychiatry. Practice parameter for the assessment and treatment of children and adolescents with suicidal behavior. *J Am Acad Child Adolesc Psychiatry*. 2001;40(Suppl 7):24S–51S.

American Psychiatric Association. Practice guideline for the assessment and treatment of patients with suicidal behaviors. *Practice guidelines for the treatment of psychiatric disorders compendium*, 2nd ed. Arlington: American Psychiatric Publishing; 2004.

Baldessarini RJ, Finklestein S, Arana GW. Predictive power of diagnostic tests. In: Flach F, ed. *Psychobiology and psychopharmacology*. New York: Norton Publishers; 1988.

Baldessarini RJ, Pompili M, Tondo L. Suicide in bipolar disorder: Risks and management. *CNS Spectr*. 2006;11:465–471.

Ballas C. How to write a suicide note: Practical tips for documenting the evaluation of a suicidal patient. *Psychiatr Times*. 2007;5:51–58.

Battaglia J, Robinson DG, Citrome L, et al. The treatment of acute agitation in schizophrenia. *CNS Spectr*. 2007;12(Suppl 11):1–16.

Beck AT, Brown G, Berchick RJ, et al. Relationship between hopelessness and ultimate suicide: A replication with psychiatric outpatients. *Am J Psychiatry*. 1990;147:190–195.

Brent DA, Perper JA, Moritz G, et al. Familial risk factors for adolescent suicide: A case-control study. *Acta Psychiatr Scand*. 1994;89:52–58.

Busch KA, Clark DC, Fawcett J, et al. Clinical features of inpatient suicide. *Psychiatr Ann*. 1993;23:256–262.

Centers for Disease Control. *Web-based injury statistics query and reporting system*. National Center for Injury Prevention and Control. Available at: http://www.cdc.gov/ncipc/wisqars/. Accessed September 1, 2007.

Cheng ATA, Chen THH, Chen CC, et al. Psychosocial and psychiatric risk factors for suicide: Case-control psychological autopsy study. *Br J Psychiatry*. 2000;177:360–365.

Cooper J, Kapur N, Dunning J, et al. A clinical tool for assessing risk after self-harm. *Ann Emerg Med*. 2006;48:459–466.

Coryell WH. Clinical assessment of suicide risk in depressive disorder. *CNS Spectr*. 2006;11:455–461.

Currier GW, Allen MH. Physical and chemical restraint in the psychiatric emergency service. *Psychiatr Serv*. 2000;51:717–719.

Davidson RJ, Putnam KM, Larson CL. Dysfunction in the neural circuitry of emotion regulation—a possible prelude to violence. *Science*. 2000;289:591–594.

De Fruyt J, Demyttenaere K. Rapid tranquilization: New approaches in the emergency treatment of behavioral disturbances. *Eur Psychiatry*. 2004;19:243–249.

D'Orio B. Reducing risk associated with seclusion and restraint. *Psychiatr Times*. 2007;24:48–52.

Dubin WR. Pain disorders. In: Stoudemire A, ed. *Clinical psychiatry for medical students and residents*, 3rd ed. Philadelphia: LippincottWilliams & Wilkins; 1998.

Goldsmith SK, Pellmar TC, Kleinman AM, et al. *Reducing suicide: A national imperative*. Washington, DC: The National Academies Press; 2002.

Gould MS, Greenberg T, Velting DM, et al. Youth suicide risk and preventive interventions: A review of the past 10 years. *J Am Acad Child Adolesc Psychiatry*. 2003;42:386–405.

Hawton K. Suicide and attempted suicide. In: Paykel ES, ed. *Handbook of affective disorders*, 2nd ed. New York: Guilford Press; 1992.

Jacobs DG, Brewer ML. Application of the APA practice guidelines on suicide to clinical practice. *CNS Spectr*. 2006;11:447–454.

Joiner TE, Walker RL, Rudd MD, et al. Scientizing and routinizing the assessment of suicidality in outpatient practice. *Prof Psychol Res Pr*. 1999;30:447–453.

Kipps CM, Fung V, Grattan-Smith P, et al. Movement disorder emergencies. *Mov Disord*. 2005;20: 322–334.

Krakowski M. Violence and serotonin: Influence of impulse control, affect regulation and social functioning. *J Neuropsychiatry Clin Neurosci*. 2003;15:294–305.

Lambert MT, Bonner J. Characteristics and six-month outcome of patients who use suicide threats to seek hospital admission. *Psychiatr Serv*. 1996;47:871–873.

Lesch KP, Merschdorf U. Impulsivity, aggression and serotonin: A molecular psychobiological perspective. *Behav Sci Law*. 2000;18:581–604.

Lewis LM. No-harm contracts: A review of what we know. *Suicide Life Threat Behav*. 2007;37:50–57.

Linehan MM, Comtois KA, Murray AM, et al. Two-year randomized controlled trial and follow-up of dialectical behavior therapy versus therapy by experts for suicidal behaviors and borderline personality disorder. *Arch Gen Psychiatry*. 2006;63:757–766.

Mann JJ, Currier D. Prevention of suicide. *Psychiatr Ann*. 2007;37(5):331–339.

Mann JJ, Waternaux C, Haas GL, et al. Toward a clinical model of suicidal behavior in psychiatric patients. *Am J Psychiatry*. 1999;156:181–189.

Mann JJ, Apter A, Bertolote J, et al. Suicide prevention strategies: A systematic review. *JAMA*. 2005; 294:2064–2074.

Meyers J, Stein S. The psychiatric interview in the emergency department. *Emerg Med Clin North Am*. 2000; 18:173–183.

Molnar BE, Berkman LF, Buka SL. Psychopathology, childhood sexual abuse and other childhood adversities: Relative links to subsequent suicidal behaviour in the United States. *Psychol Med*. 2001;31:965–977.

National Institute of Mental Health. *Suicide in the United States: Statistics and prevention*. Available at: http://www.nimh.nih.gov/publicat/harmsway.cfm. Accessed September 15, 2007.

Oquendo MA, Currier D, Mann JJ. Prospective studies of suicidal behavior in major depressive and bipolar disorders: What is the evidence for predictive risk factors? *Acta Psychiatr Scand*. 2006;114:151–158.

Paris J. Chronic suicidality among patients with borderline personality disorder. *Psychiatr Serv*. 2002;53: 738–742.

Piechniczek-Buczek J. Psychiatric emergencies in the elderly population. *Emerg Med Clin North Am*. 2006;24:467–490.

Porter RS, Kaplan JL. *Suicidal behavior. The merck manual*. Available at: http://www.merck.com/ mmpe/index.html. Last modified November 2005.

Posner K, Melvin GA, Stanley B, et al. Factors in the assessment of suicidality in youth. *CNS Spectr*. 2007; 12:156–162.

Rives W. Emergency department assessment of suicidal patients. *Psychiatr Clin North Am*. 1999;22(4): 780–787.

Rocca P, Villari V, Bogetto F. Managing the aggressive and violent patient in the psychiatric emergency. *Prog Neuropsychopharmacol Biol Psychiatry*. 2006;30:586–598.

Roy A, Fauman BJ. Psychiatric emergencies. In: Sadock BJ, Sadock VA, eds. *Kaplan and Sadock's comprehensive textbook of psychiatry*, 8th ed. Philadelphia: Lippincott Williams & Wilkins; 2004.

Rudd MD, Berman AL, Joiner TE, et al. Warning signs for suicide: Theory, research, and clinical applications. *Suicide Life Threat Behav*. 2006;36:255–262.

Sadock BJ, Sadock VA. *Kaplan and Sadock's synopsis of psychiatry*, 9th ed. Philadelphia: Lippincott Williams & Wilkins; 2003.

Sadock BJ, Sadock VA. *Kaplan and Sadock's comprehensive textbook of psychiatry*, 8th ed. Philadelphia: Lippincott Williams & Wilkins; 2004.

Sailas E, Fenton M. Seclusion and restraint for people with serious mental illnesses. *Cochrane Database Syst Rev*. 2000;2:CD001163.

Schulsinger F, Kety SS, Rosenthal D, et al. A family study of suicide. In: Schou M, Stromgren E, eds. *Origin, prevention and treatment of affective disorders*. New York: Academic Press; 1979.

Simon RI, Shuman JD. The standard of care in suicide risk assessment: An elusive concept. *CNS Spectr*. 2006;11:442–445.

Stern TA, Lagomasino IT, Hackett TP. Suicidal patients. In: Cassem NH, ed. *Massachusetts general hospital handbook of general hospital psychiatry*. St. Louis: Mosby; 1997.

Swann AC. Neuroreceptor mechanisms of aggression and its treatment. *J Clin Psychiatry*. 2003; 64(Suppl 4):S26–S35.

United States Preventive Services Task Force. Screening for suicide risk: Recommendation and rationale. *Ann Intern Med*. 2004;140:820–821.

Welton R. The management of suicidality: Assessment and intervention. *Psychiatry*. 2007;4:25–34.

Williams ER, Shepherd SM. Medical clearance of psychiatric patients. *Emerg Med Clin North Am*. 2000;18:185–198.

Yildiz A, Sachs GS, Turgay A. Pharmacological management of agitation in emergency settings. *Emerg Med J*. 2003;20:339–346.

Caring for Special Populations with Mental Illness

Caring for Children and Adolescents with Psychiatric Disorders

"There is no such thing as a baby."
   —*D.W. Winnicott* (1987)

Winnicott's famous statement refers to the extraordinarily important and symbiotic relationship between mother and child; he felt that the infant could only be conceptualized in the context of the relationship with the primary caregiver. Winnicott is one of the most important figures in the history of child psychiatry, so his words have special meaning. Unlike adults, children cannot be assessed alone. Unless they have permission and view it essential to evaluation and treatment, general psychiatrists typically do not involve their patients' employers, parents, spouses, or siblings in care. However, child psychiatrists cannot effectively perform their job without an intricate understanding of the people (parents, siblings, teachers), systems (social services, legal, schools), and dynamics (family, peer relationships) involved in a child's life. They must also have a firm understanding of normal child development, as well as a keen eye for discerning pathologic conditions that need treatment. As a result, clinicians who work with children and adolescents need specialized training to best care for this population. Unfortunately, there is a severe shortage of fully trained child and adolescent psychiatrists in the United States (American Academy of Child and Adolescent Psychiatry, 1999).

This chapter outlines a general approach to psychiatric evaluation and ongoing treatment in children and adolescents. In addition to discussing childhood development, the chapter will focus on establishing rapport with children and teens, strengthening the therapeutic alliance, working productively with other providers, and finding ways to successfully manage parental involvement in treatment. Finally, this chapter will address aspects of treatment such as confidentiality, assent versus consent, and countertransference issues that differ from psychiatric practice with an adult population.

THE INITIAL EVALUATION

Determining the Scope of the Consultation

Mental health providers who care for children must work collaboratively with the other systems involved in children's lives. Often, the first task is to determine for whom one is "working." Sometimes the child psychiatrist acts as a consultant to the parents. At others, the psychiatrist is a consultant to the pediatrician, the school, the court, or other community supports. The child psychiatrist's involvement and approach may vary based on the setting (Dulcan et al., 2003).

One of the most vital questions the child psychiatrist must consider when evaluating a child is to determine who the patient is. With rare exceptions, most children and adolescents do not request an appointment with a child psychiatrist. It is important for the child psychiatrist to understand who initiated the referral and why. Did the school insist on the evaluation due to hyperactivity and inattention, or are the parents becoming frustrated with temper tantrums or defiant behavior? Has the evaluation been ordered by the court as a condition of allowing a parent to maintain custody? Overwhelmingly, adults bring children in for treatment because they are worried about them and want help. However, even the most loving families may have dynamics that interfere with a child's function. It is important to normalize this—every family

A CASE OF INVESTIGATING FAMILY DYNAMICS

Previously a B-student, 13-year-old Sam presents with declining grades and failure to hand in his homework. He has become the "class clown." He cannot keep track of his assignments but refuses any assistance from his parents, who complain that he will not do chores or sit with them for dinner. Mrs. Smith notes that Sam was always "running like a train" yet a sweet and affectionate child, but Mr. Smith sees Sam as oppositional and knows he can do better but just does not want to and needs punishment. Mrs. Smith disagrees, sensing that Sam feels terrible about himself because he cannot meet his parents' or teachers' standards. After an initial evaluation over two sessions, Dr. Christopher finds that Sam meets clinical criteria for attention-deficit/hyperactivity disorder. Sam feels relieved and is ready to engage in a behavioral plan and willing to try a course of stimulants. Mr. Smith accuses Mrs. Smith of being "soft" on Sam and perpetuating his problems. Mrs. Smith claims Mr. Smith is insensitive and worsening Sam's low self-esteem. Dr. Christopher spends a number of meetings helping to resolve their conflict over Sam and uncovers marital difficulties over finances and Mr. Smith's excessive work and absence from the home. The Smiths agree to engage in marital therapy and to have Sam work with Dr. Christopher on the proposed treatment plan.

has stresses and unique issues beyond its particular strengths. Sometimes the adults involved in a child's life have unrealistic expectations of the child at his or her developmental stage. Other times, families are undergoing transitions, such as a move or a divorce, which may manifest in a child's maladaptive behavior. Similarly, a parent may be struggling with a mood or anxiety disorder, and the child's worry about this is causing behavioral problems. Of course, a child may also begin to exhibit concerning symptoms in the absence of any family or social stresses. Many behavioral disorders in childhood have biological origins; this can sometimes be the phenotypic expression of a genetic vulnerability that runs in families or the result of a medical problem. In these situations the family may be severely taxed in caring for a child or adolescent who displays problems with thoughts, feelings, or actions. In all cases, it should be remembered that there is a delicate and universal interplay among the biological, psychological, and social-environmental forces affecting the life of a child and family. A clinician can respectfully inquire about all of the facets of a child's world and, when appropriate, suggest that more support for the parent and child may enable them to be more effective.

The Importance of Establishing an Alliance with the Child and Family

Beyond developing a basic understanding of all the biopsychosocial issues at play for an individual patient, child psychiatrists face a daunting task. They need to earn the trust of the child or adolescent as well as that of the family. No matter how strong the therapeutic alliance between the child and clinician, parents will not bring their child to an appointment if they do not trust the clinician. The child psychiatrist must approach both the child and family in an empathic, nonjudgmental manner but also, despite the need for good rapport, must not be afraid to point out problems and suggest mechanisms for change when necessary. Particularly in the realm of behavioral problems, this process is often received by the child and parent with feelings of guilt, shame, anxiety, and/or anger. Therefore, it is important that child psychiatrists convey that their job is not to place blame but to help families understand why their children are struggling and to provide options for effective treatment (Rauch, 2000).

Structuring the Initial Interview

Before the Meeting

The first interview is very important. The clinician will need more time than is typically allotted for an adult diagnostic psychiatric evaluation. In some cases, more than one session is needed to complete the evaluation. It is often helpful to prepare parents for this beforehand. They should be instructed to bring in results from previous evaluations, health records, psychological testing, and individualized educational plans. Many child psychiatry clinics mail parents a detailed questionnaire before the appointment so clinicians have easy access to information during and after the session. It is also important to have parents sign a release of information allowing the clinician to contact the important people involved in the child's care (e.g., pediatrician, teacher, court, social services worker). It is very important that a child's legal custodian accompany the child to the appointment. Ideally, both parents should attend the interview, although this may not be possible.

During the Interview

The actual interview can be adapted to the clinical situation. It is often most helpful to meet with both parents and child together for a few minutes to determine the circumstances prompting the referral and their expectations of the evaluation. What are their concerns, hopes, or fears of the evaluation or outcome? Are they looking for medication management? Are they hoping for behavioral interventions? The clinician can explain the structure of the evaluation at this time (see Table 27-1). This is also an opportune time to observe interactions between the parents and the child. How do they get along? Is the child expressive? Do the parents encourage the child to communicate his or her concerns, or do they dominate the conversation with their own agenda? Are the parents excessively anxious? If the child is aged 5 years or older, it is a good idea to interview the parent and child separately. Children should be given the option of being interviewed first or speaking with the psychiatrist after the parents. Most adolescents want to tell their story first, but it helps to be flexible. A very socially anxious child may not want his or her parents to leave the room for the first few sessions. This is acceptable and gives important clinical information that the clinician can use over time. A provider's willingness to be flexible will likely put the child and the parents at ease. Over time, the clinician can gently challenge the child to meet for a few minutes with the parent outside the door, then in the waiting room, and so on.

Meeting with the child or adolescent

When meeting with young children, it is important to make them feel comfortable. The office should be pleasant and large enough for play. Toys of various kinds should be displayed so the children feel at ease and understand that this is not the same kind of visit as going to the pediatrician for a well-child checkup or, worse, an immunization. When conducting interviews with children, it is very important to keep in mind their developmental stage. School-aged children, for example, may be "rule" oriented and rather concrete in their thinking; they may worry about being "bad" or concerned about the approval of their parents or doctor. Adolescents, on the other hand, are more cognitively advanced and able to appreciate abstract ideals and values. They are often struggling with separation from their family as they work on issues of personal identity and independence. Although school-aged children are used to being brought places by their parents and may accept this as a matter of course, adolescents may consider this an intrusion on their time and activity and feel like a hostage. With young children, it is often helpful to get down on the floor with them to play with blocks or to draw a picture (Gilliam and Mayes, 2007). Kids will often start talking once they are occupied with a game or a drawing. Start out by making small talk or by inquiring about innocuous topics. Ask about favorite toys, games, music, or other activities. Asking younger children to draw a picture of their family and then asking them to tell

---

TABLE 27-1	**Elements of the Initial Evaluation Establishing the Consultation Question**
Introductory meeting with both parents and child present	
Interview and assessment of child alone, including mental status examination	
Interview of parent(s) alone	
Closing meeting with both parents and child present	
Rating scales, neuropsychological testing	
Assessing need for further diagnostic testing (e.g., brain imaging, phlebotomy, electroencephalogram)	
Contacting collateral sources	
Preliminary biopsychosocial formulation	
Meeting with parents and child to discuss recommendations and treatment plan	

a story about the picture can really help the clinician gather a lot of history. If the child had three wishes, for what would he or she wish? The clinician can also ask why the child thinks he or she is there, who is most concerned, and if the child thinks he or she needs help. In general, for all interviews, it is important to ask about the main domains of a child's life: home, school, peers, and play (Moss and Racusin, 2007).

Meeting with an adolescent is a little trickier. In light of the noted developmental issues, it is often useful to begin asking why the adolescent feels he or she is there. Asking questions in a lighthearted manner may put the adolescent at ease and show that the clinician really wants to understand the adolescent's point of view, regardless of what his or her parents say. Have "fidget toys" like stress balls available if needed. Sometimes it is easier for an adolescent to talk while playing catch or drawing. It can also be really helpful for clinicians to "play dumb" when interacting with teenagers, letting adolescents teach them about music, pop culture, and computers (Pataki et al., 2005). It helps adolescents reveal their sense of mastery and identity and gives clinicians insight into the adolescents' world. Discussions about favorite video games, Web sites, and text messaging, for example, can provide rich material for the session (Kutner and Beresin, 2000).

When the child is comfortable, the clinician should pursue a thorough assessment of the full range of the *Diagnostic and Statistical Manual of Mental Disorders,* Fourth Edition, Text Revision (DSM-IV-TR), diagnoses using developmentally appropriate language and a conversational, nonthreatening tone. Depending on the age of the child, this may be done with the parents present. As with adult patients, the child psychiatrist will perform a mental status examination, including appearance, orientation, eye contact, speech, psychomotor activity, mood, affect, thought process, thought content, intelligence, insight, and judgment (Lewis and King, 2007). It is important to keep the child's developmental stage in mind when assessing mental status. For example, it would be very appropriate for a 6-year-old to exhibit concrete thought processes but concerning to observe the same in an 18-year-old.

Meeting with the parents

The meeting with the parents is a time to gather a detailed medical, developmental, and psychosocial history (American Academy of Child and Adolescent Psychiatry, 1995, 1997). Ask about gestation and delivery, developmental milestones, and history of previous medical and behavioral difficulties such as encopresis, enuresis, or separation anxiety. Behavioral problems such as difficulties with mood, anxiety, aggression, impulsivity, relationships, and academic achievement should be explored. The interviewer should ask about any concerns involving serious risks, such as suicidal behavior or use of substances, and any history of trauma, including physical or sexual abuse. What is the child like temperamentally? What are the child's strengths? What do they like best about their child?

A CASE OF INITIALLY INTERVIEWING AN ADOLESCENT

Evan, a 17-year-old male, presents with his parents for an evaluation. Dr. Jones meets with them for a few minutes to gather some information and senses that Evan is not happy to be there. He sits with his arms crossed, mumbles one-word answers to questions, and is very irritable and sarcastic with his parents. Dr. Jones suggests that Evan spend some time talking alone before having his parents join the discussion. Evan rolls his eyes and says, "Whatever." Once his parents leave the room, Dr. Jones smiles and asks Evan about his symptoms. Evan sighs and says, "You tell me, you are supposed to be the doctor. Besides, my parents are going to tell you everything that is wrong with me." Dr. Jones puts down the notepad and says, "It seems as if you would rather be somewhere else, and that you are frustrated with having to be here. What would you be doing if you were not here right now?" Evan replies tersely, "I would be at track practice." Dr. Jones asks a number of low-stress questions about Evan's running, extracurricular activities, hobbies, and social life. Evan picks up a stress ball and begins to toss it in the air as he speaks. Soon he seems more relaxed, and Dr. Jones seamlessly transitions into more specific questions about Evan's understanding of the reason for the visit and the symptoms that he has been experiencing.

This meeting is also a time for parents to share concerns that they might be hesitant to address in the child's presence and to give insight into issues that the child may not know about, such as a grandparent's alcoholism, marital discord, or a cousin's suicide attempt. This can also be a time to reassure parents that the clinician's job is not to lay blame or to compete for the child's affection but to understand what is going on for the child so that everyone involved can develop a helpful treatment plan together. In talking with both adolescents and their parents, it is essential to be specific and complete. Families will answer even the most sensitive questions openly and honestly when they trust the clinician and understand the rationale for asking.

After the Interview—Gathering Additional Information

After the interview is complete, ask permission to talk with collateral sources (see Table 27-2) and then invite the family back within a week or two to discuss impressions and recommendations for the treatment approach. The clinician may also request that parents, teachers, or the child complete formalized rating scales to assist in diagnosis and ongoing monitoring. Neuropsychological testing may also be indicated and may help clarify a diagnostically challenging picture. Similarly, the child psychiatrist should assess the need for additional diagnostic tests such as head imaging or blood work. If there is concern that a medical illness is causing psychiatric symptoms, referrals should be made to the appropriate specialist (Kaplan and Sadock, 1998). Families generally like to hear that the clinician is being thoughtful and thorough before recommending an intervention, especially one involving medication.

The family can come back within a week or two, contact the pediatrician, school-based supports, community supports, and previous providers to let them know that psychiatry is involved and to gather any additional information that may still be missing after discussion with the family. Often, these people can be valuable sources of information, especially since some of them may have known the family for many years. Social service workers can give insight into concern about abuse or neglect, and court-appointed clinicians may be able to give an objective account of an acrimonious divorce or custody dispute. It is especially important to speak with school-based clinicians or teachers. As Freud (1961) said, the definition of psychological health is "to love and to work." For kids, school is their job, and it is important to know how they are doing from both academic and social perspectives. Children may be hesitant to tell providers and parents that they do not have friends or that they are being bullied or teased, often because they feel embarrassed or ashamed. Significant discrepancies in functioning between home and school warrant close attention.

Of course, there may be situations in which a child needs more immediate intervention. If hospitalization is necessary, the child psychiatrist can make a referral to an inpatient unit or escort the family to the emergency room to ensure the child's safety while arrangements are made.

TABLE 27-2   Sources of Collateral Information
Parents
Extended family members
Teachers
School principal
Guidance counselor
Clergy
Previous psychotherapist, psychiatrist
Pediatrician
Specialty medical providers
Social services case worker
Guardian ad litem
Probation officer

A CASE OF EVALUATING A CHILD

Dr. Smith is asked to evaluate Sally, an 8-year-old child hospitalized with cystic fibrosis. Sally has no psychiatric history, but the medical team has been concerned that she may be depressed. She cries frequently, sleeps poorly, and has temper tantrums when working with the respiratory therapist. Despite being fully toilet trained, Sally has had several wetting accidents. There is nothing to suggest a medical cause for her symptoms. Dr. Smith meets with Sally in her room. Per treatment recommendations for her illness, Sally has not been allowed to spend time in the recreation room with other patients, and before entering her room, all providers need to gown and glove. Her parents are very involved in her care but need to work and care for her siblings. On interview, Sally is cooperative, easily engaged, and does not appear depressed. Sally's parents deny any previous concern about mood or anxiety problems and have not noticed any concerning behaviors in the hospital when they are present. Dr. Smith suspects that Sally's symptoms are related to the isolating nature of her admission and recommends that her parents bring in her favorite items from home so that her hospital room feels more comfortable, that extended family members and friends take turns visiting her when her parents are not able to be there, and that there be as much consistency as possible with medical staff. Several days later, Sally seems brighter and more engaged.

BIOPSYCHOSOCIAL FORMULATION

Once all the relevant data have been collected, it is generally most helpful to formulate the case using a biopsychosocial model (see Table 27-3). This model takes normal cognitive/social/emotional development, genetic predisposition, and family dynamics into account in addition to psychopathology (Jellinek and McDermott, 2004). An example follows.

A 13-year-old female presents with depression, anxiety, and significant weight loss in the context of a number of stressors, including her family's move to a new state and her father's gastric bypass surgery. Her mother has a history of obsessive-compulsive disorder (OCD), and her younger brother is autistic. Her parents are extremely concerned and have been trying to force her to eat, although this typically results in fighting.

Bio: This young woman has a family history of anxiety disorders and pervasive developmental disorder, both of which tend to occur more frequently in the family members of patients diagnosed with eating disorders. Starvation can cause the body to "shut down" to conserve energy, and the resulting fatigue, psychomotor retardation, and ruminations can resemble the neurovegetative symptoms of depression. The hormonal shifts of puberty also could put her at risk for a mood disorder.

Psycho: Puberty can be a difficult time due to changes in body size and shape, which can trigger a disturbance in body image. Adolescents also begin to separate and individuate from their families during puberty, which may be difficult for this adolescent due to her mother's anxiety disorder and her father's recovery from surgery. In addition, relationships between fathers and daughters can change around puberty, and she may perceive the loss of a significant supportive relationship.

Social: With the move, this young woman will need to adjust to a new town and school and re-create a social network at an age that can be challenging, especially for girls. She may also be hypersensitive to weight concerns from exposure to societal and cultural expectations of thinness that may be at odds with her natural body composition. She may also be particularly concerned about weight due to her father's struggles with obesity. Further, she may be worried about caring for her mother's OCD, her brother's autism, and her father's postsurgical follow-up.

This case could be approached in a number of ways. This adolescent may recover quickly as she makes friends at her new school and not need any additional intervention. She may benefit from weekly psychotherapy to discuss her concerns about body image and fear that she will become obese like her father, or she may need a serotonin reuptake inhibitor to best address the mood and anxiety symptoms. Her parents may need help to manage anxiety and support her with her meal plan without being too intrusive or engaging her in a power struggle. They may need

TABLE 27-3	**Elements of the Biopsychosocial Formulation**
Biological predisposition to mental illness: family history of a mood, anxiety, or psychotic disorder; presence of a medical illness that may cause psychiatric symptoms; history of a head trauma	
Psychological factors: developmental transitions (cognitive and moral development), family dynamics, personality structure, resiliency	
Social and environmental factors: recent transition such as a move; loss of an important family member, teacher, or friend; poverty; legal issues; out-of-family placement	

guidance about care for other family members. Finally, family therapy may be useful in providing a forum to explore the multiple problems in the family.

The child psychiatrist's job is to come up with an initial approach that seems workable for the family and to involve the appropriate people if he or she is not able to fulfill each role (e.g., a family therapist or an adult psychiatrist to treat the mother's OCD). The child psychiatrist also needs to be willing to reformulate the case over time and from different perspectives as more information becomes available. For example, what appears to be an eating disorder may prove to be a mood or anxiety disorder, requiring a different therapeutic approach.

PRIVACY AND CONFIDENTIALITY

Adolescents must feel as though they have privacy in the meeting so that they are willing to be open and honest, but child psychiatrists cannot promise complete confidentiality (Ascherman and Rubin, 2008). It is important to bring this up in the beginning of the meeting, with both the parent and child present. Tell them that it is important for all parties to feel that they can be honest and that, for the most part, the clinician will keep the content of their sessions private. However, if there is concern about safety (e.g., risk taking that places the child or others in danger, such as suicidal or homicidal behavior), the child psychiatrist may need to tell the patient's parents. Most adolescents feel comfortable with this as long as they know that this will be discussed with them before their parents are told and that they are given the option to present this information to their parents themselves. Similarly, parents need to know that the clinician is always willing to listen to information or concerns that they have about their child but that the clinician will protect their child's privacy as long as it is safe to do so.

WORKING WITH A MULTIDISCIPLINARY TREATMENT TEAM

If a child psychiatrist is providing a service such as medication management but another clinician is responsible for therapy, it is very important that all members of the treatment team communicate closely to minimize splitting and to ensure that all concerns are adequately addressed (Fritz, 2003). Most providers find it helpful to clearly define roles from the start, so that there is no question about with whom the responsibility lies. Will the therapist make the decision to hospitalize, or will the psychopharmacologist? It is of paramount importance to keep the primary care physician (by definition, the point person for the child's care) apprised of changes to the treatment plan. If the child has an eating disorder, the pediatrician may be a vital member of the team, monitoring weight, vital signs, and electrolytes. A dietitian might be involved as well.

ONGOING TREATMENT: BOUNDARIES, TRANSFERENCE ISSUES, AND DIFFICULT SITUATIONS

Ongoing treatment with a child and family is different from treating adults. In general psychiatry training, residents learn to define the treatment frame, maintain a neutral stance, and refrain from sharing personal information. Most child psychiatrists would agree that boundaries, of necessity, are a little less strict when treating children and adolescents. For example, a child may need to miss a session because of a special event at school such as a tournament or recital, or the family may need to reschedule due to another child's illness or the parent's inability to get away from work. Although it is certainly appropriate to ask families for as much consistency as possible in making sessions, being too strict is likely to result in attrition.

In addition, most parents want and need sessions to update them on their child's progress. Although confidentiality is crucial for children and adolescents, child psychiatrists usually need to talk with their patients about parent meetings and review what will be revealed. At other times, parents may contact the child psychiatrist outside of meetings and provide information about events in the child's life. The child psychiatrist must sensitively inform the parents that there needs to be discussion with the child, lest the child feel that things are going on "behind the scenes."

Other interesting clinical issues may arise as well. If an adult patient were to present a general psychiatrist with a gift, the psychiatrist would devote time discussing the meaning of the gift and interpreting this with the patient. In many cases, the psychiatrist would not accept it. When treating children, the clinician needs to be very thoughtful about such situations. Most children would be crushed if an adult refused to accept a gift. Of course, there are limits to this. It is one thing to accept a plate of cookies or a drawing, but it would be inappropriate to accept jewelry or an expensive gift certificate. Similarly, many child psychiatrists typically answer personal questions (within reason) from their patients. Otherwise, they run the risk of having patients feel shamed for having asked in the first place. It is normal for patients, especially children, to be curious about their psychiatrists. This is not to say that child psychiatrists have no boundaries. The psychiatrist may not feel comfortable answering a specific question and can simply say, for example, "That is a great question, and it is completely reasonable for you to wonder about it, but I do not feel comfortable giving out my home address." Similarly, adolescents may inquire about their doctor's history of alcohol use as a teenager or how the psychiatrist handles use of alcohol with his or her own teenagers. It is important not to overidentify with children and their families, and most child psychiatrists seek out supervision with peers or senior colleagues to make sure that their own experiences do not cloud their judgment when dealing with complicated situations (Jellinek, 1995; Klosinski, 1990).

Difficult situations definitely do arise when treating children and adolescents. At the extreme, concern for a child's safety may prompt the child psychiatrist to contact social services. A child psychiatrist is a "mandated reporter," who must report and document all suspected cases of abuse or neglect to the proper authorities (Vernick, 2002). Conflict may also arise when the parent and psychiatrist disagree about parenting techniques or when a child is caught in the midst of a difficult divorce or custody dispute. There may be cultural differences that affect treatment (Munir and Beardslee, 2001). A parent may be resistant to recommendations regarding medications or disagree with a specific diagnosis. Sometimes parents can become angry or defensive about an interaction or situation, such as lack of professional support for the use of harsh punishment when it is uncalled for in the eyes of the child psychiatrist.

It is also relatively common for parents to feel competitive with the child psychiatrist. From a parent's perspective, it can be incredibly difficult to see a child bond emotionally with another adult and reveal personal information, particularly if the parent–child relationship is strained. The child psychiatrist needs to be aware of these issues and anticipate those dilemmas whenever possible (Jellinek and Wells, 2004). It is almost always helpful for the child psychiatrist to support and empower the parents when clinically appropriate. It can also be useful to reiterate the fact that the parents know their child better than anyone and that their perspective is very helpful and valued. The child psychiatrist's job is to help the family function better, not to undermine parental decisions or compete for the child's affection (American Academy of Child and Adolescent Psychiatry, 2007).

However, in cases where a child's safety is at risk, the psychiatrist may need to act against a parent's wishes. Generally, it is best to remain calm, outline the reasons for the recommendation, and acknowledge that this may be hard for the parent to hear. Ultimately, it is helpful for the clinician to verbalize that the decision to call social services or hospitalize a child against the parent's wishes is not a punishment, but an attempt to keep the child safe.

Maintaining a good relationship with the family is a crucial part of a child psychiatrist's work. Frequency of contact with parents can vary based on the clinical picture. Some parents like to join the first or last 5 minutes of each session; others like to set up a dedicated family meeting every month. Still others prefer to communicate by phone between sessions. It is helpful

A CASE OF A PARENT RESISTING TREATMENT RECOMMENDATIONS

Susie is a 16-year-old whose father has been absent since she was 5 years old due to substance abuse, bipolar disorder, and domestic violence. She broke up with her first boyfriend and in the last two months has been increasingly irritable, sleeps excessively, and is failing school. She has stayed out past curfew and once failed to come home after drinking. After a fight with her best friend, she left a note saying that she was sorry about everything. Her mother found her in her room, sedated after taking an unknown number of diphenhydramine tablets, and took her to the emergency department. Susie admitted taking six tablets, thinking she would die. The evaluating psychiatrist determined that Susie had major depression and a suicide attempt and wanted her admitted to an inpatient unit. Her mother refused, worrying that Susie would be in a place with "bad, sick kids." She also noted that because Susie took a very small number of pills, this was not really a suicide attempt. The psychiatrist noted that the situation was very serious. Considering her father's mood disorder, Susie likely had a biological depression. Further, even though the number of pills she ingested was small, Susie believed they would kill her and therefore was at high risk. Susie's mother reluctantly agreed that she be admitted.

to see what will work best for a particular child or family. Maintaining a good therapeutic alliance can help the relationship survive, even when a child or parent is not happy with a particular recommendation (Beresin, 1994). Adolescents may scream and say they hate the clinician when a parental limit is supported, but many are able to say that they understand the rationale. It can be really helpful to gently say, "I know that you do not want to do this, but I care enough about you that I am willing to have you be mad at me right now." This can be very helpful modeling for parents as well.

ASSENT AND INFORMED CONSENT

Another difference between general psychiatry and child and adolescent psychiatry is that children are not able to consent to treatment. Minor children can *assent* to therapy or psychopharmacologic interventions, but a custodial parent must make the final decision regarding care. Whenever possible, it is best to take children's concerns into account when making decisions regarding treatment and to obtain their assent (Dell et al., 2008). Adherence to medications and visits is likely to be much higher when children feel that they have some autonomy in the decision-making process.

It is also extremely important that clinicians obtain informed consent regarding treatments, particularly medication options. Children and families need to be aware of potential side effects and outcomes of all medications. Child psychiatrists should not needlessly scare parents. However, they should ensure that parents understand potential risks as well as benefits. If a child is suffering from depression and would benefit from a serotonin reuptake inhibitor, the child psychiatrist needs to discuss recent media attention, the concerns about agitation and suicidal ideation, and the importance of close follow-up as the medication is initiated and titrated (Whittington et al., 2005). Children should understand the importance of telling an adult if they experience a worsening of symptoms or an increase in irritability or mood lability that may suggest medication-related activation. Parents should understand the need to let the child psychiatrist know immediately if this happens, so that the child can be reevaluated promptly and an intervention can be made. At the same time, parents and children should be made aware of the targeted symptoms of depression and report regularly on progress. Generally, parents and children handle these expectations very well, particularly if they are confident that the child psychiatrist is going to be available to them for consultation if needed.

PREVENTION

In addition to discussing medication side effects, family stresses, and peer relationships, the child psychiatrist can play an important role in prevention. Clinicians have a unique opportunity to discuss media literacy, peer pressure, sexual activity, and drug use in a safe setting (Villani et al., 2005). Psychiatrists can provide psychoeducation, act as a sounding board for negotiating developmental tasks, and mediate areas of conflict between parents and children. Kids will often bring up difficult dilemmas on their own. The end goal is for the child psychiatrist to listen empathically, reassure children that they are capable of making good decisions, and help them figure out the best approach to solving a problem. In general, the child psychiatrist is an aid to children and adolescents and families in monitoring and modulating development.

CONCLUSION

Clearly, psychiatrists who care for children and adolescents and their families face a lot of challenges. However, it is not unusual for former patients to stop by the clinic to say hello or to update the provider on their progress by letter or phone. Most child and adolescent psychiatrists are able to stay invested in their work because it is incredibly satisfying to know that one has had a positive impact on a child's overall growth and development.

Clinical Pearls

- Parents know their children best and can be an asset to treatment when the relationship is collaborative. Help them feel validated and understood.
- Never promise a child or adolescent absolute confidentiality. Children need to understand that the clinician must involve a parent or guardian should any concern about safety arise.
- Make children and adolescents feel that their input is welcome and valued when making treatment decisions. This can increase likelihood of proper adherence to the treatment plan.
- Be flexible when clinically appropriate. If a socially anxious child wants to reschedule a session because she has been invited to a birthday party and is excited to attend, let her!
- Children may report elaborate fantasies or unusual experiences that are usually more appropriately attributed to normal development rather than a psychotic process.
- It is important for child psychiatrists to clarify their role before evaluating new patients. To whom is the clinician consulting? What are the expectations and hopes (e.g., medications, therapy, and recommendations to court)?
- Do not be afraid to ask sensitive questions. Inquire about substance use, sexual activity, history of trauma, or abuse.

Self-Assessment Questions and Answers

27-1. A mother brings her 12-year-old daughter for evaluation, stating that she has been "out of control" and "needs medications to stop lying." On further questioning, the child denies any symptoms indicative of a mood or anxiety disorder and substance use. She admits that she sometimes lies about her after-school activities, because she wants to hang out with friends. Her mother would prefer that she attend an after-school religious program. What should the child psychiatrist recommend?

A. Call the minister for an "intervention."

B. Convince the adolescent that she would be happier if she obeyed her mother.

C. Psychotherapy for oppositional behavior.

D. Reassure the mother respectfully that this behavior is developmentally appropriate.

E. Start a serotonin reuptake inhibitor.

The child psychiatrist's primary role is to help facilitate a discussion between the child and her mother. Adolescents begin to individuate from the family and tend to place more importance on peer relationships. This can cause tension between parent and child but also prepares the child to be independent. The best parental approach is to allow the young adolescent some autonomy while maintaining firm limits on behavior that is developmentally inappropriate. It is also important for the teenager to appreciate that lying does not foster trust. The best approach for the child is to discuss her interests openly with her mother and engage in productive negotiation. As she proves her competence and ability to handle increased responsibility, her mother can relax the rules gradually and safely. The psychiatrist can relay this to both parent and child in a manner that normalizes the behavior. While making sure to respect family values, the psychiatrist can help them work out a compromise that might allow the child to have time with friends after school if she agrees to attend religious classes at an alternate time. *Answer: D*

27-2. A 16-year-old female presents for her weekly therapy appointment wearing a bandage over her left forearm. When questioned about it, she tries to hide the bandage, saying "It's nothing." She eventually admits that she cut herself with a razor blade after an argument with her boyfriend. She reports that this was an attempt to relieve tension after the fight and denies any suicidal ideation. She has been secretly cutting on a regular basis for the last 6 months. When asked if her parents know, she says, "No! They would not understand; they will just get mad. Besides, you said that these sessions were private!" The best course of action is to:

A. Bring it up again at the next session.
B. Hospitalize her immediately.
C. Offer to help her tell her parents in a group setting.
D. Reassure her, and then call her parents as soon as she leaves the session.
E. Respect her confidentiality.

The child psychiatrist can respect a patient's privacy as much as possible but cannot guarantee confidentiality, particularly when there are acute safety concerns. After making sure there is no immediate medical danger (e.g., assessing the need for sutures and inquiring about her last tetanus shot), the psychiatrist must perform a careful evaluation to rule out acute safety risk. In this case, the patient is clear that the cutting is related to emotion regulation rather than an intent to kill herself. Nonetheless, cutting can be dangerous, because patients not intending to harm themselves can inadvertently cut too deep. Further, the cutting may indicate worsening of a current mood or anxiety disorder and herald potential suicidal behavior. The clinician should explain to the adolescent that the goal is to keep her safe and that her parents need to know that this has been happening. They can tell the parents together so that they can fully discuss the situation and the parents can ask questions. They can then work together to reassess the current treatment plan, focusing on skills training so that she can

access more effective coping strategies when upset or overwhelmed. *Answer: C*

27-3. A 15-year-old boy presents to a clinic with his parents for evaluation of depression. He endorses depressed mood, irritability, hypersomnia, psychomotor retardation, and guilty ruminations. He denies suicidal ideation or substance use. He had previously seen another child psychiatrist who recently moved away; until a month ago, he had been taking fluoxetine on a somewhat sporadic basis. His mother reports that it is sometimes a struggle to persuade him to take medication as prescribed. Her son interrupts, "I hate that stuff and I won't take it!" The child psychiatrist should:

A. Diagnose depression and resume fluoxetine at the previous dose.
B. Diagnose oppositional defiant disorder and add clonidine to his medication regimen.
C. Meet with him separately to determine why he does not wish to resume fluoxetine.
D. Remind him that his parents are his legal guardians and the ones who decide regarding his care.
E. Start a different serotonin reuptake inhibitor.

Although it is true that the parent or legal guardian ultimately has the final say regarding treatment options for a minor child, it is very important to involve the adolescent in conversations about medication options. Children and adolescents often have valid concerns about taking medication; when they feel that they have been heard, they are far more likely to adhere to the treatment plan. One might discover that this young man is worried about the stigma associated with taking psychotropic medication. On the other hand, he may have difficulty swallowing pills and might prefer to take fluoxetine elixir. He may be having sexual side effects that he has been too embarrassed to report to his parents or his previous provider. Finally, the provider may discover that the fluoxetine was associated with increasing irritability or mood lability that might be concerning for underlying bipolar disorder. Listening to the child or adolescent can help guide treatment most appropriately and lead to better adherence to treatment. *Answer: C*

27-4. A single mother brings her 4-year-old son to the clinic for ongoing treatment of temper tantrums and poor frustration tolerance. His preschool teacher reports that she does not see many temper tantrums during the day, which is very structured. In addition, his maternal grandmother, who baby-sits until his mother returns from work, notes rare outbursts. However, his mother reports severe daily meltdowns, which often occur in public settings. Because the mother finds these situations embarrassing, she will try to appease him with promises of candy or toys. The child psychiatrist discusses the importance of structure and consistency with limits when caring for young children and recommends that she not "give in" to the child during these outbursts, because this is inadvertently reinforcing negative behavior. As the child psychiatrist begins to describe a behavioral plan designed to reward good behavior, the mother interrupts, "Oh, so now you think I am a bad parent too? I am not going to take this from someone who probably does not even have kids. Do not judge me until you have been in my shoes!" What is the child psychiatrist's most appropriate response?

A. "It must be incredibly frustrating to feel as though I am criticizing you. Let's talk more about that."

B. "It is none of your business whether I have kids. I am a medical doctor with specialized training in child and adolescent psychiatry!"

C. "You clearly have some issues. Do you have your own psychiatrist?"

D. "You are right; I do not have kids. I am sure you are doing the best you can."

E. "Oh, you poor thing. Do you want me to talk to anyone for you?"

Many parents (and children) are curious about the child psychiatrist's background. Clearly, one does not need to be a parent to understand and treat children. However, it is very normal for parents to feel as though the psychiatrist will be better able to understand the family if he or she has children. Sometimes parents can feel defensive when getting feedback from the child psychiatrist. Parents care about their children and want others to think well of them. They may also be sensitive about their child-rearing techniques, many of which were probably modeled by their own parents. It is important for the clinician to remain calm and resist the urge to become defensive or engage in an unproductive argument. The provider should also refrain from overidentifying with a parent. It is best to maintain an empathic and nonshaming approach. The mother *may* benefit from a referral for parental guidance or individual therapy at some point, but it would be best to broach the subject when she is calm and willing to consider it. *Answer: A*

27-5. A 17-year-old female with no known psychiatric history is brought to the emergency department by police on a Friday night after she ran onto the football field during a high school game and proceeded to take off her clothes. She is unkempt, smells strongly of tobacco, and makes poor eye contact. Her speech is pressured and disorganized, and she reports that she has not slept all week. She is paranoid and appears to be responding to internal stimuli. Her serum toxicology screen is positive for marijuana, which she admits to using over the last week so she could "just chill out." The emergency department staff called her parents, who have arrived. They are very concerned but are adamant to take her home right away. Her father is convinced that someone "slipped her a Mickey" and that she will be fine after a good night's sleep. How should the consulting psychiatrist proceed?

A. Allow her parents to take her home with the understanding that they bring her back to the emergency department if she does not improve.

B. Arrange for inpatient psychiatric hospitalization.

C. Ask a hospitalist to admit her to the medical service instead of the psychiatry service so that the parents are more comfortable.

D. Call the police back and report the parents for medical neglect.

E. Start an antipsychotic and instruct the parents to follow up in the child psychiatry clinic within a month.

This teenager is at imminent risk to self and others due to severe, untreated psychosis. Although it is always preferable for the parents and child to agree to treatment, sometimes concern for patient safety compels the child psychiatrist to hospitalize a child involuntarily. Hospitalization on the medical ward would be inappropriate in this case because it is an unlocked setting and the nursing staff does not have experience safely containing a manic and psychotic patient. Treatment with antipsychotic and/or mood stabilizing medications will almost certainly be necessary in this case, as will medical clearance in the emergency department before psychiatric admission. She may have been exposed to toxic and/or hallucinogenic substances in the marijuana that may be affecting the clinical picture. If her parents continue to resist after a thorough discussion about psychiatric illness and the need for treatment, the team may need to involve social services regarding concern for medical neglect. *Answer: B*

References

American Academy of Child and Adolescent Psychiatry. Practice parameters for the psychiatric assessment of children and adolescents. *J Am Acad Child Adolesc Psychiatry*. 1995;34:1386–1402.

American Academy of Child and Adolescent Psychiatry. Practice parameters for the psychiatric assessment of infants and toddlers. *J Am Acad Child Adolesc Psychiatry*. 1997;36(Suppl):21S–36S.

American Academy of Child and Adolescent Psychiatry. *Access to treatment for children and adolescents with mental illness: Children's mental health workforce shortage.* 1999. Available at http://www .aacap.org/galleries/LegislativeAction/workforce.doc (accessed 3/1/08).

American Academy of Child and Adolescent Psychiatry. Practice parameters for the assessment of the family. *J Am Acad Child Adolesc Psychiatry*. 2007;46(7):922–937.

Ascherman LI, Rubin S. Current ethical issues in child and adolescent psychotherapy. *Child Adolesc Psychiatr Clin N Am*. 2008;17(1):vii–viii, 21–35.

Beresin EV. Developmental formulation and psychotherapy of borderline adolescents. *Am J Psychother*. 1994;48(1):5–29.

Dell ML, Vaughan BS, Kratochvil CJ. Ethics and the prescription pad. *Child Adolesc Psychiatr Clin N Am*. 2008;17(1):ix, 93–111.

Dulcan M, Martini R, Lake M. Evaluation and treatment planning. *Concise guide to child and adolescent psychiatry*, 3rd ed. Washington, DC: American Psychiatric Publishing; 2003.

Freud S. In: Strachey J, ed. *Civilization and its discontents*. New York: Norton Publishers; 1961.

Fritz GK. Promoting effective collaboration between pediatricians and child and adolescent psychiatrists. *Pediatr Ann*. 2003;32(6):383, 387–389.

Gilliam WS, Mayes LC. Clinical assessment of infants and toddlers. In: Martin A, Volkmar F, Lewis M, eds. *Lewis' child and adolescent psychiatry: A comprehensive textbook*, 4th ed. Philadelphia: Lippincott Williams & Wilkins; 2007.

Jellinek MS. Professional identity: May the force be with us . . . always. *J Am Acad Child Adolesc Psychiatry*. 1995;34(3):387–388.

Jellinek MS, McDermott JF. Formulation: Putting the diagnosis into a therapeutic context and treatment plan. *J Am Acad Child Adolesc Psychiatry*. 2004;43(7):913–916.

Kaplan HI, Sadock BJ, eds. Child psychiatry: Assessment, examination, and psychological testing. In: *Synopsis of psychiatry*, 8th ed. Philadelphia: Lippincott Williams & Wilkins; 1998.

Klosinski G. Questions of guidance and supervision at the beginning of psychotherapy in children and adolescents. *Psychother Psychosom*. 1990;53(1-4):80–85.

Kutner L, Beresin EV. Reaching out: Mass media techniques for child and adolescent psychiatrists. *J Am Acad Child Adolesc Psychiatry*. 2000;39(11):1452–1454.

Lewis M, King RA. Psychiatric assessment of infants, children, and adolescents. In: Martin A, Volkmar F, Lewis M, eds. *Lewis' child and adolescent psychiatry: A comprehensive textbook*, 4th ed. Philadelphia: Lippincott Williams & Wilkins; 2007.

Moss NE, Racusin GR. Psychological assessment of children and adolescents. In: Martin A, Volkmar F, Lewis M, eds. *Lewis' child and adolescent psychiatry: A comprehensive textbook*, 4th ed. Philadelphia: Lippincott Williams & Wilkins; 2007.

Munir KM, Beardslee WR. A developmental and psychobiologic framework for understanding the role of culture in child and adolescent psychiatry. *Child Adolesc Psychiatr Clin N Am*. 2001;10(4):667–677.

Pataki C, Bostic JQ, Schlozman SC. The functional assessment of media in child and adolescent psychiatric treatment. *Child Adolesc Psychiatr Clin N Am*. 2005;14(3):555–570.

Rauch PK. Supporting the child within the family. *J Clin Ethics*. 2000;11(2):164–168.

Stein MT, Jellinek MS, Wells RD. The difficult parent: A reflective pediatrician's response. *J Dev Behav Pediatr*. 2003;24(6):434–437.

Vernick AE. Forensic aspects of everyday practice: Legal issues that every practitioner must know. *Child Adolesc Psychiatr Clin N Am.* 2002;11(4):905–928.

Villani SV, Olson CK, Jellinek MS. Media literacy for clinicians and parents. In: Beresin EV, Olson CK, eds. *Child psychiatry and the media*, Vol. 14. Child and Adolescent Clinics of North America; 2005:523–554.

Whittington CJ, Kendall T, Pilling S. Are the SSRIs and atypical antidepressants safe and effective for children and adolescents? *Curr Opin Psychiatry.* 2005;18(1):21–25.

Winnicott DW. *The child, the family, and the outside world.* Reading: Addison-Wesley; 1987.

CHAPTER 28

James L. Levenson

Psychiatric Care for the Medically Ill

The goals of this chapter are to examine the sources and consequences of psychiatric symptoms and disorders specific to medical patients and the physician's corresponding responsibilities and opportunities for treatment. This chapter is grounded in the biopsychosocial model of illness (see Stoudemire's 1998 *Human Behavior: An Introduction for Medical Students* and Chapters 4 and 31 of this book). Major psychiatric disorders that are often encountered in the medical setting are also discussed elsewhere in this book, including delirium, dementia, and other cognitive disorders (Chapter 8), substance abuse (Chapter 9), mood disorders (Chapter 11), anxiety disorders (Chapter 12), somatoform disorders (Chapter 13), and personality disorders (Chapter 20).

This chapter focuses on special aspects of psychiatry in medical practice not discussed in depth in the earlier chapters. First, an overview is provided of psychiatric disorders in medical patients. Second, psychological and emotional reactions to physical illness are discussed, including the management of these reactions in the general medical setting. Third, the nature of grief and mourning and the dying patient are considered. Fourth, drugs and medical disorders that can produce psychiatric symptoms are reviewed. Finally, guidelines are provided to evaluate patients' competency and obtain psychiatric consultation.

PSYCHIATRIC DISORDERS IN MEDICAL PATIENTS

Psychiatric disorders are common in medical patients, although the measured frequency varies depending on the criteria used. A reasonable estimate would be that 25% to 30% of medical outpatients and 40% to 50% of general medical inpatients have diagnosable psychiatric disorders (see Table 28-1). The most common psychiatric syndromes in medical outpatients are depression, anxiety, somatoform disorders, and substance abuse (Norton et al., 2007; Schneider and Levenson, 2008) and, in medical inpatients, disorders associated with cognitive impairment (delirium, dementia, etc.), depression, and substance abuse (Bressi et al., 2006; Rothenhausler, 2006).

Psychiatric diagnoses are likely to be found in patients with multiple unexplained physical symptoms and in those who are high utilizers of medical services. Most physicians underdiagnose and undertreat psychiatric disorders in the medically ill (Lecrubier, 2007). This is unfortunate because (a) many patients with serious psychiatric illnesses depend on primary care physicians, not mental health professionals, for their mental health care (Regier et al., 1993); (b) without recognition and intervention, coincident psychopathology increases medical care utilization and costs (Saravay, 2006); and (c) there are effective interventions for psychiatric disorders in the medically ill (Blumenfield and Strain, 2006; Levenson, 2005).

There are a number of reasons why many patients with psychiatric disorders are seen by primary care and other nonpsychiatric physicians rather than mental health professionals. Some are fearful of being stigmatized as mentally ill, and some prefer to confide in an already familiar, trusted figure. The primary reason may be problems of access, such as inadequate available mental health services (especially in rural areas) or lack of knowledge regarding how to find them. Insurance barriers include less generous reimbursement for mental health care (higher costs for patients) and more restrictive "gate keeping" by managed care.

The presence of psychiatric disorders alongside medical disorders adversely affects clinical outcomes and raises health care costs. Psychopathology in general is associated with a longer length of hospital stay and more utilization of outpatient services (Saravay, 2006). Depression results in higher morbidity and mortality in several medical disorders (e.g., myocardial infarction,

TABLE 28-1	Percentage of Prevalence of Selected Psychiatric Disorders[a]		
	Community	**Primary Care Patients**	**Medical Inpatients**
All psychiatric disorders	15–20	25–30	40–50
Mood disorders	11	10–30	20–35
Major depression	10	5–16	5–10
Dysthymia	2.5	5–10	—
Bipolar disorder	1	1	1
Anxiety disorders	17	10–20	20–30
Panic disorder	2	3–6	—
Generalized anxiety disorder	5	5–10	—
Obsessive-compulsive disorder	1	1–3	—
Somatoform disorders	—	10–20	2–5
Alcohol abuse or dependence	10	5–20	5–20
Cognitive disorders before age 65	1	—	15–20
Cognitive disorders after age 65	5–10	15–20	30–50

[a]Sources include Kessler et al., 1994; Spitzer et al., 1994.

chronic renal failure). Medically ill patients with delirium have a higher mortality rate and stay in the intensive care unit longer than those without delirium, and they are more likely to remove their own tubes and assault their caregivers. Patients with somatization are especially high users of medical care, while remaining among those least satisfied with their care. Psychopathology erodes medical outcomes and raises health care costs through a variety of mechanisms. Psychiatric comorbidity decreases functional capacity, amplifies somatic symptoms, decreases motivation and adherence, promotes maladaptive risk behaviors, delays seeking health care, and strains doctor–patient relationships.

Fortunately, there are a range of effective interventions for psychiatric disorders in the medically ill. First, effective intervention requires improved recognition. The presence of a consultation-liaison psychiatrist enhances identification of psychopathology in the medically ill (Meadows et al., 2007). There are also many useful screening instruments for psychopathology in medical settings, such as the PRIME-MD-Patient Health Questionnaire, the CAGE for alcohol abuse/dependence, and the Mini-Mental Status for Examination for cognitive dysfunction.

Psychiatric interventions with demonstrated effectiveness in the medically ill include psychiatric medication, individual or group psychotherapy, and consultation–liaison interventions. For example, cognitive behavioral therapy and antidepressants for major depression in diabetic patients can improve their glycemic control (Lustman et al., 1998; Lustman et al., 2000). Group therapy has improved quality of life in cancer patients (Goodwin et al., 2001). A consultation–liaison psychiatrist's feedback to primary care physicians regarding how to better manage their patients with somatization disorder dramatically reduced their patients' (inappropriate) utilization of health care resources (Smith et al., 1986).

COMMON PSYCHOLOGICAL REACTIONS TO MEDICAL ILLNESS AND TREATMENT

Extensive reviews of psychological reactions to illness can be found elsewhere (Groves, 1978; Groves and Muskin, 2005; Kahana and Bibring, 1964). Here regression and dependency, anxiety, depression, denial, nonadherence, discharges against medical advice, and doctor-shopping will be reviewed briefly.

Regression and Dependency

Regression, a return to more childlike patterns of behavior and feeling, is a universal human reaction to illness. Sick patients wish to be comforted, cared for, and freed from the responsibilities of adult life. In moderation this is adaptive, because ill patients must give up some control and accept some dependency on others. Regression is problematic when it becomes more extreme. It is difficult to care for a patient who has minimal pain tolerance, cannot tolerate being alone, or is infantile, overly needy, whining, and easily upset or frustrated.

Not all patients regress in the same fashion. The varieties of regression are similar to the developmental phases of early childhood. Like young infants, some regressed patients are overdependent and seem to want "feeding" on demand, constantly pushing the nurses' call button in the hospital or, as outpatients, telephoning the physician too much. They let others make decisions, complain petulantly about their care, and avoid sharing responsibility.

Other regressed patients resemble children in the "terrible twos." They have an excessive need to control their medical care in the hospital environment and get into struggles over less critical elements of their care. They may have tantrums over getting their way and tend to be perfectionistic and intolerant of any irregularities, disarray, or tardiness.

Like many 3- to 4-year-olds, some patients who regress need to feel powerful and admired. They tend to be aggressive and narcissistic, oblivious to the needs of other patients around them. They may be sexually provocative, particularly if the illness has assaulted their sense of self-esteem and power (e.g., acute paraplegia, myocardial infarction).

These developmental descriptions of regression are illustrations that do appear as described but also at milder, more easily tolerated levels. When ill, we all regress more or less on needing to be cared for, control and order, and bolstering of self-esteem. Some patients find such regression comfortable (ego-syntonic), particularly if it elicits comforting responses from those around them. Others are very uncomfortable with their regression (ego-dystonic), feeling embarrassed at the unexpected emergence of childlike feelings or actions.

Sources of Regression and Dependency

As noted, moderate regression is adaptive. In the face of illness, adults hope to receive the nurturance, reassurance, and care provided by parents during childhood. Patients who regress behaviorally to an extreme often have preexisting psychopathology, particularly personality disorders. Those who use a narrow range of inflexible defenses become more helpless and regressed when serious illness overwhelms them. Patients who find regression too comfortable have usually received significant secondary gain from previous illnesses. Those who suffered serious deprivation in childhood, with emotionally or physically absent or dysfunctional parents, may experience the care of physicians and nurses as the only nurturing experiences they have ever

A CASE OF ADAPTIVE DENIAL

A 60-year-old man was admitted to the hospital after hemorrhaging from his mouth following dental work in which his dentist cauterized his gums. He was discovered to have profound thrombocytopenia secondary to lymphoma. Chemotherapy was initiated, with adverse effects, including hair loss and severe leucopenia. The patient wore his own clothes during the hospitalization and had weights brought in from home so he could maintain his exercise routine. He bragged of having the strength of a much younger man. The patient's son was a third-year medical student and at the patient's bedside were medical books he had borrowed from his son, but all first-year books (biochemistry, anatomy, physiology). Psychiatric consultation was sought because of the patient's denial; he did not acknowledge having a malignant disease. When asked why he was in the hospital, he said "first it was a platelet problem, then a white cell problem, and then to prevent infections, they bring me here for powerful antibiotics." He also denied hair loss, though it was fairly obvious he was wearing a toupee.

This case illustrates adaptive denial. This patient could not tolerate being conscious of having a life-threatening illness. He tried to maintain his normal manner of dress and exercise routine, asserting his masculine strength, defending against feeling vulnerable. The denial was adaptive because it did not interfere in his getting the needed chemotherapy. Note that he also used an intellectual defense, reading his son's textbooks to become more informed, but sticking with the "normal" books of the first year of medical school, avoiding the "pathological" books of the second year.

had. As adults, they unconsciously yearn to re-create this experience and so may regress excessively when ill.

Intervention for Regression and Dependency

When regression is marked, physicians and nurses become impatient and angry, especially with those patients who they feel should not act "childishly" (e.g., patients who are health care professionals). As with other reactions to illness, physicians should avoid scolding or shaming patients (a parallel regression in the physician). Instead, the physician can explain to the patient that feeling more dependent or needy is part of an expected reaction to illness. Patients who make repeated, unreasonable, or unrealistic demands may require behavioral limit setting. While tolerating some necessary regression, the physician takes steps to mobilize the patient physically and emotionally to participate in treatment and rehabilitation. Psychiatric consultation should be sought if regression is too great or persists too long, creating significant interference in treatment, distress for the patient, or unnecessary invalidism.

Anxiety

Anxiety occurs with the same symptoms in the medically ill as in healthy individuals, but a correct diagnosis is more difficult with coexistence of physical disease because the signs of anxiety may be misinterpreted as those of physical disease, and *vice versa*. Many somatic pathophysiological phenomena share symptoms with anxiety states, such as tachycardia, diaphoresis, tremor, shortness of breath, or abdominal or chest pain. Panic attacks present with so many prominent somatic symptoms that they are routinely misdiagnosed as a wide variety of physical illnesses. On the other hand, autonomic arousal and anxious agitation in a medically ill patient may be prematurely attributed by the physician to "reactive anxiety," when they also can be signs of a pulmonary embolus, cardiac arrhythmia, or hyperthyroidism.

Physicians tend to become desensitized in working with seriously ill patients and may lose sight of the spectrum of normal anxiety reactions. For example, having diagnosed diabetes mellitus in an asymptomatic young adult patient, the physician may assume that a diagnosis of "just chemical diabetes" ought not to cause too much anxiety. The physician may not notice that the patient is frightened, or if the physician does notice, she or he may conclude that the patient is responding with pathological anxiety. The patient may be thinking about serious complications (amputations, blindness, kidney failure) witnessed in relatives with the disease, leading to more anxiety than the physician expected.

Sources of Anxiety

There are many reasons for anxiety in the medically ill patient. Different individuals will react to the same diagnosis, prognosis, treatment, and complications with widely varying concerns. Patients may be very aware of some fears but simultaneously affected by less conscious ones. Ideally, the physician explores concerns with the patient by inquiring about those aspects of the illness that are causing anxiety and observing the patient's behavior.

Fear of death frequently occurs during the course of an illness, but not necessarily in proportion to the severity of disease. Many other factors may magnify or diminish this fear (e.g., previous losses, religious beliefs, personality, intractable pain, and previous experiences in the medical care system, including witnessing other patients' deaths). Although for some patients with minor illness the fear of death can be overwhelming, for others, with major or even terminal illness, it may be less important than other fears.

Fear of abandonment ("separation anxiety") occurs in the medically ill as the fear of being alone. It may occur under the same circumstances that give rise to the fear of death, but here an individual is less concerned about the end of life and more concerned with the thought of being separated from loved ones. For some individuals who are immature, overly dependent, or overwhelmed, being hospitalized may itself precipitate acute separation anxiety. The patient must leave the security of home, family, and friends for the impersonal and anonymous institution of the modern hospital.

Closely related to separation anxiety is the fear of strangers ("stranger anxiety"). Visiting a physician when ill requires a patient to answer personal questions and to be physically examined by and put one's trust in (usually) previously unknown physicians and other members of the health care team. As patients become more acutely ill or face a terminal illness, the fear of abandonment tends to be much greater than the fear of strangers. The sick and dying very rarely wish to be left alone. Not recognizing how important they have become to their patients, residents and interns are often surprised at how anxious and depressed some patients become when it comes time for physicians to rotate to a new service each month. What has become routine for the house staff is a repetitive source of anxiety and depression for patients.

The morbidity and disability caused by physical disease produce a number of other fears. The fear of loss of, or injury to, body parts or bodily functions includes fear of amputations, blindness, and mutilating scars and is particularly highly charged when directed at the genitalia ("castration anxiety"). The fear of pain is universal, but the threshold varies greatly among individuals. Some patients experience intense fear of loss of control. They may also fear that they will no longer be able to manage a career, family, or other aspects of their life. Directed inwardly, individuals may be frightened by loss of control over their own bodies, including fear of incontinence or metastasis. Closely related is the fear of dependency. Here, it is not so much the loss of control of one's body or life that frightens the patient but having to depend on others. For some, this fear of dependency is part of a more general fear of intimacy. Certain individuals (particularly those with schizoid, avoidant, paranoid, and some compulsive personalities) are frightened of getting close to people in any setting. Physical illness is very threatening to them because they must allow physicians and nurses to penetrate the interpersonal barriers they have constructed.

Finally, some patients experience guilty fears ("superego anxiety") related to their anticipation that others will feel angry or disappointed with them. This is particularly common with illnesses attributable to patients' habits (e.g., smoking, diet, alcohol) and in situations in which patients have not adhered to physicians' advice. Some patients may feel their illness is a punishment from God or has some special punitive significance for past "sins."

Consequences of Anxiety

Some degree of anxiety is adaptive during physical illness because it alerts the individual to the presence of danger and the need for action. An appropriate and tolerable amount of anxiety helps patients get medical help and adhere to physicians' recommendations. The total absence of anxiety may be maladaptive, promoting a cavalier attitude of minimizing disease and the need for treatment. In most such cases, however, the absence of anxiety is only an apparent one—the patient is often extremely anxious unconsciously and is resorting to defenses like denial (see subsequent text) in order not to be overwhelmed by the illness. Too much anxiety is also maladaptive, leading to unnecessary invalidism. Becoming paralyzed with fear of disease progression or relapse, such patients give up functioning occupationally, socially, and/or sexually. In most diseases, a modicum of anxiety is expectable and adaptive, but occasionally even a normal amount of anxiety can pose some risk. For example, immediately after an acute myocardial infarction, significant anxiety-associated increases in heart rate and blood pressure may be considered dangerous and warrant treatment.

Intervention for Anxiety

To address anxiety, the physician should first explore the particular patient's fears. If the physician wrongly presumes to know why the patient is anxious without asking, then the patient is likely to feel misunderstood. Facile, nonspecific reassurance can undermine the physician–patient relationship, because the patient is likely to feel that the physician is out of touch with and not really interested in what he or she is actually feeling.

Knowing the patient's specific fears leads the physician to appropriate therapeutic interventions. Unrealistic fears can be reduced by cognitive interventions. For example, the patient who is frightened of having intercourse after a heart attack can be reassured that it is unnecessary to give up sex. Fears of closeness can be reduced by taking extra care to respect the patient's privacy. When fears of pain, loss, or injury to body parts are not unrealistic, it is helpful for the physician to emphasize the ways in which medical care can reduce suffering and enhance functioning through rehabilitation. Physicians should tell patients about disease-specific support organizations for patients and families, which provide a continuing antidote for anxiety.

When clarifying the patient's anxieties and intervening in one of these ways is insufficient, the judicious, short-term use of benzodiazepines may be helpful (see Chapters 12 and 22);

however, drug therapy for anxiety is no substitute for the reassurance and support that can be provided through the doctor–patient relationship. Antianxiety medication may be appropriate for new symptoms of anxiety that have been precipitated by an identifiable recent stressor (e.g., hospitalization). Because such anxiety is often temporary, benzodiazepines are usually preferable to antidepressants because the former provide immediate benefits. In most cases, benzodiazepines for anxiety in the medically ill should be time limited (usually 1 to 3 weeks), because tolerance and dependence may develop with long-term use. If benzodiazepines are abruptly discontinued after sustained use, significant withdrawal symptoms may occur, including rebound anxiety and insomnia, agitation, psychosis, confusion, and seizures. Although benzodiazepines are relatively safe in the medically ill, their most common side effect, sedation, may intensify confusion in delirium and dementia, suppress respiratory drive in severe pulmonary disease, and interfere with optimal participation by patients in their medical care. Sustained use of benzodiazepines or other sedatives may aggravate depression. Antianxiety medication prescribed during a medical hospitalization should not be automatically continued after discharge.

In deciding whether psychiatric consultation and intervention are required, it is important to distinguish normal, expectable anxiety from more serious "pathological" anxiety. Anxiety is usually a symptom of a psychiatric disorder when it remains unrealistic or out of proportion, despite the physician's clarification and reassurance, as described earlier. Other signs that anxiety requires psychiatric intervention are sustained disruption of sleep or gastrointestinal functions, marked autonomic hyperarousal (tachycardia, tachypnea, sweating), and panic attacks. Psychiatric consultation should also be requested when anxiety fails to respond to low doses of benzodiazepines, is accompanied by psychosis, or renders patients unable to participate in their medical care (including those who threaten to leave against medical advice).

Depression

In addition to clinical psychiatric depressions, depressed states in the medically ill may include grief, sadness, demoralization, fatigue, exhaustion, and psychomotor slowing. The same pitfalls of under- or overdiagnosis described for anxiety also occur with depression. On one hand, the vegetative signs and symptoms of depression (e.g., anorexia, weight loss, weakness, constipation, insomnia) may be incorrectly attributed to a physical etiology and lead the physician to undertake unnecessary diagnostic evaluations. On the other hand, the physician must also guard against prematurely concluding that somatic symptoms are due to depression, because an occult

A CASE OF ANXIETY

Mr. A, a 62-year-old married accountant with coronary artery disease, was referred for psychiatric evaluation because he declined coronary artery bypass surgery (CABG) despite strong recommendations by his cardiologist, who perceived that his resistance was not from lack of information or understanding.

Mr. A had no acute psychiatric symptoms but several lifelong phobias, including claustrophobia. His coronary artery disease was severe, with two myocardial infarctions, recurrent ventricular arrhythmias, and continuing angina despite maximal medical management. Past medical history included infectious complications and multiple pulmonary emboli after orthopedic operations.

Mr. A had a long written list of arguments for and against surgery and other variables that could influence the decision and outcome. His analysis was well informed, accurate, flexible, and appropriate, but it had not enabled him to reach a decision. He knew this was taking much longer than average but thought it could not be resolved another way. The psychiatrist told Mr. A that she was impressed with the thoroughness with which he had considered all aspects of the surgery and that she was confident in his ability to make the right decision. Mr. A soon called his cardiologist and had successful CABG.

Mr. A could have had a number of fears related to his cardiac disease and CABG but was consciously preoccupied with the fear of making the wrong decision. His obsessional style was largely adaptive in his chosen occupation and used here to cope with his anxiety. Confronted with a major health care decision and mindful of complications he had suffered previously, he was paralyzed in his decision making. An understanding of the focus and sources of his anxiety facilitated resolution of the impasse.

medical disease (e.g., malignancy) may be missed. Desensitization to illness and suffering may make physicians unaware of, or impatient with and intolerant of, normal depressive reactions. Physicians sometimes err in the other direction and regard a serious (and treatable) coexisting psychiatric depression as merely a "normal" response to physical illness.

Sources of Depression

Medically ill patients feel sad or depressed about many of the same issues discussed earlier under anxiety. When a feared event has not yet taken place, patients are anxious; when the loss or injury has already occurred, the patient becomes depressed. Therefore, depression may arise secondary to loss of relationships, loss of body parts or functions, loss of control or independence, chronic pain, or guilt. Hospitalization, which results in separation of the patient from loved ones, is a potential source for depression, especially for young children and mothers of infants. Medical illness also may reawaken dormant grief and sadness when the patient recalls a parent or sibling who died from the same disease the patient has. Patients who cannot express anger, either because they have always had difficulty doing so or because they are afraid of offending those with whom they are angry (e.g., physicians), are at higher risk for depression.

Another explanation for depression in the medically ill is learned helplessness, a behavioral model derived from animal experiments. When repeatedly exposed to painful or other aversive stimuli while being prevented from controlling or escaping from such stimulation, many species become passive, withdrawn, and unmotivated. In patients, the course of physical illness, particularly multiple relapses, relentless progression, and/or treatment failure, may produce a very similar state of helplessness, giving up, and the perception that one has no control over one's fate. Both experimentally and clinically, learned helplessness can be reduced by increasing the person's sense of control (Lawrence-Smith and Sturgeon, 2006). Physicians may unwittingly add to some patients' helplessness by not actively eliciting patients' participation and preferences in decision making about their health care.

Consequences of Depression

In the face of disease and disability, patients frequently feel discouraged, dejected, and helpless and need physicians who are able and willing to listen to such feelings. When feelings of sadness become too great and demoralization or clinical depression occurs, maladaptive consequences may ensue, including poor adherence, poor nutrition and hygiene, and giving up prematurely. If severe, patients may become actively or passively suicidal (e.g., a transplant patient who deliberately misses doses of maintenance immunosuppressive drugs). Recognizing these serious consequences helps the physician distinguish pathological depression from normal depressive reactions, including grief (see subsequent text).

Intervention for Depression

As with the anxious patient, the first step for the physician in addressing depression is to listen and understand. Physicians can help patients by encouraging them to openly express sadness and grief related to illness and loss. Physicians should avoid premature or unrealistic reassurance or an overly cheerful attitude, because this tends to alienate depressed patients, who feel that their physician is insensitive and either does not understand or does not want to hear about their sadness. Physicians should provide specific and realistic reassurance, emphasize a constructive treatment plan, and mobilize the patient's support system. For patients who seem to be experiencing learned helplessness, enabling them to have a sense of more control over their illness will be helpful. Physicians can accomplish this by encouraging patients to express preferences about their health care, giving them more control over the hospital and nursing routines, and emphasizing active steps they can undertake, rather than just passively accepting what others prescribe for them. Patients who are demoralized before beginning treatment or who are at the start of major treatment (e.g., transplantation, amputation, dialysis, chemotherapy, colostomy) can benefit from speaking with successfully treated patients who have had the same disorder.

Normal depressive reactions to illness must be differentiated from pathological depression, which requires psychiatric consultation and intervention (e.g., antidepressants, psychotherapy). Patients experiencing normal degrees of depression retain their abilities to communicate, make decisions, and participate in their own care when encouraged to do so. Depression usually constitutes a psychiatric disorder when depressed mood, hopelessness, worthlessness, withdrawal, and vegetative symptoms (e.g., insomnia, anorexia, fatigue) are persistent *and* out of proportion to coexisting medical illness. Urgent psychiatric referral should always be obtained when the patient is thinking about suicide (see subsequent text) or has depression with psychotic symptoms. Psychiatric consultation should also be obtained if less serious depression fails to improve with the physician's support and reassurance and becomes prolonged, if an antidepressant has been tried and found ineffective, or if patients remain too depressed to participate in their own health care and rehabilitation. The treatment of depression is discussed from the biological standpoint in Chapters 22 and 24, and psychotherapy for depression is discussed in Chapter 23.

Assessing Suicide Risk in Medical Patients

All physicians should be able to screen patients for suicide risk in the medical setting. Chapter 26 addresses assessment of suicide in the emergency setting. Suicide is a common preventable cause of death in the medically ill, and patients frequently drop hints to their physicians about suicidal impulses or plans. Chronic illness and chronic pain are risk factors for suicide. The physician's concern should increase when other risk factors are present (Bostwick and Levenson, 2005; Copsey Spring et al., 2007), including major mood disorder, alcoholism, schizophrenia, disorders associated with impaired cognition, recent loss of a loved one, divorce, loss of a job, or a family history of suicide.

Whenever patients appear depressed or despondent, physicians should explicitly ask about suicidal feelings and plans (see Chapter 30 in Schneider and Levenson, 2008). Physicians are sometimes reluctant because they fear that they will "put ideas into the patient's head" or offend the patient. Others simply are not sure how to ask. The great majority of patients who are experiencing suicidal thoughts are relieved to discuss them with a caring physician. The physician should ask gradually and directly, with a series of questions like: How bad have you been feeling? Have you ever felt bad enough to not go on with life? Have you ever thought of doing something about it? What did you think of doing? Ominous signs indicative of serious suicide risk include the following:

The motive behind the suicidal wish is entirely self-directed, with no apparent intent to influence someone else.

Detailed suicide plans are contemplated over an extended period of time.

Lethal means have been considered by and are available to the patient.

A suicide attempt was made in an isolated setting where the individual was unlikely to be discovered.

The individual is putting affairs in order, such as making out a will, reviewing life insurance coverage, or giving away prized possessions.

Hints or direct statements are made about feeling suicidal. Spontaneous statements like "I am going to kill myself" should never be dismissed as "just talk" but always carefully and thoroughly explored by the primary physician.

The presence of any suicidal ideation, with or without any attempt, is an indication for psychiatric consultation, and it is the physician's responsibility to ensure that it is obtained. Physicians must also guard against unwittingly providing the means for suicide: for significantly depressed patients, physicians should prescribe all medications that are dangerous if overdosed in carefully monitored, small supplies (usually 1 week at a time) or arrange for a responsible family member to dispense the patient's medication daily.

Denial

Denial is a defense mechanism that reduces anxiety and conflict by blocking conscious awareness of thoughts, feelings, or facts that an individual cannot face. Denial is common in the medically ill but varies in its timing, strength, and adaptive value. Some patients are aware of what is wrong with them but consciously suppress this knowledge by avoiding thinking about or discussing it. Others cope with the threat of being overwhelmed by their illness by unconsciously repressing it and thereby remain unaware of their illness. Physicians may sometimes misperceive as deniers patients whose lack of awareness stems from not having been sufficiently informed about and/or not understanding the nature of their disease.

Although denial of physical disease may accompany and be a symptom of a major psychiatric disorder (e.g., schizophrenia), outright denial also occurs in the absence of other significant psychopathology. Marked denial, in which the patient emphatically refuses to accept the existence or significance of obvious symptoms and signs of a disease, may be seen by the physician as an indication that the patient is "crazy," because the patient seems impervious to rational persuasion. In the absence of other evidence of major psychopathology (e.g., paranoid delusions), such denial is not often a sign of psychosis but, rather, a defense against overwhelming fear.

Denial also occurs as a direct consequence of disease of the central nervous system, commonly in dementia along with other cognitive deficits and, rarely, as an isolated finding with parietal lobe lesions (anosognosia).

Sources of Denial

Denial is a defense mechanism used in the face of intolerable anxiety or unresolved conflict. The medically ill patient, threatened with any of the fears outlined earlier, may resort to denial. Individuals who deny other life stresses, such as marital or occupational problems, are particularly likely to use denial in the face of clinical illness. Denial is also common in individuals who are threatened by the dependency associated with illness, for whom the sick role is inconsistent with their self-image of potency and invulnerability.

To avoid fear and conflict, the patient may deny all or only part of the disease and its consequences. Some will deny that they are ill at all; others will accept the symptoms but deny the particular diagnosis (usually displacing it to a more benign organ system, e.g., interpreting angina as indigestion), the need for treatment, or the need to alter lifestyle.

Consequences of Denial

Denial is not always a pathologic defense and may serve several adaptive purposes (Vos and de Haes, 2007). When denial occurs as part of the initial shock upon learning of a serious diagnosis or complication, it allows the individual sufficient time to adjust to the bad news and avoid overwhelming, full, immediate awareness. A lesser, continuing degree of denial helps patients function without being overly preoccupied with full consciousness of the morbidity or mortality associated with their diseases.

The adaptive value of denial may vary, depending on the nature or stage of illness. For example, myocardial infarction and sudden death may occur when denial prevents an individual with symptoms of coronary artery disease from acknowledging the symptoms and promptly seeking medical care. Those who delay going to the hospital after the acute onset of coronary symptoms have greater morbidity and mortality. Physicians seldom have an opportunity to affect denial at that stage of illness (that is, before seeking medical care), except by educating the general public and patients who appear at higher risk. Moderate denial during hospitalization may be very adaptive, perhaps even reducing morbidity and mortality in some diseases (Levenson et al., 1989). If not excessive, such denial reduces anxiety but does not prevent the patient from accepting and cooperating with medical treatment.

Denial after hospital discharge may also be helpful or harmful. Too little denial may leave the patient flooded with fears of disability and death and result in unnecessary invalidism. However, excessive denial may result in the patient's rushing back to full-time work, disregarding the rehabilitation plan, ignoring modifiable risk factors, and adopting a cavalier attitude toward medication or other treatment.

Intervention for Denial

When a patient's denial does not preclude cooperation with treatment, the physician should leave it alone. The physician does have an ethical and professional obligation to ensure that the patient has been informed about the illness and treatment. Following that, if the patient accepts treatment but persists in what seems an irrationally optimistic outlook, the physician should respect the patient's need to use denial to cope. For some, the denial is fragile, and the physician must judge whether the defense should be supported and strengthened or whether the patient would do better by giving up the denial to discuss fears and receive reassurance from the physician. The physician should never support denial by giving the patient false information but, rather, encourage hope and optimism in the patient.

When denial is extreme, patients may refuse vital treatment or threaten to leave against medical advice (see "Discharges Against Medical Advice" in subsequent text). Here, the physician must try to help reduce denial, but not by directly assaulting the patient's defenses. Because such desperate denial of reality usually reflects intense underlying anxiety, trying to scare the patient into cooperating will intensify denial and the impulse to flight. A better strategy for the physician is to avoid directly challenging the patient's claims, while simultaneously reinforcing concern for the patient and maximizing the patient's sense of control. Involving family members should be considered, because they may be more successful in convincing the patient that accepting medical care is in the patient's best interests. Psychiatric consultation is very helpful in cases of extreme or persistent maladaptive denial and should always be obtained if the denial is accompanied by symptoms of a major psychiatric disorder (see also Chapters 5 and 14 in Stoudemire, 1998).

Nonadherence

Nonadherence with medical treatment is a frequent behavioral response to medical illness. It may occur in up to 90% of those receiving short-term medication regimens and probably averages approximately 50% in the drug treatment of patients with chronic disease (Gold and McClung, 2006; Winnick et al., 2005). Misled both by wishful thinking and stereotypes of the nonadhering patient, physicians generally underestimate its occurrence. Nonadherence is common in patients who poorly understand their treatment, are hostile to medical care, have major psychiatric disorders, and flatly deny their illness; however, nonadherence also occurs in "ideal" patients and is not confined to any socioeconomic or ethnic group. Physicians are also misled because patients overestimate their adherence when asked. They may be embarrassed by their failure to stick to the regimen, frightened of the consequences (such as angering their physician), or unconscious of the problem. The physician will more likely get accurate information by asking about adherence in a friendly, nonjudgmental way, without any threats, accusations, or anger. The physician should not shame or infantilize the patient through scolding or patronizing.

Labeling a patient as "noncompliant" implies that the physician's recommendations are entirely correct, but sometimes our instructions are unnecessary, debatable, or even wrong. Physicians must also avoid concluding nonadherence whenever there is unexplained failure of the patient to respond to the usual treatment. This may be an appropriate time to suspect nonadherence, but the physician should not reach a conclusion without evidence.

A patient is noncompliant when the patient and physician both share the belief that treatment is warranted, but the patient fails to follow through; however, physicians must remember that patients have their own value and belief systems that guide their actions. Scientific principles and the medical literature are not as compelling for most patients as they are for physicians. Religious beliefs, cultural values, and the patient's own theories of causation and treatment, which may be culture bound or idiosyncratic, all influence patient responses to physicians' recommendations.

Nonadherence is not a monolithic behavior. While some patients are globally noncompliant, others are only noncompliant with a particular aspect of treatment. Some have difficulty keeping appointments; others, with taking medication. Many have difficulty complying with recommended changes in habits or lifestyle, including patterns of work and sleep, smoking, diet, and exercise. Others may follow recommendations coming from one trusted doctor (often a primary care physician), while ignoring the advice of unfamiliar consultants. Some individuals are only intermittently noncompliant (for example, only during periods of depression).

Sources of Nonadherence

As suggested earlier, preexisting beliefs the patient has about diagnosis and treatment are a major source of deviation from the treatment plan (Chia et al., 2006; Phatak and Thomas, 2006). Many ethnic subcultures have their own traditional theories of disease and therapy that may influence how members take medications. Such patients tend to hide their beliefs from physicians who are not members of the same ethnic or cultural group because the patients think their beliefs will not be accepted or they are embarrassed to acknowledge "old-fashioned," "superstitious" ideas. A similar phenomenon is seen with those who believe various "counterculture" theories of disease, like homeopathy or naturopathy, and followers of religions that practice faith healing. Some patients have deep and powerful beliefs about the right and wrong way to treat their illness, based on past personal or family experience. If a severe side effect has previously occurred with dire consequences or, alternatively, the patient knows someone who did well despite refusing treatment, the physician may find the patient very reluctant to accept treatment.

Nonadherence is more likely to occur when the treatment regimen is too complex (i.e., multiple drugs on different dosage schedules), expensive, inconvenient, or long term or requires alteration of lifestyle. Misunderstanding or lack of knowledge may be the most common source of apparent nonadherence. Physicians widely overestimate patients' understanding of the reasons for treatment, the method and schedule prescribed, and the consequences of not following through. Physicians tend to assume that they are understood by patients, when they often are not, especially by patients of low literacy. One study showed that 77% of patients misinterpreted prescriptions specifying dosing instructions in hourly intervals (e.g., every 6 hours) (Hanchak et al., 1996). Other investigators found that rates of correct interpretation of prescription warning labels ranged from 0% to 78.7% in adults with low literacy (Wolf et al., 2006).

The previously described emotional and defensive reactions to illness (anxiety, depression, denial, and regression) are also major causes of nonadherence. Patients may be frightened by the treatment itself or simply avoid carrying out the treatment or change in habit because it reminds them of the feared disease. Patients who are depressed may do a poor job of following treatment recommendations because of poor concentration, low motivation, pessimism, or acting out suicidal feelings. Individuals who need to feel strongly in control of their lives may get into struggles with physicians over adherence as a way of maintaining a sense of power over their lives and disease.

Consequences of Nonadherence

Nonadherence results in inadequate treatment, poor follow-up, and failure to reduce risk factors, with consequent increased morbidity and mortality. Nonadherence also causes much frustration and consternation for the physician and strains the doctor–patient relationship. A vicious circle may be established in which the patient, finding that the physician becomes angry over incomplete adherence, volunteers less and less information about it. The physician in turn feels increasingly upset that the patient seems to be ignoring instructions and is not being forthright.

Intervention for Nonadherence

Trying to scare patients into adherence is rarely successful. Patients who are noncompliant because they are already frightened will become even more anxious and resistant. Physicians should inform patients of the consequences of not following recommendations, but preferably by emphasizing the benefits of treatment. Positive reinforcement to motivate behavior is almost always more effective than negative reinforcement or punishment, a truism well established in behavioral psychology. Scolding, shaming, or threatening seldom has a beneficial effect. It is also important to maintain a nonjudgmental, nonpunitive attitude when a patient confesses nonadherence, so that the patient will be open about deviations later in the course of treatment.

Physicians can also enhance adherence by careful attention to treatment recommendations. The regimen should be simplified by minimizing the number of drugs and the times per day they need to be taken. Even the most highly motivated patients will have difficulty if they must take one drug every 4 hours, one drug three times a day, and two others every morning, one on an empty stomach and the other only after eating. When a regimen remains necessarily complex, the physician should help the patient determine which aspects of treatment are most important. It is also helpful to implement the complex regimen gradually, adding one drug at a time, and to tailor dosage schedules to the patient's lifestyle. Adherence is also enhanced by incorporating the patient's preferences, which may be based on realistic factors (e.g., differing side effect profiles) or less objective beliefs (e.g., the drug that the patient's sister did well on).

Physicians should also exercise some restraint pursuing therapeutic goals. Although physicians have an ethical responsibility to maximize patients' health, therapeutic perfectionism fails to recognize that, for a particular patient, other values may counterbalance some aims of treatment. Physicians have an ethical responsibility to respect the individual patient's autonomous wishes and not ignore them in the pursuit of an ideal therapeutic outcome. Compromise with the patient is not only ethically justified but also a practical way of enhancing adherence with the most essential aspects of treatment.

Psychiatric consultation is appropriate whenever nonadherence appears linked to a major psychiatric disorder. Consultation may also be very helpful whenever physician and patient are at a standoff, although the physician should not expect the psychiatrist to compel the patient to become compliant. Instead, the psychiatrist helps arbitrate the dispute by eliciting the patient's values and motivation, recognizing psychological factors that may be interfering like anxiety or a personality disorder, and repairing misunderstandings in the patient's relationship with the primary physician (Cohen-Cole and Levinson, 1998).

Discharges Against Medical Advice

Leaving the hospital against medical advice (AMA) might be viewed as a drastic extension of nonadherence. Approximately 1% of all general hospital discharges are AMA. Patients who leave this way have many different motives. Some have psychological reactions to illness so intense that they try to flee (e.g., a patient phobic about undergoing general anesthesia who leaves AMA the night before surgery). Some patients are angry, feeling mistreated, misinformed, ignored, or insulted by medical or nursing staff members. Such perceptions may conform to actual experience, may be distortions arising from a patient's disordered personality, or more often may be both. Any patient who suddenly, and for no apparent reason, wishes to leave during the first few days of hospitalization may be dependent on alcohol, nicotine, or other substances. Agitation and irritability may reflect early withdrawal symptoms, and the patient may wish to leave the hospital to gain access to the substance of abuse and avoid further withdrawal. Another segment of potential AMA discharges are patients who are delirious or demented. If the physician has not recognized that the patient has cognitive dysfunction, the patient's attempt to leave the hospital may be misperceived as rationally motivated when, instead, it results from the patient's confusion and misperception of reality.

The direct consequence of AMA discharges is the disruption or cessation of medical care. Such discharges are rarely if ever amicable, leaving patients, physicians, and other hospital staff resentful, hurt, and indignant. Rather than approaching the widening breach in the relationship as something to be repaired, physicians and staff may respond in a legalistic and bureaucratic manner. Patients may in turn become more upset, feeling further misunderstood and not cared for.

When a patient first expresses the intention of leaving the hospital AMA, the physician should not coerce, threaten, or try to scare the patient into remaining. The first step is to try to restore the alliance by listening to the patient's grievances, giving them legitimate consideration, and trying to work out compromises. Suspected withdrawal syndromes should be appropriately treated. If the patient still wishes to leave, the physician should calmly explain the potential consequences and emphasize the benefits further hospitalization can offer.

If these initial steps do not lead to constructive negotiations, psychiatric consultation is indicated. The actual AMA form used by many hospitals should not be overvalued: although it serves an administrative purpose, it is unnecessary and is insufficient to protect against future lawsuits. The physician's ethical and legal obligation in such a situation is to ensure that the patient is making an informed choice. The patient's reasons for leaving and the physician's concerns that have been communicated to the patient should be documented in the patient's chart. If it appears that the patient is incapable of understanding the need for continued treatment due to mental illness, severe medical illness, or both, this too should be documented, and the possibility of involuntary medical treatment should be considered.

Doctor-Shopping

Physicians commonly encounter patients who appear to be shopping around for medical care, either visiting a succession of doctors or several simultaneously for the same complaints. Some are patients with strong psychological motivations for staying in the sick role (e.g., those with somatization disorder). Others may be seeking a particular diagnosis, treatment approach, or personality style in their physician and will continue searching until they find it. A few are unconsciously gratified by frustrating and defeating the efforts of physicians (e.g., those with factitious disorder, a variant of which is called *Munchausen syndrome*—see Chapter 13). Of course, there are also those who shop around because they have received bad medical care elsewhere and/or have an illness that has defied correct diagnosis. Certain medical and psychiatric diagnoses are notorious for eluding diagnosis, and it is not unusual for the patient to have visited many physicians before being correctly diagnosed. Panic disorder has been often misdiagnosed as various medical illnesses because of the prominent somatic symptoms; myasthenia gravis, in its early stages, is often mistaken for "stress" or depression because routine physical and laboratory examinations are normal.

On first seeing a patient who appears to have been doctor-shopping, the physician should carefully and objectively consider the chief complaint and previous evaluation and treatment. The physician should not pursue extensive diagnostic evaluation or aggressive treatment solely because of strong pressure from the patient to "do something!" There is neither an ethical nor a legal obligation to duplicate workups when they are not clinically indicated. Were the patient's evaluation and treatment elsewhere adequate? Were they optimal? What led the patient to change physicians? Some patients are shopping around not because they want more procedures but because they are looking for a physician who will spend adequate time listening to them.

In all such cases, one should temper enthusiasm with moderation. The physician should not tell the patient that there is nothing wrong nor be overconfident, promising to certainly find out what is wrong and take care of it. This is particularly important for patients who have visited several good physicians and are still frustrated. Acknowledging the limitations of medicine is often better than promising too much. Psychiatric consultation is indicated if the physician suspects underlying primary psychopathology, such as depression or panic disorder. The physician must recognize that many doctor-shoppers may refuse psychiatric consultation, particularly those who are receiving substantial secondary gain by staying in the sick role. Doctor-shopping is also discussed in the context of the somatoform disorders in Chapter 13.

NORMAL AND PATHOLOGICAL GRIEF

Normal Grief

Grief is the psychological response to loss. We are most familiar with grief following the death of a loved one, but analogous reactions follow other losses (e.g., body parts or functions, independence, affection). Grief and the mourning process, through which grief is resolved, follow a typical course with recognizable manifestations (see Figure 28-1) (Brown and Stoudemire, 1983).

Psychological symptoms of grief begin with an initial state of shock and disbelief, followed by painful dejection, despair, helplessness, protest, and anger. Social dysfunction occurs with loss of interest in life's activities, social withdrawal, apathy, and inertia. Whereas some individuals retreat into silent sadness, others are affectively very demonstrative and cry. Somatic symptoms accompanying grief include insomnia; anorexia and weight loss; tightness in the throat, chest, or abdomen; and fatigue.

The initial phase of shock and numbness lasts for days and is followed by a period of preoccupation with the deceased. During the day, thoughts focus on recalling the life of the deceased and one's relationship with the deceased. Anger, jealousy, and resentment about the lost loved one may resurface, along with guilt over unresolved conflicts and regret over missed opportunities. The living may experience self-blame, wishing they had acted or felt differently in the past, ruminating over why they have been the ones to survive, and wondering if they should have done something more during the terminal illness. Sleep is delayed by these obsessive thoughts and often interrupted by dreams about the deceased. Fleeting hallucinations may occur in which the dead seem to appear at one's bedside or in a crowd or call out, usually the name of the living.

The length and intensity of the phases of shock and preoccupation are affected by the suddenness of the death. When there has been no warning, the period of shock and disbelief is prolonged and intense; when death has been long expected, much of the mourning process may occur while the loved one is still alive, leaving an anticlimactic feeling after the death. In normal grief, the intensity of symptoms gradually abates, so that by 1 month after the death, the mourner should be able to sleep, eat, and function adequately at work and at home. Crying and feelings of longing and emptiness do not disappear, but are less intrusive. By 6 to 12 months most normal life activities will have been gradually resumed. For major losses, the grieving process continues throughout life, with the reappearance of the symptoms of grief on anniversaries of the death or other significant dates (family holidays, wedding anniversaries, birthdays). "Normal" reactions demonstrate a wide range of variability, and there is not a "right way" to mourn applicable to everyone (e.g., not all must verbalize their feelings of grief).

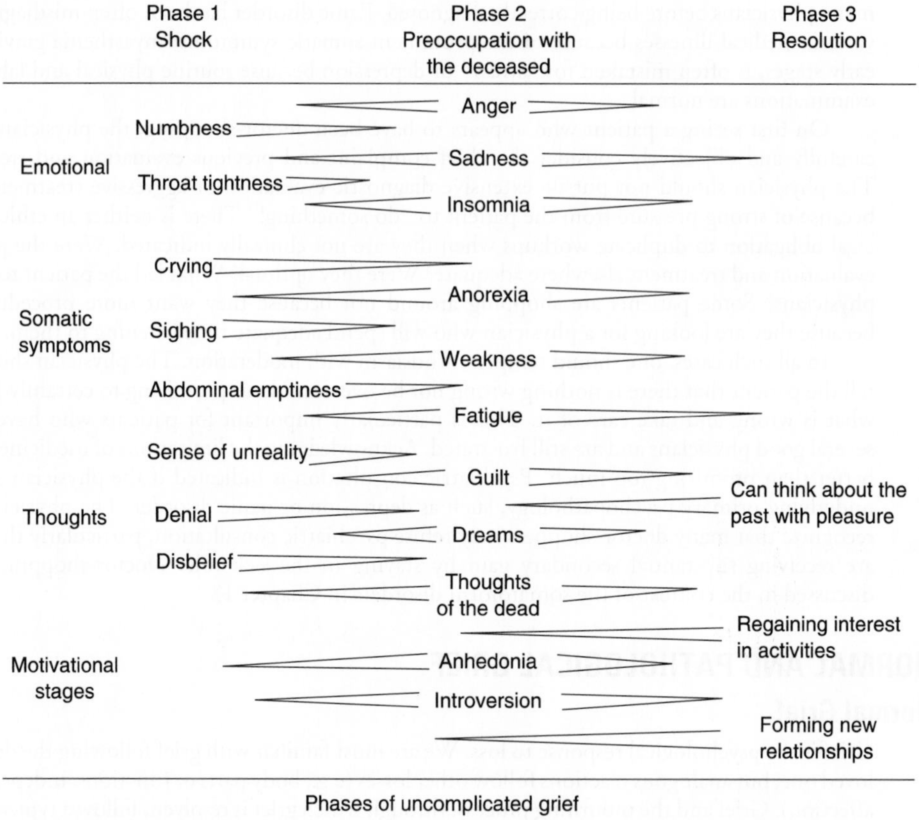

	Phase 1 Shock	Phase 2 Preoccupation with the deceased	Phase 3 Resolution
Emotional	Numbness Throat tightness	Anger Sadness Insomnia	
Somatic symptoms	Crying Sighing Abdominal emptiness	Anorexia Weakness Fatigue	
Thoughts	Sense of unreality Denial Disbelief	Guilt Dreams Thoughts of the dead	Can think about the past with pleasure
Motivational stages		Anhedonia Introversion	Regaining interest in activities Forming new relationships

Phases of uncomplicated grief

FIGURE 28-1. Phases of grief. (Reproduced with permission from Brown and Stoudemire, 1983.)

The type or cause of death can greatly influence the character of grief and mourning. Grief is least likely to be complicated following anticipated deaths of elderly patients with diseases without social stigma. Those mourning a victim of suicide or homicide usually have more anger, angst, religious conflicts, and guilt. Anger toward a family member or close friend who has committed suicide is particularly difficult to "metabolize" in the mourning process. Grief following a death from human immunodeficiency virus/acquired immunodeficiency syndrome (HIV/AIDS) may be complicated by fear, shame, hopelessness, sexual conflicts, recrimination, isolation, and stigma. Disasters may result in multiple deaths and community upheaval and disorder, with the grieving process simultaneously both disrupted by social chaos and facilitated by communally shared feelings. Loss of an infant to sudden infant death syndrome (SIDS) results in especially intense shock and grief. The parents must also face questions regarding the possibility of abuse or neglect. Even though there is no abuse in most apparent cases of SIDS, grieving parents often blame themselves for not somehow preventing the death. A neonatal death is a loss of hopes, dreams, plans, and a relationship that has already started unilaterally in the parents' minds. Although usually not quite as intense, similar grief follows miscarriage, stillbirth, termination of pregnancy for severe congenital abnormality, and even at the point of prenatal diagnosis of such an abnormality.

Grief and mourning also occur following losses other than deaths. Grief follows loss of body parts (e.g., amputation, mastectomy) and loss of bodily functions (e.g., blindness, paraplegia). Caregivers for a patient with Alzheimer disease experience grief long before the patient's death because "his personality died long before he did." Even the loss of time may produce grief, such as an individual who overcomes long-standing substance abuse and then in abstinence feels the full weight of wasted years.

The experience of grief changes developmentally over the life span. Although young children usually do not fully comprehend death's permanence, they certainly experience grief. Sleep disturbance, developmental regression (e.g., enuresis), behavior problems, and magical thinking are common. Older children and adolescents have a fuller understanding of death; decline in school performance, strained peer relations, sleep disturbance (especially hypersomnia), and acting out are common. Young adults have full intellectual comprehension of death, but denial of death's personal relevance is typical. At this stage of life, grief over the death of an elderly relative is very different from grief over the unexpected death of a peer, the latter breaking through the defensive denial of death. For the elderly, accumulating experiences of loss and death are desensitizing; grief and mourning become more ritualized and less intense. This easing of the intensity of grief is offset against increasing loneliness, as well as closer identification with the deceased—older individuals think "that could have been me," whereas the younger reassure themselves "that was not me."

Distinguishing Grief from Depression

Many of the psychological, social, and vegetative symptoms of depression also occur in grief (see Table 28-2). Distinguishing them is important for physicians, for the indicated interventions are quite different. As noted, in normal grief, severe symptoms should abate after several months, while in depression, symptoms persist longer. Although wishes to join the deceased are normal in acute grief, frank suicidal ideation (especially with a plan) is not and points to a major depression. Transient hallucinatory experiences occur with grief, but not more sustained psychotic symptoms indicative of a psychotic depression (e.g., delusions of decay, nihilism, irrational guilt). Crying and intense feelings of sadness and loneliness occur in both grief and depression, but in grief, they occur as pangs interspersed with periods of more normal feeling; in depression, they are more continuous. Self-reproach is experienced in both, but not equivalently. In grief, self-blame is focused on the deceased, including what one could have done differently. The depressed are primarily negative about themselves, feeling worthless, guilty, and helpless, not just in regard to the deceased. Finally, grief and depression respond differently to intervention. The grieving welcome emotional support from others, congregate with them, and feel better after ventilating their feelings. Those who have major depression tend to withdraw from reassurance and feel worse when encouraged to ventilate.

Pathological Grief

In some individuals, grief and mourning do not follow the normal course. Grieving may become too intense or last too long; be absent, delayed, or distorted; or result in chronic complications. Risk factors for pathological grief in the mourner include sudden or terrible deaths, an ambivalent relationship with or excessive dependency on the deceased, traumatic losses earlier in life, social isolation, and actual or imagined responsibility for "causing" the death. Grief that is too intense or prolonged exceeds the descriptions given of normal grief and can lead to an inability to function occupationally or socially for months. Absent or delayed grief occurs when the feelings of loss

TABLE 28-2	**Distinguishing Grief from Major Depression**[a]	
	Grief	**Major Depression**
Time course	Severe symptoms $\geq$1–2 months	Longer
Suicidal ideation	Usually not present	Often present
Psychotic symptoms	Only transient visions or voice of the deceased	May have sustained depressive delusions
Emotional symptoms	Pangs interspersed with normal feelings	Continuous pervasive depressed mood
Self-blame	Related to deceased	Focused on self
Response to support and ventilation	Improvement over time	No change or worsening

[a]Depressive *symptoms* are a pervasive part of the grief response, and a clear delineation of grief versus depression is not always possible.

would be too overwhelming and so are repressed and denied. Such avoidance or repression of affect tends to result in the later onset of much more prolonged and distorted grief and in a higher risk for developing a major depression, especially at later significant anniversaries. Physicians should be careful not to assume that grief is absent just because the individual is quiet and not affectively demonstrative. This may be a matter of personal or cultural style; what counts is the individual's internal experience of grief.

Grief that is still symptomatic 1 year after the death is called *chronic grief* and occurs in approximately 10% of grief reactions. Some chronic persistence of active mourning is expectable after the closest losses (child, spouse, or life partner) but is considered abnormal if the mourner is unable to eventually resume full social and occupational functioning. Risk factors for chronic grief include major unresolved conflicts with the deceased, overdependence, dysfunctional individual personalities, or families characterized by chronic hostility. Chronic grief may evolve into a chronic depression; the boundary between them is not sharp.

Anticipatory grief is grief experienced in anticipation of a death, sometimes long before the terminal phase of an illness. For example, asymptomatic patients who learn they are HIV positive may experience a full-blown grief reaction, with an acute sense of a shortened future, although it may be years before any illness develops. Anticipatory grief is not necessarily pathological but would be considered so when it promotes "giving up/given up" feelings or the grief inappropriately interferes with adaptation to life, medical treatment, or planning for death.

Distorted grief occurs when any one facet of grieving becomes disproportionate in magnitude or duration. *Survival guilt* refers to the feeling that one does not deserve to have outlived the deceased and is especially common in those who have shared a traumatic experience with the deceased (e.g., same organ transplant program, airplane crash, or concentration camp). It is normal in moderation but can become so pronounced that the survivors remain too guilty to ever return to full lives.

Some degree of identification with the deceased is also normal. Grief is partly resolved through intensification of traits shared with or admired in the deceased and the treasuring of special inherited possessions. When conscious or unconscious identification is too strong, it leads to a variety of maladaptive outcomes. The living may abdicate personal life or identity to pursue the interests of the deceased. Through a process of conversion, mourners may develop symptoms identical to those of the loved one's illness. When denial of the loss is very pronounced, there may be an attempt to maintain the deceased's room and belongings entirely unchanged.

Prolonged pathological grief often results in chronic complications, including major depression, substance dependency, hypochondriasis, and increased morbidity and mortality from physical disease.

The Physician's Role

Physicians are in a critically important position to identify and help manage grief, especially if they have long-established relationships with patients and their families. During the acute phase of shock following a death, the physician can help the family accept the reality of the loss and provide a calm and reassuring presence that facilitates both the release of emotion and the planning necessary by those grieving. The physician must sit down, not stand, when talking with anyone experiencing acute grief; otherwise, the physician will be perceived as too busy or uncomfortable or eager to leave. Patients frequently seek out their personal physicians when they are acutely suffering from grief and often focus on the somatic manifestations. The physician can explain the normal symptoms and process of grief and mourning and reassure patients that they are not "losing their minds" (a common fear, especially if vivid nightmares or fleeting hallucinatory phenomena have been experienced). Family members who wish to see the body of the deceased in the hospital should be allowed (but never pressured) after the physician prepares them for any distortion of appearance due to the fatal disease, accident, or treatment.

The physician's role in the management of grief has expanded in importance in recent years. The physician should address resuscitation status, advance directives, and related treatment issues with patients who are competent and with the families of patients who are not. Besides the medical, ethical, and legal reasons for doing so, there are psychological benefits in making patients and families feel heard, respected, and able to contribute to terminal care. Discussion regarding the patient's wishes (e.g., organ donation) is another vital responsibility of physicians that may provide a source of hope and meaning in the face of senselessness and despair.

Physicians should resist the temptation to sedate the individual suffering from acute grief, because this tends to delay and prolong the mourning process. Antidepressants should not be prescribed for acute grief but, rather, reserved for a possible subsequent major depression. If insomnia is severe and does not spontaneously improve after several days, a brief course of a hypnotic may be prescribed, but extended use will be more harmful than beneficial.

THE DYING PATIENT

Helping dying patients is a major responsibility of the physician. Kubler-Ross (1969) drew professional attention to this long-neglected subject 40 years ago and described a model of five sequential stages that characterize the typical response to impending death: denial, anger, bargaining, depression, and acceptance. As we have learned more, there does not appear to be a unique, correct, or necessarily sequential order to this process. Individual patients will experience each of these reactions (and others) in varying degrees, combinations, and sequences. How a patient copes with the knowledge that she or he has a fatal illness generally reflects the style used to cope with other life stresses. A compulsive patient may become obsessed with statistical prognostic information, while a histrionic one exhibits dramatic emotional outbursts. Usual coping styles may become exaggerated or markedly change. Some variability in patients' psychological responses to dying derives from the nature of the illness (e.g., acute versus chronic, occult vs. easily visible) and beliefs about the illness (e.g., viewing the illness as a punishment).

Cultural and religious background profoundly influences how patients respond when they learn they are dying. Knowing this background is important for the physician, but it can also be misleading, as the prospect of death may produce abrupt changes in the patient: an agnostic may become deeply religious; a lifelong skeptic of medicine may become obsessed with medical progress; patients who have been very distant from their families may seek to reunite; and those who have been close may begin to withdraw from their relationships in anticipation of ultimate separation. Most patients take comfort through some form of sustaining hope, including hopes for miraculous cures, new medical discoveries, resolution of personal conflicts or alienated relationships before death, leaving a legacy, or something as simple as enough improvement to leave the hospital briefly and walk in the garden.

Physicians' Reactions to the Dying Patient

Physicians' reactions are also important in the management and support of the dying patient. The dying patient may make the physician feel like a failure, because treatment has been ineffective and it appears that there is nothing more to offer the patient. The physician's feeling of failure is especially likely to occur with younger patients because it is harder for the physician to resort to fatalistic rationalizations (e.g., "she lived a full life" or "he died due to the inevitable progression of old age"). Even experienced physicians feel sad if the dying patient has become well known to them. Sadness in the physician is also likely if the physician is reminded of a personal loss in his or her own life.

Sadness, helplessness, and a feeling of failure in the physician may interfere with optimal care in a number of ways. The physician may avoid the patient, spend little or no time with the patient while on rounds, and rationalize this behavior as not wanting to disturb the patient. Avoidance is particularly unfortunate because most patients have a fear of dying alone and the physician is less available to provide specific comfort-care measures. The secure belief that the physician's attention will continue unceasingly until death is a benefit to patients often underestimated by physicians. Support through human contact often is most meaningful and invaluable to the patient precisely when technological treatment options have been exhausted.

Some physicians take an overly cheerful approach in an effort to instill hope. When cheerfulness is excessive, it alienates patients, who contrast their fate with that of the seemingly happy physician, and creates a gulf between them. Believing that they ought to be truthful, some physicians are overly blunt and announce to the patient, "Nothing more can be done; we have done everything we can think of." This message robs patients of hope. It is possible to be truthful without being so disheartening. Some physicians have difficulty accepting that further treatment is useless and resort to excessive heroics, needlessly prolonging death. Finally, many well-meaning physicians, sensing a patient's need to talk about dying, may prematurely refer the patient to a psychiatrist, social worker, or chaplain. At best, the patient will take the referral as a sign that the physician is uncomfortable discussing these issues; at worst, the patient may worry that the physician thinks there is something wrong with how the patient is reacting or that the feelings are too unimportant for the physician's attention. Most patients prefer talking about death and dying directly with their primary physician.

Intervention for the Dying Patient

How to inform a patient of a grave diagnosis and prognosis is part of the art of medicine. Taking into account the patient's intellectual abilities and emotional and physical state, the physician must gauge how much to tell and at what rate. The questions the patient asks are an indicator of whether the physician is going too fast or slow. Important information may require repetition within the same session and over several visits. Shock induced by the initial pronouncement may interfere with the patient's registering other needed information. Physicians must balance their truth-telling obligation with some respect for differences in how much patients want to know about the details of a grave prognosis.

Another important responsibility for the physician is to discuss the patient's preferences and values regarding future treatment decisions, particularly those involving the termination of aggressive treatment. This should not be raised too quickly after the patient has been first told of a serious diagnosis, both because the patient may be too overwhelmed to participate meaningfully in such a discussion and because the patient may misinterpret the discussion as a sign that the physician is ready to give up. However, physicians tend to err in delaying such discussion until the patient's illness has progressed to the point when it can no longer be avoided. Unfortunately, by then the patient may no longer be competent and the physician will feel less certain that the patient's preferences have not been unduly influenced by physical discomfort, family pressure, or financial worries. This problem is avoidable by initiating discussion before the final stages of illness. Physicians should also allow the patient the opportunity to include family members in the discussion.

In the face of serious illness, physicians feel better doing something. Anticipating a patient's inevitable and impending death, physicians should focus on what can be done. Quality of life during the process of dying can be significantly improved through adequate pain control (which is often underprescribed), attention to bowel and bladder function, hygiene, sleep, and other comfort measures. For some patients, comfort is the primary goal, while other patients may be willing to sacrifice some comfort for greater mobility and the chance to even briefly leave the hospital. Physicians should encourage patients to make wills and put their affairs in order with legal assistance, help mobilize the patient's support system, and discuss options like hospice care.

Patients with grave illnesses often have questions about what to tell their children. Most children do not develop a firm concept of the finality of death until between ages 8 and 11, but children, like adults, vary in the intellectual and emotional maturity necessary to comprehend death. Patients and families should be urged to gauge their answers by the nature of their children's questions. Questions spontaneously asked by a child of any age should be answered truthfully in language the child can understand. The adult should indicate his or her continued availability for further questions and comfort. Should children attend funerals? If the child wishes to go, this wish should be respected and supported. If the child appears very reluctant or refuses, this too should be respected. When in doubt, it is probably helpful for the child to attend, as funerals are rituals that have evolved in our cultures to help us collectively deal with death.

As noted, psychiatric consultation should not be sought prematurely as a substitute for direct conversation between patient and physician. Psychiatric consultation is indicated for the terminally ill patient when suicidal ideation appears, for assistance with management of intractable pain or delirium, and for the emergence of major unresolved emotional conflicts.

The fundamental fear of dying patients is usually not the fear of death itself, but the fear of being abandoned or deserted by others, including their physician, and dying alone. Perhaps the most reassuring comment that a physician can make to a patient with a terminal illness is, "No matter what happens, we are in this together, and I will stick by you. As long as you are ill, I will be here to help you with whatever comes, including making sure you will be comfortable and kept out of pain."

DRUGS THAT CAUSE PSYCHIATRIC SYMPTOMS

Drugs used to treat medical illnesses frequently cause psychiatric symptoms or side effects through a variety of mechanisms. Most drugs at toxic levels produce signs of central nervous system disturbance, including drugs that are normally benign with few side effects, such as aspirin. Certain medications frequently cause psychiatric symptoms even at therapeutic drug dosages (e.g., interferon). Symptoms may occur through a direct effect of the drug on the central nervous system (e.g., lidocaine), a metabolic effect of the drug (e.g., hypokalemia caused by thiazide diuretics), or drug interactions. Some drugs may precipitate an underlying psychiatric disorder in vulnerable patients, such as isoniazid-induced depression (through its inhibition of monoamine oxidase) or sympathomimetic-induced panic attacks. Physicians must be vigilant for the possibility of psychiatric side effects induced by medications the patient may be taking without the doctor's knowledge, particularly if the patient is doing this surreptitiously and embarrassed to tell the physician (e.g., the excessive use of over-the-counter nasal decongestants or inhalers).

Table 28-3 shows many of the drugs that can cause psychiatric symptoms. Most of these can cause a wide variety of symptoms, influenced by the patient's premorbid psychopathology and personality style, metabolic status, and preexisting central nervous system pathology. When the effect on the brain is mild to moderate, many of the listed drugs can cause anxiety, depression, sleep disorders (insomnia, hypersomnia, nightmares), and sexual dysfunction. When severe, psychosis (schizophreniform, manic, depressive), delirium, or dementia may occur and sometimes seizures and coma. For a more detailed review see *The Medical Letter*, 2002.

MEDICAL DISORDERS THAT CAUSE PSYCHIATRIC SYMPTOMS

Many medical disorders produce psychiatric symptoms as part of their pathophysiology, sometimes as the initial presentation of the disease. Here we focus on psychiatric symptoms that are a consequence of the disease process itself through either direct effects on the central nervous system or derangement in metabolism or homeostatic regulatory mechanisms. Some diseases cause a wide range of different neuropsychiatric symptoms in different individuals, largely determined by which areas of the brain have been affected by the disease, and other diseases commonly cause specific psychiatric symptoms (see Table 28-4). Although most of these also can cause a range of symptoms, they typically present with the indicated psychiatric syndromes. Symptoms and signs in other organ systems serve as clinical clues to help the clinician suspect a particular cause, but psychiatric symptoms may precede the onset of other clinical signs in most disorders.

When a patient presents with unexplained psychiatric symptoms, certain clues should heighten the physician's suspicions that an underlying medical disorder may be responsible, such as when:

1. Psychiatric symptoms increase and decrease in concert with prominent physical symptoms
2. "Vegetative symptoms" of an apparent psychiatric disorder are disproportionately greater than psychological symptoms (e.g., a patient with a 50-lb weight loss and only mild depressive ideation is unlikely to have major affective disorder explain the weight loss)
3. Significant cognitive abnormalities are present in the mental status examination, particularly changes in level of consciousness, attention, and memory
4. Age of onset or course of psychiatric illness is very atypical (e.g., new onset of "schizophrenia" in an 85-year-old)
5. There are objective findings of central nervous system disease (e.g., pathological reflexes; abnormal electroencephalogram, computed tomography scan, or magnetic resonance image; or changes in spinal fluid)

As with drug-induced psychiatric symptoms, medical illnesses may cause mild to moderate changes in affect, personality, sleep, or sexual function, which can be easily missed or misattributed. When severe, medical illnesses produce psychosis, delirium, or dementia, which are less likely to be missed but the nature or causation of which may still be misinterpreted (see Chapter 8).

TABLE 28-3	Drugs That May Cause Psychiatric Symptoms[a]

Depression

Antihypertensives (especially reserpine, methyldopa, clonidine)[a]	Indomethacin (and other nonsteroidal anti-inflammatory drugs)
Amphotericin B	Antineoplastic drugs
Corticosteroids[a]	Procarbazine
Anticonvulsants	Tamoxifen
Sedative-hypnotics[a]	Vinblastine
Oral contraceptives	Asparaginase
Antipsychotics	Ethionamide
Metoclopramide	Acetazolamide
Interferon-α[a]	Isotretinoin

Mania

Corticosteroids[a]	Dopamine agonists
Sympathomimetics (especially nonprescription decongestants and bronchodilators)	Antidepressants
Isoniazid	Zidovudine (AZT)
Tramadol	Stimulants

Anxiety

Sympathomimetics[a]	Stimulants
Theophylline[a]	Antidepressants (selective serotonin reuptake inhibitors [SSRIs])[a]
Caffeine[a]	Sedative-hypnotics (withdrawal)[a]

Psychosis (Hallucinations or Delusions)

Anticholinergics[a]	Antiviral drugs
Antihistamines (cimetidine, ranitidine, diphenhydramine, etc.)	Acyclovir
Antiarrhythmics (especially lidocaine, tocainide, mexiletine, quinidine)	Vidarabine
	Interferon
Dopamine agonists[a]	Zidovudine (AZT)
L-dopa	Podophyllin
Bromocriptine	Antineoplastic drugs
Amantadine	Asparaginase
Corticosteroids[a]	Methotrexate
Digitalis	Vincristine
Antidepressants	Cytarabine
Opiates	Fluorouracil
Meperidine	Disulfiram
Pentazocine	Sympathomimetics
Antimalarials	Metrizamide
Anticonvulsants	Methysergide
β-Blockers	Baclofen
	Cycloserine
	Cyclosporine
	Interleukin (IL-Z)

[a]Denotes especially "high-risk" drugs for causing symptoms in question.

The physician should also keep in mind those diseases that do not produce psychopathology *per se* but may be mistaken for it. Recurrent pulmonary emboli or paroxysmal supraventricular tachycardia may be misdiagnosed as anxiety or panic attacks because of episodic autonomic arousal. Early myasthenia gravis is often mistaken for depression or a conversion disorder because the clinician finds a normal examination in a patient who complains of weakness and fatigue whenever working too hard. Multiple sclerosis may be misdiagnosed as conversion disorder

TABLE 28-4 Psychiatric Presentation of Selected Medical Disorders

	Psychiatric Presentation	Clinical Clues	Screening Diagnostic Evaluation[a]
Endocrine Disorders			
Hypothyroidism	Retarded depression (± psychosis)	Weight gain, fatigue, cold intolerance, hoarseness, bradycardia, constipation, hair loss	TSH
Hyperthyroidism	Anxiety, panic attacks, agitated depression (often retarded in the elderly)	Tremor, tachycardia, heat intolerance	TSH
Hyperadrenalism (Cushing)	Depression or mania	Hypertension, diabetes, hirsutism, moon facies, weight gain	Dexamethasone suppression test
Hypoadrenalism (Addison)	Depression	Postural hypotension, nausea, vomiting, skin pigmentation, weight loss	Cosyntropin stimulation test
Metabolic Disorders			
Hypoglycemia	Anxiety, panic attacks	Sweating, tachycardia, headache	Blood glucose during symptoms
Hypokalemia	Depression	Weakness, ECG changes	Serum K^+
Hyponatremia	Depression, psychosis	Weakness, nausea, vomiting, seizures	Serum Na^+
Hypercalcemia	Retarded depression	Weakness, nausea, confusion	Serum Ca^{2+}
Hypocalcemia	Anxiety	Tremor, tetany, paresthesias	Serum Ca^{2+}
Hypermagnesemia	Retarded depression	Hypotension, nausea, vomiting	Serum Mg^{2+}
Hypomagnesemia	Anxiety, psychosis	Tremor, tetany	Serum Mg^{2+}, Ca^{2+}
Hypophosphatemia	Depression	Weakness, paresthesias	Serum PO_4^{2-}
Vitamin B_{12} deficiency	Psychosis, dementia	Megaloblastic anemia, peripheral neuropathy, myelopathy (but may occur in absence of these)	Serum B_{12}
Hepatic encephalopathy	Confusion, psychosis	Asterixis, jaundice	Liver function tests, serum NH_3
Uremia	Depression, dementia	Anemia, nausea, edema	BUN, creatinine
Porphyria (acute intermittent)	Psychosis	Episodic abdominal pain with nausea and vomiting, constipation, neuropathy	Blood and urine porphyrin screen
Lead poisoning	Personality change, depression	Colic, anemia, peripheral neuropathy	Serum FEP
Neurologic Disorders			
Normal pressure hydrocephalus	Depression, dementia	Gait apraxia, urinary incontinence	CT or MRI scan
Multiple sclerosis	Depression	Multiple intermittent neurologic symptoms over time	Neurologic evaluation, MRI, CSF (oligoclonal bands)
Huntington disease	Personality disorder, psychosis	Movement disorder, family history	Neurologic examination
Parkinson disease	Depression, dementia	Bradykinesia, tremor, rigidity	Neurological examination
Wilson disease	Psychosis	Movement disorder, liver disease, Kayser-Fleischer rings	Slit lamp examination, serum ceruloplasmin

Continued

TABLE 28-4 *Continued*

	Psychiatric Presentation	Clinical Clues	Screening Diagnostic Evaluation[a]
Neoplastic Disorders			
Pancreatic cancer	Depression	Weight loss, abdominal pain	Abdominal CT or MRI scan
Paraneoplastic limbic encephalitis (usually associated with small cell carcinoma of the lung)	Psychosis, dementia	Seizures, fluctuating course	EEG, lumbar puncture
Infectious Diseases			
Infectious mononucleosis	Depression	Lymphadenopathy, hepatosplenomegaly, sore throat, malaise	CBC, monospot
Viral hepatitis	Depression	Anorexia, fatigue, jaundice, malaise, hepatomegaly	Liver function tests, serologies
Encephalitis	Psychosis	Fever, seizures	EEG, lumbar puncture
Whipple disease	Depression, dementia	Diarrhea, weight loss, arthritis, lymphadenopathy	Malabsorption studies, small bowel biopsy

[a]TSH, thyroid-stimulating hormone; RIA, radioimmunoassay; BUN, blood urea nitrogen; FEP, free erythrocyte protoporphyrin; CT, computed tomography; MRI, magnetic resonance imaging; CSF, cerebrospinal fluid; EEG, electroencephalogram; CBC, complete blood count.

because the pattern of the patient's symptoms seems changing and inconsistent and does not conform to simple neuroanatomical localization.

COMPETENCY

When a patient refuses diagnostic procedures or treatment or seems unable to make medical care decisions, physicians often question whether the patient is competent. Strictly speaking, "competency" is a legal concept and is determined by the court; physicians, including psychiatrists, render opinions about competency, based on their clinical assessment of the patient's mental status. What physicians must decide is whether the patient appears to have the capacity to participate in rational and reasoned decision making (President's Commission for the Study of Ethical Problems in Medicine and Biomedical and Behavioral Research, 1982). Is limited intelligence, a psychiatric disorder, or a medical disease preventing the patient from thinking rationally about medical care? Most determinations of this kind are made by clinicians at bedside; their frequency and the need for timely resolution make it impractical to seek judicial action on every case.

Although psychiatric consultation is often requested to help determine if the patient is competent, primary physicians can determine themselves in most cases whether the patient possesses sufficient capacity for a particular decision. Does the physician actually suspect impaired mental capacity, or do the patient and the physician simply disagree? The test of whether a patient possesses the capacity to participate in health care decision making is a simple, functional one: does the patient understand the particular decision at hand? First, the physician must ensure that the patient has been fully informed. Then, the following questions should be asked, taking into account that patients will answer in their own words, not in "medically correct" terms:

1. Can the patient describe what the physician believes is wrong with the patient?
2. Does the patient understand the diagnostic procedure or treatment proposed and the reasons for it?
3. Does the patient understand any alternative procedures or treatments that may exist?
4. Does the patient understand the risks and benefits of each course of action, including the consequences of refusing treatment?
5. Is the patient able to use the information rationally and express a choice?

If the answer is yes to all of these questions, the patient possesses the capacity for making the decision. To be viewed as competent, the patient does not necessarily have to have a good reason (in the eyes of the treatment team) for disagreeing with the physician, but the patient must be able to demonstrate an understanding of the physician's advised plan.

Since this clinical competency test focuses on particular proposed treatments, it is possible that some patients may be judged able to make some but not all decisions or that their ability varies over time. Others may be so mentally impaired that it is obvious they entirely lack decision-making capacity.

Some patients will give answers that demonstrate their ability to understand what the physician has said, but they will persist on an irrational course, based on psychotic delusional thinking. This too may be grounds for a determination of lack of capacity and indicates the need for psychiatric consultation, which is also helpful if the primary physician remains unsure of the patient's level of understanding, there is disagreement among the physicians caring for the patient, or legal action is considered likely.

If the physician determines that the patient does not possess sufficient capacity, a surrogate decision maker will be required. If the surrogate is a family member, as it is in most circumstances, this usually does not necessitate going to court. A court-appointed guardian may be necessary when the family members remain intractably divided over health care decisions, when they appear unable to act in the best interests of the impaired patient, or when there are no family available or willing to serve as the surrogate decision maker.

PSYCHIATRIC CONSULTATION

From the other parts of this chapter, it is evident that there are many reasons for a physician to seek psychiatric consultation. Unfortunately, some physicians are reluctant or do not ask very effectively. Some fear that seeing a psychiatrist will upset the patient, who may feel that the physician thinks he or she is crazy. Others approach patients with the belief that all medical pathology should be absolutely ruled out before considering psychological explanations for symptoms. It is certainly reasonable to avoid prematurely concluding that a patient's symptoms are psychogenic, but the relentless pursuit of a physical etiology is costly, exposes patients to unnecessary risks, reinforces a disregard for psychological factors by the patient, and neglects treatable psychiatric disorders.

Some physicians hesitate to obtain psychiatric consultation simply because they are unsure how to tell the patient. It is a mistake to ask for consultation without telling the patient, since this makes it more likely that the patient will misunderstand the physician's intentions. If not told, patients may well wonder if their physician thinks them mentally ill or believe that their physician is frustrated and wants to transfer their care to someone else. Several studies have demonstrated that when patients are informed by physicians of the purpose of a psychiatric consultation, the great majority have little difficulty accepting it.

The physician should explain that the psychiatrist is a consultant who will advise the patient and the physician and that the physician is still the primary doctor committed to helping the patient recover. The specific purpose for the consultation should be explained in terms the patient can understand (e.g., "Besides having heart failure, your spirits seem very low. I would like to have our psychiatrist see if there is anything we can do to help you feel better emotionally, as well as physically").

The physician should always formulate a specific question or problem for which the consultant's help is desired (see Table 28-5). If the physician is unsure whether psychiatric consultation would be helpful, the physician should discuss the concern with the consultant. Occasionally, the physician may anticipate problems in persuading the patient to see a psychiatrist. Here too, discussion with the consultant ahead of time will be helpful. With careful explanation and a respectful approach, a skilled psychiatric consultant can persuade the great majority of patients who initially refuse consultation to agree to be interviewed.

When the patient has unexplained symptoms, physicians should avoid either/or thinking (i.e., considering the symptoms as either physical or psychological). Otherwise, the physician may be misled into thinking too narrowly about causation. Physicians should never diagnose by exclusion (i.e., conclude that symptoms must be psychogenic because physical and laboratory

TABLE 28-5	Common Indications for Psychiatric Consultation
Suicidal ideation or behavior	
Verbal threats or dangerous behavior	
Psychosis (hallucinations, delusions, thought disorder)	
Need for psychiatric medication or change of dose	
Psychiatric disorder in need of treatment	
Psychiatric disorder complicating medical illness	
Psychiatric symptoms thought to be caused by medical illness	
Psychiatric symptoms thought to be due to medication	
Competency evaluations	
Nonadherence, discharges against medical advice (AMA)	
Significant problems in doctor−patient relationship (or nurse−patient relationship)	
Evaluation of cognitive dysfunction (delirium, dementia)	

examinations have revealed only "normal" results). A medical disease may still be present. Psychiatric diagnoses should be made on the basis of positive criteria, not solely on the absence of identifiable physical pathology. In evaluating symptoms of unclear causation, when the physician suspects the possibility of psychogenic origin, psychiatric consultation should not be delayed until the end of the diagnostic evaluation. Such delays are unfortunate because they leave little time for psychiatrists to do their job, reinforce the patient's (possibly false) belief that the symptoms are physical, promote unnecessary diagnostic testing, and leave the patient with the implied message that the physician is at a loss and giving up the patient to the care of a psychiatrist.

Even when symptoms clearly appear due to conversion, somatization, or hypochondriasis, the physician should never tell the patient, "There is nothing wrong" or "It is all in your head." Patients experience such remarks as humiliating and insulting, and consequently, the doctor−patient relationship is seriously strained. Instead, patients can be reassured that extensive diagnostic testing has not turned up any grave or malignant etiology for their illness and that it appears they have a physical symptom exacerbated by stress for which help is available.

Indications for Psychiatric Referral

Although patients often bring psychiatric and psychosocial problems to their primary care physicians, some should be referred for primary management and treatment by psychiatrists (and/or other mental health professionals). Nonpsychiatric physicians will individually vary in expertise and desire to manage psychiatric disorders themselves, but some general rules guide who should be referred.

Patients with depression who are suicidal, psychotic, or so depressed that they cannot maintain normal daily functioning should be referred to a psychiatrist, as should those who have failed to improve with standard antidepressant therapy. Depressed individuals with a personal or family history of bipolar illness should be referred to a psychiatrist for evaluation for mood-stabilizing medications. Patients with severe, incapacitating anxiety disorders and anxiety disorders with a history of substance abuse should be referred to a psychiatrist. Patients with chronic phobias, obsessive-compulsive disorders, or agoraphobia should be referred to a mental health clinician with expertise in behavioral therapy. Schizophrenia, mania, and other psychoses should be managed by psychiatrists. Anorexia nervosa and bulimia usually require involvement of a primary care physician, psychiatrist, and psychotherapist. Dementia requires psychiatric management primarily when behavioral complications like psychosis, depression, or severe agitation develop.

Nicotine dependence usually can be managed by primary care physicians, although referral to a substance-abuse specialist is indicated for intractable abuse despite serious medical complications.

Addiction to alcohol, sedatives, or illicit drugs is best treated through referral to specialized (usually outpatient) substance-abuse treatment programs.

Severity of illness is not the only factor that may indicate the need for referral. Time constraints prevent most primary care physicians from providing more than very limited counseling. Psychological problems requiring further attention should be referred to a mental health professional. In addition, some patients are not comfortable discussing adjustment and relationship problems with their primary care physician (especially if this physician also cares for other members of the same family), so even "minor" problems sometimes require referral to a mental health professional.

CONCLUSION

In this chapter, the sources and consequences of psychiatric symptoms and disorders in medical and surgical patients encountered by all physicians in clinical practice, and physicians' corresponding responsibilities and opportunities for improving management of their patients, have been reviewed. Both psychiatric disorders and the range of psychological and emotional reactions to physical illness can profoundly affect the doctor–patient relationship. This is particularly important in the context of grief and mourning and the dying patient. Physicians must also be cognizant of medical disorders and medications that can produce psychiatric symptoms. Finally, guidelines have been provided to evaluate patients' competency and how to obtain psychiatric consultation.

Clinical Pearls

- The most common psychiatric syndromes in medical outpatients are depression, anxiety, somatoform disorders, and substance abuse.
- The most common psychiatric syndromes in medical inpatients are cognitive disorders, depression, and substance abuse.
- Anxiety in the medically ill takes many forms, including fears of death, abandonment, strangers, loss of or injury to body parts or bodily functions, pain, loss of control, dependency, and intimacy.
- The great majority of patients who are experiencing suicidal thoughts are relieved to discuss them with a caring physician.
- Nonadherence may occur in up to 90% of those receiving short-term medication regimens and averages about 50% in the drug treatment of patients with chronic disease.
- Nonadherence is more likely to occur when the treatment regimen is too complex, expensive, inconvenient, or long term or requires alteration of lifestyle.
- If a patient wants to leave the hospital against medical advice (AMA), the physician's key responsibility is to ensure that the patient is making an informed choice. The critical documentation is notation of the patient's reasons for leaving and the physician's concerns that have been communicated to the patient, not the AMA form.
- Physicians should resist the temptation to prescribe sedatives for the individual suffering from acute grief, since this tends to delay and prolong the mourning process.
- The fundamental fear of dying patients is usually not the fear of death itself, but the fear of being abandoned or deserted by others, including their physician, and dying alone.
- An underlying medical disorder as the etiology of psychiatric symptoms should be considered when (a) psychiatric symptoms appear with prominent physical symptoms; (b) "vegetative symptoms" are disproportionately greater than psychological symptoms; (c) significant cognitive abnormalities are present in the mental status examination; (d) age of onset or course of psychiatric illness is very atypical; (e) there are objective findings of central nervous system disease.
- The key elements of capacity for health care decision making include awareness, comprehension, ability to use information rationally, and ability to express a choice.
- It is a mistake to ask for psychiatric consultation without telling the patient.

Self-Assessment Questions and Answers

28-1. In a regressed, medically ill, hospitalized adult patient who is overly demanding of the nurses' attention, the most appropriate initial intervention is to:

A. Explain that feeling needy is part of an expected reaction to illness.

B. Ignore the patient's attention-seeking behavior.

C. Interpret the patient's underlying fear of abandonment.

D. Prescribe antianxiety medication.

E. Scold the patient for acting childishly.

Regression is a universal human reaction to illness. Physicians should avoid scolding or shaming patients but instead explain that feeling more dependent is part of an expected reaction to illness. Patients who make repeated, unreasonable, or unrealistic demands may require behavioral limit-setting and mobilization physically and emotionally to participate in treatment and rehabilitation. Psychiatric consultation should be sought if regression significantly interferes in treatment, distresses the patient, or results in unnecessary invalidism. *Answer: A*

28-2. Mastectomy is recommended for a woman with newly diagnosed breast cancer, but she is too scared to proceed. The most appropriate initial intervention is to:

A. Advise her to discuss it with her husband.

B. Ask her what she fears.

C. Explain that mastectomy is likely to be curative in her case.

D. Explain that reconstructive surgery can restore her body image.

E. Reassure her that mastectomy is a safe surgery with very small risk.

Medically ill patients have many reasons for anxiety and different patients will react to the same diagnosis, prognosis, treatment, and complications with different concerns. Ideally, the physician explores concerns with the patient by inquiring about those aspects of the procedure that are causing anxiety and observing the patient's behavior. *Answer: B*

28-3. A 70-year-old man's wife died 3 months ago. Which of the following characteristics most suggests that he has major depression rather than normal grief?

A. Pervasive self-blame

B. Restless sleep

C. Tearfulness when her name is mentioned

D. Transient visions of his wife

E. Wishing to be reunited after death

Wishes to join the deceased are normal in acute grief, as are transient hallucinatory experiences and crying. Self-reproach is experienced in both grief and depression, but not equivalently. In grief, self-blame is focused on the deceased. The depressed are primarily negative about themselves, feeling worthless, guilty, and helpless, not just in regard to the deceased. *Answer: A*

28-4. Which of the following best describes the determination of whether a patient has capacity to make a specific medical decision?

A. The determination of capacity requires input from the patient's family.

B. The determination of capacity requires a judge.

C. The determination of capacity requires a psychiatrist.

D. Primary physicians can determine capacity themselves in most cases.

E. Patients lacking capacity for one medical decision lack capacity for all medical decisions.

Although psychiatric consultation is often requested to help determine if the patient is competent, primary physicians can determine themselves in most cases whether the patient possesses sufficient capacity for a particular decision. Some patients may be judged able to make some but not all decisions or their ability may vary over time. If the physician determines that the patient does not possess sufficient capacity, a surrogate decision maker is required, and if the surrogate is a family member, this usually does not necessitate going to court. Most determinations of this kind are made by clinicians at bedside; their frequency and the need for timely resolution make it impractical to seek judicial action on every case. *Answer: D*

28-5. Which of the following is the most common cause of patient nonadherence with medication?

A. Counterculture theories of disease

B. Denial

C. Depression

D. Doctor-shopping

E. Misunderstanding or lack of knowledge

Physicians widely overestimate patients' understanding of the reasons for treatment, the method and schedule prescribed, and the consequences of not following through, assuming that they are understood by patients when they often are not. *Answer: E*

References

Blumenfield M, Strain JJ, eds. *Psychosomatic medicine*. Philadelphia: Lippincott Williams & Wilkins; 2006.

Bostwick JM, Levenson JL. Suicidality. In: Levenson JL, ed. *American psychiatric publishing textbook of psychosomatic medicine*. Washington, DC: American Psychiatric Publishing; 2005:219–234.

Bressi SK, Marcus SC, Solomon PL. The impact of psychiatric comorbidity on general hospital length of stay. *Psychiatr Q*. 2006;77:203–209.

Brown JT, Stoudemire GA. Normal and pathological grief. *JAMA*. 1983;250:378–382.

Chia LR, Schlenk EA, Dunbar-Jacob J. Effect of personal and cultural beliefs on medication adherence in the elderly. *Drugs Aging*. 2006;23:191–202.

Cohen-Cole SA, Levinson RM. The biopsychosocial model in medical practice. In: Stoudemire A, ed. *Human behavior: An introduction for medical students*. Lippincott Williams & Wilkins; 1998:22–63.

Copsey Spring TR, Yanni LM, Levenson JL. A shot in the dark: Failing to recognize the link between physical and mental illness. *J Gen Intern Med*. 2007;22:677–680.

Gold DT, McClung B. Approaches to patient education: Emphasizing the long-term value of adherence and persistence. *Am J Med*. 2006;119(4 Suppl 1):S32–S37.

Goodwin PJ, Leszcz M, Ennis M, et al. The effect of group psychological support on survival in metastatic breast cancer. *N Engl J Med*. 2001;345:1719–1726.

Groves MS, Muskin PR. Psychological responses to illness. In: Levenson JL, ed. *American psychiatric publishing textbook of psychosomatic medicine*. Washington, DC: American Psychiatric Publishing; 2005:67–90.

Groves JE. Taking care of the hateful patient. *N Engl J Med*. 1978;298:883–887.

Hanchak NA, Patel MB, Berlin JA, et al. Patient misunderstanding of dosing instructions. *J Gen Intern Med*. 1996;11:325–328.

Kahana RJ, Bibring GL. Personality types in medical management. In: Zinberg NE, ed. *Psychiatry and medical practice in a general hospital*. Madison: International Universities Press; 1964:108–123.

Kessler RC, McGonagle KA, Zhao S, et al. Lifetime and 12-month prevalence of DSM-III-R psychiatric disorders in the United States. Results from the National Comorbidity Survey. *Arch Gen Psychiatry*. 1994;51:8–19.

Kubler-Ross E. *On death and dying*. London: Macmillan; 1969.

Lawrence-Smith G, Sturgeon D. Treating learned helplessness in hospital: A reacquaintance with self-control. *Br J Hosp Med*. 2006;67:134–136.

Lecrubier Y. Widespread underrecognition and undertreatment of anxiety and mood disorders: Results from 3 European studies. *J Clin Psychiatry*. 2007;68(Suppl 2):36–41.

Levenson JL, Mishra A, Hamer R, et al. Denial and medical outcome in unstable angina. *Psychosom Med*. 1989;51:27–35.

Levenson JL, ed. *American psychiatric publishing textbook of psychosomatic medicine*. Washington, DC: American Psychiatric Publishing; 2005.

Lustman PJ, Griffith LS, Freedland KE, et al. Cognitive behavior therapy for depression in type 2 diabetes mellitus: A randomized, controlled trial. *Ann Intern Med*. 1998;129:613–621.

Lustman PJ, Freedland KE, Griffith LS, et al. Fluoxetine for depression in diabetes: A randomized double-blind placebo-controlled trial. *Diabetes Care*. 2000;23:618–623.

Meadows GN, Harvey CA, Joubert L, et al. Best practices: The consultation-liaison in primary-care psychiatry program: A structured approach to long-term collaboration. *Psychiatr Serv*. 2007;58:1036–1038.

Norton J, De Roquefeuil G, Boulenger JP, et al. Use of the PRIME-MD patient health questionnaire for estimating the prevalence of psychiatric disorders in French primary care: Comparison with family practitioner estimates and relationship to psychotropic medication use. *Gen Hosp Psychiatry*. 2007;29:285–293.

Phatak HM, Thomas J III. Relationships between beliefs about medications and nonadherence to prescribed chronic medications. *Ann Pharmacother*. 2006;40:1737–1742, Epub 2006 Sep 19.

Regier DA, Narrow WE, Rae DS, et al. The de facto U.S. mental and addictive disorders service system. Epidemiologic catchment area prospective 1-year prevalence rates of disorders and services. *Arch Gen Psychiatry*. 1993;50:85–94.

Rothenhausler HB. Mental disorders in general hospital patients. *Psychiatr Danub*. 2006;18(3–4): 183–192.

Saravay SM. Interventions, outcomes, and costs. In: Blumenfield M, Strain JJ, eds. *Psychosomatic medicine*. Philadelphia: Lippincott Williams & Wilkins; 2006:867–880.

Schneider RK, Levenson JL. *Psychiatry essentials for primary care*. Philadelphia: American College of Physicians; 2008.

Smith GR Jr, Monson RA, Ray DC. Psychiatric consultation in somatization disorder: A randomized controlled study. *N Engl J Med*. 1986;314(22):1407–1413.

Spitzer RL, Williams JBW, Kroenke K, et al. Utility of a new procedure for diagnosing mental disorders in primary care: The PRIME-MD 1,000 study. *JAMA*. 1994;272:1749–1756.

Stoudemire A, ed. *Human behavior. An introduction for medical students*, 2nd ed. Philadelphia: Lippincott Williams & Wilkins; 1998.

The Medical Letter. Drugs that may cause psychiatric symptoms. *Med Lett Drugs Ther*. 2002;44:59–62.

Vos MS, de Haes JC. Denial in cancer patients, an explorative review. *Psychooncology*. 2007;16:12–25.

Winnick S, Lucas DO, Hartman AL, et al. How do you improve adherence? *Pediatrics*. 2005;115: e718–e724.

Wolf MS, Davis TC, Tilson HH, et al. Misunderstanding of prescription drug warning labels among patients with low literacy. *Am J Health Syst Pharm*. 2006;63:1048–1055.

29

Vinay P. Saranga and David Bienenfeld

Caring for Elders with Mental Illness

In a census completed at the turn of the 21st century, roughly 13% of the U.S. population (approximately 35 million people) was 65 years old or older (Federal Interagency Forum on Aging Related Statistics, 2000). The elderly are at increased risk for social stressors including retirement, widowhood, and physical infirmity. Aging individuals therefore bring to their physicians problems that occur in a multilayered context. The features of clinical syndromes are often different in older patients, and therapy frequently requires modification. The examination of geriatric psychopathology and its treatment best begins with a perspective on normal aging.

AGING AND THE LIFE CYCLE

Erikson (1959) proposed that psychological development continued throughout life in a series of predictable life crises. In his outline, elderly adults have to deal with the crisis of *integrity versus despair*. Their struggle is to reevaluate their lives and to accept their roles during life (and the meaning of their relationships with others). They learn to own responsibility for their actions and to accept the things that might not be pleasant but cannot be changed. If they cannot do so, they are left with the despair of knowing that the unacceptable aspects of their lives cannot be undone.

The range of life stressors confronting the aging individual is broad. Friends and relatives become ill and die, children grow up and move away, retirement is often mandatory, and physical health may fail. To deal with such a wide array of stressors, one must mobilize a multitude of coping strategies. These strategies, the *defense mechanisms*, are the ways that people process the data from the environment to maintain emotional stability. The individual whose earlier life has allowed him or her to adopt many kinds of defense mechanisms is better able to weather these stressors without psychological symptoms than one who has come to use only a narrow range of coping skills (Bienenfeld, 1990).

COGNITION AND AGING

Aging affects processing, learning, memory, and intelligence. Processing is the translation of stimuli into usable neural signals. Learning is the acquisition of skills and information. Memory is the storage and retrieval of that information. Intelligence is the capacity to manipulate and apply available knowledge (Bienenfeld, 1990). The most predictable age-related finding in the realm of cognition is a reduction in processing speed (Spar and LaRue, 2006). Older groups perform much worse than younger ones on tests of processing speed.

Because learning requires the retention of data into a small "compartment" of memory for just a few seconds before further processing, the reduction in processing speed effectively limits the capacity of this store, leading to a cascade of memory deficits downstream. Executive function is defined as the system of control over virtually all other cognitive functions. It includes planning, abstraction, cognitive flexibility, recognition of rules, selecting relevant information, and initiating appropriate actions. It is typically measured by tools such as card sorting tests and tests of abstract associations. This function declines in late life, but executive losses are directly proportional to processing speed, not to age (Crawford et al., 2000; Rabbitt and Lowe, 2000). Not only pure memory but a wide variety of functional capacities, including activities of daily living, driving, and mobility, diminish as a function of processing speed (Wood et al., 2005). Additionally, older individuals are more vulnerable to distraction when trying to learn information than are younger ones (Grégoire, 2001; Spar and LaRue, 2006).

Memory is not a singular function, and its parts are variably affected by aging. Immediate (or short-term) memory holds a small amount of information, the size of approximately seven digits, for a few seconds. In general, the capacity of this store is not affected by age, but processing speed and vulnerability to distraction play a significant role in making it less efficient. Working memory allows one to manipulate the data from immediate memory, and to process them for further storage. Its capacity is directly affected by diminished processing speed with increasing years. Working memory encodes data for long-term storage. Because of the learning deficits described earlier, it declines moderately with age, although its total storage capacity is stable. Remote, or long-term, memory is more variably affected by aging. Information put into long-term store appears to remain intact, but retrieval mechanisms may become less efficient. New information put into long-term memory is similarly filed less efficiently, making subsequent retrieval unreliable (Craik, 2006). Elements of personal history are least vulnerable to long-term memory effects of aging (Spar and LaRue, 2006). Verbal memory consistently declines with age. Spatial memory, as measured by location of pieces on a chess board or objects on a map or in the real environment, also becomes less effective with age (Shaw, 2006). Explicit memory, as evidenced in pure verbal recall, is more severely affected by aging than is implicit memory, which drives learned motor tasks (Spar and LaRue, 2006). The compartments of memory are shown in Table 29-1.

The most long-accepted model for describing and explaining the effects of aging on intelligence is Horn and Cattell's 1966 model of fluid and crystallized intelligence. Crystallized intelligence is the accumulated body of knowledge about one's world, and the skills used to function in it. Fluid intelligence includes the "processes of reasoning in the immediate situation in tasks requiring abstracting, concept formation and attainment" (Horn and Cattell, 1966). When common intelligence instruments such as the Wechsler Adult Intelligence Scale are measured grossly against age, results are inconsistent and unrevealing. When subsets of the scales are separated, verbal scores, which reflect crystallized intelligence, remain stable, and even increase modestly. Subsets that require novel thinking and manipulation of knowledge, reflected in performance scores, decline gradually from early adulthood; these functions are representative of fluid intelligence. Crystallized intelligence (facts and knowledge) is the product of experience, and fluid intelligence (manipulation and abstraction) depends on neural factors that decline with age; the model is useful and consistent (Bienenfeld, 1990; Grégoire 2001).

Many of the declines in cognitive function described earlier seem to be less dramatic in individuals of higher educational achievement. Common wisdom holds that continued intellectual engagement in late life is somehow protective against loss of memory and intellect. More specifically, higher levels of education are associated with less severe declines in verbal scores on intelligence tests, but measures of fluid intelligence seem equally vulnerable regardless of education (Compton et al., 2003). Processing speed is not at all protected by higher levels of education. Rather, better educated elders are able to compensate for inevitable reductions in capacity by mobilizing other intellectual resources (Compton et al., 2000).

Functional brain imaging is consistent with the psychometric findings. In tasks of verbal recall, young adults will remember the details as well as the essence of a story. Older adults become more likely to omit details but retain the gist. Positron emission tomography (PET) and

TABLE 29-1   Compartments of Memory

Compartment	Characteristics	Age-Related Changes
Immediate memory (short-term)	Seven digits, few seconds	Vulnerable to distraction and reduction of processing speed
Working memory (intermediate)	Processes immediate memory for storage	Total capacity stable; declines moderately with processing speed
Remote memory (long-term)	Infinite capacity, permanent retention	Storage and retrieval mechanisms less efficient

(Craik, 2006; Spar and LaRue, 2006.)

functional magnetic resonance imaging (fMRI) show that younger adults tend to localize activity for such tasks, but with increasing age, the cortical representations become more diffuse. This effect may represent either compensation by recruiting or a dedifferentiation. Dedifferentiation is comparable to the intellectual patterns of younger children who may identify all pets as "doggy" or all vehicles as "car" (Craik, 2006).

EVALUATION

Although much of the psychiatric evaluation of the elderly is similar to any psychiatric evaluation, some features require special consideration. See Chapters 3 to 6 for detailed information on the psychiatric evaluation. Because of the breadth of the evaluation and the slower response time of some elderly patients, it may often last more than an hour. The physician also must be flexible enough to conduct the interview in stages if it becomes clear that the patient cannot tolerate an extended interview (Sadavoy and Lazarus, 2004; Silver and Herrmann, 2004).

Because geriatric patients are often referred to physicians by family members or other health professionals, collateral information is essential. Family members often can detail changes in behavior that are not otherwise available. Reassurance of ongoing communication and cooperation with the patient's primary physician is often helpful. Not only do examiners ask the patient about past psychiatric symptoms but they also inquire about expectable life stressors and transitions, such as departure of children from the home and retirement. Knowing the types of coping skills mobilized in these transitions allows the clinician to assess the potential coping skills brought by the patient to the current situation (Sadavoy and Lazarus, 2004; Silver and Herrmann, 2004).

PSYCHIATRIC DISORDERS IN THE ELDERLY

Although the diagnostic criteria for adult mental disorders do not rely on age, clinical diagnosis in geriatric psychiatry entails some particular features. The physician who cares for the elderly confronts presentations of common disorders that change over the course of life as well as disorders that increase in incidence with age.

Dementia, Delirium, and Other Cognitive Disorders

See Chapter 8 for a full discussion of dementia, delirium, and other cognitive disorders.

Mood Disorders

Depression

Among the elderly in the general community, only 1% met criteria for major depression (Koenig and Blazer, 2007). Less severe depression, however, is much more common, with conservative estimates of subsyndromic depression in the range of 11% to 16% of Americans age 65 or older (Teresi et al., 2001). Approximately one fourth or more of nursing home residents who are elderly meet criteria for major depression (Gerety et al., 1994). In primary care settings around the world, 15% or more have some depressive disorder, although most of the cases are neither recognized nor treated by the physician (Whooley et al., 2000). Depressed elders are functionally disabled by their mood disorder and use significantly more primary care medical resources than their nondepressed cohort. For individuals with almost any medical condition, the presence of depressive symptoms is associated with significantly reduced survival (Alexopoulos, 2004).

Besides the discomfort and disability caused by the depressive symptoms alone, the risk of suicide also increases greatly in those with depression. For those older than age 65, the risk of death by suicide is approximately twice what it is for the population as a whole. The rate for suicide in males climbs from approximately age 65 with no plateau; for women, it peaks between 50 and 65 years of age. Part of this increase is attributable to the increased lethality of the elderly person's suicide attempt. Before the age of 50, only one in eight (13%) who attempts suicide actually kills himself or herself with the attempt. After age 65, that completion rate approaches one in two (50%)! The elderly suicide tends to use more lethal means, communicates the intent less frequently, and is less likely than the younger person to use suicide threats and gestures as tools for manipulating others (Bienenfeld, 1990).

Depression may be difficult to diagnose in the elderly patient, with reasons ranging from denial of symptoms to pseudodementia to not responding to medication. Therefore, the use of diagnostic criteria may be difficult in elderly patients with some depressive disorders (Koenig and Blazer, 2007). Additionally, the clinical presentations may change with age. As noted earlier, primary care physicians only recognize the condition in a fraction of their affected patients. It is fairly rare, for example, that an elderly patient will give as a chief complaint, "I am depressed." Much more commonly, the patient will describe vague somatic complaints, decreased energy, sleep difficulties, memory disturbances, anxiety, or "nerves." Somatic complaints, in fact, are the predominant way in which elderly patients present their depression or anxiety. Pain, weakness, and gastrointestinal disturbances are the most frequent avenues of presentation. Even someone with numerous neurovegetative complaints may deny depression or sadness but admit to feeling "down" or "blue" (Alexopoulos, 2004; Silver and Herrmann, 2004).

A wide variety of cardiovascular, pulmonary, endocrine, and neurologic diseases, most of which increase in prevalence with aging, can present with depressive symptoms such as fatigue, anorexia, and decreased functioning. Depression also can be induced or mimicked by numerous medications commonly used in the elderly, including antihypertensives, benzodiazepines, corticosteroids, and cimetidine. It is equally hazardous to attribute problems in appetite, energy, sleep, or concentration to either depression or medical causes alone. An appropriate evaluation should be conducted to assess accurately the physical status of the depressed patient in regard to medical illness, including relevant aspects of the history, physical examination, laboratory tests, and radiologic procedures (Alexopoulos, 2004).

Clinicians must be aware of normal changes of aging, including difficulty initiating sleep, decreased appetite, and lethargy, making it difficult to elicit true depressive symptoms in the elderly (Koenig and Blazer, 2007). Patients with depression may present with memory impairment resembling dementia (formerly called *pseudodementia* but more properly termed *dementia syndrome of depression*) (Folstein and McHugh, 1978). Patients with depression seem to have quicker onset and shorter duration of cognitive symptoms, as well as fluctuating symptoms. Depressed patients will not try to hide their memory problems as dementia patients would (Wells, 1979). One must not ignore the possibility of comorbid depression and dementia, since depression may occur in approximately one fifth of patients with cognitive impairment (Reifler et al., 1982).

At least 70% of depressed elderly patients who are given an adequate trial of antidepressant medication will recover from the index major depressive episode (Koenig and Blazer, 2007). Even in elderly patients with treatment-resistant depression, approximately half of the patients improved within 15 months of receiving either electroconvulsive therapy or antidepressant medication, with up to 71% showing clinical improvement after 4 years (Stoudemire et al., 1993).

Bereavement

In people 65 years old or older in the United States, 15% of men and 45% of women have been through bereavement of a spouse. Because women live longer than men, women spend a longer

A CASE OF GERIATRIC DEPRESSION

A 72-year-old woman is referred by her primary care physician (PCP). She had been complaining for many months to the PCP of fatigue and insomnia. She had been presenting a shifting variety of aches and pains. She had looked and sounded nervous to the PCP, who prescribed low doses of lorazepam. If anything, her fatigue got worse with the medication. She came to see the psychiatrist only reluctantly, saying, "I'm not crazy." She admitted to anhedonia and diminished motivation. She denied being "depressed," but admitted to being "worried about lots of little things."

Careful history uncovered no prior similar episodes, and there were no major recent stressors despite the patient's constant worry. The psychiatrist initiated sertraline at 25 mg per day. After 2 weeks, the patient was overly sedated, and medication was changed to venlafaxine extended release, 37.5 mg per day. After 2 weeks, her fatigue improved, and her activity level increased. By the fourth week, her mood had lifted noticeably and lorazepam was tapered and discontinued.

time in widowhood (Centers for Disease Control and Prevention, 2002). Approximately half of the elderly widows do well with minimal distress both before and after the spouse's death, but approximately 16% become "chronic grievers" (Bonnano et al., 2004). Elderly widows and widowers should improve their social network to decrease risk of mortality, because poor socialization after losing a spouse is associated with a poorer prognosis (Gallagher-Thompson et al., 1993).

Although uncomplicated bereavement (normal grieving) is not a psychopathological condition, grieving individuals may experience, transiently, depressive symptoms such as anorexia and insomnia in the context of their situational sadness. Normal grieving generally starts with a period of shock that lasts a few weeks or less, characterized by emotional numbing and even brief episodes of denial. Next comes a period of preoccupation with thoughts of the lost loved one and symptoms including crying, fatigue, and withdrawal. This phase may easily last a year or much longer in older widows and widowers and may recur on the lost person's birthday, the wedding anniversary, or the anniversary of the death. Finally, preoccupation gives way to resolution, as somatic and depressive symptoms diminish and the survivor regains interest in social and individual activities. These phases are similar at all ages, but in the elderly, somatic symptoms are often predominant expressions of the emotional distress, and the phases may take much longer to progress and resolve than at younger ages (Horowitz, 1986).

Mania

Although bipolar disorder usually begins in the third or fourth decade of life, episodes usually persist into old age. Additionally, first onset of mania in the sixth or even seventh decade may be observed. Compared with younger manic patients, older individuals are more likely to be irritable than euphoric and paranoid rather than grandiose. Older patients are more likely than younger ones to present with dysphoric mania or a mixed episode, a constellation in which there is pressure of speech, flight of ideas, and hyperactivity but thought content is as morbid and pessimistic as that of a patient with typical major depression (Koenig and Blazer, 2007). Bipolar disorder is present in one tenth to one fourth of elderly patients with mood disorders (Wylie et al., 1999).

Psychotic Disorders

Schizophrenia

Most elderly patients with schizophrenia developed their illness between ages 20 and 40. Only 7% of schizophrenias are first diagnosed after age 60 and only 3% after age 70 (Harris and Jeste, 1988). Aging affects the clinical appearance of schizophrenia, particularly producing a blunting of the positive symptoms, such as delusions and hallucinations. Residual delusions and hallucinations become less bizarre and more monotonous. The negative symptoms, including social withdrawal, apathy, and blunted affect, become more apparent (Cohen, 1990).

Although the numbers are small, some individuals do develop schizophrenia after their 50s and into their 60s, a condition formerly labeled *paraphrenia*. These individuals are more likely to be women than men. The clinical presentation usually centers on persecutory delusions and generally does not include a formal thought disorder (Jeste et al., 2004). Late-onset schizophrenics tend to function better premorbidly than early-onset schizophrenics (Jeste and Dolder, 2007).

Delusional Disorders

Delusional disorders generally begin in mid to late life. In the elderly, the delusions most often involve persecutory or somatic themes. Medications are only marginally successful at stopping the delusions but do tend to decrease their intensity and lessen the chance of the patient's acting on them. Psychotherapy generally does not produce good results, because the beliefs are unshakably true to the patient, who sees little motivation for therapy (Jeste et al., 2004).

Anxiety and Somatoform Disorders

Anxiety

Among mental health disorders in the elderly, the most common are those of the anxiety spectrum (Blazer et al., 1991). Because medical conditions, such as bladder incontinence, make it difficult for some elderly to leave the home, a careful assessment should be made before diagnosing an elderly patient with agoraphobia. Social phobia may be difficult to diagnose also, because elderly people may avoid situations in which any physical abnormality (tremors) may be noticed and because it fluctuates and sometimes goes into remission. Obsessive-compulsive disorder in the elderly often presents as frequent medical appointments for excessive physical problems (Beyer, 2007).

Elderly patients should be carefully assessed for post-traumatic stress disorder, because some may have served in World War II or been through the Holocaust (Sutker et al., 1993). Most panic attacks of late onset have been associated with medical conditions (Hassan and Pollard, 1994; Raj et al., 1993). Anxiety may be the cause of many elderly patients' physical complaints, such as nausea and weakness, for which they would seek help from a primary care doctor (White et al., 1986). Anxiety may also lead to or worsen cardiac problems (Kawachi et al., 1994). Symptoms of anxiety may be caused by medications prescribed to the elderly (Beyer, 2007).

As a symptom and diagnosis, anxiety is common in the elderly. Ten percent to 20% of the elderly complain of anxiety severe enough to warrant a visit to a physician. On self-rating scales, 27% of individuals in their 60s and 29% older than age 70 report significant anxiety symptoms.

Upward of 70% of elderly individuals with major depression will also experience considerable anxiety. Situational anxiety originating from any one of the many psychosocial changes experienced by the elderly can manifest as an adjustment disorder with predominant anxiety symptoms. Numerous medical illnesses also can cause anxiety symptoms. When elderly patients complain of anxiety, depression should be at the top of the clinician's differential diagnosis (Flint, 2004).

Somatoform Disorders

Like those with primary anxiety disorders, most patients with somatoform disorders begin to experience them well before late life. Although somatizing behavior, including the expression of anxious and depressive symptoms as somatic complaints, may increase with aging, new-onset somatoform disorders are uncommon in old age. Delusional disorders with predominately somatic symptoms occur in the elderly, but in these conditions, the complaints are more bizarre and lack the initial plausibility of those voiced in somatoform disorders. In those individuals with persistent somatoform disorders that started earlier in life, the particular complaints, especially in somatization disorder and hypochondriasis, may change over the course of middle age and late life. Elderly patients with somatization disorder will focus less on sexual function and more on gastrointestinal distress. Elderly hypochondriacs may voice the unfounded conviction that they have a dementia. Hypochondriacal complaints are extremely common as secondary symptoms of depression in the elderly (Agronin, 2007).

Substance Abuse

Alcoholism

Although alcoholism has no clear definition in any age-group, it is clear that alcohol abuse is a common problem in the elderly. Five percent of the elderly population in the community may meet the criteria for alcohol dependence, and twice as many drink alcohol in an abusive fashion. According to self-reports, 10% to 20% of the elderly drink daily, up to 25% have 5 to 7 drinks a week, and 7% to 8% have between 12 and 21 drinks a week. One fifth of elderly medical and psychiatric patients may be problem drinkers, as are as many as 45% of patients admitted to acute geriatric psychiatric units (Liberto et al., 1992).

Despite this evidence of continued problem drinking throughout life, the actual incidence in cross-sectional studies declines sharply after the age of 70. Possible reasons for this decrease include an increased mortality in problem drinkers at ages younger than 70 and the distinct difficulties of recognizing alcohol abuse in elders (Atkinson, 2004).

Because of the alterations in ethanol metabolism that accompany aging, a given amount of alcohol will produce a higher blood alcohol level in an older person than in a younger one. Additionally, the brain and other organs become increasingly sensitive to the effects of alcohol. As a result, it is fairly common for a person to maintain a constant level of alcohol consumption over many years and only begin to have problems such as confusion, depression, or hepatic dysfunction after age 60 (Offsay, 2007).

It is currently recommended that geriatric patients should only have one standard drink per day and never any more than two standard drinks at any one time. Clues to a geriatric alcohol problem can be very vague and difficult to recognize but include auto accidents, elevated amounts of anxiety, cognitive impairment, changes in sleep, difficulty maintaining hygiene, falling or bruising frequently, gastrointestinal problems such as bleeding, and disturbances in gait. The elderly tend to be more receptive to receiving help with their alcohol problem if the concerns are coming from their family members, so a family meeting may be of benefit if resistance occurs (Offsay, 2007).

Confounding the recognition of alcoholism in the elderly is the fact that many of the diagnostic criteria for alcohol abuse and dependence involve features that may not apply to aging individuals. Largely because of retirement, the elderly are not likely to suffer occupational problems due to their drinking. They are also less likely to suffer legal consequences. Changes in their behavior such as confusion, self-neglect, malnutrition, and depression may be improperly dismissed as "normal" aging (Bienenfeld, 1990). Using standardized screening tests also may be ineffective. The Michigan Alcoholism Screening Test—Geriatric (MAST-G) version, an adaptation of a widely used screening instrument, is both simple and sensitive in older populations (Babor et al., 1992).

Compared with elderly people who do not abuse alcohol, those who do are more likely to commit suicide, live alone, and have serious health problems such as hepatic, pulmonary, and cardiovascular diseases. Fifteen percent of those elderly who present to emergency rooms with depression or confusion develop these conditions as a result of alcohol use (Atkinson, 2004).

Four out of five geriatric patients who abuse alcohol and have evidence of depression are experiencing a depression due to their alcohol use. Up to 60% of older alcoholics will fit the criteria for dementia. They suffer difficulty because of the direct toxic effects of alcohol on the central nervous system or exacerbations of other causes of dementia. Alcohol can exacerbate the changes in sleep and sexual function that normally accompany aging. It can also interact with more than 150 prescribed medications, including anticoagulants, phenytoin, sedatives, and antidepressants (Bienenfeld, 1990).

Treatment of elderly alcoholics is similar to the treatment of their younger counterparts with only slight differences. Detoxification will more frequently require hospitalization because of concern for autonomic and cardiovascular instability. Because of the particular risk of delirium, it is also generally recommended that elderly alcoholics not receive prophylactic benzodiazepines unless they have a history of complicated alcohol withdrawal. If these agents are required, lorazepam and oxazepam are generally preferred because of their rapid hepatic oxidation. Disulfiram, which can be used to discourage alcohol consumption in younger patients, is not recommended in the elderly because it may react with numerous drugs besides alcohol, and the elderly can experience severe and even life-threatening reactions. Naltrexone has been found to be safe and efficacious in the elderly (Oslin et al., 1997; Oslin et al., 2002). Geriatric alcoholics also benefit from Alcoholics Anonymous meetings as well as supportive psychotherapy to treat their problem (Offsay, 2007).

Abuse of Other Substances

The use of illicit drugs such as narcotics and hallucinogens is not generally a significant problem in the elderly. Much more common is the abuse of prescription and over-the-counter (OTC) medications. The average American senior takes approximately three prescription medications per day; fewer than one in five takes none and more than one in five takes five or more different prescription drugs daily. People 75 years of age and older take an average of 7.9 prescription drugs per person per day (Ennis and Reichard, 1997). The elderly often will have multiple providers who are not fully aware of what other medications are being prescribed. Because some elderly individuals tend to hoard pills, trade medications, and take their medications in a nonprescribed manner, the situation is ripe for abuse (Atkinson, 2004).

OTC medications also represent a problem for the elderly. Sixty-nine percent of people older than 65 years take at least one OTC medication a day. The average US senior takes 1.8 OTC medications daily. Many of these can interact with alcohol or other medications that the patient is taking. Because these medications are not prescribed, many people do not consider them drugs and will not volunteer them when asked about medications. The most common OTC classes used are analgesics, laxatives, and nutritional supplements. OTC cold remedies often include ingredients that can induce delirium (such as sleeping pills that have anticholinergic effects), as can nonsteroidal anti-inflammatory drugs. Laxatives, which are taken weekly by one third of the population older than 65 years, can result in diarrhea, malabsorption, and even hypokalemia. The

---

A CASE OF PARANOID PERSONALITY DISORDER

A 69-year-old man had lived a fairly isolated life and had generally been suspicious of most people. He had only taken odd jobs for cash to avoid registering his name with any public entity or paying taxes. He deliberately remained homeless to limit contacts with others and minimize official records of himself. Now, weakened by various illnesses, he is repeatedly brought to the emergency department by police. He is usually hostile and uncooperative. He resents any questions and accuses his doctors of being responsible for his ailments.

The psychiatric consultant made no attempt to argue with the patient's suspicions and, in fact, acknowledged how threatening the system could feel. She asked if he would welcome some medication to help him relax, but he refused. As she continued to meet with him regularly though briefly, she began to strategize with him how he might minimize the intrusions posed by the authorities, and presented tactics of collaboration as means to maintain his autonomy.

---

practitioner is therefore well advised to inquire about OTC medications in evaluating the elderly patient (Bienenfeld, 1990; Hanlon, 2001). See Chapter 9 for a full discussion of substance-related disorders.

Personality Disorders

The basic characteristics of individuals with personality disorders are evident early in adult life and manifest in long-standing patterns of maladaptive perception, communication, and behavior. People do not develop personality disorders in late life, but the characteristic features of these disorders do change over time within individuals. In general, the behavior of individuals with narcissistic, borderline, and histrionic personality disorders becomes less intense with age. Some belated maturation may occur, impulsive actions may become incompatible with the geriatric lifestyle, and early mortality from hazardous behaviors may eliminate those with the most severe personality pathology (Abrams and Sadavoy, 2004).

Before making a new diagnosis of a personality disorder in an older patient, one should assess carefully and treat aggressively axis I disorders, particularly depressive disorders and substance abuse. The influence of a hostile environment in which the patient may live might temper the clinician's interpretation of ideas that sound unusually suspicious. Psychotherapy (see subsequent text) is the optimal treatment for personality disorders at any age; in late life, it is particularly important to make sure the therapeutic goals of the therapy are matched to the patient's resources and life circumstances (Abrams and Bromberg, 2007).

TREATMENT

Pharmacotherapy

Although caution must be used whenever medications are prescribed, there are some special considerations in the use of psychotropic medications in the elderly. Because most elderly psychiatric patients will already be receiving some medication for somatic disorders, their drug regimens may become quite confusing, and the clinician must carefully consider the possible drug interactions and additive side effects of any proposed new medication. Additionally, nonadherence becomes a problem when the reasons for the medication and the prescribed dosing schedule are poorly understood. Cognitive impairment may mandate that a third-party set up or administer the medications (Meyers and Young, 2004).

Certain alterations in metabolism and sensitivity occur with aging. There is a decrease in the lean body mass and total body water along with an increase in body fat. These changes decrease the volume of distribution of hydrophilic drugs such as alcohol and increase the volume of distribution of lipophilic drugs such as benzodiazepines, accounting for the relative increase in blood alcohol content and the decreased clearance of benzodiazepines in the elderly user. Hepatic metabolism decreases, in general, with age, as does the production of albumin. The former effect results in a generalized slowing of hepatic clearance and the latter effect can cause a relative increase in the free fraction of drugs such as tricyclic antidepressants, which are largely protein bound. Receptor sensitivity seems to change with age, causing older patients to be more sensitive to the therapeutic and adverse effects of medications (Meyers and Young, 2004).

Antipsychotic Medications

Even in the elderly population, the atypical antipsychotics are considered first-line treatment for psychosis (Rapoport et al., 2005). They have a smaller risk of extrapyramidal symptoms and tardive dyskinesia than the typical antipsychotics. Smaller doses of antipsychotics are generally used in the elderly compared to younger populations (Jeste and Dolder, 2007). Risperidone has been the most studied atypical antipsychotic in the elderly (Alexopoulos et al., 2004). Current dosage recommendations for risperidone are between 0.5 mg and 2 mg a day for elderly patients with dementia and less than 4 mg a day for elderly patients without dementia (Mulsant and Pollock, 2007). The advantages of risperidone are its small amount of sedation or anticholinergic effect. Quetiapine is currently the first-line agent in the elderly with Parkinson disease, Lewy body dementia, or tardive dyskinesia, due to its low risk of extrapyramidal side effects (Alexopoulos et al., 2004; Poewe, 2005). Clozapine is minimally used in the elderly due to its serious side effect profile (Mulsant and Pollock, 2007). Aripiprazole and ziprasidone are currently considered second-line agents in the elderly due to very minimal studies in this age-group (Alexopoulos et al., 2004).

Mood Stabilizers

Aging bipolar patients continue to require treatment because they can experience both manic and depressive episodes throughout their life. The elderly are more sensitive to the effects of lithium but can often be managed with serum levels of 0.4 to 0.7 mEq/L. The decrease in renal functioning that occurs with aging slows the elimination of lithium, increasing its half-life from 18 hours at age 20 to 36 hours by age 70 (Jenike, 1989). As a result, the serum lithium levels of an elderly patient can be two or even three times higher than a younger patient's after taking equal doses of the medication. The elderly are more sensitive to the toxic effects of lithium and can experience difficulty with doses that are considered routine in younger patients. Patients should be periodically assessed for tremor, nausea, diarrhea, and memory deficits. Numerous drugs that the elderly commonly use, such as nonsteroidal anti-inflammatory drugs and thiazide diuretics, can also raise the serum lithium level and induce lithium toxicity (Mulsant and Pollock, 2007).

Because lithium can be so problematic to use in the elderly, anticonvulsants, such as valproate and carbamazepine, have become increasingly accepted agents for mania in the elderly (Mulsant and Pollock, 2007). These drugs may be useful in those elderly patients who cannot tolerate lithium or for whom lithium has lost some of its prophylactic benefit. Generally, valproate is much better tolerated than carbamazepine and is more likely to maintain its benefit without breakthrough symptoms of mania (Meyers and Young, 2004). Anticonvulsants have also been used to manage dementia-related agitation (Mulsant and Pollock, 2007). Mania related to neurologic diseases may respond better to anticonvulsants (Shulman, 1997).

The use of atypical antipsychotics as mood stabilizers is quite variable due to limited data in elderly manic patients. However, some clinicians prefer to reserve these agents for augmentation purposes in order to limit side effects (Satlin et al., 2005). Olanzapine has been approved by the U.S. Food and Drug Administration (FDA) for use in bipolar mania, and risperidone has been found to be useful as an augmenting agent along with a mood stabilizer (Meyers and Young, 2004; Tohen et al., 1996).

Antidepressant Medications

For depression in the elderly, the selective serotonin reuptake inhibitors (SSRIs) have assumed a place as the first-line agents. In general, they are well tolerated by the elderly. The preferred SSRIs at this time in the elderly are sertraline, citalopram, and escitalopram (Alexopoulos et al., 2001; Mulsant et al., 2001). SSRIs may also be helpful in treating dementia-related agitation and psychosis (Nyth and Gottfries, 1990; Nyth et al., 1992; Pollock et al., 1997; Pollock et al., 2002). In the elderly, SSRIs should be started at half the lowest efficacious dose and then doubled 1 week later (Mulsant and Pollock, 2007). There is no evidence that any one SSRI is more effective than another. Clinicians generally base their choices on side effects. When agitation or insomnia is prominent, selection of a more sedating antidepressant is sensible; when retardation and fatigue are principal features, more activating agents may be chosen (Jacobson et al., 2007).

The newer antidepressants, including venlafaxine, bupropion, mirtazapine, duloxetine, and nefazodone, should be used with caution in the elderly due to limited research in this population (Oslin et al., 2003; Rabins and Lyketsos, 2005). Venlafaxine, bupropion, and mirtazapine are second-line agents in the elderly (Alexopoulos et al., 2001). Bupropion has stimulant properties in many patients and almost no cardiovascular side effects and should be used before psychostimulants for long-term treatment (see subsequent text) (Jacobson et al., 2007).

Tricyclic antidepressants are third-line agents to treat depression in the elderly, with monoamine oxidase inhibitors being fourth line, because both have significant side effect profiles (Mottram et al., 2006; Mulsant et al. 2001; Wilson and Mottram, 2004). Of the many tricyclic antidepressant side effects that occur in the elderly, two of the more troubling are confusion, which often is related to the anticholinergic effect, and hypotension due to antiadrenergic and muscarinic effects, which can result in dangerous and even life-threatening falls. Caution must be exercised in the use of monoamine oxidase inhibitors, because they can cause autonomic instability (Jacobson et al., 2007).

Trazodone (a heterocyclic antidepressant) has little anticholinergic effect, moderate antia-drenergic effect, and significant sedative effects. It can be useful in the depressed patient with significant agitation, anxiety, or insomnia. Most clinicians view trazodone as a relatively "weak" antidepressant in which high doses, which elderly patients may not tolerate, are needed to achieve a therapeutic response (Jacobson et al., 2007).

Psychostimulants such as dextroamphetamine and methylphenidate are used by some physicians in the treatment of their elderly depressed patients. These medications can be used to treat those patients who have prominent medical illnesses or who display prominent lethargy and apathy. One of the great benefits of these medicines is the rapidity of their therapeutic activity. Although stimulants improve depressive symptoms quickly in many individuals, their effect on the core depressive illness has never been demonstrated, and their long-term usefulness is controversial (Jacobson et al., 2007; Mulsant and Pollock, 2007).

Antianxiety Medications and Sedative-Hypnotics

The SSRIs and venlafaxine are currently first-line agents for anxiety in the elderly (Mulsant and Pollock, 2007). Chronic use of benzodiazepines has been associated with an increased risk of cognitive impairment, falls, and fractures of the hip (Sorock and Shimkin, 1988).

Buspirone is a nonbenzodiazepine anxiolytic that has demonstrated safety and efficacy in the elderly. It differs from the benzodiazepines clinically in that it may take 3 to 6 weeks of therapy before the patient's anxiety diminishes. Elderly patients appear to require the same dosages of buspirone as younger patients, approximately 15 to 40 mg a day given in divided doses (Fernandez et al., 1995).

Newer benzodiazepine-1 (BZ-1) receptor-specific sedative-hypnotics such as zolpidem, eszopiclone, and zaleplon, as well as the melatonin-stimulating agent ramelteon, are both safe and effective in the aged. They may have less propensity to induce confusion than traditional, nonspecific benzodiazepines (Cotroneo et al., 2007).

Electroconvulsive Therapy

Electroconvulsive therapy (ECT) may be used in depressed elderly patients in whom medication trials have failed, who have had significant side effects to medications, or who have exhibited significant self-harming behavior (Koenig and Blazer, 2007). Elderly patients respond just as well to ECT as younger patients (Stoudemire et al., 1995). Spinal x-rays are particularly important in elderly women due to possible osteoporosis, leading to compression fractures (Koenig and Blazer, 2007).

Psychotherapy

For much of the early history of psychiatry, elderly patients were not considered appropriate candidates for psychotherapy because individuals older than age 40 were seen as too close to death and too rigid in their personality structure to benefit. As the scope of psychotherapy has broadened, the prospect of treating elderly patients has been reexamined. In fact, the aging process brings about a number of challenges and issues that could be best dealt with by psychotherapy (Bienenfeld, 1990).

Aging persons need to deal with their changing environments and shifting societal expectations. Retirement, changes in financial status, the loss of loved ones, and decreased social support can threaten the elderly person. The patient also may experience changes in the family role as parent, grandparent, and spouse or widow/widower. Those who obtained self-esteem from their work roles or their roles as parents must begin to find other sources for this esteem. Dependency issues begin to surface as aging individuals find themselves less able to control their environment. Failing health and approaching death also are universal issues that will need to be dealt with in some way. In addition, advancing age can bring an increased awareness of abilities that were not utilized, goals that were not actively pursued, or personality features that were left underdeveloped (Sadavoy and Lazarus, 2004).

Grief and loss are central issues in much of the psychotherapy of older persons. The therapeutic task is to identify the particular meaning of the loss to the individual and to find less distressing ways to cope. For example, a man who is embittered in his retirement may come to discover through therapy that he had tied his entire sense of self-worth to his business accomplishments. He then can use the psychotherapy as a forum for exploring other sources of self-esteem. From a more behavioral perspective, the objective is to redirect energy and activity to pursuits more likely to foster emotional recovery so that the same retiree might be encouraged to participate in community activities or to engage regularly with his grandchildren (Sadavoy and Lazarus, 2004).

Cognitive therapy (or cognitive behavioral therapy, CBT) has proved effective with older patients just as it has with younger adults, for depression as well as anxiety, particularly around somatic issues. Goal setting, a critical early step in CBT, must be realistic enough to warrant likely success. Limitations of processing speed and its resultant influence on memory and abstraction, as noted earlier, may demand a slower pace of therapy, with more need for repetition (Koder et al., 1996).

Group therapy directly lessens the elder's sense of isolation. The patient is encouraged to practice social and communicative skills in a nonthreatening environment. Feedback concerning communication and behavior is received from peers and not just from the therapist, who might be significantly younger than the patient. The group environment also tends to increase self-esteem by allowing the patient to help others with their problems. To be an appropriate member, the patient must be able to make meaningful relationships, motivated to participate in the group, and cognitively able to follow the conversation and group interactions (Leszcz, 2004).

Despite the increased mobility of society, families continue to play a pivotal role in the lives of the elderly. Families therefore can be a part of the therapy and more than just sources of information. The clinician can help the family identify and clarify problems and frame them into manageable terms. A statement such as "My children do not care for me" may be reformulated as "I wish you would visit me more often." Solutions then are crafted in measurable dimensions to address the mutually identified problem (Mintzer et al., 2004).

Typically, too, children overcome the loss of parents more quickly than elders recover from the loss of spouses. There may come a period months after a death when the adult children avoid contact with the still-grieving parent or make comments such as "You should be over that by now." Education to families about the time course of grieving in later life can prevent the mourning from becoming complicated by guilt and isolation from family (Gwyther, 2007; Zisook et al., 2004).

SUMMARY AND CONCLUSIONS

Even in the absence of dementing conditions that become more common in late life, aging brings about numerous effects on memory, most of which derive from the progressive loss of processing speed. The psychiatric evaluation of the aging patient requires accommodations for slowing and for sensory impairment, as well as liberal use of collateral sources of information.

Psychiatric illnesses look different in older individuals. Depression becomes more easily confused with both anxiety and mania. Substance abuse disorders become more difficult to recognize because of age-related changes in metabolism.

The guiding principle for pharmacotherapy is "start low, go slow." Psychotherapy remains an indispensable element of treatment for psychiatric disorders in late life.

Clinical Pearls

- The effects of aging on crystallized and fluid intelligence make older people less "sharp" but more "wise."
- Any acute or subacute change in an elderly person's cognition is pathological and merits careful evaluation, and should not be dismissed as "normal aging."
- Major depression and anxiety in the elderly are frequently secondary to physical illness, drug effects, and alcohol use.
- Because of age-related changes in physiology, a person can begin to have alcohol-related problems with mood or cognition in late life while consuming the same amounts he or she did without adverse effects when younger.
- Most medications should be started in the elderly at doses between one third and one half of the starting dose in young adults, and dosages should be advanced more slowly.
- Older adults are just as likely to benefit from psychotherapy as younger persons.

Self-Assessment Questions and Answers

29-1. The change in cognitive function most widely demonstrated, and which lies at the root of most other age-related changes in cognition, is:

A. Diminished crystallized intelligence
B. Reduced processing speed
C. Reduced short-term memory
D. Reduced long-term memory
E. Vulnerability to distraction

The reduction in processing speed with increasing age lies at the heart of most other cognitive deficits. It limits the capacity and speed of short-term memory, which cascades into intermediate memory. Long-term memory is not inherently affected by age, although older people use less efficient strategies of storage and retrieval. Vulnerability to distraction is present, but is not nearly as central as diminished processing speed. Crystallized intelligence increases with age (Spar and LaRue, 2006). *Answer: B*

29-2. Compared to younger patients with bipolar disorder, older bipolar patients:

A. Are less likely to experience mixed episodes
B. Are more likely to be irritable than euphoric
C. Have shorter depressed episodes
D. Require higher doses of lithium
E. Respond less well to anticonvulsant mood stabilizers

Older manic patients are more likely to be irritable or paranoid than euphoric or grandiose. Depressed periods lengthen and euthymic intervals shorten with age. Older bipolar patients usually need lower doses of lithium, and respond just as well to anticonvulsants as do younger ones (Koenig and Blazer, 2007; Mulsant and Pollock, 2007). *Answer: B*

29-3. Which of the following conditions is most likely to produce anxiety symptoms in older individuals?

A. Alcohol abuse
B. Chronic obstructive pulmonary disease
C. Delirium
D. Depression
E. Post-traumatic stress disorder

Depression is the most common cause of anxiety symptoms in late life. Approximately 70% of depressed elders endorse anxiety symptoms, and over one third of all those with anxiety meet criteria for depression. All the conditions listed can cause anxiety, but none is as likely as depression (Flint, 2004). *Answer: D*

29-4. Which of the following pharmacokinetic changes is a common effect of aging?

A. Blood–brain barrier becomes less permeable.
B. Blood flow to liver and kidney increases.
C. Body fat comprises a larger percentage of body mass.
D. Glomerular filtration rate decreases.
E. Intestinal absorption decreases.

With normal aging, body mass decreases in general, but the fluid compartment shrinks while the fat compartment either grows or remains stable. Drugs distributed to the water compartment reach higher blood levels, while those distributed to fatty stores exhibit longer elimination half-lives. In the absence of disease, hepatic and renal blood flow do not diminish significantly, nor does glomerular filtration rate. The blood–brain barrier becomes more permeable with age (Meyers and Young, 2004). *Answer: C*

29-5. With increasing age, which of the following changes is most likely to be observed in persons with personality disorders?

A. Affect becomes more labile.
B. Impulsive behaviors become less common.
C. Legal troubles become increasingly serious.
D. Substance abuse becomes less likely.
E. Suicide gestures become more frequent.

As persons with personality disorders age, some maturation occurs and behaviors become less impulsive and disruptive; affective swings remain unchanged or become milder. Although such individuals remain at significant risk for completed suicide, suicidal gestures decrease with age. Abuse of alcohol remains common in older persons with personality disorders (Abrams and Sadavoy, 2004). *Answer: B*

References

Abrams RC, Bromberg CE. Personality disorders in the elderly. *Psychiatr Ann.* 2007;37(2):123–127.

Abrams RC, Sadavoy J. Personality disorders. In: Sadavoy J, Jarvik LF, Grossberg GT, et al., eds. *Comprehensive textbook of geriatric psychiatry,* 3rd ed. New York: W.W. Norton & Co.; 2004:701–722.

Agronin ME. Somatoform disorders. In: Blazer DG, Steffens DC, Busse EW, eds. *Essentials of geriatric psychiatry,* 1st ed. Washington, DC: American Psychiatric Publishing; 2007:207–218.

Alexopoulos GS. Late-life mood disorders. In: Sadavoy J, Jarvik LF, Grossberg GT, et al., eds. *Comprehensive textbook of geriatric psychiatry,* 3rd ed. New York: W.W. Norton & Co.; 2004:609–653.

Alexopoulos GS, Katz IR, Reynolds CF III, et al. Pharmacotherapy of depression in older patients: A summary of the expert consensus guidelines. *J Psychiatr Pract.* 2001;7:361–376.

Alexopoulos GS, Streim J, Carpenter D, et al. Expert consensus panel for using antipsychotic drugs in older patients: Using antipsychotic agents in older patients. *J Clin Psychiatry.* 2004;65(Suppl 2):5–104.

Atkinson RM. Substance abuse. In: Sadavoy J, Jarvik LF, Grossberg GT, et al., eds. *Comprehensive textbook of geriatric psychiatry,* 3rd ed. New York: W.W. Norton & Co.; 2004:723–762.

Babor TF, de la Fuente JR, Saunders J, et al. *AUDIT: The alcohol use disorders identification test: Guidelines for use in primary health care.* Geneva, Switzerland: World Health Organization; 1992.

Beyer JL. Anxiety and panic disorders. In: Blazer DG, Steffens DC, Busse EW, eds. *Essentials of geriatric psychiatry,* 1st ed. Washington, DC: American Psychiatric Publishing; 2007:193–205.

Bienenfeld D, ed. *Verwoerdt's clinical geropsychiatry,* 3rd ed. Baltimore: Lippincott Williams & Wilkins; 1990.

Blazer DG, George LK, Hughes D. The epidemiology of anxiety disorders: An age comparison. In: Salzman C, Lebowitz BD, eds. *Anxiety in the elderly: Treatment and research.* New York: Springer; 1991: 17–30.

Bonnano GA, Wortman CB, Nesse RM. Prospective patterns of resilience and maladjustment during widowhood. *Psychol Aging.* 2004;19:260–271.

Centers for Disease Control and Prevention. *U.S. life tables, 2002.* Hyattsville: National Center for Health Statistics; 2002. Available at http://www.cdc.gov/nchs/data/dvs/life2002.pdf. Accessed April 8, 2008.

Cohen CI. Outcome of schizophrenia into later life: An overview. *Gerontologist.* 1990;30:790–797.

Compton DM, Bachman LD, Brand D. Working memory and perceptual speed mediation of age-associated changes in cognition within a sample of highly-educated adults. *North Am J Psychol.* 2003;5(3):451–478.

Compton DM, Bachman LD, Brand D, et al. Age-associated changes in cognitive function in highly educated adults: Emerging myths and realities. *Int J Geriatr Psychiatry.* 2000;15:75–85.

Cotroneo A, Gareri P, Nicoletti N, et al. Effectiveness and safety of hypnotic drugs in the treatment of insomnia in over 70-year-old people. *Arch Gerontol Geriatr.* 2007;44(1):121–124.

Craik FIM. Brain-behavior relations across the lifespan: A commentary. *Neurosci Biobehav Rev*. 2006;30: 885–892.

Crawford JR, Bryan J, Luszcz MA, et al. The executive decline hypothesis of cognitive aging: Do executive deficits qualify as differential deficits and do they mediate age-related memory decline? *Aging Neuropsychol Cogn*. 2000;7(1):9–31.

Ennis KJ, Reichard RA. Maximizing drug compliance in the elderly: Tips for staying on top of your patients' medication use. *Postgrad Med*. 1997;102:211–213, 218, 223–224.

Erikson EH. *Identity and the life cycle*. New York: International Universities Press; 1959.

Federal Interagency Forum on Aging Related Statistics. *Older Americans 2000: Key indicators of well-being*. Washington, DC: Federal Interagency Forum on Aging Related Statistics; 2000.

Fernandez F, Levy JK, Lachar BL, et al. The management of depression and anxiety in the elderly. *J Clin Psychiatry*. 1995;56(2):20–29.

Flint AJ. Anxiety disorders. In: Sadavoy J, Jarvik LF, Grossberg GT, et al., eds. *Comprehensive textbook of geriatric psychiatry*, 3rd ed. New York: W.W. Norton & Co.; 2004:687–699.

Folstein MF, McHugh PR. Dementia syndrome of depression. In: Katzman R, Terry RD, Bick KL, eds. *Alzheimer's disease: Senile dementia and related disorders (Aging Vol. 7)*. New York: Raven Press; 1978:87–92.

Gallagher-Thompson D, Futterman A, Farberow N, et al. The impact of spousal bereavement on older widows and widowers. In: Stroebe MS, Stroebe W, Hansson R, eds. *Handbook of bereavement*. Cambridge: Cambridge University Press; 1993:227–239.

Gerety MB, Williams JW Jr, Mulrow CD, et al. Performance of case-finding tools for depression in the nursing home: Influence of clinical and functional characteristics and selection of optimal threshold scores. *J Am Geriatr Soc*. 1994;42:1103–1109.

Grégoire J. What factors underlie the aging effects on WAIS-R and WAIS-III subtests? *Int J Gastrointest Cancer*. 2001;1(3-4):217–233.

Gwyther LP. Working with the family of the older adult. In: Blazer DG, Steffens DC, Busse EW, eds. *Essentials of geriatric psychiatry*, 1st ed. Washington, DC: American Psychiatric Publishing; 2007: 357–374.

Hanlon JT, Fillenbaum GG, Ruby CM, et al. Epidemiology of over-the-counter drug use in community dwelling elderly. *U S Perspect Drugs Aging*. 2001;18(2):123–131.

Harris MJ, Jeste DV. Late onset schizophrenia: An overview. *Schizophr Bull*. 1988;14:39–55.

Hassan R, Pollard CA. Late-life-onset panic disorder: Clinical and demographic characteristics of a patient sample. *J Geriatr Psychiatry Neurol*. 1994;7:86–90.

Horn JL, Cattell RB. Refinement and test of the theory of fluid and crystallized general intelligence. *J Educ Psychol*. 1966;57:253–270.

Horowitz MJ. *Stress response syndromes*. Northvale: Aronson; 1986.

Jacobson SA, Pies RW, Katz IR. *Clinical manual of geriatric psychopharmacology*. Washington, DC: American Psychiatric Publishing; 2007:141–258.

Jenike MA. *Geriatric psychiatry and psychopharmacology: A clinical approach*. Chicago: Year Book Medical Publishers; 1989.

Jeste DV, Dolder CR. Schizophrenia and paranoid disorders. In: Blazer DG, Steffens DC, Busse EW, eds. *Essentials of geriatric psychiatry*, 1st ed. Washington, DC: American Psychiatric Publishing; 2007:177–192.

Jeste DV, Dunn LB, Lindamer LA. Psychoses. In: Sadavoy J, Jarvik LF, Grossberg GT, et al., eds. *Comprehensive textbook of geriatric psychiatry*, 3rd ed. New York: W.W. Norton & Co.; 2004: 655–685.

Kawachi I, Sparrow D, Vokonas PS, et al. Symptoms of anxiety and risk of coronary heart disease: The Normative Aging Study. *Circulation*. 1994;90:2225–2229.

Koder DA, Brodaty H, Ansety KJ. Cognitive therapy for depression in the elderly. *Int J Geriatr Psychiatry*. 1996;11:97–101.

Koenig HG, Blazer DG. Mood disorders. In: Blazer DG, Steffens DC, Busse EW, eds. *Essentials of geriatric psychiatry*, 1st ed. Washington, DC: American Psychiatric Publishing; 2007:145–176.

Leszcz M. Group therapy. In: Sadavoy J, Jarvik LF, Grossberg GT, et al., eds. *Comprehensive textbook of geriatric psychiatry*, 3rd ed. New York: W.W. Norton & Co.; 2004:1023–1054.

Liberto JG, Oslin DW, Ruskin PE. Alcoholism in older persons: A review of the literature. *Hosp Community Psychiatry*. 1992;43:975–984.

Meyers BS, Young RC. Psychopharmacology. In: Sadavoy J, Jarvik LF, Grossberg GT, et al., eds. *Comprehensive textbook of geriatric psychiatry*, 3rd ed. New York: W.W. Norton & Co.; 2004:903–992.

Mintzer J, Lebowitz B, Olin JT, et al. Family issues in mental disorders of late life. In: Sadavoy J, Jarvik LF, Grossberg GT, et al., eds. *Comprehensive textbook of geriatric psychiatry*, 3rd ed. New York: W.W. Norton & Co.; 2004:1055–1070.

Mottram P, Wilson K, Strobl J. Antidepressants for depressed elderly. *Cochrane Database Syst Rev.* 2006;(1):CD003491; DOI: 10.1002/14651858:CD003491.

Mulsant BH, Alexopoulos GS, Reynolds CF III, et al. The PROSPECT Study Group. Pharmacological treatment of depression in older primary care patients: The PROSPECT algorithm. *Int J Geriatr Psychiatry.* 2001;16:585–592.

Mulsant BH, Pollock BG. Psychopharmacology. In: Blazer DG, Steffens DC, Busse EW, eds. *Essentials of geriatric psychiatry*, 1st ed. Washington, DC: American Psychiatric Publishing; 2007:293–336.

Nyth AL, Gottfries CG. The clinical efficacy of citalopram in treatment of emotional disturbances in dementia disorders: A Nordic multicentre study. *Br J Psychiatry.* 1990;157:894–901.

Nyth AL, Gottfries CG, Lyby K, et al. A controlled multicenter clinical study of citalopram and placebo in elderly depressed patients with and without concomitant dementia. *Acta Psychiatr Scand.* 1992;86:138–145.

Offsay J. Treatment of alcohol-related problems in the elderly. *Ann Long Term Care Clin Care Aging.* 2007;15:39–44.

Oslin DW, Liberto JG, O'Brien J, et al. Naltrexone as an adjunctive treatment for older patients with alcohol dependence. *Am J Geriatr Psychiatry.* 1997;5(4):324–332.

Oslin DW, Pettinati H, Volpicelli JR. Alcoholism treatment adherence: Older age predicts better adherence and drinking outcomes. *Am J Geriatr Psychiatry.* 2002;10(6):740–747.

Oslin DW, Ten Have TR, Streim JE, et al. Probing the safety of medications in the frail elderly: Evidence from a randomized clinical trial of sertraline and venlafaxine in depressed nursing home residents. *J Clin Psychiatry.* 2003;64(8):875–882.

Poewe W. Treatment of dementia with Lewy bodies and Parkinson's disease dementia. *Mov Disord.* 2005;20(Suppl 12):S77–S82.

Pollock BG, Mulsant BH, Rosen J, et al. Comparison of citalopram, perphenazine, and placebo for the acute treatment of psychosis and behavioral disturbances in hospitalized, demented patients. *Am J Psychiatry.* 2002;159:460–465.

Pollock BG, Mulsant BH, Sweet R, et al. An open pilot study of citalopram for behavioral disturbances of dementia. *Am J Geriatr Psychiatry.* 1997;5:70–78.

Rabbitt P, Lowe C. Patterns of cognitive aging. *Psychol Res.* 2000;63:308–316.

Rabins PS, Lyketsos CG. Antipsychotic drugs in dementia: What should be made of the risks? *JAMA.* 2005;294:1963–1965.

Raj BA, Corvea MH, Dagon EM. The clinical characteristics of panic disorder in the elderly: A retrospective study. *J Clin Psychiatry.* 1993;54:150–155.

Rapoport M, Mamdani M, Shulman KI, et al. Antipsychotic use in the elderly: Shifting trends and increasing costs. *Int J Geriatr Psychiatry.* 2005;20(8):749–753.

Reifler BV, Larson E, Henley R. Coexistence of cognitive impairment and depression in geriatric outpatients. *Am J Psychiatry.* 1982;39:623–626.

Sadavoy J, Lazarus LW. Individual psychotherapy. In: Sadavoy J, Jarvik LF, Grossberg GT, et al., eds. *Comprehensive textbook of geriatric psychiatry*, 3rd ed. New York: W.W. Norton & Co.; 2004:993–1022.

Satlin A, Liptzin B, Young RC. Diagnosis and treatment of late-life bipolar disorder. In: Salzman C, ed. *Clinical geriatric psychopharmacology*, 4th ed. Philadelphia: Lippincott Williams & Wilkins; 2005.

Shaw RM. Age-related change in visual, spatial and verbal memory. *Aust J Aging.* 2006;25(1):14–19.

Shulman KI. Disinhibition syndromes, secondary mania and bipolar disorder in old age. *J Affect Disord.* 1997;46:175–182.

Silver IL, Herrmann N. Comprehensive psychiatric evaluation. In: Sadavoy J, Jarvik LF, Grossberg GT, et al., eds. *Comprehensive textbook of geriatric psychiatry*, 3rd ed. New York: W.W. Norton & Co.; 2004:253–279.

Sorock GS, Shimkin EE. Benzodiazepine sedatives and the risk of falling in a community-dwelling elderly cohort. *Arch Intern Med.* 1988;148:2441–2444.

Spar JE, LaRue A. *Clinical manual of geriatric psychiatry.* Washington, DC: American Psychiatric Publishing; 2006.

Stoudemire A, Hill CD, Morris R, et al. Long-term outcome of treatment-resistant depression in older adults. *Am J Psychiatry*. 1993;150:1539–1540.

Stoudemire A, Hill CD, Morris R, et al. Improvement in depression-related cognitive dysfunction following ECT. *J Neuropsychiatry Clin Neurosci*. 1995;7:31–34.

Sutker PB, Allain AN Jr, Winstead DK. Psychopathology and psychiatric diagnoses of World War II Pacific theater prisoner of war survivors and combat veterans. *Am J Psychiatry*. 1993;150:240–245.

Teresi J, Abrams R, Holmes D, et al. Prevalence of depression and depression recognition in nursing homes. *Soc Psychiatry Psychiatr Epidemiol*. 2001;36:613–620.

Tohen M, Zarate CA, Centorrino F, et al. Risperidone in the treatment of mania. *J Clin Exp Psychopathol Q Rev Psychiatry Neurol*. 1996;57:249–253.

Wells CE. Pseudodementia. *Am J Psychiatry*. 1979;136:895–900.

White LR, Cartwright WS, Cornoni-Huntley J. Geriatric epidemiology. *Annu Rev Gerontol Geriatr*. 1986;6:215–311.

Whooley MA, Stone B, Soghikian K. Randomized trial of case-finding for depression in elderly primary care patients. *J Gen Intern Med*. 2000;15(5):293–300.

Wilson K, Mottram P. A comparison of side effects of selective serotonin reuptake inhibitors and tricyclic antidepressants in older depressed patients: A meta-analysis. *Int J Geriatr Psychiatry*. 2004;19(8):754–762.

Wood KM, Edwards JD, Clay OJ, et al. Sensory and cognitive factors influencing functional ability in older adults. *Gerontology*. 2005;51:131–141.

Wylie ME, Mulsant BH, Pollock BG. Age of onset in geriatric bipolar disorder: Effects on clinical presentation and treatment outcomes in an inpatient sample. *Am J Geriatr Psychiatry*. 1999;7:77–83.

Zisook S, Shuchter SR, Dunn LB. Grief and bereavement. In: Sadavoy J, Jarvik LF, Grossberg GT, et al., eds. *Comprehensive textbook of geriatric psychiatry*, 3rd ed. New York: W.W. Norton & Co.; 2004:579–608.

Psychiatric Research and Its Application to the Care of Patients

SECTION

V

Psychiatric
Research and Its
Application to the
Care of Patients

Research Advances in Neuroscience and Psychiatric Genetics

There has never been a more exciting time in the development of our biological understanding of the etiology of psychiatric illness and our understanding of how genetic variability can influence responses to treatment. It is now generally agreed that virtually all psychiatric illnesses are best described as being "complex" genetic illnesses wherein products of multiple susceptibility genes interact in ways that lead to the expression of psychiatric symptoms. Importantly, critical epigenetic interactions also influence gene expression. Ultimately, salient experiential stressors precipitate clinical dysfunction presumably as a consequence of epigenetic mechanisms.

This is also a time of great progress in the development of functional neuroimaging. Progress in neuroimaging has been accelerated by the production of higher resolution images of the brain. This greater resolution has made it possible to more precisely define variation in functional activity and to measure the chemical signatures of psychiatric illnesses by focusing on increasingly smaller structural volumes of the brain.

As a consequence of these scientific advances, innovative strategies for translating these findings into clinical practice have emerged. The development of transcranial magnetic stimulation, vagal nerve stimulation, and deep brain stimulation represents translational efforts to use new research insights in neuroscience to improve the care of patients in clinical practice.

Although both genetic analyses and neuroimaging advances promise to provide a better understanding of psychiatric illness, the primary focus of this chapter is to consider molecular genetic insights into the etiology of psychiatric illness and review how new tools, such as pharmacogenomic clinical testing, can guide psychiatrists in their management of psychotropic medications.

The clarification of how gene variability results in the expression of complex illnesses has been accelerated by recent advances in genome-wide scanning. However, new insights into how specific gene variants interact with the effects of early environmental stressors have been among the most important findings of the last decade.

GENETIC SUSCEPTIBILITY ASSOCIATED WITH THE DEVELOPMENT OF PSYCHIATRIC ILLNESS

For many years, ongoing psychiatric research projects have collected DNA samples in well-characterized clinical samples with the goal of identifying what were hoped to be a relatively small number of genes associated with the onset of each of the major psychiatric illnesses. Over the last decade, it has become increasingly clear that the expression of most psychiatric illnesses is the result of multiple gene products interacting in a manner that leads to symptomatic behavior. These insights have led to a conceptual reevaluation of the taxonomy of psychiatric illness (Jensen et al., 2006). A shift is now occurring to move the diagnosis process away from an exclusively categoric approach, which has been the dominant paradigm of the last half of the 20th century. Currently, a more dimensional approach is beginning to emerge that challenges the traditional definitions of psychiatric illnesses.

Schizophrenia

A major research enterprise has been put into place to identify the genes associated with the onset of schizophrenia. Evidence now supports the position that multiple genes actually increase

TABLE 30-1	Genes Thought to Be Associated with Susceptibility to Selected Mental Disorders and Behaviors	
Mental Disorder or Behavior	**Genes**	**Chromosome Locus of Gene**
Schizophrenia	COMT (catechol-O-methyltransferase)	22q11
	DAOA (D-amino acid oxidase activator)	13q33.2; 13q34
	DISC1 (disrupted in schizophrenia 1)	1q42
	GRM3 (glutamate receptor, metabotropic 3)	7q21-22
	NRG1 (neuregulin 1)	8p12
	RGS4 (regulator of G-protein signaling 4)	1q23.3
Depressive illness	TPH2, NTPH (tryptophan hydroxylase 2)	12q21.1
	MDD1 (major depressive disorder)	12q22-q23.2
	HTR2A (5-hydroxytryptamine [serotonin] receptor-2A)	13q14-q21
	MDD2 (major depressive disorder 2)	15q25.3-q26.2
	SLC6A3 (dopamine transporter gene)	5p15.3
	SLC6A4 (serotonin transporter gene)	17q11.1-q12
Suicidal ideation, suicidal behavior	GRIA3 (glutamate receptor, ionotropic, AMPA 3)	Xq25-q26
	GRIK1 (glutamate receptor, ionotropic, kainate 1)	21q22.11
	GRIK2 (glutamate receptor, ionotropic, kainate 2)	6q16.3-q21
	HTR1B (5-hydroxytryptamine [serotonin] receptor 1B)	6q13
	HTR2A (5-hydroxytryptamine [serotonin] receptor 2A)	13q14-q21
	HTR2C (5-hydroxytryptamine [serotonin] receptor 2C)	Xq24
	MAOA (monoamine oxidase A)	Xp11.3
	SCN8A (sodium channel, voltage gated, type VIII, α-subunit)	12q13
	SLC6A4 (serotonin transporter gene)	17q11.1-q12
	TPH1 (tryptophan hydroxylase 1 [tryptophan 5-monooxygenase])	11p15.3-p14
	TPH2 (tryptophan hydroxylase 2)	12q21.1
	VAMP4 (vesicle-associated membrane protein 4)	1q24-q25
Alcohol dependence	ADH1A (alcohol dehydrogenase 1A)	4q21-q23
	ADH1B (alcohol dehydrogenase 1B)	4q21-q23
	ADH1C (alcohol dehydrogenase 1C)	4q21-q23
	ADH4 (alcohol dehydrogenase 4)	4q21-q24; 4q22
	ALDH2 (aldehyde dehydrogenase 2)	12q24.2
	CYP2E1 (cytochrome P450, family 2, subfamily E, polypeptide 1)	10q24.3-qter
	DRD4 (D4 dopamine receptor gene)	11p15.5
	OPRM1 (opioid receptor, μ 1)	6q24-q25
	SLC6A4 (serotonin transporter gene)	17q11.1-q12

NTPH, neuronal tryptophan hydroxylase; AMPA, amino-3-hydroxy-5-methyl-4-isoxazole propionate.

the vulnerability for all psychotic illnesses, including schizophrenia. The goal of this research has become the identification of different groups of susceptibility genes (Harrison and Weinberger, 2005; Weinberger, 2006). Table 30-1 provides a list of some genes that have variant alleles which have been associated with schizophrenia. Evidence now exists that some of these genes, such as D-amino acid oxidase activator (*DAOA*), are also linked to the onset of bipolar disorder. Variations in many of the genes have been associated only with schizophrenia in certain groups of patients. For example, neuregulin 1 (*NRG1*) has primarily been shown to be associated with schizophrenia in northern European samples. In contrast, variants in other susceptibility genes, such as disrupted in schizophrenia (*DISC1*), have been associated with schizophrenia in quite different parts of the world.

Depression

Variations in many susceptibility genes also have been associated with the onset of depressive illness (Table 30-1). Still other genes have been linked to the specific symptoms of depressive illness, such as suicidal ideation and behavior. As a consequence of these studies, it has become increasingly clear that having high-risk alleles of these vulnerability genes does not necessarily result in the development of clinical symptoms. However, patients who do have these at-risk alleles are more likely to become clinically depressed after exposure to environmental stressors.

Caspi et al. (2003) reported a gene–environment interaction that was demonstrated by their analyses of the Dunedin longitudinal study in New Zealand. One of their key findings was an association between early child maltreatment and a later increased risk of developing depression in young adults who had the "short form" of serotonin transporter gene (*SLC6A4*). Patients with this form of *SLC6A4* produce less serotonin transporter protein than do individuals who have two copies of the long form of *SLC6A4*. This results in less available serotonin transporter protein in the neuronal cleft, which appears to increase the likelihood of developing depressive symptoms. Individuals with less effective reuptake of serotonin are now believed to be less "resilient" to stress and consequently more vulnerable to environmental stressors.

This same research team has described a similar gene–environment interaction relationship involving the monoamine oxidase A gene (*MAOA*) (Caspi et al., 2002). Two common versions of the *MAOA* have been well studied. A higher incidence of psychiatric problems has been reported in children with the less active form of the gene, but again, only if they were exposed to abusive situations in their first 4 years of life.

Association studies have demonstrated that variations in several genes have been associated with an increased risk of suicidal behavior and completed suicide (Table 30-1). These include the serotonin transporter gene (*SLC6A4*), one of the tryptophan hydroxylase genes (*TPH2*), and several genes that code for the receptors of serotonin or glutamate. Many of these association studies were conducted with small regional populations and will require further replications before the development of a molecular diagnostic tool to provide an estimate of suicidal risk.

Alcohol Dependence

The development of alcohol dependence has also been linked to variations in vulnerability genes. It has long been known that the children of parents with alcohol dependence are more likely to develop drinking problems (Schuckit, 1972). However, the specific vulnerability genes have only recently been identified. Table 30-1 lists some of the known alcohol susceptibility genes.

The alcohol dehydrogenase gene (*ADH*) and the acetaldehyde dehydrogenase gene (*ALDH*) produce enzymes that play a primary role in alcohol metabolism. Variations in these two genes have been associated with different levels of risk for alcohol dependence. Largely as a consequence of variability in these two genes, it is estimated that some individuals are able to metabolize alcohol four times more rapidly than others.

Seven versions of the *ADH* gene all produce alcohol dehydrogenase. This redundancy in coding capacity suggests that this enzyme is important for survival. One function of alcohol dehydrogenase is to metabolize alcohol to acetaldehyde. Two high-activity variants are associated with rapid conversion of alcohol to acetaldehyde. The first is a variant of the *ADH1B* gene known as the **47His version*. The second is a variant of the *ADH1C* gene known as the **349Ile version*. Each of these two variants is considered to be a protective factor for alcohol dependence. A promoter region variant of a third alcohol dehydrogenase gene, *ADH4*, has also been associated with a different level of risk for alcohol dependence based on the rate of metabolism of alcohol.

There are also several versions of the ALDH. The *ALDH2* gene has a clinically important *2 allele that produces a completely inactive form of acetaldehyde dehydrogenase. Individuals with the *2 allele have difficulty metabolizing acetaldehyde and are less likely to become alcohol dependent, because they develop a "flushing" reaction due to a buildup in the serum of acetaldehyde. This *2 variant is common in Asian populations.

Another relevant gene for alcohol metabolism is the cytochrome *P450 2E1* gene (*CYP2E1*), which codes for an enzyme that plays a role in a secondary pathway of alcohol metabolism.

However, *CYP2E1* can become quite important in individuals who are heavy drinkers because it has the capacity to be upregulated, which results in a large increase in the rate of alcohol metabolism and, therefore, more tolerance to alcohol consumption. The *1D allele of *CYP2E1* is associated with increased inducibility and, consequently, alcohol dependence.

Two gene variants have been linked to improved response to anticraving medication. Specifically, the 118G variant of the μ-opioid gene has been associated with a better response to naltrexone (Anton et al., 2008). Similarly, patients with the 7-repeat allele of the dopamine type 4 receptor gene (*DRD4*) have been demonstrated to have a better response to olanzapine, which is an antagonist of both the *DRD2* and *DRD4* receptors (Hutchison et al., 2006).

CLINICAL PHARMACOGENOMIC TESTING

It is well recognized that patients vary in their response to specific medications. An explanation for some of this variability is the differential function of drug metabolizing enzyme genes, which influence the biological availability of most psychotropic drugs. Using microarray genotyping strategies, it is now possible to predict the clinical drug metabolizing phenotypes of patients based on easily defined genetic variations. Pharmacogenomic testing has been most widely studied and utilized related to the many variations of the cytochrome *P450 2D6* gene. Many psychotropic medications are either primarily or substantially metabolized by the 2D6 enzyme. Table 30-2 lists the commonly prescribed psychotropic medications that are 2D6 substrates.

CYP2D6 Genotyping

The predicted *2D6* drug metabolizer phenotype of a given patient is directly related to the amount of functional enzyme that the patient is able to produce.

Pharmacogenomics promises to be particularly important for the creation of more evidence-based decision making in the selection and dosing of psychotropic medication (Pickar, 2003). Four traditional drug metabolizing phenotypes have been established. The "normal" *2D6* phenotype, also referred to as the *extensive phenotype*, is defined by the response of a patient to a 2D6 substrate when a patient has two normal copies of the *2D6* gene.

The poor 2D6 metabolizing enzyme genotype is defined as a patient who does not have even one fully functioning copy of the *2D6* gene. The intermediate 2D6 metabolizer phenotype is defined as a patient who has only one functional gene but has a second copy of the gene that is either totally or partially inactive. These individuals are usually able to metabolize 2D6 substrate medications at lower doses.

The fourth drug metabolizing genotype category is designated as the ultrarapid metabolizer phenotype. Although multiple genetic variations can lead to enhanced drug metabolism, the most common condition is to have three or more functional copies of the *2D6* gene. This results in the production of a large quantity of the 2D6 enzyme and a rapid clearing of substrate medication (Weinshilboum, 2003; Dalen et al., 1998).

The most obvious clinical benefit of cytochrome *P450 2D6* genotyping is the identification of patients who have the poor metabolizer phenotype. In theory, these individuals should either be given medications that are not primarily 2D6 substrate compounds or use 2D6 substrate medication in very low doses to avoid toxic reactions and adverse side effects. The other category of patients to identify so as to minimize ineffective treatment is the ultrarapid drug metabolizer phenotypes, because these individuals will very rapidly clear 2D6 substrate medications from their system and therefore be unable to achieve a therapeutic response.

CYP2C19 Genotyping

Another important drug metabolizing enzyme gene that has been available for clinical use for several years is the cytochrome *P450 2C19* gene. Table 30-2 shows the most common 2C19 substrate antidepressant medications.

CYP1A2 Genotyping

The cytochrome *P450 1A2* gene (*CYP1A2*) is now available for clinical testing. Both inactive and enhanced alleles have been demonstrated. The most common antidepressant substrates are described in Table 30-2.

TABLE 30-2	Antidepressant Substrates		
	Antidepressants Metabolized by Enzyme		
CYP450 Enzymes	**Primarily**	**Substantially**	**Minimally**
2D6	Fluoxetine Paroxetine Venlafaxine	Amitriptyline Duloxetine —	Citalopram Sertraline —
2C19	Citalopram Clomipramine Escitalopram	Nortriptyline Sertraline —	Venlafaxine — —
1A2	Fluvoxamine	Duloxetine Imipramine	Mirtazapine —

Serotonin Transporter Genotyping

The serotonin transporter gene (*SLC6A4*) produces the serotonin transporter protein that is the target of the selective serotonin reuptake inhibitors. This transporter protein is involved in the regulation of the availability and reuptake of serotonin. An insertion/deletion variant in the promoter region of the serotonin transporter gene has been shown to affect the transcription of this gene and appears to modulate the response of patients to treatment with these antidepressant medications (Rasmussen and Werge, 2007). There are essentially two variant classes. The short form has a 14-unit sequence in the promoter, while the long form has 16 units. Most versions of the long form are more active. Patients with the long form have been shown to be more likely to respond to selective serotonin reuptake inhibitors, and their response is more rapid (Serretti et al., 2007).

Variants in the second intron that are caused by variable nucleotide repeats (VNTR) are also associated with treatment response. The 9-repeat version is the most active, and the 10-repeat version is the least active. These intronic variants have been shown to predict medication response independently (Mrazek et al., 2008).

Serotonin 2A Receptor Genotyping

Currently, the primary clinical utility of genotyping the serotonin 2A receptor gene (*5HT2A*) is to identify variability in response to psychotropic medications. The T102C variation of *5HT2A* was first shown to be associated with a differential response to paroxetine (Murphy et al., 2003). Specifically, patients with two copies of the C allele at this location had more side effects and were more likely to discontinue using paroxetine when compared to patients with two copies of the T allele. More recently, a single nucleotide polymorphism (SNP) variant in the second intron of the gene with the reference SNP (rs) identification of rs7997012 was shown to predict a better response to citalopram (McMahon et al., 2006).

The Introduction of Algorithmic Guidance to Enhance Clinical Decision Making

As more associations between individual gene variations and medication responses have been demonstrated, the challenge of how to interpret the clinical implications of having multiple genetic variations has increased. Not only are there multiple variants within a gene but variations in multiple genes also affect response to the same drugs. A good example is the calculation of the implications of having variants in both the *SLC6A4* gene and the *5HT2A* gene. Presumably, a patient with enhancing variants in both genes is highly likely to respond very well to citalopram. Conversely, individuals with variants in these two genes that decrease their activity are less likely to respond positively to citalopram. What is more difficult to predict is how a patient with an enhancing variant in one gene and a problematic variant in the other gene will respond to citalopram. Table 30-3 represents four variants in these genes that are associated with differential response to citalopram.

A patient with two long insertion/deletion promoter variants of *SLC6A4* and two copies of the allele 1 variant of SNP rs7997012 in *5HT2A* would be expected to respond well to escitalopram.

TABLE 30-3	Enhancing and Problematic Variants of *SLC6A4* and *5HT2A*	
Genotypic Variant	**Enhanced Response**	**Reduced Response**
SLC6A4		
Insertion/deletion promoter variant	Long/long	Short/short
Second intron VNTR variant	9/9	10/10
5HT2A		
T102C SNP	T/T	C/C
rs7997012 SNP	1/1	2/2

VNTR, variable nucleotide repeats; SNP, single nucleotide polymorphism.

Conversely, a patient with two short insertion/deletion promoter variants of *SLC6A4* and two copies of the allele 2 variant of SNP rs7997012 in *5HT2A* is not likely to respond positively to escitalopram. However, further studies will be necessary to define the relative probabilities of response, given the many possible heterozygotic genotypes.

FUNCTIONAL NEUROIMAGING

The goal of functional neuroimaging is to use currently available innovative neuroimaging technology to measure aspects of brain function. Studies using functional technologies are being primarily used to better understand the relationship between variations in brain activity in discrete regions in the brain that have been linked to specific mental functions. Although neuroimaging has been used primarily as a research tool by cognitive neuroscientists, clinical applications are being developed.

Innovative methods that will be reviewed in this chapter include magnetic resonance spectroscopy (MRS), functional magnetic resonance imaging (fMRI), and positron emission tomography (PET).

PET and fMRI essentially measure changes related to blood flow. Given that measurable changes in hemodynamics occur at a relatively slow rate, these technologies are generally used to measure the location of a neural event rather than to document its time course. Traditional functional studies focus on determining the anatomic distribution of patterns of brain activity that have been associated with specific tasks. However, defining the interactions of multiple brain regions and the neural networks that connect the regions to one another will be necessary to more effectively characterize the complex expression of psychiatric symptoms.

Magnetic Resonance Spectroscopy

Proton 1H-MRS is an *in vivo*, noninvasive brain imaging technique that can detect alterations of brain biochemistry in patients who may have completely normal structural magnetic resonance imaging (MRI) studies. The resonance frequency of six metabolites on the 1H-MRS spectrum can now be reliably quantified. These include *N*-acetyl aspartate (NAA), which has been considered a marker of gray matter neuronal viability. Both glutamate (Glu) and glutamine (Gln) can be measured and represent the level of excitatory amino acid concentration. At the 1.5-T level of resolution, the composite peak of both Glu and Gln is reported and referred to as the *Glx peak*. Creatine (CR) and phosphocreatine are considered measures of energy utilization. The creatine signal is a relative stability and consequently has been used as an internal standard. Choline (Cho) is a composite of glycero- and phosphocholine and believed to reflect intracellular signal transduction. Finally, myo-inositol (mI) is an important component of the phospho-inositol second messenger system.

A series of MRS studies have reported associations between decreased glutamate concentration in the anterior cingulate and left dorsolateral prefrontal cortex in patients with major depressive disorder (Auer et al., 2000; Mirza et al., 2004; Rosenberg et al., 2004; Yildiz-Yesiloglu and Ankerst, 2006). Even more interestingly, normalization of glutamate level in these regions of interest has been associated with treatment response. This has been true of treatment with medication (Sanacora et al., 2002), electroconvulsive treatment (Michael et al., 2003; Pfleiderer et al., 2003), and transcranial magnetic stimulation (Luborzewski et al., 2007). MRS studies have also demonstrated abnormalities of glutamate and glutamine concentration in patients during their first episode of schizophrenia. Specifically, the level of glutamine has been shown to be higher in the left anterior cingulate cortex and the thalamus (Theberge et al., 2002). Of perhaps even greater interest, similar increases in the glutamate/glutamine peak have been demonstrated in adolescents who have been determined to be at high genetic risk for the development of schizophrenia when compared to adolescents at lower genetic risk (Tibbo et al., 2004). Although these findings demonstrate the potential clinical utility of MRS studies, further research using MRS is still needed to clarify key variables affecting variations in glutamate and glutamine levels before MRS testing is likely to become adopted in clinical settings.

Functional Magnetic Resonance Imaging

fMRI measures the hemodynamic changes that are related to neural activity in the brain. Given that changes in blood flow and blood oxygenation in the brain are closely linked to neural activity, when neurons are activated, oxygen carried by hemoglobin in red blood cells is consumed. Therefore, oxygen utilization is related to enhanced blood flow to regions of increased neural activity. However, a short interval of time is required following the stimuli for the response to occur.

A blood-oxygen-level–dependent (BOLD), fMRI methodology is used to measure changes in regions of the brain that reflect increases or decreases in activity (Turner and Jones, 2003). Neurons require an external source of energy to activate. The hemodynamic response is measurable because blood releases oxygen more quickly in active neurons than in inactive neurons. The difference in magnetic susceptibility is calculated between oxyhemoglobin and deoxyhemoglobin. These changes generate a magnetic signal variation, which is detected using an MRI scanner. Statistical methods have been developed to reliably identify those regions of the brain which change in response to exposure to a stimulus.

An interesting example of the sensitivity of fMRI has been demonstrated by measures of response to emotional processing of salient stimuli. More visceral emotional stimuli that are fearful in nature have been associated with activity in the amygdala, anterior cingulate, and limbic structures. In contrast, cognitive tasks that require intense concentration have been associated with increased activity in the dorsal regions of the cortex and attenuation of activity in the amygdala. It has been further demonstrated that complex stimuli, which have emotional content but require cognitive processing, involve both limbic and cortical regions. This pattern of response suggests the activation and regulatory modulation of a neural network (Keightley et al., 2003).

Positron Emission Tomography

PET is a nuclear imaging technique that produces a three-dimensional image of functional processes within the brain. This technology detects pairs of γ rays emitted indirectly by a positron-emitting radioisotope. Images of metabolic activity are then reconstructed by computer-based algorithms.

Completing a PET scan requires exposure of the patient to a radioactive tracer isotope. As the tracer decays, positrons are emitted. The tracer isotope is injected into the patient's bloodstream and after a period of 30 to 60 minutes, metabolically active molecules become concentrated in specific regions of the brain. At that point, the patient is placed in the scanner and the concentration and distribution of the tracer are measured. The molecule most commonly used for this purpose is fluorodeoxyglucose (FDG).

PET scans have not yet been used to diagnose complex psychiatric illnesses. However, increased uptake of [^{18}F] fluorodopa has been demonstrated in the ventral striatum in patients with schizophrenia and supports the hypothesis that the presynaptic striatal dopamine dysfunction plays a role in the expression of symptoms (McGowan et al., 2004). Similarly, studies of patients at risk for the development of schizophrenia have also found striatal dopamine overactivity when compared with age-matched controls (Howes et al., 2006). PET studies in depressed patients also have been used to study treatment response. Characteristic patterns of glucose metabolism have been associated with depressed patients who have responded to both venlafaxine and cognitive behavioral therapy (Kennedy et al., 2007).

Neuroimaging Endophenotypes

Identification of the genetic determinants of complex brain-related disorders continues to be a challenge, and it is well demonstrated that psychiatric illnesses represent a significant economic and public health burden (Uhl and Grow, 2004). However, one potential reason for the delay in identifying specific genes associated with psychiatric disorders is the relative lack of emphasis on the study of quantitative endophenotypes that index disease risk. An endophenotype is a heritable trait that is associated with a complex illness (Walters and Owen, 2007). Imaging methods are being successfully applied in a wide range of psychiatric disorders so as to develop insights into the pathophysiology of these illnesses. There is evidence that many psychiatric disorders have demonstrated disturbances in brain function. These include addictions (Thompson et al., 2004), attention-deficit/hyperactivity disorder (Sowell et al., 2003), and schizophrenia (Cannon et al., 2002), which have all been associated with alterations in demonstrated variable brain functioning.

CONCLUSIONS

The use of genotyping to guide clinical prescribing is now feasible, and the clinical utility of these tests has improved as a consequence of ongoing research defining the implications of variations in pharmacokinetic drug metabolizing genes and pharmacodynamic target genes. The immediate goal of research exploring the potential benefit of diagnostic genotyping is to find genes associated with an increased risk of the development of psychiatric illnesses. Progress in linking gene variation with clinical diagnosis is still limited to increasing awareness of the probability of having an illness rather than being able to definitively make a specific diagnosis.

Functional neuroimaging is still a research tool limited to helping investigators better understand how biological variability is associated with diagnosis and treatment. However, MRI spectroscopy is now able to demonstrate specific areas of the brain that are implicated in the development of major depressive disorder and schizophrenia. An immediate research objective is to extend the use of this form of neuroimaging to provide specific indications for the selection of treatments.

References

Anton RF, Oroszi G, O'Malley S, et al. An evaluation of mu-opioid receptor (OPRM1) as a predictor of naltrexone response in the treatment of alcohol dependence: results from the Combined Pharmacotherapies and Behavioral Interventions for Alcohol Dependence (COMBINE) study. *Arch Gen Psychiatry*. 2008;65:135–144.

Auer DP, Putz B, Kraft E, et al. Reduced glutamate in the anterior cingulate cortex in depression: An *in vivo* proton magnetic resonance spectroscopy study. *Biol Psychiatry*. 2000;47:305–313.

Cannon TD, Thompson PM, van Erp TG, et al. Cortex mapping reveals regionally specific patterns of genetic and disease-specific gray-matter deficits in twins discordant for schizophrenia. *Proc Natl Acad Sci U S A*. 2002;99:3228–3233.

Caspi A, McClay J, Moffitt TE, et al. Role of genotype in the cycle of violence in maltreated children. *Science*. 2002;297:851–854.

Caspi A, Sugdnen K, Moffitt T, et al. Influence of life stress on depression—moderation by a polymorphism in the 5-HTT gene. *Science*. 2003;301:386–389.

Dalen P, Dahl ML, Ruiz ML, et al. 10-Hydroxylation of nortriptyline in white persons with 0, 1, 2, 3, and 13 functional CYP2D6 genes. *Clin Pharmacol Ther*. 1998;63:444–452.

Harrison P, Weinberger D. Schizophrenia genes, gene expression, and neuropathology: On the matter of their convergence. *Mol Psychiatry*. 2005;10:40–68.

Howes OD, Montgomery AJ, Asselin MC, et al. The pre-synaptic dopaminergic system before and after the onset of psychosis: Initial results from an ongoing [^{18}F]fluoro-DOPA PET study. *Schizophr Res*. 2006;86:s11.

Hutchison KE, Ray L, Sandman E, et al. The effect of olanzapine on craving and alcohol consumption. *Neuropsychopharmacology*. 2006;31:1310–1317.

Jensen PS, Knapp P, Mrazek DA. *Toward a new diagnostic system for child psychopathology: Moving beyond the DSM*. New York: The Guilford Press; 2006.

Keightley ML, Winocur G, Graham SJ, et al. An fMRI study investigating cognitive modulation of brain regions associated with emotional processing of visual stimuli. *Neuropsychologia*. 2003;41:585–596.

Kennedy SH, Konarski JZ, Segal ZV, et al. Differences in brain glucose metabolism between responders to CBT and venlafaxine in a 16-week randomized controlled trial. *Am J Psychiatry*. 2007;164:778–788.

Luborzewski A, Schubert F, Seifert F, et al. Metabolic alterations in the dorsolateral prefrontal cortex after treatment with high-frequency repetitive transcranial magnetic stimulation in patients with unipolar major depression. *J Psychiatr Res*. 2007;41:606–615.

McGowan S, Lawrence AD, Sales T, et al. Presynaptic dopaminergic dysfunction in schizophrenia: A positron emission tomographic [^{18}F]fluoro-DOPA PET study. *Arch Gen Psychiatry*. 2004;61:134–142.

McMahon FJ, Buervenich S, Charney D, et al. Variation in the gene encoding the serotonin 2a receptor is associated with outcome of antidepressant treatment. *Am J Hum Genet*. 2006;78:804–814.

Michael N, Erfurth A, Ohrmann P, et al. Metabolic changes within the left dorsolateral prefrontal cortex occurring with electroconvulsive therapy in patients with treatment resistant unipolar depression. *Psychol Med*. 2003;33:1277–1284.

Mirza Y, Tang J, Russell A, et al. Reduced anterior cingulate cortex glutamatergic concentrations in childhood major depression. *J Am Acad Child Adolesc Psychiatry*. 2004;43:341–348.

Mrazek DA, Rush AJ, Biernacka JM, et al. SLC6A4 variation and citalopram response. *Am J Med Genet B Neuropsychiatr Genet*. 2008 July 10. [Epub ahead of print].

Murphy GM, Kremer C, Rodrigues HE, et al. Pharmacogenetics of antidepressant medication intolerance. *Am J Psychiatry*. 2003;160:1830–1835.

Pfleiderer B, Michael N, Erfurth A, et al. Effective electroconvulsive therapy reverses glutamate/glutamine deficit in the left anterior cingulum of unipolar depressed patients. *Psychiatry Res*. 2003;122:185–192.

Pickar D. Pharmacogenomics of psychiatric drug treatment. *Psychiatr Clin North Am*. 2003;26:303–321.

Rasmussen HB, Werge TM. Novel procedure for genotyping of the human serotonin transporter gene-linked polymorphic region (5-HTTLPR)—a region with a high level of allele diversity. *Psychiatr Genet*. 2007;17:287–291.

Rosenberg DR, Mirza Y, Russell A, et al. Reduced anterior cingulate glutamatergic concentrations in childhood OCD and major depression versus healthy controls. *J Am Acad Child Adolesc Psychiatry*. 2004;43:1146–1153.

Sanacora G, Mason GF, Rothman DL, et al. Increased occipital cortex GABA concentrations in depressed patients after therapy with selective serotonin reuptake inhibitors. *Am J Psychiatry*. 2002;159:663–665.

Serretti A, Kato M, De Ronchi D, et al. Meta-analysis of serotonin transporter gene promoter polymorphism (5-HTTLPR) association with selective serotonin reuptake inhibitor efficacy in depressed patients. *Mol Psychiatry*. 2007;12:247–257.

Schuckit MA. Family history and half-sibling research in alcoholism. *Ann N Y Acad Sci*. 1972;197:121–125.

Sowell ER, Thompson PM, Welcome SE, et al. Cortical abnormalities in children and adolescents with attention-deficit hyperactivity disorder. *Lancet*. 2003;362:1699–1707.

Theberge J, Bartha R, Drost DJ, et al. Glutamate and glutamine measured with 4.0 T proton MRS in never-treated patients with schizophrenia and healthy volunteers. *Am J Psychiatry*. 2002;159:1944–1946.

Thompson PM, Hayashi KM, Simon SL, et al. Structural abnormalities in the brains of human subjects who use methamphetamine. *J Neurosci*. 2004;24:6028–6036.

Tibbo P, Hanstock C, Valiakalayil A, et al. 3-T proton MRS investigation of glutamate and glutamine in adolescents at high genetic risk for schizophrenia. *Am J Psychiatry*. 2004;161:1116–1118.

Turner R, Jones T. Techniques for imaging neuroscience. *Br Med Bull*. 2003;65:3–20.

Uhl GR, Grow RW. The burden of complex genetics in brain disorders. *Arch Gen Psychiatry*. 2004;61:223–229.

Walters JT, Owen MJ. Endophenotypes in psychiatric genetics. *Mol Psychiatry*. 2007;12:886–890.

Weinberger DR. New directions in psychiatric therapeutics. *NeuroRx*. 2006;3:1–2.

Weinshilboum R. Inheritance and drug response. *N Engl J Med*. 2003;348:529–537.

Yildiz-Yesiloglu A, Ankerst DP. Neurochemical alterations of the brain in bipolar disorder and their implications for pathophysiology: A systematic review of the *in vivo* proton magnetic resonance spectroscopy findings. *Prog Neuropsychopharmacol Biol Psychiatry*. 2006;30:969–995.

Epidemiology Research in Psychiatry

HOW MANY PEOPLE HAVE A PSYCHIATRIC DISORDER?

Epidemiologic studies of the prevalence of psychiatric disorders describe how many individuals in a population have a psychiatric disorder. From this data, lifetime risk for a psychiatric disorder is determined. But why are these numbers important to anyone working in health care? Three reasons: psychiatric disorders are common; they exhibit symptoms that may be misinterpreted as medical conditions, leading to inaccurate diagnosis and treatment; and in an individual with a medical condition, they may interfere with response to the treatment of the medical disorder.

Kessler et al. (2007) reported the lifetime prevalence and projected lifetime risk of four groups of *Diagnostic and Statistical Manual*, Fourth Edition (DSM-IV), and International Statistical Classification of Disease and Related Problems (ICD-10) psychiatric disorders for Africa, the Americas, Asia, Europe, and the Middle East, including any anxiety, mood, impulse control, and substance use disorders. Lifetime prevalence and projected lifetime risk were also determined for any psychiatric disorder among the populations studied. In the United States, lifetime prevalence for any of these disorders was approximately one in every two individuals, and lifetime risk was 55.3%. Outside the United States, lifetime prevalence for any psychiatric disorder ranged from one in eight to one in three individuals, and lifetime risk ranged from 19.5% to 55.2%.

The United States has both the highest lifetime prevalence and potential risk in nearly all psychiatric groups of disorders. This difference was initially thought to be from a liberal threshold for diagnosing psychiatric disorders in U.S. epidemiologic studies. However, Haro et al. (2006) found that this was not a bias and that the results depict what would be found with standardized clinical diagnostic measures. The prevalence for these groups of major psychiatric disorders continues to support that psychiatric disorders commonly occur in the U.S. population. The lifetime prevalence of a psychiatric disorder is also common in other populations worldwide.

The common occurrence of psychiatric disorders poses a problem for clinicians. Many psychiatric disorders have somatic symptoms such as weight loss, poor energy, or pain. Not accounting for the possibility of a psychiatric disorder in the presentation of these symptoms leads the unsuspecting clinician to focus diagnosis and treatment only on medical etiologies. Alternatively, a psychiatric disorder as an explanation for the patient's complaint may be dismissed as "not a legitimate reason" for a symptom such as pain. This perception is changing. In recent decades, awareness has improved identification of psychiatric disorders in the differential diagnosis of pain, which has progressed from the "it is all in your head" explanation to an accepted differential diagnosis with algorithms for effective treatment. Once marginalized by the medical community, education and surveillance of psychiatric symptoms are changing the perception of psychiatric disorders by nonpsychiatrists.

Psychiatric disorders may exhibit symptoms of medical conditions, but they also worsen the presentation of existing medical conditions. Untreated depression in chronic medical conditions such as diabetes mellitus worsens prognosis through increased morbidity and mortality. Ultimately, identification of a comorbid psychiatric disorder may explain why first-line treatment is not improving the patient's condition (American Diabetes Association, 2007). The complication of a comorbid psychiatric disorder also affects primary psychiatric disorders. A substance use disorder co-occurring in depressive, anxiety, and personality disorders worsens outcome. Ultimately, awareness of the prevalence of psychiatric disorders aids clinicians in understanding prognosis and the outcome for their patients presenting with either medical or psychiatric conditions.

EPIDEMIOLOGY, THE *DIAGNOSTIC AND STATISTICAL MANUAL,* AND PSYCHIATRY

The relationship of epidemiology to mental illness is similar to its relationship with other medical disciplines. However, U.S. psychiatry defines itself in its study of psychopathology through the DSM, originally published by the American Psychiatric Association in 1952. It is regularly updated, with six versions of the four editions: DSM-I (American Psychiatric Association, 1952), DSM-II (American Psychiatric Association, 1968), DSM-III (American Psychiatric Association, 1980), DSM-III-revised (American Psychiatric Association, 1987), DSM-IV (American Psychiatric Association, 1994), and DSM-IV-text revision (TR) (American Psychiatric Association, 2000). DSM-III set the standard for what would be the modern version by using specific diagnostic criteria. DSM's relationship to epidemiology beckons discussion.

Readers of DSM-IV-TR should not view its epidemiology solely as the measure and reporting of prevalence and incidence rates of psychiatric disorders. Regrettably, this is the perception of epidemiology held by many physicians, residents, and medical students because other medical disciplines refine epidemiologic discussion in compendium texts to disease frequency and distribution. The definitions of epidemiology range from narrow to broad descriptions. A narrow view of epidemiology is the study of disease distribution in populations. *A Dictionary of Epidemiology* (Last, 2001) more broadly defined epidemiology as "the study of the distribution and determinants of health-related states or events in specific populations and the application of this study to control of health problems." These definitions all share the study of the distribution of disease as a core theme. This may explain how so many come to define epidemiology as a quantifying discipline in the study of illness.

The relationship of psychiatry to epidemiology includes not just the frequency of disorders but also the definition and classification of a disorder along with the etiology and management within a population. For all of these features, however, the inability to describe a psychiatric disorder undermines any attempt to measure its frequency distribution. Counting the number of cases of a psychiatric disorder before knowing what a case is is analogous to putting the cart before the horse.

Along with defining a case, the classification of a case into categories sharing similar symptoms and/or causes cannot be neglected in the pursuit of a diagnosis. Nosology, the classification of disease, serves as the starting point for identifying the disorder by achieving an understanding of a patient to justify a diagnosis. Case classification and definition are not new concepts in the study of mental illness. Their history dates back more than 2,500 years.

THE PREVALENCE OF PSYCHIATRIC DISORDERS IN THE COMMUNITY

The study of mental illness begins with knowing how many may be afflicted. The discussion of rates of disease in DSM-IV-TR and other psychiatry references includes descriptions of the prevalence and incidence of a disease. These are different measures, but both are fractions of specific populations. How these fractions are defined explains how prevalence and incidence differ.

Prevalence is a measurement of the number of cases of a disease in the population at a specific time over the number of persons in the population at the same specified time. It is frequently expressed as X number per 1,000. Prevalence is a cross-sectional measure, that is, a head count at a particular point in time. This slice-in-time count of those in the population with the diagnosis right now is the point prevalence. Period prevalence establishes a length of time, such as the last 5 years, and asks individuals if they have the disease. It should not be confused with incidence. With period prevalence, those who have the disease are counted in both the numerator and the denominator, because the affected are counted as part of the whole population. Incidence rates count those with a new onset of the disease during a period of time in the numerator whereas the denominator includes those at risk of developing the disease for the period of time studied. For that period of time counting new cases, someone who is affected cannot be counted as both a new case and someone at risk of developing a case. There must be some measure of time for new cases to occur and be counted to have a measure of incidence.

Prevalence can be derived from incidence, but caveats must be met to work both into a single equation. First, the duration of the disease is needed. The rates of disease are not changing, and the migration in is equal to the migration out in the population. In DSM-IV-TR, point prevalence is most commonly cited but incidences are included for some disorders. What matters more than the measure itself is the way the measure was obtained. Both prevalence and incidence rates are best performed in a sample of individuals that can describe the general population.

PREVALENCE, POPULATION STUDIES, AND STUDIES WITH CLINICAL PATIENTS

To describe the prevalence rate of a psychiatric disorder or just a symptom among the general population, a research study needs to be able to generalize its results. Generalizability means that the results found in the study of a population sample can be applied to the reference population. Does the reference population mean the general population? The reference population may target the general population, or it may be a more selective population of interest, such as all women with female orgasmic disorder or children aged 2 to 10 years with childhood disintegrative disorder. The population of interest, or the group of people meant to be studied, is determined by the investigators when the study is being developed. The general population is the target population in most cases to determine prevalence of a disorder. The study sample of individuals who will participate in the study is recruited to match the reference population as closely as possible.

Not all studies that determine prevalence of a disorder can collect potential participants for a count from the general population. Although this approach has many advantages, the limitation is how many individuals would need to be included to study rare disorders. For example, a rare disorder that may occur in 1 for every 10,000 individuals quickly consumes the study's resources to find enough individuals to accurately describe the disorder within the entire population.

Methods for completing larger studies have improved, but investigators seeking to answer how many in the general population have a rare disorder turn to locations where these individuals are more likely to be found. For psychiatric disorders, records from hospitals and clinics are a potential source. The advantage is that these locations will have the documentation to begin the search to count the occurrence of a disorder; however, limitations also exist for this source of participants for a study of prevalence. A variety of influencing factors, also known as *biases*, may affect who is seen in the hospital or clinic. The individuals seen may not represent an even distribution across socioeconomic status or geographic area. A major medical center may see several individuals with the same rare illness, but that is because their disorder is severe, thereby skewing the results so that morbidity and possibly mortality appear higher than what naturally occurs in the general population. Many more factors would affect the count such as availability and quality of records and whether the records are designed for a study of prevalence. These biases are considered in the development of a study of prevalence so that adjustments can be made to correct for them, but ideally it would be helpful in more common disorders like depression to count how many affected individuals are found within a representative sample of the general population.

In recent years, study procedures have improved to allow for determining prevalence rates from a general population sample. In the next section, some of the major studies that measure prevalence will be discussed.

SELECTED STUDIES OF PSYCHIATRIC SYMPTOMS AND DISORDERS

The National Comorbidity Survey Replication

The Epidemiologic Catchment Area (ECA) study determined the prevalence of DSM-III mental disorders in the United States from 1980 to 1985 (Robins and Regier, 1991). The ability to generalize the results of the ECA on a broader scale was limited. The next major U.S. epidemiologic study of mental illness was the National Comorbidity Survey (NCS), which analyzed a nationally representative U.S. sample from 1990 to 1992 based on DSM-III-R (Kessler et al., 1994). The next major mental illness epidemiologic survey was the National Comorbidity Survey Replication (NCS-R), a representative community household survey of the prevalence and correlates of mental disorders in the United States. The questions were based on DSM-IV. The NCS-R was designed to investigate and expand the assessment of the prevalence of mental disorders beyond the baseline NCS (Kessler and Merikangas, 2004). It measured prevalence and evaluated mental health treatment in terms of minimal adequacy according to recommendations and guidelines from the American Psychiatric Association and the Agency for Healthcare Research and Quality. The NCS-R set out to not only count but also to describe how treatment is provided and its outcome.

Two additional minority-specific psychiatric epidemiology studies are linked to the NCS-R: the National Survey of American Life (NSAL) and the National Latino and Asian American Study (NLAAS). These studies were also conducted using nationally representative samples and include diagnostic, pharmacologic, and service-use modules that are consistent with the NCS-R, as well as scales that measure culture-specific constructs among the minority groups.

The National Institute of Mental Health (NIMH) Collaborative Psychiatric Epidemiology Surveys (CPES) provides data on prevalence, factors affecting and associated with prevalence, and risk factors of mental disorders among the general population and minority groups.

Unlike most disabling physical diseases, mental illness begins very early in life. Half of all lifetime cases begin by age 14; three fourths by age 24. Therefore, mental disorders are the chronic diseases of the young. For example, anxiety disorders often begin in late childhood, mood disorders in late adolescence, and substance use disorders in the early 20s. Unlike heart disease or most cancers, young people with mental disorders suffer disability when they are in the prime of life, when they would normally be the most productive. The risk of mental disorders is substantially lower among people who have matured past the high-risk age range. Prevalence increases from the youngest age-group (ages 18 to 29) to the next oldest age-group (ages 30 to 44) and then declines, sometimes substantially, in the oldest group (ages 60 years and older). Females have higher rates of mood and anxiety disorders, whereas males have higher rates of substance use and impulse control disorders (Kessler et al., 2005a; Wang et al., 2005).

As described earlier, mental disorders are quite common in the United States; the 1-year prevalence of mental disorders is 26.2%. However, many of these cases are mild or will resolve without formal interventions (Kessler et al., 2005a).

Individuals with one mental disorder are at a high risk for having at least one additional comorbid disorder. Nearly half of those with one mental disorder met criteria for two or more disorders. Higher comorbidity led to greater severity of mental illness.

The four most common disorders found by the NCS-R in rank order of their 12-month period prevalence are specific phobia, 8.7%; social phobia, 6.8%; major depressive disorder, 6.7%; and attention-deficit/hyperactivity disorder, 4.1% (Kessler et al., 2005b).

Bipolar, substance use, and obsessive-compulsive disorders form the highest proportion of seriously disabling cases for a 1-year prevalence. The most prevalent 12-month disease categories in rank order of their period prevalence are anxiety disorders, 18.1%; mood disorders, 9.5%; impulse control disorders, 8.9%; and substance use disorders, 3.8%.

The most common disorders based on lifetime prevalence are anxiety disorders, 28.8%; mood disorders, 20.8%; impulse control disorders, 24.8%; and substance use disorders, 14.6% (Kessler et al., 2005a).

In most cases of impulse control, substance use, and anxiety disorders, age of onset falls into a narrow range. Most cases of impulse control disorder occur between ages 7 and 15 years; substance use disorders, ages 18 and 27 years; anxiety disorders, ages 6 and 21 years; and lastly, mood disorders, ages 18 to 43 years. Individuals with comorbid disorders tend to have had an earlier onset of the first disorder than those who only have one mental disorder.

A limitation of the NCS-R is that prevalence rates were drawn from households but limited in representing the entire population. It did not include homeless and institutionalized (nursing homes, group homes) populations. In addition, the study did not assess some rare and clinically complex psychiatric disorders, such as schizophrenia and autism, because a household survey is not the most efficient study design to identify and evaluate those disorders. The problem with failing to identify a rare or clinically complex psychiatric disorder is that such a disorder may be the source for other symptoms and an incorrect disorder could instead be identified as the symptoms' source in the study. The diagnostic criteria of many psychiatric disorders include the clause "is not better accounted for by. . . ." This means that when considering one diagnosis, it is important to make certain the symptoms are not due to another disorder that may present similarly but is diagnostically different. With this diagnostic caveat, it may be difficult to determine if the suspected diagnosis is due to a diagnosis that cannot be identified by the survey.

The National Survey on Drug Use and Health

The National Survey on Drug Use and Health (NSDUH) is the primary source of information on the prevalence, patterns, and consequences of alcohol, tobacco, and illegal drug use and abuse in the general U.S. civilian, noninstitutionalized population ages 12 and older. It was previously known as the *National Household Survey on Drug Abuse* (NHSDA). The NSDUH survey, conducted annually, produces drug and alcohol use incidence and prevalence estimates. Periodically, additional information is collected in the survey on special topics of interest such as serious mental illness, criminal behavior, treatment, mental health issues, and attitudes about drugs. It also provides estimates of prevalence for drug use and serious mental illness by state.

NSDUH is currently conducted by the Substance Abuse and Mental Health Services Administration (SAMHSA) Office of Applied Studies. SAMHSA is the leading federal agency for improving access to quality substance abuse prevention, addiction treatment, and mental health services in the United States. SAMHSA makes the NSDUH findings available to the public annually.

NSDUH is conducted annually in all 50 states plus the District of Columbia. The results of surveys ranging from 1994 to the present are available to the public online at http://www.oas.samhsa.gov/p0000016.htm. Although it might be tempting to provide the latest statistics and insights into their meaning, this would only be a replication of the work completed by the SAMHSA. SAMHSA provides exceptional resources to address these questions. Recent excerpts are shown in Table 31-1.

The Centers for Disease Control and Prevention Studies

The mission of the Centers for Disease Control and Prevention (CDC) is "to promote health and quality of life by preventing and controlling disease, injury, and disability" (www.cdc.gov). The CDC works with many partners throughout the nation and the world to monitor health, detect and investigate health problems, conduct research to enhance prevention, develop and advocate sound public health policies, implement prevention strategies, promote healthy behaviors, foster safe and healthful environments, and provide leadership and training. The steps needed to accomplish this mission are founded on scientific excellence, requiring well-trained public health practitioners and leaders dedicated to high standards of quality and ethical practice. The online data collections CDC WONDER are useful to psychiatry and epidemiology.

TABLE 31-1 Excerpts from the Recent National Survey on Drug Use and Health
Of the 61.6 million persons aged 12 or older who in 2006 smoked cigarettes in the last month, 57.7% (35.5 million) met the criteria for nicotine dependence
Persons aged 12 or older who were dependent on nicotine were more likely than those who were not nicotine dependent to have engaged in alcohol use (61.7% vs. 49.1%), binge alcohol use (40.1% vs. 20.1%), and heavy alcohol use (14.9% vs. 5.5%) in the last month
In 2006 approximately 3.1 million persons aged 12–25 (5.3%) had ever used an over-the-counter cough and cold medication to get high (i.e., used it nonmedically). Approximately 1 million persons aged 12–25 (1.7%) had used an over-the-counter cough and cold medication to get high in the last year
The rate of alcohol use disorder was more than twice as high among adults who had experienced a major depressive episode (16.2%) compared with adults who had not experienced a major depressive episode in the last year (7.3%)
In 2003–2004, last month alcohol use rates for persons aged 12–20 were the lowest in Utah (18.6%) and Tennessee (22.3%) and the highest in North Dakota (42.7%) and South Dakota (39.1%)

SAMHSA, Substance Abuse and Mental Health Services Administration.

CDC WONDER is the Wide-ranging ONline Data for Epidemiologic Research. Developed by the CDC, it is an integrated information and communication system for public health. CDC WONDER promotes information-driven decision making by placing timely, useful facts in the hands of public health practitioners and researchers. It also provides the general public with access to specific and detailed information from the CDC through the Internet. It speeds and simplifies access to public health information for state and local health departments, the Public Health Service, and all academic communities and is valuable in providing statistics for public health research, decision making, priority setting, program evaluation, and resource allocation.

Using the CDC WONDER site allows one to search for and read published documents on public health concerns, including reports, recommendations and guidelines, articles and statistical research data published by CDC, as well as reference materials and bibliographies on health-related topics. One can also look up statistics.

Unlike the NCS-R and NSDUH, the WONDER site contains information ascertained from many public health data sources. The CDC designed WONDER so that specific details concerning data collection methodology, latest updates, summary of references, and frequently asked questions are linked to the data source of interest. The WONDER data are ready for use in desktop applications such as word processors, spreadsheet programs, or statistical and geographic analysis packages. File formats available include Web pages, chart and map images, and spreadsheet files. All of these facilities are menu driven, and require no special computer expertise.

The CDC WONDER reports national results for U.S. health statistics and, similar to the NSDUH, the CDC WONDER site constantly changes as new health statistics are added throughout the year. The medical student is encouraged to start at http://wonder.cdc.gov/Welcome.html and select from the A to Z listing of sites at http://wonder.cdc.gov/WelcomeA.html or from the topics at http://wonder.cdc.gov/WelcomeT.html to begin exploring the available information.

The World Health Organization Studies

The World Health Organization (WHO) directs and coordinates authorities for health within the United Nations system. The WHO developed the International Statistical Classification of Disease and Related Problems, known as *ICD-10*. ICD-10 is the international diagnostic standard from which criteria are used in many epidemiologic studies, including those involving mental illness. ICD-10 and DSM-IV-TR have been written to share many criteria and diagnoses. The WHO is responsible for providing leadership on global health matters, shaping the health research agenda, setting norms and standards, articulating evidence-based policy options, providing technical support to countries, and monitoring and assessing health trends. It sees the health of people as key to socioeconomic progress. Poverty and health are linked, with the worsening of one a detriment to the other. The WHO develops health programs to target groups caught in this cycle by strengthening health systems, securing and protecting groups from outbreaks, and optimizing their strategic planning through multiple partnerships and implementation of health policies. Partnership across private and public as well as national and international sectors is required to achieve these goals. The WHO uses its results-based management approach to measure performance against expected results.

The WHO collects data and statistics. As with the CDC, these data include psychiatric and neurologic disorders, including unipolar depressive disorders (equivalent to DSM-IV-TR's major depressive disorder), bipolar affective disorder, schizophrenia, epilepsy, alcohol use disorders, Alzheimer disease and other dementias, Parkinson disease, multiple sclerosis, drug use disorders, post-traumatic stress disorder, obsessive-compulsive disorder, panic disorder, insomnia (primary), and migraine. The listings of prevalence for these disorders are available at http://www.who.int/healthinfo/bodestimates/en/index.html. World statistics also include the rates of tobacco, drug, and alcohol use; suicides; and homicides. The results of World Health Surveys are available for analysis at http://surveydata.who.int/index.html and the survey itself is available at http://www.who.int/healthinfo/survey/instruments/en/index.html.

The impact of mental illness and related disorders is broad and, for some disorders, devastating. Worldwide, 450 million people are affected by mental, neurologic, or behavioral problems, and the rate is steadily rising. In spite of existing knowledge about effective treatments for most psychiatric disorders, huge gaps in treatment and resources exist. Furthermore, data from the WHO *Mental Health Atlas 2005* show a tremendous human resource gap in the developing regions of the world.

An estimated 873,000 people commit suicide every year, which represents 1.4% of the global burden of disease. The proportion of the global disease burden due to suicide varies regionally, from 0.2% in Africa up to 2.6% in the Western Pacific Region. Suicide among young people is of significant concern: in some regions, suicide is the third leading cause of death among those aged 15 to 35 years. Suicide is the leading cause of death for this age-group in China and the second in Europe. The WHO estimated in 2002 that 154 million people globally suffer from depression and 25 million from schizophrenia. Alcohol use disorders affect 91 million people and drug use disorders, 15 million.

Barriers to effective treatment include lack of recognition of the seriousness of mental illness and lack of understanding about the benefits of services. Policy makers, insurance companies, health and labor policies, and the public at large all discriminate between physical and mental problems (WHO, 2001a,b,c). Most middle- and low-income countries devote <1% of their health expenditure to mental health (WHO, 2003). Consequently, mental health policies, legislation, community care facilities, and treatments for people with mental illness are not given the priority they deserve (Saxena et al., 2002, 2003; WHO, 2001d). The student is encouraged to visit the WHO archive at http://www.who.int/bulletin/volumes/en/ and review the bulletins available. Volume 4 of 2000, a bulletin on psychiatric epidemiology, can be found online at http://whqlibdoc.who.int/bulletin/2000/Number%204/. More recent findings are available at http://surveydata.who.int/index.html.

GENERAL LIMITATIONS OF EPIDEMIOLOGIC STUDIES

All studies have limitations. Limitations are the boundaries for the conclusions to be drawn from the results of the study. Researchers determine a study's limitations from the facts known about the type of study, the population being studied, and the study methods used.

Studies are categorized based on when participant data were collected. A retrospective study looks back in time, analyzing data already collected such as medical records. A prospective study collects data within a predefined sample of participants. One limitation of a retrospective study is the investigators' access to only the data available in the records. A prospective study allows investigators to pick what types of data to collect before the study begins. A prospective study is not limited like a retrospective study in the type of data collected, but still limitations exist. Although the investigators have control over what data they collect, the data may still have limitations.

The sample of individuals chosen to be in a study are sought to represent a population, either the whole population or a segment of the population (e.g., adult women). Prospective studies have more control over selecting study participants compared with retrospective studies because the recruitment is guided to collect enough study participants across different groupings (e.g., socioeconomic status, race, and age range), so that the study sample closely matches the population of interest. Sometimes a prospective study cannot recruit enough individuals of a particular section of a group (e.g., Asian women aged 20 to 29 years), so adjustments are made in the analysis. The adjustment will weight the underrepresented portions of a particular group to match the target number for the statistical analysis of the study. It is a means to compensate for the limitation that the study could not collect a truly representative sample of the population of interest. This limitation needs to be mentioned in the published report so readers know that adjustments were needed.

Limitations in the method of a prospective study are in how and what data are collected. The study of a prevalence of a disorder requiring large numbers of participants may be hampered by the ability to reach and interview all the study participants. Interviewing a study participant face-to-face at his or her household is the gold standard. The logistics of doing household, face-to-face interviewing have a cost. Collecting interviews for a prevalence study that requires 1,000 study participants to receive a structured diagnostic interview may take a daunting amount of time. Consider that a structured diagnostic interview takes 2 to 6 hours to complete. There is travel time for the interviewer. Some study participants may drop out of the study. The interviewer needs time to check and score the findings. So a study may require tens of thousands of hours of work. To limit the amount of time, household, face-to-face interviewing may be substituted with

TABLE 31-2 Online Resources of Selected Studies in Psychiatric Epidemiology

Online Site	Brief Description	Main Site Location	Quick Reference Lookup Tables	Statistical Analysis for Online Research
National Comorbidity Survey Replication	Prevalence and correlates of mental illness—United States	http://www.hcp.med.harvard.edu/ncs/	http://www.icpsr.umich.edu/CPES/	http://www.icpsr.umich.edu/CPES/
The National Survey on Drug Use & Health	Prevalence and correlates of drug use—United States	http://www.oas.samhsa.gov/nhsda.htm	http://www.oas.samhsa.gov/nhsda.htm	https://www.icpsr.umich.edu/ICPSR/
Centers for Disease Control and Prevention—CDC WONDER	Morbidity and mortality of behavioral and health problems—United States	http://wonder.cdc.gov/	http://wonder.cdc.gov/WelcomeT.html	https://www.icpsr.umich.edu/ICPSR/
World Health Organization	Morbidity and mortality of behavioral and health problems—International	http://www.who.int/research/en/	http://www.who.int/globalatlas/dataQuery/default.asp http://www.who.int/healthinfo/statistics/regions/en/index.html	https://www.icpsr.umich.edu/ICPSR/

other means of collecting information such as by telephone or computer. The limitation is that these other methods of collecting information do not match the gold standard of a face-to-face interview, and the investigators need to explain how the chosen method will affect the results. For example, not everyone owns a telephone; some study participants are wary of answering questions on a computer versus speaking to a person they have met; and study participants of higher socioeconomic status are more likely to have Internet access to participate in an online study compared with those of lower status. The investigators need to explain the differences unique to their method of data collection and justify that the method did not limit the study.

The type of data collected in a study itself may influence the study participant answering questions. As idyllic a pursuit as research may be, asking questions about a person's life remains an invasion of privacy and needs to be protected. Protections must be in place during and after the study to ensure that the study participant feels secure and is secure that answering questions will not lead to reprisals by others. Investigators receive specific training in the protection of their study participants before they can begin any human research. Some topics of research remain fraught with challenges, especially sexual health and substance use. Knowing if the study participant is forthcoming in responding to questions is a potential study limitation.

To further address these circumstances, studies undergo review by an institutional review board (IRB) for approval before starting. IRBs are mandated to ensure that studies protect the participants. The investigators must answer questions from the IRB on how they will meet the expectations of collecting accurate data and protecting the study participants. The goal for the investigators and the IRB is to address potential study flaws before the work begins rather than try to fix problems after the study. Such potential limitations also must be described in the discussion of the publication so that the reader understands it was anticipated before the study began.

ACCESSING EPIDEMIOLOGIC STUDY RESULTS THROUGH THE INTERNET

As described earlier, epidemiologic studies have implemented new approaches in data collection that accommodate previous limitations such as in recruiting study participants when determining rates of a psychiatric disorder. The availability of the data and the results of these studies have improved through the Internet. The four groupings of studies—the NCS-R, NSDUH, CDC, and WHO—all provide online results. Table 31-2 lists the sites and Web addresses for finding results. Most sites provide "lookup" or reference tables of the study results. These interactive tables allow the user to determine the prevalence of a disorder or its symptom for groups within a population by using combinations of variables like age, race, or gender. For example, what is the rate of suicide thinking among male African American high school sophomores? The answer comes from the Youth Risk Behavior Surveillance System at the CDC through this link http://apps.nccd.cdc.gov/yrbss/index.asp, under Unintentional Injuries and Violence. Other sites offer even more detailed results through online analysis, which can conduct statistical analysis of collected data and give results that may not have even been previously published. This provides a rich opportunity for students to develop research projects of their own interests.

CONCLUSION

Epidemiology and psychiatry have mutually benefited from the advancements of research and information technology. Medical students have access to research data and the means to conduct research to answer their own questions. Reading remains critical to understand mental illness and psychiatry. Psychiatry epidemiology has taken a step forward for the first generation of the Internet by providing interactive research tools and the data to help students find answers.

References

American Diabetes Association. Standards of medical care in diabetes—2007. *Diabetes Care*. 2007;30 (Suppl 1):S4–S41.

American Psychiatric Association. *Diagnostic and statistical manual of mental disorders*, 1st ed. Washington, DC: American Psychiatric Association; 1952.

American Psychiatric Association. *Diagnostic and statistical manual of mental disorders*, 2nd ed. Washington, DC: American Psychiatric Association; 1968.

American Psychiatric Association. *Diagnostic and statistical manual of mental disorders*, 3rd ed. Washington, DC: American Psychiatric Association; 1980.

American Psychiatric Association. *Diagnostic and statistical manual of mental disorders*, 3rd ed (revised). Washington, DC: American Psychiatric Association; 1987.

American Psychiatric Association. *Diagnostic and statistical manual of mental disorders*, 4th ed. Washington, DC: American Psychiatric Association; 1994.

American Psychiatric Association. *Diagnostic and statistical manual of mental disorders*, 4th ed (revised). Washington, DC: American Psychiatric Association; 2000.

Haro JM, Arbabzadeh-Bouchez S, Brugha TS, et al. Concordance of the Composite International Diagnostic Interview Version 3.0 (CIDI 3.0) with standardized clinical assessments in the WHO World Mental Health surveys. *Int J Methods Psychiatr Res*. 2006;15:167–180.

Kessler RC, Angermeyer M, Anthony JC, et al. Lifetime prevalence and age-of-onset distributions of mental disorders in the World Health Organization's World Mental Health survey initiative. *World J Biol Psychiatry*. 2007;6(3):168–176.

Kessler RC, Berglund PA, Demler O, et al. Lifetime prevalence and age-of-onset distributions of DSM-IV disorders in the National Comorbidity Survey Replication (NCS-R). *Arch Gen Psychiatry*. 2005a;62(6): 593–602.

Kessler RC, Chiu WT, Demler O, et al. Prevalence, severity, and comorbidity of twelve-month DSM-IV disorders in the National Comorbidity Survey Replication (NCS-R). *Arch Gen Psychiatry*. 2005b;62(6): 617–627.

Kessler RC, McGonagle KA, Zhao S, et al. Lifetime and 12-month prevalence of DSM-III-R psychiatric disorders in the United States: Results from the National Comorbidity Survey. *Arch Gen Psychiatry*. 1994;51:8–19.

Kessler RC, Merikangas KR. The National Comorbidity Survey Replication (NCS-R): Background and aims. *Int J Methods Psychiatr Res*. 2004;13(2):60–68.

Last, JM, ed. *A dictionary of epidemiology*, 4th ed. New York: Oxford University Press; 2001.

Robins LN, Regier DA, ed. *Psychiatric disorders in America: The Epidemiologic Catchment Area Study*. New York: The Free Press; 1991.

Saxena S, Maulik PK, O'Connell K, et al. Mental health care in primary community settings: Result from WHO's Project Atlas. *Int J Methods Psychiatr Res*. 2002;48:83–85.

Saxena S, Sharan P, Saraceno B. Budget and financing of mental health services: Baseline information on 89 countries from WHO's Project Atlas. *J Ment Health Policy Econ*. 2003;6:135–173.

Wang PS, Berglund PA, Kessler RC, et al. Failure and delay in initial treatment contact after first onset of mental disorders in the National Comorbidity Survey Replication (NCS-R). *Arch Gen Psychiatry*. 2005;62(6):603–613.

World Health Organization. *Atlas: country profiles on mental health resources*. Geneva: World Health Organization; 2001a.

World Health Organization. *Atlas: mental health resources in the world 2001*. Geneva: World Health Organization; 2001b.

World Health Organization. *The world health report 2001. Mental health: new understanding, new hope*. Geneva: World Health Organization; 2001c.

World Health Organization. *Mental health policy project: policy project: policy and service guidance package—executive summary*. Geneva: World Health Organization; 2001d.

World Health Organization. *Investing in mental health*. Geneva: World Health Organization; 2003.

CHAPTER 32

John H. Coverdale and Paul Haidet

Practicing Evidence-Based Psychiatry

The principles and practices of evidence-based medicine (EBM) are core to the practice of psychiatry. Psychiatrists, as all physicians, are obliged to practice in accordance with the intellectual standard of EBM, a standard that was articulated by John Gregory (1724 to 1773). Gregory called on medicine to be based on experience, or on the rigorously collected results of natural and designed experiments (McCullough, 1997, 1998). This reliance on evidence, now called *EBM,* is a cornerstone of the fiduciary relationship and enables patients to trust their psychiatrists intellectually (McCullough, 1997, 1998).

The practice of EBM is a lifelong directed learning process integrally linked to providing optimal care for patients. It is founded on the science of epidemiology and its application to practice. Therefore, the reader should seek to develop an understanding of epidemiologic design and analysis in order to facilitate an understanding of the importance of the strengths and weaknesses of individual studies. Although a discussion of epidemiologic design and analysis is beyond the scope of this chapter, the McMaster Clinical Epidemiology Group has published structured guides for appraising epidemiologic studies (Guyatt et al., 1993, 1994; Jaeschke et al., 1994a,b; Laupacis et al., 1994; Levine et al., 1994; Oxman, et al., 1994; Oxman, et al., 1993).

An important starting point is to ask what the evidence is for a particular view or statement. We encourage the reader to practice asking questions on clinical rounds and to challenge their own or others' beliefs. Because there is an overwhelming number of such opportunities, one challenge is to determine the questions of greatest interest or importance and to manage one's time devoted to pursuing evidence. Developing a team approach to asking questions and to comprehensive resolution of questions can help with time efficiency and is a tremendously enriching learning experience.

EBM can be more in depth and useful for clinical decision making than the discussion sections often found in cited articles or materials (including this book) (Horowitz, 2003). EBM also rejects the notion of accepting conclusions in scientific papers as the final word without first independently assessing their validity and the strength of the papers' results (Straus et al., 2005). Finally, EBM can challenge the hierarchical structure of learning in medicine in that, with adequate training, medical students can become equal to residents and attendings in questioning and critically evaluating evidence (Grimes, 1995).

Our goal for this chapter is briefly to review some of the processes of EBM, particularly as they apply to treatment studies, because they likely answer the most commonly asked questions in psychiatry. We will use the structured guides for appraising epidemiologic treatment studies provided by the McMaster Clinical Epidemiology Group for this purpose. We will illustrate this process with a case example and hope to learn some psychiatry along the way as well.

THE EVIDENCE-BASED MEDICINE PROCESS

As demonstrated in Table 32-1, there are four steps to EBM (Rosenberg and Donald, 1995). Practitioners should begin by formulating a clear question to a clinical problem. Questions can relate to treatment, diagnosis, prognosis, ethics, harm, or economics.

Second, practitioners should search the literature for the best evidence. The strongest evidence usually includes well-conducted systematic overviews, meta-analyses, or well-conducted randomized controlled trials (RCTs). Other study designs include case–control, cohort, and case series. A relatively full discussion of the structure and advantages/disadvantages of the various designs is available elsewhere (Grimes, 2002). In general, though, systematic reviews,

TABLE 32-1	**Four Steps to Evidence-Based Medicine (EBM)**

1. Formulating a clear question to a clinical problem
2. Searching the literature for the best evidence
3. Evaluating the evidence for its validity and utility
4. Implementing the valid and important findings into clinical practice

meta-analyses, and randomized trials, if rigorously conducted, are subject to less bias or methodological problems that can distort the results.

The third step is to appraise the evidence for its validity, strength, and applicability. This step allows psychiatrists to judge the adequacy of the conclusions of the paper in light of the initial specific question(s), the study design, and the methodological processes.

Finally, psychiatrists should integrate the evidence with available resources and clinical expertise and apply the evidence to practice. In general, the practice of psychiatry will improve if this step is achieved on a large scale. The entire process, then, requires medical students and psychiatrists to be open to new scientific evidence, as Gregory counseled, as opposed to rigid adherence to entrenched methods that may or may not be backed by evidence (Coverdale, 2007).

CASE STUDY

In the major portion of this chapter, we will present a case study on psychosocial interventions for patients with schizophrenia and the critical appraisal of an article in order to demonstrate the processes of critical appraisal.

Background

Psychosocial interventions for schizophrenia are those that aim to incorporate primary care providers (including family members) into treatment and are based on the stress–vulnerability model, which emphasizes the importance of various psychosocial stressors in patients' lives. In addition to biological and genetic vulnerabilities, such stressors are determinative of prognosis (Falloon and Shanahan, 1990). Interventions have been devised that aim to reduce stress in the lives of patients and primary care providers by strengthening natural coping mechanisms and by integrating evidence-based psychopharmacologic approaches, including education, managing early warning signs, and teaching problem-solving strategies, communication, and social skills (Falloon et al., 1998). A central underpinning of these strategies is to involve the family. Falloon and Shanahan (1990), originators of the methods of psychosocial treatment in schizophrenia, emphasized how families are the most valuable resource in promoting the long-term health and welfare of their members.

With this background, we will select and appraise one randomized controlled trial concerning the validity and utility of adding psychosocial interventions to medications in managing patients with schizophrenia.

> A 20-year-old university student living with her parents presents to an outpatient clinic with a second episode of auditory hallucinations and paranoid delusional beliefs. The first episode had occurred approximately 9 months before. She was otherwise well and had no significant past medical history. She had a history of occasional marijuana use. The clinician wonders whether psychosocial interventions would be effective in improving outcomes.

Step 1: Formulating the Question

Clear questions that are useful for integrating evidence into practice are written in four parts. For intervention studies, these parts are patient group, intervention, comparison group, and outcome, also abbreviated as PICO. For studies that explore whether certain elements are risk factors for illness, the risk factor is substituted for the intervention in the four-part format. For our case, we are interested in psychosocial interventions; therefore, a structured four-part question might read as follows:

P: In patients with schizophrenia,
I: How does psychosocial rehabilitation (including psychoeducation, managing early warning signs, family therapy, communication, and social skills training),
C: Compared to case management (treatment as usual [TAU]),
O: Prevent relapse (specifically, frequency of illness episodes and rehospitalization rates)?

Step 2: Searching the Literature

Most clinicians are familiar with PubMed, a web-based resource for searching the MEDLINE database maintained by the US National Library of Medicine. However, other databases contain useful evidence that may not exist in MEDLINE. An exhaustive list of databases is beyond the scope of this chapter, but we provide some examples that we have found useful. The Embase database includes more medical articles from Europe than PubMed. The Cochrane databases include rigorously conducted systematic reviews or overviews as well as a register of controlled trials. Additional databases for psychiatry searches include PsychInfo and PsychLit.

The four-part question sets up the search strategy by identifying the key search terms. For our case, MEDLINE (years 1980 to present) and the Cochrane Controlled Trials Register were referred. Search terms included *schizophrenia, relapse prevention*, and *controlled trials*. Combining *schizophrenia* and *relapse prevention* resulted in 480 hits, but when these were combined with *controlled trials*, the number of hits was 120. In order to be fairly sure that all relevant articles were identified, we conducted several searches using a combination of terms. The entire process of searching and reviewing abstracts takes less time than you think once you become experienced with it. It is important to mention here that adding search terms to reduce the number of hits to a very small list (e.g., 5 to 10 hits) is likely to miss relevant articles.

We found the following article: Herz MI, Lamberti JS, Mintz J, et al. A program for relapse prevention in schizophrenia: A controlled study. *Arch Gen Psychiatr*. 2000;57:277–283. We suggest that readers will be greatly enhanced by obtaining this article for reference purposes.

Step 3: Evaluating the Evidence for Validity and Utility

Brief Elements of the Study

The study can be described in terms of its four PICO parts:

P: The study population consisted of 82 outpatients aged 19 to 60 years with schizophrenia or schizoaffective disorder according to the *Diagnostic and Statistical Manual of Mental Disorders, Third Edition, Revised* (DSM-III-R) (American Psychiatric Association, 1987).
I: The main intervention studied was psychosocial treatment approaches (psychoeducation, prodromal symptoms monitoring and early relapse intervention, weekly group therapy and multifamily groups). The group getting the intervention is called the *program for relapse prevention* (PRP) group.
C: The comparison group received biweekly individual supportive therapy and this group is called the *TAU* group.
O: The outcomes measured were relapse and rehospitalization.

In the following sections we will critique the validity and utility of this article's evidence using questions drawn from the RCT validity questions outlined in Table 32-2 related to study population and time period, composition of the study's two experimental groups, and measurement of critical aspects of the study groups and the outcomes that occurred. These questions can provide a framework to assess the validity of many types of studies in the medical literature. In addition, in Tables 32-3 and 32-4 we offer some questions specific to diagnostic test studies and systematic reviews.

TABLE 32-2	**Assessing the Validity of a Randomized Control Trial**

1. Did the trial address a clearly focused issue?
2. Was the assignment of patients to treatment randomized?
3. Were the groups similar at the start of treatment?
4. Were patients, health workers, and study personnel blind to treatment?
5. Aside from the experimental intervention, were the groups treated equally?
6. Were all the patients who entered the trial properly accounted for at its conclusion?
7. Were outcomes clearly defined and replicable?
8. Was measurement of outcomes sufficient between comparison groups?
9. Was follow-up sufficiently long?

The Study Population and Time Period
Who are the study participants? From which source population are they drawn?

It is important to begin by looking carefully at who was recruited to be in the study and what differences exist between the study population and the patient to whom the results will be applied. If there are differences on critical factors that could affect the outcome for one patient, then the study may not be completely applicable (or *generalizable*, in the language of EBM). Our study of interest enrolled patients attending a community support program at the University of Rochester Department of Psychiatry. Eligible patients were identified through reviews of the medical records, and therapists were asked to approve their recruitment into the study.

What were the inclusion and exclusion criteria?

An examination of the criteria that the investigators used to select participants provides a further check on whether the study can be generalized to one's patient. Studies that are widely inclusive tend to be more generalizable than less inclusive studies. In addition, the investigators should provide a sensible rationale for the inclusion and exclusion criteria. For our study, inclusion criteria were specified as (a) aged 19 to 60 years, (b) schizophrenia or schizoaffective disorder based on a structured instrument used for diagnostic assessments, and (c) at least one hospitalization within the last 3 years and two or more lifetime hospital admissions. Exclusion criteria were evidence of organic mental disorder or marked retardation and severe drug or alcohol dependence that required inpatient treatment or detoxification. Because the exclusion criteria were not very restrictive, generalizability was enhanced.

Were the participants a representative and well-defined sample from a relevant and recognizable population?

Questioning who participated provides a final global check on whether the population was appropriate to conduct the study and whether the study will be generalizable. For the clinical scenario mentioned earlier, this study was fairly representative in that this was an outpatient group of patients with major mental disorders (schizophrenia or schizoaffective disorder) who had been hospitalized within the last 3 years. However, therapists had to approve their recruitment into the study, and no information was given on the number of those who were approved in relation to the total number who met inclusion criteria and were eligible to participate. Also of interest here is that the clinic served a population of 750,000. If the lifetime prevalence of schizophrenia

TABLE 32-3	**Assessing the Validity of a Diagnostic Test**

1. Did the clinician face diagnostic uncertainty (i.e., were the diagnostic conditions very easily identifiable or not)?
2. Was an appropriate spectrum of illness present in those with and without the disease?
3. Were the selected subjects similar to real world patients with whom the test would be used to resolve uncertainty?
4. Was there a blind comparison with a suitable independent gold standard?
5. Did all patients undergo the index test and the same reference test?

TABLE 32-4	Assessing the Validity of a Systematic Review

1. Did the review address a clearly focused question?
2. Did the authors select the right sort of studies for the review?
3. Were the important, relevant studies included?
4. Did the review's authors do enough to assess the quality of the included studies?

is a conservative 0.25%, this would suggest that the clinic should serve approximately 1,875 individuals with this disorder. There may, therefore, have been biases not mentioned in the article that were operating while including people in the study.

During what time period of follow-up were outcomes of study participants measured?

The study's timeline is an important indicator that can affect the results. In general, a study needs to have a long enough timeline so that the results will be indicative of the final outcomes, which can be expected for patients who undergo the treatment. This study lasted 18 months from the time of assignment to the treatment groups.

Composition of the Study's Experimental Groups
Was the assignment of participants to the intervention group randomized, and was the assignment to study groups concealed?

Randomization is a powerful method of making sure that separate study groups are similar at the beginning of a study. In theory, it spreads all factors evenly between the study groups, including factors called *confounders* that could impact the outcome being studied. Not only is randomization itself important, but the methods of randomization (including concealment of the study groups, called *blinding*) are critical to ensure that the study groups are similar at the outset and treated similarly during data collection. RCTs with poorly performed methods of randomization have been demonstrated to show positive results more often than RCTs with rigorous randomization, suggesting that less acceptable randomization can itself affect the results (Rosenberg and Donald, 1995).

Our study used a randomization scheme of computer-generated cards stored in sealed envelopes. However, it is not known if the sealed envelopes were sequentially numbered or opaque to prevent the experimenter from determining how participants were assigned. This is probably not, therefore, an acceptable method for concealing the results of randomization (Beller et al., 2002; Schulz, 1995).

Were the comparison groups similar at the start of the study?

It is important for the comparison groups to be as evenly matched at the beginning of the study as possible, so that the only difference between the groups is the intervention itself. If they are different in some critical way, it could be that difference (instead of the intervention) which explains any variation found in the outcomes of the study.

In our study, the groups were similar in some but not all instances. In theory, randomization should provide all subjects an equal chance to belong to either the experimental or comparison group; however, this does not always happen. On one hand, although the control groups were clearly defined and "randomized," there was a slight trend for the PRP group to have had fewer hospitalizations. On the other hand, significantly fewer PRP patients were receiving intramuscular antipsychotic medication at baseline. Few data were provided on how the groups may have differed on other important variables at baseline. For example, it is not known if there were differences in likelihood of associated affective symptoms during illness episodes, the duration of illness, associated factors such as a history of violence to self and others, or illicit drug use, particularly marijuana. Less importantly, no information was provided on medical history or family psychiatric history, although we are told that for all patients there was no evidence of organic mental disorders. The lack of baseline data about these potential confounders is a weakness of the study.

Were the participants analyzed in the groups to which they were randomized?

A commonly encountered term is *intention to treat*. This means *all* participants who were randomized to a group are included in the analysis, whether or not they completed the study. If a participant does not complete the study, that participant is assumed to have a negative outcome and counted as such in an intention to treat analysis. True intention to treat analysis should include lost to follow-up/violated protocol. Also, once randomization occurs, no participants should be changed from one group to the other—this ultimately defeats the advantages that randomization provides. In our study, participants were analyzed in the groups to which they were randomized.

Measurement of Exposures
Were the interventions clearly defined and replicable?

Sometimes an article will not clearly describe the intervention. If the intervention is not described in enough detail that the reader could replicate it, then it is impossible to know exactly what is being studied. In our study, the intervention was clearly described.

Were participants, health workers, and study personnel blind to interventions?

Blinding of the raters who do the outcome assessments is critical, especially when those outcomes have some degree of subjectivity (such as quality of life, quality of care, and adherence to clinical guidelines). Subtle biases, either conscious or unconscious, can influence the assessment of outcomes when the raters know what the study is about and in which study group each participant is. In our study, the participants were not blinded nor were the treatment team members (psychiatrist, nurse clinician or certified social worker, and case manager). The research interviewers were blinded to the group assignment, not associated with the clinical care, and instructed not to inquire about a patient's treatment during interviews. However, little information was given about what steps were taken to ensure that no communication occurred between the treatment team members and research interviewers or patients and research interviewers. In addition, the adequacy of blindness of the research interviewers was not checked.

Aside from the experimental interventions, were groups treated equally during the study?

Again, the goal is for both groups to be identical in as many ways as possible so that the intervention is the only difference between groups. The following questions can help assess whether the groups were treated equally in all ways other than the intervention:

1. Did the groups receive other interventions associated with the outcomes of interest unequally (i.e., cointervention)?
   Probably not.
2. Did some of the comparison groups receive the main intervention(s)?
   No, although we cannot definitively exclude a potential for *contamination* (a condition where patients in the control group receive some of the intervention either through study practitioners giving it to them or study patients communicating with one another) because individual supportive therapy may have included some attention to early warning signs.
3. Was compliance with interventions measured?
   Yes, by using a questionnaire with a five-point scale (1 = always, 5 = never) designed for that purpose. Noncompliance was conservatively defined as a rating of 5; however, the occasions of partial or incomplete compliance were not defined as noncompliant.

Measurement of Outcomes
Were all participants who entered the study properly accounted for and attributed at its conclusion?

It is important to check the completeness of the follow-up in the study. In this research, follow-up was good with 88% of PRP and 85% of TAU patients completing the study. However, seven

PRP and two TAU patients were noncompliant with maintenance antipsychotic medication and psychosocial treatment throughout the study.

Were outcomes clearly defined and measured the same way in all comparison groups?

In this study, the outcomes were clearly defined, and the three raters were tested for reliability at study inception and monthly intervals for the outcome measures. In addition, it is important that the measurement of subjective outcomes be done with surveys that have been previously *validated* (i.e., tested and shown to be reliable measures of the outcomes of interest). All scales, including the early warning signs questionnaire, had been previously published, which is one piece of evidence that had been tested for validity in the past. Comparisons based on data from published scales are less likely to favor the treatment group than comparisons based on unpublished scales.

Was follow-up sufficiently long to detect the important effects of the exposures on the outcomes of interest?

As discussed earlier, a study needs to be conducted over a long enough time to allow for a meaningful measure of the efficacy of the interventions. Ideally, follow-up would be longer in this case. It is not known how many of the patients had relapsed or had hospitalizations within the preceding year or 18 months or what the average relapse rate per unit of time was, and it may be that most were unlikely to relapse within this time frame.

What is the strength (utility) of the results?

In this section, we will discuss how large the difference is in outcomes between the two groups and whether this difference is clinically relevant. Sometimes a study will show a statistically significant difference that is not large enough to be clinically relevant. The statistics that we will discuss in this section allow the psychiatrist to determine the size and clinical relevance of the findings of the study.

It is useful to construct an evidence table, which includes the relative risk (RR), relative risk reduction (RRR) (for a treatment study assessing benefits), absolute risk reduction (ARR), and number needed to treat (NNT). Of these, the NNT is an especially useful statistic defined by the number of participants one would need to treat in order to achieve one positive outcome (Barratt et al., 2004). For studies assessing harms, the equivalent measure is the number needed to harm (NNH), defined as the number of participants one would need to treat in order to produce one adverse event. The following formulas apply for the construction of the evidence table, where control event rate (CER) refers to the event rate in the control group and experimental event rate (EER) refers to the event rate in the experimental or treatment group.

RR = EER/CER (ratio of the risk of an event among the treatment group to the risk among the control group)

RRR = (1 − RR) (the proportional reduction in rates of harmful outcomes between the treatment and control groups)

ARR = CER − EER (the absolute difference in rates of harmful outcomes between the experimental and control groups)

NNT = 1/ARR (the number of patients who need to be treated over a specific time period in order to achieve one good outcome)

Therefore, in our study example and considering the outcome of relapse:

CER = 14/41 = 0.341
EER = 7/41 = 0.170
RR = 0.170/0.341 = 0.499
RRR = 0.501
ARR = 0.341 − 0.170 = 0.171
NNT = 1/0.171 = 5.85.

That is, almost six patients have to be treated by the PRP method for 18 months in order for one patient to benefit by not relapsing.

Confidence intervals can be calculated for each of the estimates of effect (RRR, ARR, and NNT). They provide a measure of precision and specify the limits within which the estimates likely lie. One word about the NNT. It does not prescribe what to do. For one, impairment in the validity of the study (e.g., a significant potential for bias and confounding) will likely create higher effect sizes than normally observed. In this study, the large apparent protective effect of preventive interventions (PRP group) on relapse cannot be considered as definitive evidence of benefit, given the potential for bias in the selection and randomization processes and potential confounding. Further, the local culture of treatment, including the availability of training, provision of outreach to patients with schizophrenia, and administrative and financial considerations, can weigh as an important consideration whether to proceed.

Summary of Study

Important strengths of the study included the prior relative paucity of information on relapse prevention programs for outpatients with schizophrenia. The design was well described, including randomization to groups, and treatment groups were clearly defined. Outcome measures were also clearly defined, and the drop-out rate was low.

Important weaknesses of the study included small group numbers, a possible selection bias, and possible impairments in concealing randomization and blinding investigators. Information on potential confounders and additional outcomes was also lacking.

Step 4: Applying the Evidence to Clinical Practice

The last step, which is perhaps the most crucial, involves integrating the findings with available resources and clinical expertise. If the patient whose clinical circumstances evoked the structured four-part question meets the inclusion criteria of the selected study, the study results would more likely apply. The evidence-based practitioner should then appreciate what additional services would be required in order to meet the standards of the PRP group. This involves an understanding of administrative, financial, personnel, and training implications for the local site. Clearly, when the required changes are substantial and costly, these will require greater justification.

The appraised study has important strengths and weaknesses and should be considered alongside other studies that try to answer the same research question. It does appear to be valid (with limitations), and the NNT seems clinically important. As noted earlier, however, the NNT does not, by itself, prescribe what to do, because financial and administrative factors must also be weighed. Nevertheless, and dependent on new information becoming available, the results support the use of relapse prevention programs for managing outpatients with schizophrenia.

PRACTICING EVIDENCE-BASED MEDICINE IN PSYCHIATRIC SETTINGS

EBM is a systematic, disciplined process of asking questions, searching, critically appraising, and implementing best evidence into clinical settings. A detailed understanding of the validity and strength of results of individual studies should enable an appreciation of when to incorporate findings into practice. This is counter to the notion of treating study conclusions, or other reports of those conclusions, as authoritative. If done consistently, the EBM approach will reduce the potential for bias in the practice of psychiatry. Clearly, this is a process that can take time and underscores the importance of prioritizing questions and working with teams.

It should be appreciated that individual, critically appraised studies contain only a single element of the pertinent literature and may lose relevance as new studies appear. Therefore, students and their teams should aim to develop more than one critical appraisal on a particular topic to view each study in relation to others. Developing such critical appraisals on one topic is a step toward developing a comprehensive or systematic overview on the same topic. These are processes that together create a very high standard indeed for the practice of psychiatry.

Clinical Pearls

- EBM is a systematic, disciplined process, which is core to the practice of psychiatry.
- A key starting point is questioning the evidence for a particular view or statement.
- Questions arise from clinical problems and can relate to diagnostics, prognostics, treatments, ethics, or economics.
- Treatment questions should be formally structured into four parts: patient group, intervention (or risk factor), comparison, and outcomes.
- EBM is counter to the notion that the conclusions of scientific papers should be accepted as authoritative without critical appraisal. The highest forms of evidence are well-conducted systematic reviews, meta-analyses, and RCTs.
- RCTs should be evaluated for both the validity of evidence and strength of results.
- Three important considerations in judging the validity of a trial are the adequacy of randomization, blinding, and the presence of a control group.
- An evidence table for judging the strength or utility of results from a RCT includes the RR, ARR, and NNT.
- The critically important final step in EBM is to apply the evidence to clinical practice in relation to available resources and clinical expertise.

Self-Assessment Questions and Answers

32-1. The database that includes a collection of rigorously collated systematic reviews is:

A. Cochrane
B. Embase
C. MEDLINE
D. PsychInfo
E. PsychLit

The Cochrane databases are a rich resource for clinicians. They include a database of systematic reviews that are rigorously constructed and frequently updated. Students should get into the habit of routinely checking the Cochrane database of systematic reviews on topics of interest. *Answer: A*

32-2. The section of a research paper most useful for judging the validity of evidence is the:

A. Abstract
B. Introduction
C. Methods
D. Results
E. Conclusions

The methods section is central to determining the validity of research findings. The research question or study hypothesis drives the study design. A detailed understanding of the methods in relation to the research question will facilitate a critical appraisal of the study and deciding whether to incorporate the findings into clinical practice. *Answer: C*

32-3. Randomization protects against:

A. Confounding
B. Bias caused by dropouts

C. Bias caused by unequal treatment of groups
D. Measurement bias
E. Rater bias

Randomization, when well conducted, provides every subject with an equal chance of being in the experimental or control group. With good randomization methods, factors that could impact the outcome between groups, which are called *confounders*, are likely spread evenly between the experimental and control groups. It is important to routinely check to what degree the study groups are evenly matched for possible confounders at the beginning of the study. The methods section should describe to what degree this was achieved. *Answer: A*

32-4. The number needed to treat (NNT) is directly derived from which of the following statistics?

A. ARR
B. CER
C. EER
D. RR
E. RRR

The NNT is calculated as the reciprocal of the ARR. The ARR, in turn, is defined as CER − EER. *Answer: A*

32-5. A number needed to treat (NNT) of 10 means that:

A. For every person treated, 10 will benefit.
B. For every person harmed, 10 will benefit.

C. For every 10 people treated, 1 will benefit.

D. For every 10 people treated, 1 will be harmed.

An NNT of 10 means that 10 patients have to be treated (by the specific experimental intervention for a specified period of time) for 1 patient to benefit. *Answer: C*

References

American Psychiatric Association, *Diagnostic and statistical manual of mental disorders (DSM III-R)*, 3rd ed, Revised. Washington, DC: American Psychiatric Association; 1987.

Barratt A, Wyer PC, Hatala R, et al. Evidence-based Medicine Teaching Tips Working Group. Tips for learners of evidence-based medicine. 1. Relative risk reduction, absolute risk reduction and number needed to treat. *Can Med Assoc J*. 2004;171:353–357.

Beller EM, Gebski V, Keech AC. Randomisation in clinical trials. *Med J Aust*. 2002;177:565–567.

Coverdale J. Virtues-based advice for beginning medical students. *Acad Psychiatry*. 2007;31:339–342.

Falloon IRH, Coverdale J, Laidlaw TM, et al. OTP collaborative group. Early intervention for schizophrenic disorders. Implementing optimal treatment strategies in routine clinical services. *Br J Psychiatry Suppl*. 1998;172(Suppl):33–38.

Falloon IRH, Shanahan WJ. Community management of schizophrenia. *Br J Hosp Med*. 1990;43:62–66.

Geddes JR, Game D, Jenkins NE, et al. What proportion of primary psychiatric interventions are based on evidence from randomised controlled trials? *Qual Health Care*. 1996;5:215–217.

Grimes DA. Introducing evidence-based medicine into a department of obstetrics and gynecology. *Obstet Gynecol*. 1995;86:451–457.

Grimes DA. An overview of clinical research: the lay of the land. *Lancet*. 2002;359:57–61.

Guyatt GH, Sackett DL, Cook DJ. Users' guides to the medical literature. II. How to use an article about therapy or prevention. A. Are the results of the study valid? *JAMA*. 1993;270:2598–2601.

Guyatt GH, Sackett DL, Cook DJ. Users' guides to the medical literature II. How to use an article about therapy or prevention. B. What were the results and will they help me in caring for my patients? *JAMA*. 1994;271:59–63.

Herz MI, Lamberti S, Mintz J, et al. A program for relapse prevention in schizophrenia. A controlled study. *Arch Gen Psychiatry*. 2000;57:277–283.

Horowitz HW. A piece of my mind. Dumbing down. *JAMA*. 2003;289:1349–1350.

Jaeschke R, Guyatt GH, Sackett DL. Users' guides to the medical literature. III. How to use an article about a diagnostic test. A. Are the results of the study valid? *JAMA*. 1994a;271:389–391.

Jaeschke R, Guyatt G, Sackett DL. Users' guides to the medical literature. III. How to use an article about a diagnostic test. B. What are the results and will they help me in caring for my patients? *JAMA*. 1994b;271:703–707.

Laupacis A, Wells G, Richardson WS, et al. Users' guides to the medical literature. V. How to use articles about prognosis. *JAMA*. 1994;271:234–237.

Levine M, Walter S, Lee H, et al. Users' guides to the medical literature. V. How to use an article about harm. *JAMA*. 1994;271:1615–1619.

McCullough LB. John Gregory (1724–1773) and the invention of professional relationships in medicine. *J Clin Ethics*. 1997;8:11–21.

McCullough LB. *John Gregory (1724–1773) and the invention of professional medical ethics and the profession of medicine*. Dordrecht, The Netherlands: Kluwer Academic Publishers; 1998.

Oxman AD, Cook DJ, Guyatt GH. Users' guides to the medical literature. VI. How to use an overview. *JAMA*. 1994;272:1367–1371.

Oxman AD, Sackett DL, Guyatt GH. Users' guides to the medical literature. 1. How to get started. *JAMA*. 1993;270:2093–2095.

Rosenberg W, Donald A. Evidence-based medicine; an approach to clinical problem solving. *Br Med J*. 1995;310:1122–1126.

Schulz KF, Chalmers I, Hayes RJ, et al. Empirical evidence of bias. Dimensions of methodological quality associated with estimates of treatment effects in controlled trials. *JAMA*. 1995;273:408–412.

Straus SE, Richardson WS, Paul Glasziou, et al. *Evidence-based medicine: How to practice and teach EBM*, 3rd ed. Edinburgh: Churchill Livingstone; 2005.

INDEX

Note: Page numbers followed by f indicate a figure; t following a page number indicates tabular material